Handbook of Practice Nursing

To Ursula Shine,
who has been a great inspiration to me,
with my thanks.

Jeannett Martin

To Dr Geoffrey Smerdon,
with my thanks for his insight,
encouragement and support.

Julia Lucas

For Churchill Livingstone:

Senior Commissioning Editor: Ninette Premdas
Project Development Manager: Katrina Mather/Claire Wilson
Project Manager: Ailsa Laing
Design: Judith Wright

Handbook of Practice Nursing

Edited by

Jeannett Martin SRN PN Cert MA

Director of Clinical Leadership & Quality, Lewisham Primary Care Trust, London, UK

Julia Lucas RGN General Practice Specialist Nurse MSc

Practice Nurse Manager, Rosedean Surgery, Liskeard, Cornwall, UK

Foreword by

Monica Fletcher MSc BSc(Hons) PGCE RSCN HVDip

Chief Executive, National Respiratory Training Centres, Warwick, UK and Carolina, USA

Joan Sawyer RGN RCNT FP Cert Dip Asthma and COPD

Patient and Public Involvement Manager, Richmond & Twickenham Primary Care Trust, Richmond upon Thames, UK

THIRD EDITION

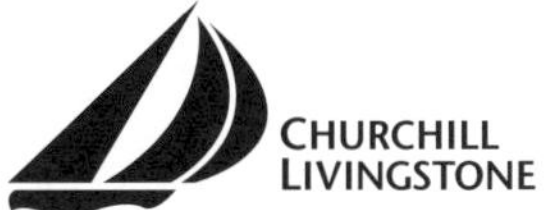

EDINBURGH LONDON NEW YORK OXFORD PHILADELPHIA ST LOUIS SYDNEY TORONTO 2004

CHURCHILL LIVINGSTONE
An imprint of Elsevier Limited

First edition 1992
Second edition 1998
Third edition 2004

ISBN 0443 07212 4

British Library Cataloguing in Publication Data
A catalogue record for this book is available from the British Library

Library of Congress Cataloging in Publication Data
A catalog record for this book is available from the Library of Congress

Note
Knowledge and best practice in this field are constantly changing. As new research and experience broaden our knowledge, changes in practice, treatment and drug therapy may become necessary or appropriate. Readers are advised to check the most current information provided (i) on procedures featured or (ii) by the manufacturer of each product to be administered, to verify the recommended dose or formula, the method and duration of administration, and contraindications. It is the responsibility of the practitioner, relying on their own experience and knowledge of the patient, to make diagnoses, to determine dosages and the best treatment for each individual patient, and to take all appropriate safety precautions. To the fullest extent of the law, neither the publisher nor the editors assume any liability for any injury and/or damage.

The Publisher

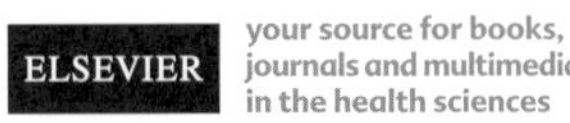

www.elsevierhealth.com

The Publisher's policy is to use **paper manufactured from sustainable forests**

Printed in China

Contents

Contributors

Liam Benison BA(Hons) MA
Editor, Practice Nursing, MA Healthcare Limited, London, UK

Tina Bishop RGN DipN(Lond) BSc(Hons) MA
Senior Lecturer, APU, Essex, UK

Rachel Booker RGN DN(Cert) HV
COPD Course Leader, National Respiratory Training Centre, The Athenaeum, Warwick, UK

Elaine Campbell RGN BSc(Hons) DipN(Lond) NP NDN Cert
Practice Nurse/Practice Nurse Mentor, Bermuda Close Surgery, Basingstoke, UK

Nancye Carr RGN BSc(Hons) Dip HS Dip CHD AMC FETC PN Cert
CHD Nurse Co-ordinator for Derwentside PCT and Visiting Scholar, University of Northumbria at Newcastle, UK

Karen Didovich
Senior Employment Relations Adviser, Employment Relations Department, Royal College of Nursing, London, UK

Linda Drake RGN BSc(Hons) MSc
Practice Nurse, Elm Lodge Surgery, London and Clinical Adviser, Southwark Primary Care Trust Public Involvement Team, London, UK

Jane Elwood SRN
Regional Trainer, Medical Research Council General Practice Research Framework and Local Research Co-ordinator, School of Health and Related Research, University of Sheffield, UK

Atie Fox BSc(Hons) Clinical Practice (Nurse Practitioner Pathway) RGN
Lecturer/Practitioner, Bournemouth University, Bournemouth and Nurse Practitioner, Family Medical Services, Poole, UK

Marilyn Gallichan MSc RGN MCGI Cert Ed
Diabetes Specialist Nurse, Bodmin Health Centre, Bodmin, Cornwall, UK

Lesley Hand MSc SRN
Practice Nurse Manager, Bungay Medical Practice and Regional Trainer, Medical Research Council, General Practice Research Framework and Professional Development Nurse, Waveney PCT, UK

Lis Hughes RGN
Practice Nurse Trainer and Menopause Nurse, Lee Bank Group Practice, Colston Health Centre, Birmingham, UK

Josie Irwin
Senior Employment Relations Adviser, Employment Relations Department, Royal College of Nursing, London, UK

Julia Lucas RGN General Practice Specialist Nurse MSc
Practice Nurse Manager, Rosedean Surgery, Liskeard, Cornwall, UK

Wendy K MacKinnon AsthmaDip(NRTC)
Specialist Practitioner (Practice Nursing), Supplementary Nurse Prescriber, Dingwall Health Centre, Ross-shire and Regional Trainer, Dingwall, UK

Jeannett Martin SRN PN Cert MA
Senior Nurse Manager, MRC General Practice Research Framework, London, UK

Vicky Padbury SRN A08
Senior Nurse in Family Planning, East Surrey Primary Care Trust, Redhill, Surrey, UK

Claire Pratt BPhil NPDip BSc(Hons) DPSN RGN ENB 928 General Practice Specialist Nurse
Practice Coach/Nurse Advisor, NHS Direct West Country and Module Teacher (Minor Illness), Plymouth University, UK

Jane Proctor SRN General Practice Nurse
Practice Nurse, Sonning Common Health Centre, Sonning Common, Reading, UK

Mags E Rees RN RM MSc
Nurse Practitioner, Cardiff Local Health Board, Cardiff, Wales, UK

Andy Shave BSc(Hons)
Clinical Nurse Manager, St Mary's Hospital, London, UK

Susan H Simpson BA(Hons) MSc RGN RNT
Nurse Consultant in Cardiac Care, Queen Elizabeth Hospital, Woolwich, UK

Janette Swift BSc RGN
Head of Clinical Governance, Specialist Practitioner Practice Nursing, Sutton and Merton Primary Care Trust, London, UK

Trisha Weller MHS RGN NDN Cert CPT DPSCHN (PN)
Head of Quality Assurance, Asthma Module Leader, National Respiratory Training Centre, The Athenaeum, Warwick, UK

Marion M Welsh RGN SCM BSc SPQ (GPN)
General Practice Nurse/Lecturer, School of Nursing, Midwifery & Community Health, Glasgow Caledonian University, Glasgow, UK

Foreword

The Handbook of Practice Nursing was originally published in 1991 and updated in 1998. As the two original nurse authors we are very excited to be invited to write the Foreword of this hardback version of the *Handbook*, 13 years on from the original publication.

At the time the first edition was published, practice nursing was certainly in its 'baby boom' and there was a degree of antagonism concerning where the specialism fitted in alongside other community nurses and GPs. How things have changed – now viewed as the bedrock of primary care services and no longer the Cinderella!

Nursing is the largest single professional group in primary care and, given the increasing demands and expectations placed on all healthcare professionals in primary care, it is essential that nurses are kept up to date in both clinical and non-clinical developments. Evidence-based practice and justification for one's actions as a health professional are essential in order to ensure the best possible care is delivered to our patients. The shift to more patient-centred care is one that nurses mainly applaud, but it requires new ways of working and new skills.

The number of practice nurses has continued to grow steadily, not at the rate we witnessed back in the late 1980s and early 1990s, but nevertheless there are now 25% more nurses employed than there were in 1991 and numbers continue to grow year-on-year. According to Department of Health statistics there were 20 983 practice nurses employed in 2002. No other area of nursing can boast such an achievement.

Practice nursing has forged ahead as a profession during this time and continues to develop new areas of skill and expertise. These are not purely in terms of both the depth and range of clinical areas, but also education, research, clinical governance and management roles. The role is more complex than ever before and there are huge expectations from the public, the government and medical and non-medical colleagues.

It is not unusual for practice nurses to be the first point of contact for people at their GP surgery for either telephone advice or face-to-face consultations; indeed it will soon be common practice across primary care services. Nurses are also taking a lead in a wide range of chronic diseases and preventative services and their role in women's health is a pivotal one in many surgeries up and down the country.

The level of knowledge required to undertake the role is far greater and more multifaceted than ever before and this *Handbook* will certainly assist nurses to carry out their role on a day-to-day basis. It will not, however, replace the need for more formal educational programmes.

Nursing services in primary care are delivered against a background of increasingly complex influences upon policy and practice. In April 2004 the new General Medical Services contract came live, and the role of the practice nurse took on another challenge. The markers embedded in this contract demand evidence of quality care. This is not to say that this is not being achieved, but it has encouraged a good deal of discussion within the whole primary care team to review the methodology and standards of care. The development of this phase of change offers still more opportunities for innovation in the models of care offered, both within the practice, and in the wider primary care arena. The shift of services and management from secondary care to primary care is demanding the creation of new ways of working, and practice nurses are key to many of these new ventures.

The diversity and breadth of knowledge demanded of the experienced practice nurse and the pace of change in general practice is providing far-reaching opportunities for career development, whether this is in clinical specialism, teaching or change-management. Practice nurses have certainly risen to the challenge of taking a pivotal role in developing and commissioning local health services in their leadership roles within primary care trusts. They have also demonstrated how well they can work within multi-professional teams, working alongside clinicians and managers. The Health and Social Care Act of 2001 makes the involvement of patients and carers in the strategic planning of the services they use mandatory, and this is reflected in this edition.

The employment of health care assistants is increasing rapidly, and the impact on services delivery will be to create opportunities for more appropriate use of practice nursing time. With this comes the further responsibility for clinical supervision of a new role. To support all of these changes, and shifts in working patterns, we are delighted to see the sections on management and professional issues expanded.

Monica Fletcher
Joan Sawyer

2004

Plate section

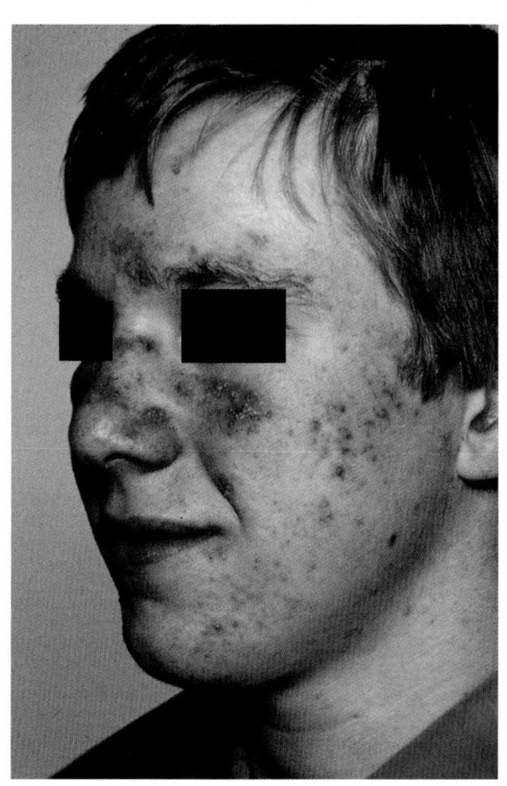

Plate 1 Acne.

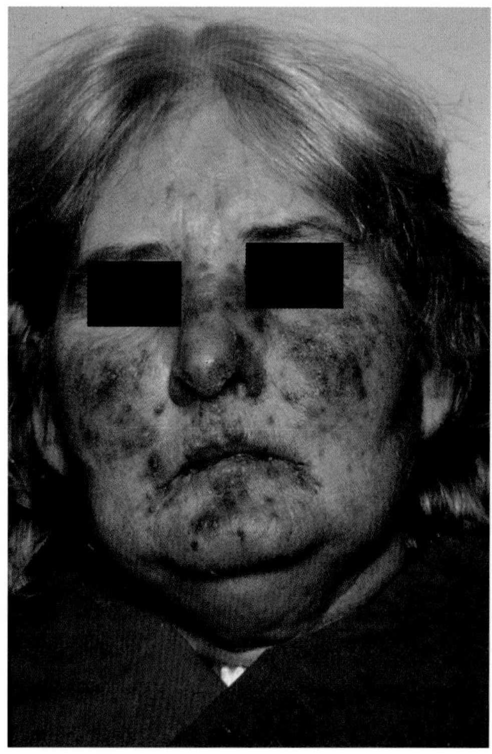

Plate 2 Rosacea.

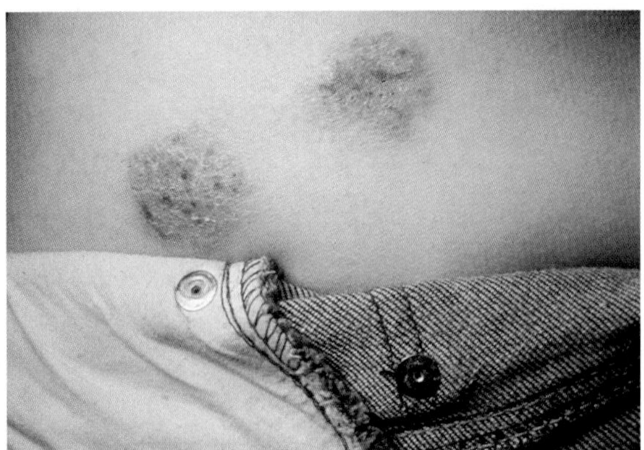

Plate 3 Allergic dermatitis.

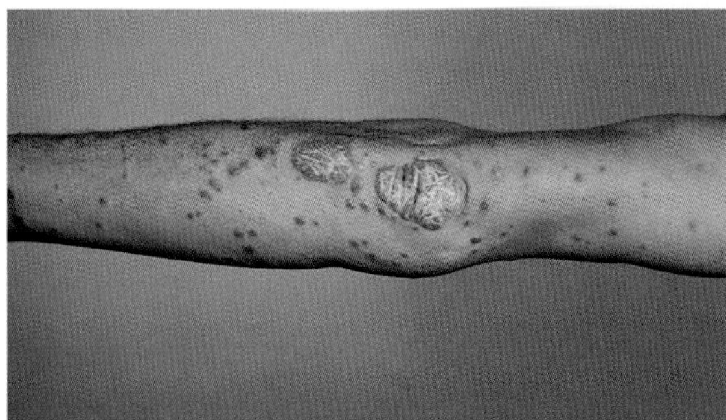

Plate 6 Plaque psoriasis.

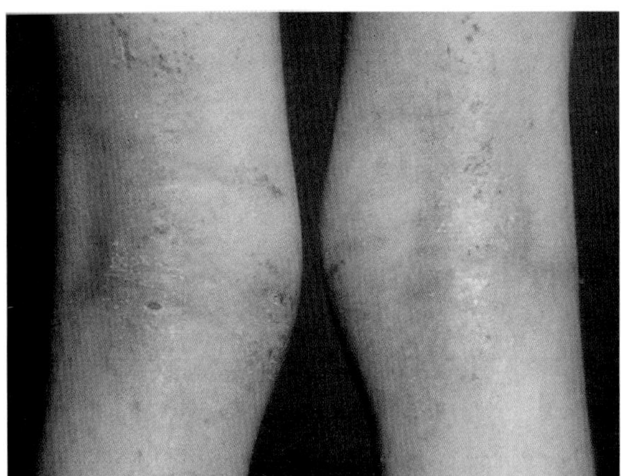

Plate 4 Atopic eczema.

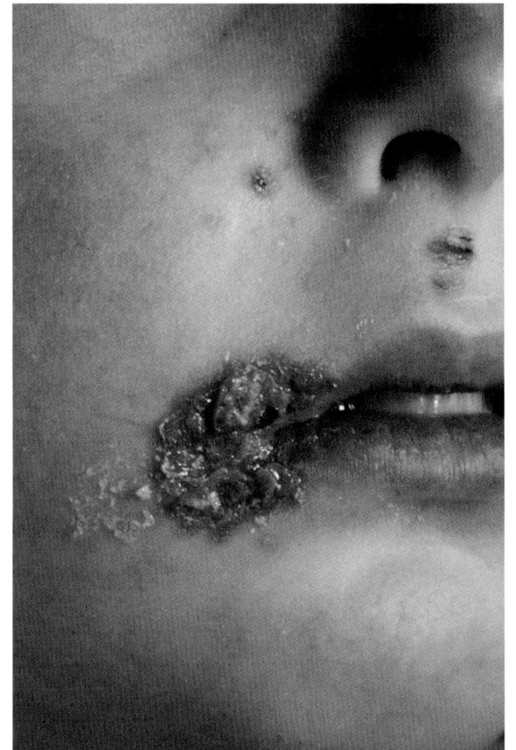

Plate 7 Impetigo.

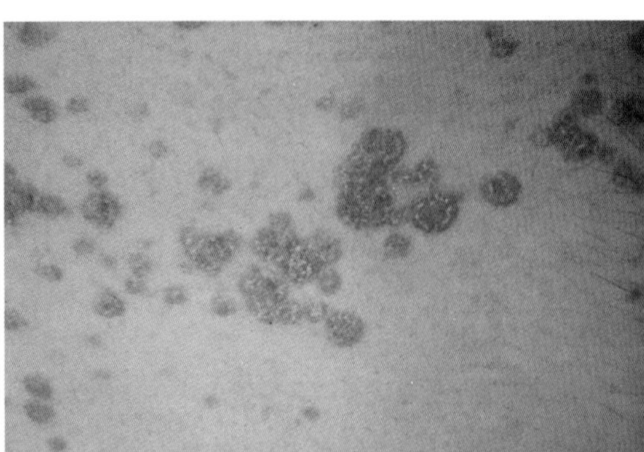

Plate 5 Guttate psoriasis.

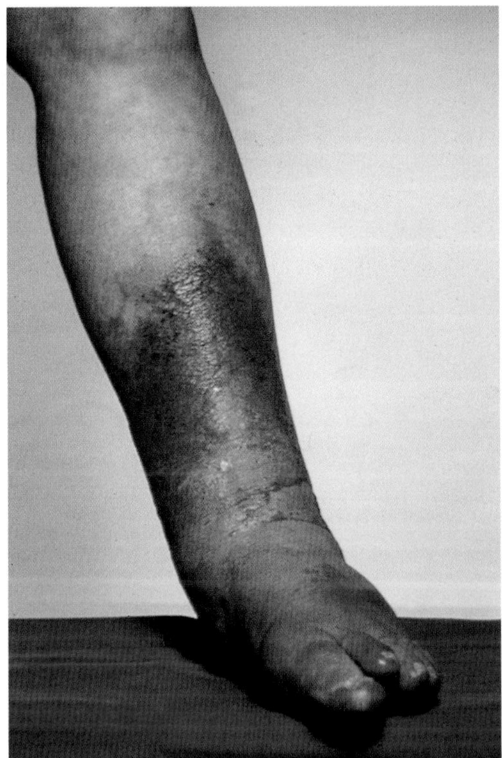

Plate 8 Cellulitis.

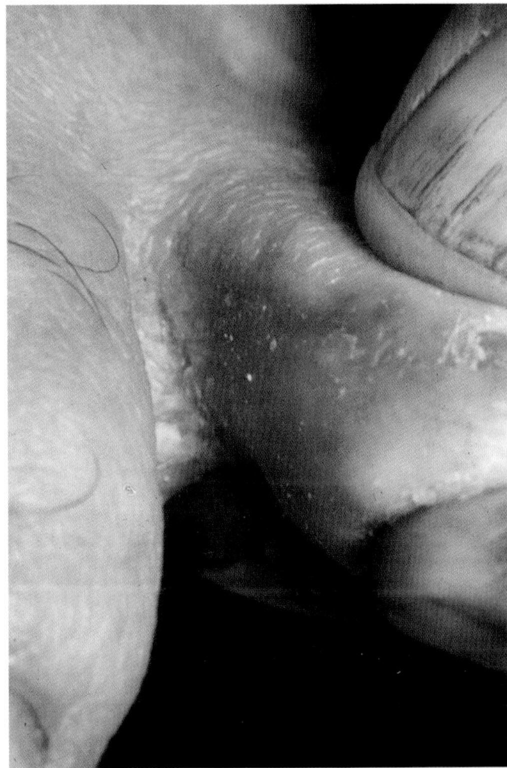

Plate 10 Tinea pedis.

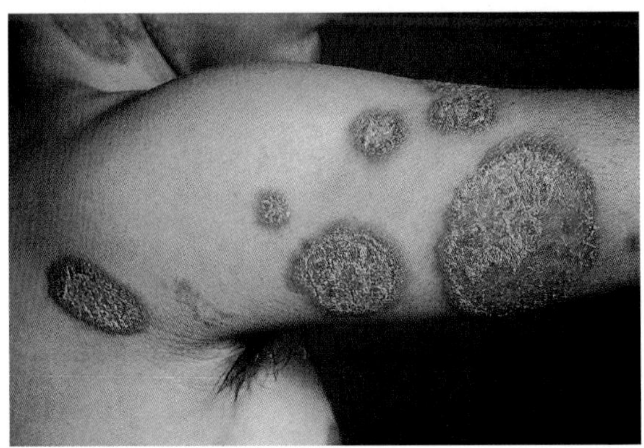

Plate 9 Tinea corporis.

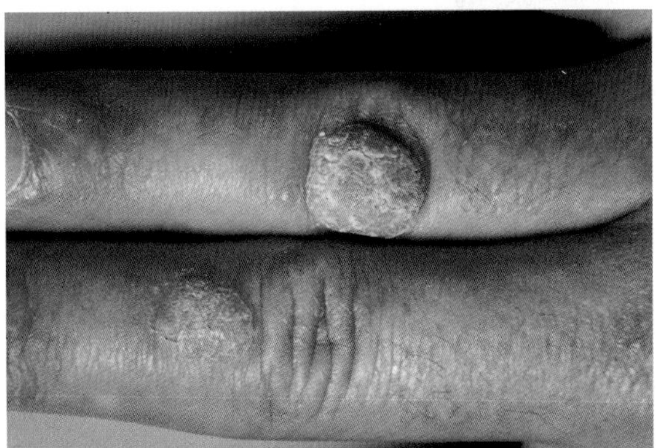

Plate 11 Warts.

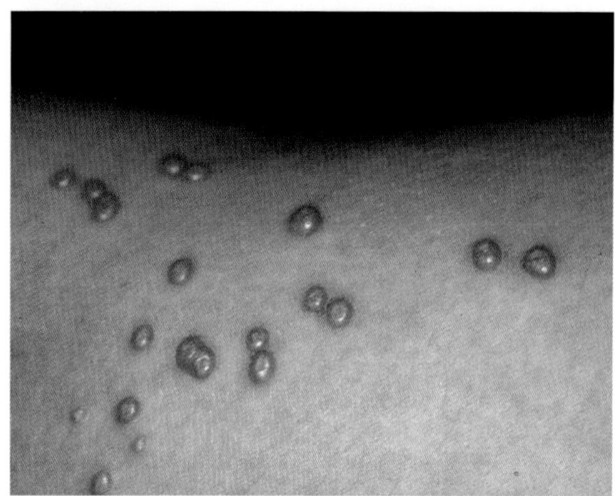

Plate 12 Molluscum contagiosum.

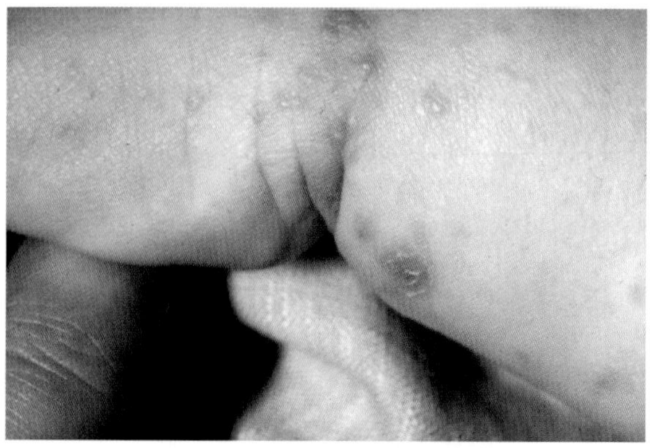

Plate 14 Scabies.

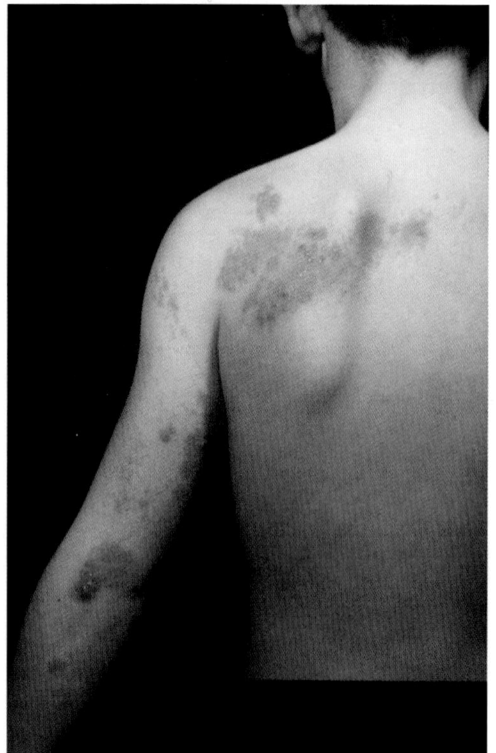

Plate 13 Herpes zoster.

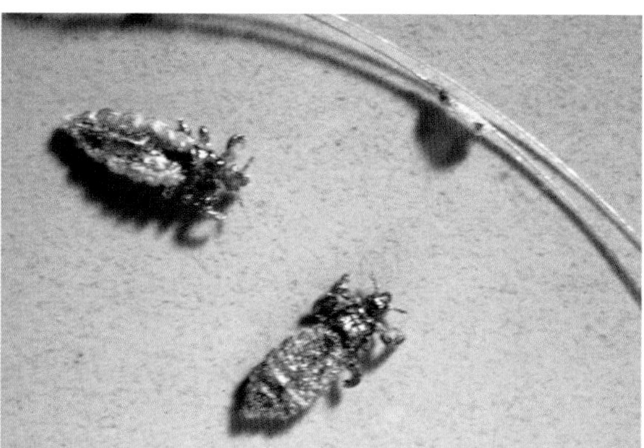

Plate 15 Head lice.

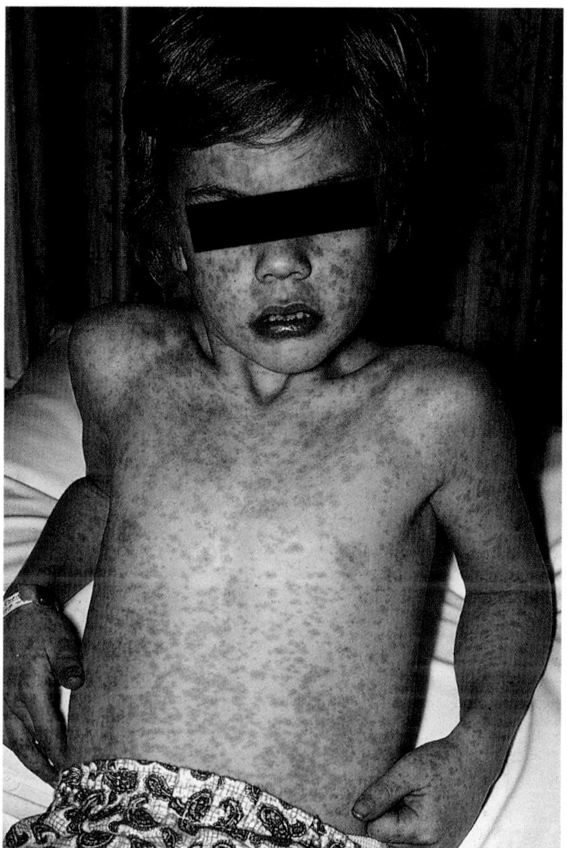

Plate 16 Measles.

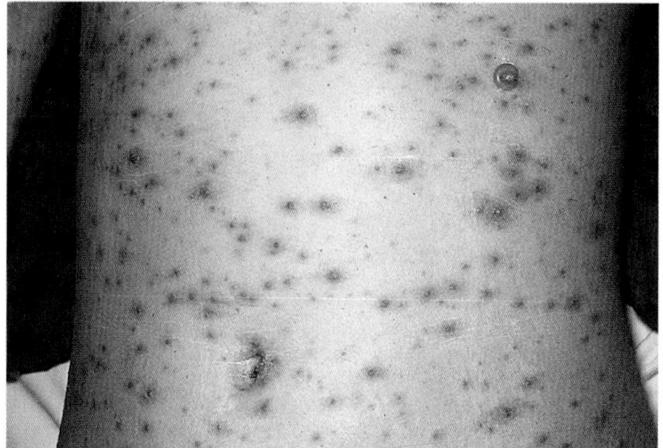

Plate 17 Chickenpox.

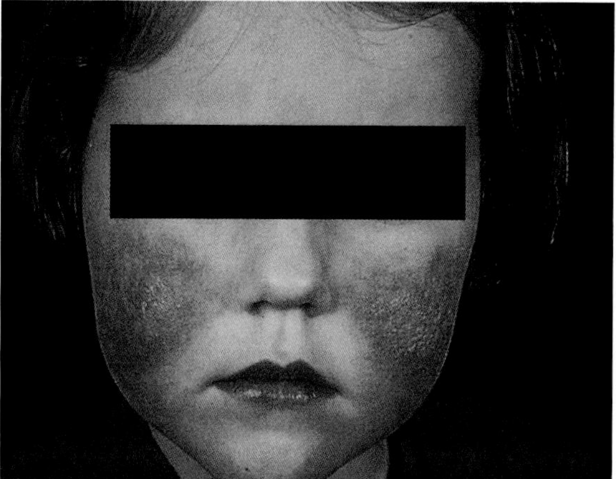

Plate 18 Slapped cheek syndrome (erythema infantum) (reproduced with permission of St John's Institute of Dermatology).

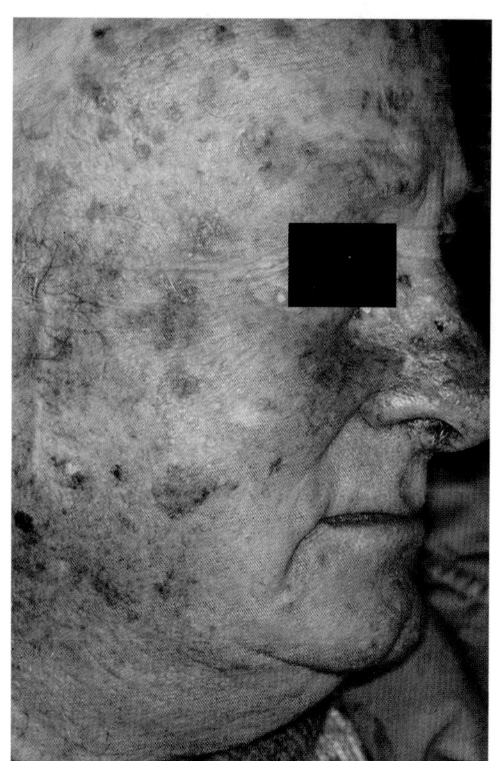

Plate 19 Actinic (solar) keratosis.

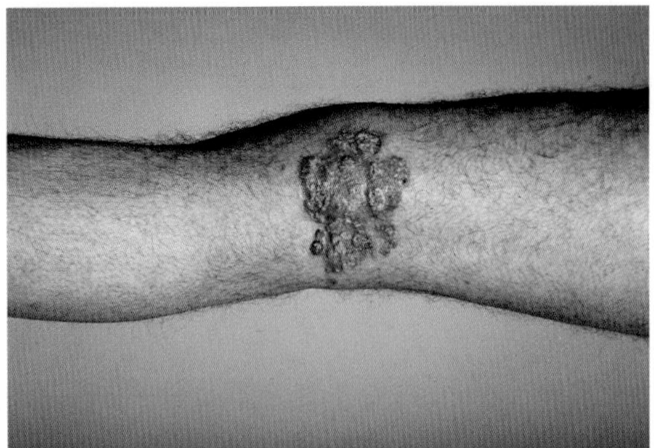

Plate 20 Bowen's disease.

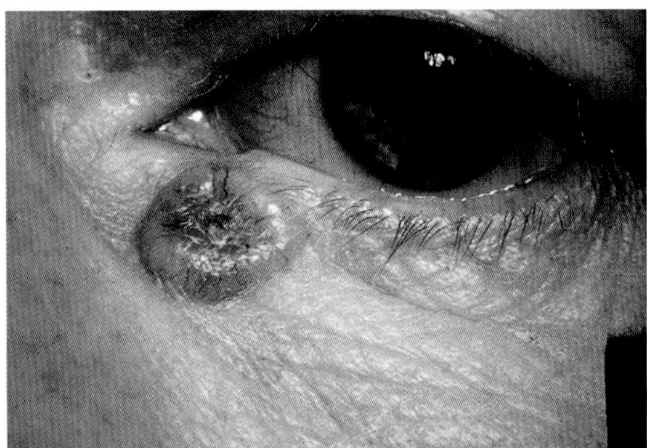

Plate 21 Basal cell carcinoma.

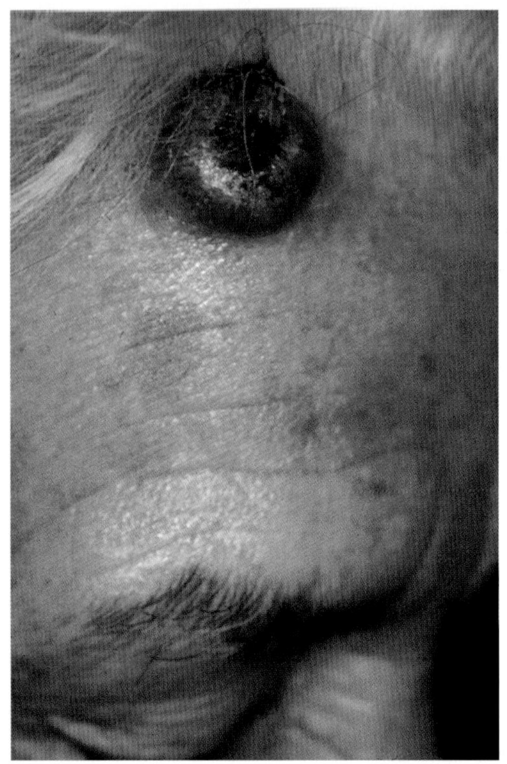

Plate 22 Squamous cell carcinoma.

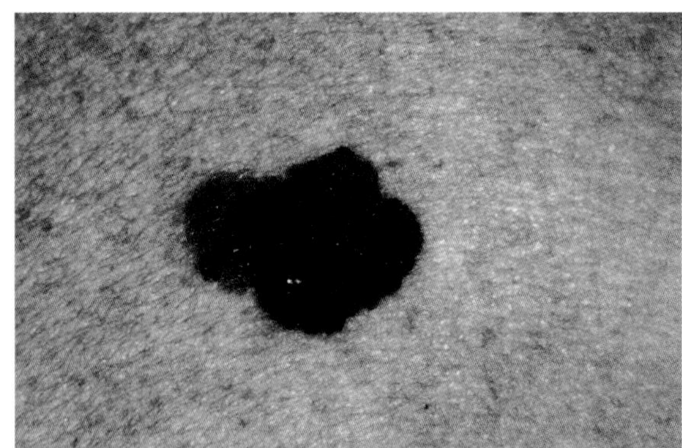

Plate 23 Malignant melanoma.

SECTION 1

Health promotion and health education

SECTION CONTENTS

Chapter 1

Women's health

Lis Hughes

CHAPTER CONTENTS

INTRODUCTION

The health needs of women are numerous and in today's society, with access to the Internet and media coverage of women's health issues, women are far better informed about their bodies and about the services available.

This chapter will give a holistic approach to a woman's health and well-being. It is known that women consult their doctor more frequently than men and they also attend with their children. For this reason there is great scope for health education among women. Illness or female problems can affect not just the woman but also her relationships, her family and her job as well as her general well-being.

Women's healthcare is changing and forms an increasing part of the practice nurse's role. With the major changes in the NHS and the evolution of primary care organizations such as primary care trusts (PCTs) practice nurses have a chance to play a lead role in the management of community care.

Women have more opportunities to make free and responsible choices and the practice nurse with her special nurse–patient relationship and her interactive skills can be a woman's advocate and support.

In dealing with women's health issues it is important that the practice nurse has a sound knowledge base and a realistic attitude to her own beliefs and values and has had adequate training in clinical skills and counselling and communication (Andrews 2001).

Everyone's health is important but there is a body of opinion that asserts that women are treated differently and unfairly within the healthcare system (Sutherland 2001). The following are examples that have been quoted (Doyal 1998).

- A woman's own experiences are often devalued in comparison with 'expert' medical knowledge.
- Women may be denied the opportunity to participate fully in treatment decisions, both medical and surgical.
- The recent reduction in community family planning and women's services has taken away some choice for some women.
- Women have to endure and negotiate the personal judgement of others when seeking fertility control and termination of pregnancy.
- Deaths from breast cancer may be unnecessarily high, due to inconsistency in the standards of specialist treatment and in women's access to treatment.
- Women may be denied the same opportunities as men for research, investigation and treatment of coronary heart disease.

In order to understand the issues around women's health it is important to have a sound knowledge of the anatomy and physiology of the female reproductive organs and the menstrual cycle.

ANATOMY AND PHYSIOLOGY OF THE FEMALE REPRODUCTIVE ORGANS

Males and females both produce *gametes* or reproductive germ cells. In the male they are spermatozoa and in the female they are ova. The gametes contain genetic material which is passed onto the offspring. In other body cells there are 46 chromosomes arranged in 23 pairs but in the gametes there are only 23, one from each pair. When the ovum is fertilized by the spermatozoon, the resulting zygote contains 23 pairs of chromosomes, one of each pair from the father and one from the mother.

The zygote embeds itself in the wall of the uterus where it develops during a 40-week gestation period prior to birth. Therefore the function of the female reproductive system is to form the ovum and, if it is fertilized, to nurture it until it is born and then feed it with breast milk until it is able to be weaned (Wilson 1990).

The female reproductive organs or genitalia are divided into external and internal organs.

The external genitalia are known collectively as the *vulva* and consist of the:

- labia majora
- labia minora
- clitoris
- vestibule
- hymen
- greater vestibular glands.

EXTERNAL GENITALIA

The *labia majora* are two folds of skin which form the boundary of the vulva. They are composed of skin, fibrous tissue and fat and a number of sebaceous glands. Anteriorly the folds join in front of the symphysis pubis and posteriorly they merge with the skin of the perineum. At puberty hair starts to grow on the mons pubis and on the lateral surfaces of the labia majora.

The *labia minora* are two smaller folds of skin inside the labia majora containing numerous sebaceous glands. They fuse posteriorly to form the fourchette. The cleft between the labia minora is the *vestibule* and opening into it are the ducts of the vestibular glands and the vagina and urethra.

The *clitoris* contains erectile tissue and corresponds to the penis in the male. It has no reproductive significance.

The *hymen* is a thin layer of mucous membrane which partially occludes the opening to the vagina.

Bartholin's glands or the greater vestibular glands lie on either side of the vaginal opening. They are the size of a pea and have ducts opening into the vestibule. They secrete mucus that keeps the vulva moist.

The *perineum* is the area from the fourchette to the anal canal. It consists of connective tissue, muscle and fat and gives attachment to the muscles of the pelvic floor.

The blood supply is by branches from the internal pudendal arteries which branch from the internal iliac arteries and external pudendal arteries that branch from the femoral arteries. Veins drain into the internal iliac veins. Lymph drainage is through the superficial inguinal nodes and the nerve supply is via branches from the pudendal nerves.

INTERNAL REPRODUCTIVE ORGANS

The internal reproductive organs lie in the pelvic cavity and consist of the vagina, uterus, two Fallopian tubes and two ovaries.

Vagina

The vagina is a fibromuscular tube lined with stratified epithelium. It connects the uterus with the external reproductive organs. It runs obliquely upwards and backwards between the bladder in front and rectum and anus posteriorly. It has an outer cover of areolar tissue, a middle layer of smooth muscle and a lining of stratified epithelium. It does not have secretory glands but the surface is kept moist by cervical secretions.

From puberty to the menopause *Lactobacillus acidophilus* microbes are normally present and they secrete lactic acid, maintaining the pH between 3.5 and 4.9. This acidity inhibits the growth of most microbes that may enter the vagina from the perineum.

Uterus

The uterus is a hollow muscular pear-shaped organ. It lies in the pelvic cavity between the bladder and the rectum in an anteverted anteflexed position. *Anteversion* is when the uterus leans forward. *Anteflexion* means that the uterus is bent forward almost at right angles to the vagina. When the woman stands upright the uterus lies in a horizontal position. The parts of the uterus are the fundus, body and cervix.

The *fundus* is the dome-shaped part of the uterus above the openings of the Fallopian tubes. The *body* is the main part. It is narrowest inferiorly at the *internal os* where it is continuous with the cervix. The *cervix* protrudes through the anterior wall of the vagina, opening into it at the *external os.*

The walls of the uterus are composed of three layers – perimetrium, myometrium and endometrium. The *perimetrium* consists of peritoneum which is distributed differently on the various surfaces of the uterus. Laterally it forms a double fold with the Fallopian tubes and it is called the *broad ligament.* It attaches the uterus to the sides of the pelvis. The *myometrium* is a thick layer of smooth muscle fibres interlaced with areolar tissue, blood vessels and nerves. The *endometrium* consists of columnar epithelium. It contains a large number of mucus-secreting tubular glands. The upper two-thirds of the cervical canal is lined with mucous membrane and the lower third is lined with squamous epithelium continuous with that of the vagina.

Supports of the uterus The uterus is supported in the pelvic cavity by surrounding organs, the muscles of the pelvic floor and ligaments that suspend it from the walls of the pelvis.

Two *broad ligaments* are formed by a double fold of peritoneum, one on each side of the uterus. They hang down from the Fallopian tubes and are attached to the sides of the pelvis. The *round ligaments* are made of fibrous tissue between two layers of broad ligament, one on each side of the uterus. They pass through the inguinal canal and end by fusing with the labia majora.

There are also two *uterosacral ligaments*, two *transcervical ligaments* and the *pubocervical fascia.*

Functions of the uterus After puberty the menstrual cycle influences changes in the uterus. Every month it prepares to receive, nourish and protect a fertilized ovum. The cycle is usually regular and lasts between 26 and 30 days. If the ovum is not fertilized a new cycle begins with a period of bleeding (menstruation).

If the ovum is fertilized the zygote embeds itself in the uterine wall which begins to relax to accommodate the growing fetus. At the end of the gestation period labour begins and is concluded when the baby is born and the placenta delivered. During labour the muscle of the fundus and body of the uterus contract intermittently and the cervix relaxes and dilates. As labour progresses the uterine contractions become stronger and more frequent. When the cervix is fully dilated the mother assists the birth of the baby by pushing during the contractions.

Fallopian tubes

The Fallopian tubes are approximately 10 cm long and extend from the side of the uterus between the body and the fundus. They are positioned in the upper border of the broad ligament and have trumpet-shaped lateral ends which penetrate the posterior wall and open into the peritoneal cavity close to the ovaries. At the end of each tube are *fimbriae* or finger-like projections. The longest are the ovarian fimbriae which are close to the ovary.

The Fallopian tubes have an outer covering of broad ligament, a middle layer of smooth muscle and are lined with ciliated epithelium.

Function of the Fallopian tubes They convey the ovum from the ovary to the uterus by peristalsis and ciliary movement. The mucus secreted by the membrane lining provides the ideal conditions for movement of ovum and sperm. Fertilization usually occurs in the Fallopian tube and the resulting zygote is moved to the uterus.

Ovaries

The ovaries are the female gonads and they lie in a shallow fossa on the lateral walls of the pelvis. Each ovary is attached to the upper part of the uterus by the *ligament of the ovary* and to the back of the broad ligament by a broad band of tissue called the *mesovarium*.

Structure and function of ovaries The ovaries have two layers of tissue. The *medulla* in the centre consists of fibrous tissue, blood vessels and nerves. The *cortex* surrounds the medulla. It has a framework of connective tissue covered by *germinal epithelium*. It contains *Graafian (ovarian) follicles* each of which contains an ovum.

Before puberty the ovaries are inactive but they already contain immature follicles. During the fertile years one ovarian follicle matures, ruptures and releases its ovum into the peritoneal cavity during each menstrual cycle.

Preovulatory phase At the beginning of each cycle the anterior pituitary gland secretes increased concentrations of follicle-stimulating hormone (FSH) and luteinizing hormone (LH). These hormones cause accelerated maturation in some ovarian follicles. The follicles secrete a high concentration of oestrogen (Guyton & Hall 1997). This stimulates growth of the endometrium and increases the production of mucus from the cervical glands. It also causes changes in the mucus, making it thinner to assist the entry of sperm (Bray et al 1999). Before ovulation occurs one of the follicles begins to outgrow the others which subsequently involute.

About 2 days before ovulation the secretion of LH by the anterior pituitary gland increases. FSH also increases and the two hormones act together to cause rapid swelling of the follicle that culminates in ovulation.

Ovulation Ovulation occurs when the follicle ruptures and the ovum is released into the abdominal cavity close to the open end of the Fallopian tube. In a woman with a 28-day cycle ovulation occurs 14 days after the onset of menstruation. During the last day before ovulation and immediately afterwards, granulosa cells still remaining in the ovary at the site of the ruptured follicle become the corpus luteum. This secretes large amounts of progesterone and some oestrogen.

Post ovulation Progesterone and to a lesser extent oestrogen cause marked development of the endometrium. This contains stored nutrients and can provide the correct conditions for a fertilized ovum. Progesterone also promotes secretory changes in the mucosal lining of the Fallopian tubes. These secretions are important as a source of nutrients for an embryo during transport to the endometrium. Progesterone also modifies cervical mucus, making it more viscous and resistant to sperm penetration. It is also progesterone which causes an increase in basal body temperature after ovulation.

During the postovulatory phase oestrogen and progesterone secreted by the corpus luteum act together to provide negative feedback effects on the secretion of FSH and LH (levels fall). These feedback effects operate directly on the anterior pituitary gland and to a lesser extent the hypothalamus, resulting in a decreased secretion of gonadotrophin-releasing hormone (GnRH).

The postovulatory fall in FSH and LH mean that no new follicles begin to grow in the ovaries. If the ovum is not fertilized the corpus luteum degenerates on approximately the 26th day of the cycle. Consequently oestrogen and progesterone levels fall and the negative feedback effects on FSH and LH secretion are removed. FSH and LH then initiate the growth of new follicles to start a new cycle.

The sudden reduction in oestrogen and progesterone levels at the end of the cycle causes involution of the endometrium and shedding of the superficial layers; this is menstruation. If fertilization and implantation occur the corpus luteum does not degenerate and menstruation does not take place.

Sometimes more than one follicle matures at a time, releasing two or more ova in one cycle. When this happens and the ova are fertilized the result is a multiple pregnancy.

Oestrogens Three oestrogens occur in the plasma of normal, non-pregnant women and these are beta-oestradiol, oestrone and oestriol.

Oestrogens, as well as causing changes to the reproductive organs, also promote the growth of bone and skeletal muscle. In the preovulatory phase of the menstrual cycle oestrogens stimulate growth of the endometrium, increase the output from the cervical glands and change the cervical mucus in ways that assist the entry of sperm (Bray et al 1999, Guyton & Hall 1997).

Oestrogen receptors have been identified in the urethra, bladder, pelvic floor muscles (Rees 1999), brain (Perry 1998), bone cells and blood vessel walls (Woolf & St John Dixon 1998).

Progestogens Progesterone is the most important of all the progestogens. In the postovulatory phase of the menstrual cycle progesterone causes a marked development of the endometrium. It also makes the cervical mucus more viscous and resistant to sperm penetration and causes an increase in basal body temperature (Bray et al 1999). Progesterone also promotes the development of the alveoli and lobules of the breasts and, with increased fluid in the subcutaneous tissue, causes the breasts to swell (Guyton & Hall 1997).

Androgens Androgens are produced in low but significant concentrations in the ovaries and adrenal cortex. They have a role to play in promotion of libido.

Physiological changes at menopause At birth the ovaries each contain about one million immature follicles but these numbers decline and at puberty they contain 300 000–400 000 follicles each. During reproductive life only about 400 follicles mature and expel ova (Bray et al 1999, Guyton & Hall 1997).

When a woman reaches approximately 45 only a few follicles remain in the ovary and the production of oestrogen declines. The menstrual cycles usually become irregular and eventually cease. The oestrogen production becomes too low to inhibit the production of FSH and LH and so after the menopause FSH and LH levels become raised. Serum levels of testosterone and androstenedione fall with declining ovarian function (WHO 1996).

MENSTRUAL DISORDERS

PREMENSTRUAL SYNDROME (PMS)

PMS exists when a woman complains of regular recurring psychological or physical symptoms or both which occur specifically during the luteal phase of the menstrual cycle and are relieved by the onset of menstruation (Wyatt et al 1999).

The symptoms can be enough to affect everyday life. Mild psychological symptoms occur in 95% of women of reproductive age but about 5% of symptomatic women complain of such severe symptoms that their lives are completely disrupted (O'Brien 1993).

In 2.5% of women the syndrome may cause depression, violence, child abuse and other anti-social and criminal behaviours (Barter 1999). It is possible that this exacerbation is due to a combination of biochemical and psychological factors.

PMS is a condition which in the past has not been taken seriously but now, as women take a more positive attitude to understanding their health, they realize just what an effect it can have on daily life.

Despite extensive research the precise cause of PMS remains uncertain and so treatment and advice are aimed at relieving the distressing symptoms rather than preventing PMS. The practice nurse can play a major role in providing advice and comfort (Andrews 2001).

Symptoms

These are less common in the early reproductive years and are more likely to occur after a first pregnancy. They can become progressively worse as a woman gets older and may merge with menopause symptoms in the perimenopause in the mid-40s.

Physical symptoms include:

- abdominal bloating and discomfort
- weight increase
- breast tenderness
- hot flushes
- muscle stiffness
- headaches and migraine
- appetite changes and cravings
- pelvic discomfort

- acne and skin blemishes
- lethargy
- constipation or diarrhoea
- clumsiness.

Psychological symptoms include:

- depression and irritability
- aggression and tension
- mood swings
- low self-esteem
- anxiety
- poor concentration
- paranoia
- loss of libido.

Behavioural symptoms include:

- absenteeism
- agoraphobia/claustrophobia
- avoidance of social activities
- alcohol binges
- chocolate binges
- criminal behaviour.

Although women usually complain about the negative effects of PMS, there are some who feel better and experience a feeling of well-being, energy and confidence (Logue & Moos 1988). The symptoms appear to be due to an exaggerated response to the fluctuating levels of oestrogen and progesterone within their normal range. Serotonin, endorphins, prostaglandins and lifestyle issues such as diet, caffeine, alcohol, exercise and stress may all contribute to PMS-type symptoms (Aiken 2000).

Assessment

Diagnosis is made by taking an accurate history of the symptoms – their duration and when they start in the menstrual cycle. Keeping a symptom and menstrual diary for 3 months can be helpful if there is any doubt about the diagnosis (Sutherland 2001).

Underlying psychological problems and previous psychiatric history should also be considered.

Blood tests are of no diagnostic value but might be helpful to exclude hypothyroidism and anaemia (Andrews 1998).

Management

Many women try a variety of self-help remedies before seeking professional help. There are also a few official self-help groups in the UK and many women have their own network of friends and family who understand the problem and exchange advice and support. This can have considerable benefit psychologically.

Treatments include lifestyle, diet and stress reduction, non-hormonal treatments and hormonal treatments.

Dietary changes Reduce salt intake, caffeine intake, alcohol, saturated fat and sugary foods. Maintain a healthy diet by increasing intake of complex carbohydrates, fruit and vegetables. Eat frequent regular meals which can prevent low blood sugar levels which may cause headaches and irritability.

Exercise and relaxation Regular exercise may increase natural endorphins and give a feeling of well-being. This combined with adequate rest and relaxation can improve a woman's self-esteem and help her cope with PMS.

Stress management Advice about making adjustments in lifestyle to avoid stressful situations can be helpful. Psychotherapy, counselling, yoga and meditation may also be helpful to some women. Sex may help as a great reliever of tension.

Non-hormonal treatments

- Alternative therapies such as aromatherapy, reflexology, herbal medicine, hypnosis, homeopathy and acupuncture may be useful in reducing stress levels and have a strong placebo effect. There are few controlled trials to show these benefits in PMS but if they help and the woman is less stressed then support should be given.

St John's wort (*Hypericum perforatum*) is increasingly popular as an antidepressant and can be purchased over the counter. The Committee on Safety of Medicines has emphasized that it can affect the absorption of some medication, especially the combined oral contraceptive pill (Ernst 1999).

- Gamma linolenic acid (evening primrose oil) is no longer available on prescription for treating mastalgia. There is no evidence that it is beneficial for other PMS symptoms.
- Pyridoxine (vitamin B6) is widely used but the daily dose should not exceed 10 mg and should be started 3 days prior to the predicted onset of PMS symptoms. There is little evidence that it has any beneficial effect. Long-term use with higher doses may lead to peripheral neuropathy (Leather et al 1993).
- Multivitamins and minerals are also promoted and may have a placebo effect combined with a sympathetic discussion with a nurse. Magnesium 200 mg in one study was shown to reduce fluid retention in mild PMS (Walker et al 1998). Royal jelly is also taken by some women with good effect.

• Prostaglandin inhibitors have an effect on the central nervous system and can treat pelvic pain, menstrual migraine, menorrhagia and dysmenorrhoea. Mefenamic acid 250–500 mg tds was demonstrated to be more effective than placebo in one study (Mira et al 1986). It should be started on day 16 of the cycle and taken with food to reduce gastrointestinal side-effects.

• Diuretics may help women who have proven weight gain and fluid retention during the luteal phase of their cycle. They should be taken on alternate days and electrolyte imbalance must be avoided. In one study spironolactone was shown to be effective for swelling and weight increase (O'Brien 1987).

• Serotonin reuptake inhibitors (SSRIs) have made a noticeable impact on treatment of PMS with underlying depression (Steiner et al 1995). Fluoxetine has the only UK licence for premenstrual dysphoric disorder (PMMD) which is a severe type of PMS affecting 8% of American women.

Hormonal treatments

• Progesterone and progestagen have not been shown to be effective in treating PMS. The use of Cyclogest suppositories for 14 days of the cycle prior to menstruation has never been supported by controlled trials.

• The combined oral contraceptive pill (COC) is a suitable treatment for PMS because it suppresses ovulation and will provide contraception and reduce bleeding. If PMS symptoms return during the pill-free week it is possible to tricycle the pill, i.e. take three packets consecutively and then have a 7-day break. If PMS symptoms are worse a change of progestogen should help.

• Oestrogen suppresses ovulation and may be given as a transdermal patch or subcutaneous implant (Watson et al 1989). Oestrogen must be opposed by progestagen for 12 days each cycle to prevent endometrial hyperplasia.

• Pregnancy is also a temporary cure for PMS but symptoms may return after childbirth.

• Danazol is a synthetic steroid and if given continuously will suppress ovulation. PMS symptoms will improve but the side-effects of hirsutism, weight gain and acne can be unpleasant. It is not recommended to be used for longer than 6 months (Halbreich et al 1991).

• GnRH analogues suppress ovulation completely and cause a medical oophorectomy. They can be given by monthly implant (Goserelin) or daily nasal spray (Buserelin). Long-term use is restricted because of the risks of osteoporosis and ischaemic heart disease.

Surgery Surgery is rare and only used in extreme circumstances. Hysterectomy and bilateral oophorectomy may be considered in the older woman with severe PMS symptoms or menorrhagia.

POLYCYSTIC OVARY SYNDROME

Polycystic ovary syndrome (PCOS) is a common condition which one in four to five women will experience. It is associated with a range of symptoms but only a few women will experience all of them (Hopkinson et al 1998).

Polycystic ovaries are usually enlarged and are characterized by:

- increased number and size of follicles
- thickened ovarian stroma producing excessive androgens
- an absence of preovulatory follicles
- ovulation failure
- disrupted FSH/LH ratio.

Presentation

PCOS has a number of clinical features ranging from gross hirsutism, obesity and amenorrhoea at one end of the scale to mild hirsutism or mild menstrual irregularity at the other end. Acne and androgenic alopecia, caused by raised serum testosterone, may also occur (Adams et al 1986, Conway et al 1989). Cushing's disease, congenital adrenal hyperplasia, androgen-secreting tumours and severe insulin resistance must be excluded before the diagnosis is made.

Menstrual disorders Menses are often irregular from menarche but irregularity may be associated with sudden weight gain or stopping the pill.

PCOS is present in:

- 26% of women with amenorrhoea
- 87% of women with oligomenorrhoea
- 20% of normal population with irregular periods
- 7% of women with regular periods.

Hirsutism Ninety-two percent of women with idiopathic hirsutism have PCOS but only 55–85% of women with PCOS are hirsute or have acne. The hirsutism appears at menarche and gradually progresses with age.

Obesity Women with PCOS are usually more obese than controls. They have an increased waist to hip ratio and a predominantly central fat deposition and this can lead to increased risk of cardiovascular disease in later life.

Subfertility Fifty percent of patients seen in endocrine clinics have PCOS. Infertility may be caused by anovulation or by high circulating levels of LH which inhibit the ovum development within the follicle and embryo implantation in the uterus if conception takes place.

Diagnosis

- History and observation.
- Abdominal and transvaginal ultrasound scan to confirm the presence of polycystic ovaries. The multiple cystic follicles have a string of pearls appearance.
- Blood tests for hormone levels. FSH is usually normal in PCOS but LH levels may be elevated in 45–70% of PCOS.
- Androgen levels usually raised are testosterone and androstenedione.
- Oestradiol levels are usually normal or raised since there is overproduction from the increased number of follicles. Also peripheral conversion of the increased androgens to oestrogens in subcutaneous fat.
- Prolactin levels may be raised in 7–11% of patients with PCOS.
- Sex hormone binding globulin (SHBG) should be checked.

Management

The symptoms of PCOS require careful management based on the needs of the individual patient.

Obesity In PCOS increasing body mass index (BMI) directly correlates with the menstrual cycle disturbance and hirsutism. Obese patients should be encouraged to lose weight as this has been shown to be the most effective way of restoring regular periods and diminishing hirsutism (Kiddy et al 1992).

Subfertility This is usually due to anovulation. Ovulation induction is unlikely if the BMI is more than 30 (RCOG 1998).

For the woman who wants to become pregnant drugs will be needed to induce ovulation and there are two types of drug available.

Clomiphene citrate This is an anti-oestrogen which stimulates endogenous FSH production and can be used for up to six cycles. There is a 40% pregnancy rate and ovulation is induced in 80% of women. Clomiphene is not given for longer than six cycles because of the possible risk of ovarian cancer. In women with very high LH levels (over 10 iu/l) there is a reduced success rate and greater chance of miscarriage.

Gonadotrophin therapy This is indicated in women who have been treated without success with clomiphene. They may have failed to ovulate, have hypersecretion of LH or a failed postcoital test due to anti-oestrogens in the cervical mucus.

This treatment should be carried out in a specialist unit with appropriate supervision and monitoring as it carries a higher risk of multiple pregnancy and ovarian stimulation.

There is a possible association between induced multiple ovulations or superovulation therapies and cancer of the ovary.

Surgical treatment Laparoscopic ovarian diathermy is now used to treat clomiphene-resistant women with PCOS. The advantages are:

- low risk of multiple pregnancies
- no risk of ovarian hyperstimulation
- no intensive ultrasound monitoring
- diathermy to one ovary leads to bilateral ovarian activity.

The disadvantages are:

- need appropriately trained gynaecologist
- unsure of minimum dose of diathermy needed.

Hirsutism This can be very distressing and tends to increase with age. The majority of women with moderate to severe PCOS resort to cosmetic measures such as bleaching, depilatory creams, waxing, shaving, electrolysis and laser therapy. In some places the latter two are available on the NHS.

Medical treatments are also available but will only modify the degree of hirsutism and may have undesirable side-effects and are not always a practical long-term solution. Cyproterone acetate in conjunction with ethinyloestrodiol (Dianette) reduces testosterone levels and helps to control excess body hair, greasy skin and acne. It produces a regular withdrawal bleed and provides contraception. It may take over a year to be effective in managing acne and hirsutism.

Menstrual disturbance Women with PCOS have an increased risk of developing endometrial cancer if they have prolonged amenorrhoea and obesity. Options for treatment include the progesterone-only pill (POP). Non-androgenic progestogens (e.g. medroxyprogesterone acetate, desogestrel and gestodene) given cyclically will produce a regular withdrawal bleed.

A 30 microgram COC will also reduce symptoms and provide a withdrawal bleed and contraception.

The Mirena intrauterine system (IUS) may also be used to provide endometrial protection as well as contraception.

Long-term health issues

Diabetes In 1999 the link between PCOS and diabetes was definitely established; 35% of women with PCOS were shown to have impaired glucose tolerance and 10% have maturity-onset type 2 diabetes.

Cardiovascular disease Obese patients with PCOS have been shown to have increased triglycerides and an abnormal lipid profile. Many are at an increased risk of atherosclerosis and cardiovascular disease in later life (Dahlgren et al 1992).

Insulin resistance Insulin resistance in PCOS has been shown to be aggravated by amenorrhoea. It is now felt that better insulin sensitivity may improve the clinical symptoms of PCOS (Taylor & Marsden 2000). Metformin, a biguanide used to treat type 2 diabetes, has recently been used in PCOS. Randomized controlled trials are currently taking place to establish the value of this drug in the management of PCOS.

Possible annual screening for women with PCOS

- Urine test for glycosuria
- Capillary blood glucose
- Glucose tolerance test if necessary
- Weight and BMI
- Menstrual history (three periods per year)
- Blood pressure monitoring
- Lipid profile
- Dietary advice

Practice nurses involved in women's health should be able to provide all the above and also be able to discuss and explain treatment options. They should have knowledge of drugs used to treat PCOS and be aware of resources available (Edwards 1999).

ENDOMETRIOSIS

Endometriosis is a chronic gynaecological condition which can affect women during their reproductive years (Chandler 2000, Farquhar 2002). Endometrial tissue is found in deposits outside the uterus where it is subject to the same hormonal changes. The common sites are the ovary, Fallopian tubes, the peritoneum, pouch of Douglas and the uterosacral and broad ligaments. Less common sites are the bladder, bowel wall, cervix, vagina, vulva, scar tissue and umbilicus. Very rarely it may be found in the pleura.

During every menstrual cycle the endometrial cells respond as they do in the uterus. As they cannot be shed into the vagina they develop into collections of blood that form cysts, patches and spots. These may grow and in some cases they can adhere to nearby organs, causing pain and inflammation.

In the ovary the bleeding may result in chocolate cysts (cysts filled with old blood). Infertility may be a consequence of endometriosis.

CAUSES

The aetiology is not known but there are many theories.

- Retrograde menstruation where the blood flows into the pelvis and Fallopian tubes during menstruation instead of out of the vagina (Liu & Hitchcock 1986).
- Possible autoimmune response.
- Cell transfer during surgery.
- Hereditary – first-degree relatives have a 6–9-fold increased risk compared to general population.
- Vascular or lymphatic transportation.
- Embryonic cells may give rise to deposits in the umbilicus by embryological migration.

SYMPTOMS

Some symptoms are cyclical and made worse by menstruation and others are present all the time.

- Dyspareunia (painful sexual intercourse), often caused by the fixing of the uterus in a retroverted position.
- Chronic pelvic pain which may occur pre- or postmenstrually (Buck 1997).
- Dysmenorrhoea may last throughout the period and become more severe towards the end.
- Menorrhagia, often with a dark bleed at the beginning of the period.
- Infertility may be the only symptom and occurs in approximately one-third of cases.
- Irregular uterine bleeding.
- Rectal pain and pain with defaecation.
- Urination pain.
- Swollen abdomen.
- Low energy level probably caused by insomnia due to pain.
- Cyclical haematuria, rectal bleeding or haemoptysis are less common.

DIAGNOSIS

- Initially pelvic examination may reveal nodularity and tenderness.
- Pelvic ultrasound may reveal presence of ovarian cyst or chocolate cyst.
- Laparoscopy will confirm the diagnosis. The deposits may be seen as tiny black spots or larger chocolate cysts.

Laparoscopy

This is a procedure carried out under general anaesthetic. The abdomen is distended with carbon dioxide through a cut in the umbilicus. A laparoscope is inserted into the abdomen where areas of endometrial tissue can be seen. Any other pathology can be excluded at this stage by laparoscopy.

TREATMENT

Can be medical or surgical and the aim is to relieve pain, improve fertility if desired and to reduce or remove areas of endometrial cells. It will be influenced by the woman's age, the extent and severity of the disease and the possible desire for a pregnancy.

Medical treatment

Non-steroidal antiinflammatory drugs (NSAIDs) such as ibuprofen or mefenamic acid can be used to relieve pain. They have an antiprostaglandin effect and reduce vasoconstriction and uterine contractions but they do not have any effect on endometrial cells.

Combined oral contraceptive pill

Given continuously for 3 months (tricycling), this may be successful especially when contraception is also needed. Spotting and breakthrough bleeding may occur.

Progestogens

Medroxyprogesterone, norethisterone or dydrogesterone, given in high enough doses, will have the same hormonal effect as a pregnancy and suppress ovulation. The side-effects may be fluid retention, breast tenderness, nausea, irregular bleeding and PMS-type symptoms.

Gonadotrophin-releasing hormone (GnRH) analogues

These reduce the natural production of oestrogen and cause endometrial cells to shrink. They prevent GnRH being released from the hypothalamus. Side-effects are menopausal symptoms such as hot flushes and sweats and loss of bone density after 6 months of use.

GnRH analogues used to treat endometriosis are:

- Buserelin nasal spray 150 μg into each nostril 3 times daily
- Naferelin nasal spray 200 μg twice daily
- Leuprorelin 3.75 mg s.c. or i.m. as a single dose in the first 5 days of the cycle and then every 28 days for a maximum of 6 months
- Goserelin 3.6 mg implant into anterior abdominal wall every 28 days.

Danol

This androgen-decreasing GnRH may be used for up to 9 months if the side-effects can be tolerated. It can be very effective in controlling endometriosis. The possible side-effects include weight gain, depression, acne, mood swings, libido loss, muscle cramps, hirsutism and headaches.

Alternative therapies

These may help with some symptoms such as mood swings, vaginal dryness, muscle cramps and breast pain. Oil of evening primrose and vitamin B6 are thought to be the most beneficial but as with most alternative therapies, there are no research studies to support their use.

Surgical treatment

Conservative surgery aims to remove active disease and restore normal pelvic anatomy. Laparoscopy using ablative laser or diathermy techniques and microsurgery and enucleation of chocolate cysts may be carried out in some centres where the gynaecologists are skilled in these techniques.

Hysterectomy and bilateral salpingo-oophorectomy may be the final option for a woman who has experienced pain for many years and for whom other treatments have failed. This may be a relief but there is also the chance of regret for lost fertility, especially in the younger woman. It is important that these women have the appropriate hormone replacement therapy.

MENOPAUSE

DEFINITION

The menopause is ovarian failure due to loss of ovarian follicular function accompanied by oestrogen deficiency, resulting in permanent cessation of menstruation and loss of reproductive function (Utian 1999).

Natural menopause is acknowledged to have occurred after 12 months of amenorrhoea. The average age for menopause is 51 years, with the age range being 45–55 years.

Perimenopause is the time around the menopause, starting with the first clinical signs of menopause – longer cycles with heavier and longer bleeding which are due to a decline in ovarian follicular function. Vasomotor symptoms also start to occur, e.g. hot flushes and night sweats.

Post menopause is after a period of 12 consecutive months since the last menstrual period.

Menopausal transition is the period of time before the final menstrual period when variations in the cycle are experienced.

The *climacteric* is defined as the transition from reproductive to non-reproductive state and the menopause is an event which takes place during that time.

Premature menopause or premature ovarian failure (POF) occurs before the age of 45 and premature menopause can occur before the age of 40 in 1% of women (Chamberlain 1995). Women who smoke experience their menopause 2 years earlier than non-smokers (Coope 1997).

Induced menopause is defined as the cessation of menstruation which follows either surgical removal of the ovaries or ablation of ovarian function by chemotherapy, radiotherapy or GnRH analogue. In the absence of surgery, induced menopause may be either temporary or permanent (Rees & Purdie 2002).

The menopause is a natural event and is not an illness although some of the consequences can be distressing. It often coincides with other major life events which can be a problem. These may be:

- children leaving home
- coping with elderly parents and relatives
- relationship changes and divorce
- concern about possible redundancy
- acceptance of failed expectations of life
- accepting the end to fertility
- looming retirement.

As a contrast it may be anticipated in a positive way:

- no more periods
- no risk of unplanned pregnancy
- greater self-confidence
- greater self-esteem
- fewer responsibilities and more time for relaxation
- in some cultures postmenopausal women have a higher social status.

A woman's life expectancy now means that she could be in the postmenopausal state for at least 30 years. It is thus important that women should be well informed about menopause and its consequences. The practice nurse is an ideal person to give accurate and unbiased information.

SYMPTOMS

Vasomotor symptoms:

- hot flushes
- night sweats
- palpitations
- headaches.

Psychological symptoms:

- mood swings
- panic attacks
- depression
- poor concentration and memory loss
- anxiety and loss of confidence
- libido loss and sexual difficulties.

Urogenital symptoms:

- vaginal dryness leading to dyspareunia
- vulval and vaginal atrophy
- vaginitis
- bladder dysfunction and urethral syndrome
- uterovaginal prolapse
- stress incontinence.

Other symptoms may include joint and muscle pain and aches, thinning of hair and skin and brittle nails.

LONG-TERM EFFECTS

The long-term effects of oestrogen deficiency can be osteoporosis and cardiovascular disease.

Osteoporosis

As oestrogen levels fall bone turnover is increased, leading to imbalance between bone formation and resorption. The result is skeletal loss, leading to osteoporosis in which bone strength is compromised and predisposes to fracture (NIH 2000). This can have huge financial and personal health implications.

Cardiovascular disease

Myocardial infarction and stroke are unusual in women before the menopause but cardiovascular disease becomes the most common cause of death in women over the age of 60. Women have a 3.4-fold risk of atherosclerosis after a natural menopause (Stevenson 1996).

DIAGNOSIS

If the woman is in her early 40s or 50s the diagnosis can be made by symptoms and history. Some menopause symptoms can be confused with other conditions:

- dysfunctional uterine bleeding
- pregnancy
- exercise-induced amenorrhoea
- thyroid or adrenal disorder.

Measurement of FSH is helpful when:

- premature menopause is suspected
- the woman has had a hysterectomy with conservation of ovaries.

An FSH above 30 iu/l is diagnostic of menopause.

MANAGEMENT

Healthy lifestyle advice may be helpful.

- Smoking cessation.
- Dietary advice – balanced diet with at least 700 mg calcium and avoidance of caffeine and hot spicy foods which may trigger hot flushes.
- Regular exercise such as walking, dancing, swimming or tennis.
- Alcohol in moderation with some alcohol-free days.
- Relaxation and stress reduction will improve coping strategies.
- Counselling may help with life events which are causing concern.
- Weight control and the advice that the majority of women are heavier at menopause than they were 20 years ago, with a change in shape.

Participation in the breast and cervical screening programmes every 3 years should be encouraged. Routine breast examinations are no longer advocated but the woman should be encouraged to be breast aware.

Monitoring of blood pressure and BMI should be carried out regularly.

HORMONE REPLACEMENT THERAPY (HRT)

HRT will relieve hot flushes and night sweats and improve vaginal atrophy and help with some of the other short-term symptoms associated with the menopause (Rees & Purdie 2002). It will have a positive effect on bone density by delaying the skeletal loss which occurs at and after the menopause (Whitehead & Godfree 1992). Recent research has shown that HRT increases the risk of venous thromboembolism and breast cancer. Contrary to earlier observational studies, trials have shown no beneficial effect on cardiovascular disease (MHRA 2003).

HRT consists of a wide range of preparations and a regime may have to be individualized for some women with adjustments made to standard doses and routes.

HRT usually consists of oestrogen and progestogen which are packed together with instructions for use. Women who have had a hysterectomy can have oestrogen alone whereas women with an intact uterus need to have progestogen as well as oestrogen. This is to prevent endometrial hyperplasia which can occur with unopposed oestrogen (Grady et al 1995). The progestogen may be given sequentially or continuously and the oestrogen is given continuously.

The commonest types of progestogen are:

- medroxyprogesterone acetate
- dydrogesterone
- norethisterone
- levonorgestrel.

The dose and strength will vary from product to product. There is a comprehensive list in the Monthly Index of Medical Specialities (MIMs) and this is updated regularly.

In the perimenopause whilst periods are still occurring or within 12 months of the last period, HRT is given cyclically and this may be monthly or 3 monthly and resulting in a regular bleed. In the postmenopausal phase, i.e. more than 1 year after the last period, continuous combined treatment may be given. The use of a gonadomimetic (Tibolone) may be recommended as an alternative to conventional HRT at this time. These products are described as no bleed or 'period free' but initially irregular bleeding may occur and the woman should be warned about this possibility.

Routes of administration

- Oral
- Transdermal (patches or gel)
- Subcutaneous implant
- Nasal spray
- Vaginal (cream, ring, pessary or tablet)

Oestrogen

Can be:

- an implant inserted subcutaneously into the lower abdomen, buttocks or thigh
- oral, either alone or with a progestogen, continuously or sequentially
- gel
- transdermal patch, either alone or with a progestogen continuously or sequentially
- vaginal cream, pessary, tablet or a ring.

The oestrogen in HRT is made from naturally occurring products and is very different from the synthetic oestrogen used in the COC pill.

Progestogen

Can be:

- oral, alone or with oestrogen
- transdermal patch combined with oestrogen
- IUS system which is a levonorgestrel-releasing device awaiting licence for use as HRT.

Testosterone

Administered via an implant and is used to improve libido.

Gonadomimetics

These are synthetic steroids which have mixed oestrogenic, progestogenic and androgenic actions. Tibolone has a licence for libido improvement and is being used increasingly for women who have had breast cancer. It is taken continuously without progestogen and is for women who are postmenopausal as it is period free.

Starting HRT

This will vary from woman to woman and depends on her individual reasons for wanting HRT. Some start in the perimenopause to relieve symptoms and others delay starting until they are older especially if they are concerned about osteoporosis prevention. It is never too late to start.

Investigations prior to starting HRT

- Weight/height BMI
- Blood pressure
- Cervical smear if due
- Breast awareness and encouragement to attend for mammography when appropriate
- Serum cholesterol if appropriate
- Lifestyle advice
- Pelvic examination only if clinically indicated
- Urinalysis

Monitoring

- Bleeding pattern
- Symptom relief
- Blood pressure
- Breast awareness

CONTRACEPTION AND SEXUAL HEALTH

Following the Teenage Pregnancy Report in 1999, focus has now turned to the wider issues of sexual health and the publication of The National Strategy for Sexual Health and HIV. This identifies a much bigger role for primary care in the delivery of sexual health services. Implementing the strategy will have far-reaching implications for practice nurses and it is essential that they have undertaken appropriate training for the advice and care that they provide. The code of professional conduct (NMC 2002) stresses that nurses must be aware of their limitations and seek to rectify any gaps in their knowledge base. Nurses must be aware that poor sexual health has an impact on an individual's sense of worth and well-being.

The ability to respond positively to the needs of diverse clients and the demand for proactive sexual health promotion, health education and health protection mean that all nurses working in primary care will need to have a working knowledge of sexual health (Belfield 1999a,b, Guillebaud & Hannaford 1998).

If a practice is unable to provide the appropriate services the practice nurse must be able to supply leaflets and help the patient to access the service required.

The extension to nurse prescribing is the most exciting and innovative development for nurses working in the field of reproductive and sexual health. The extended formulary includes almost every method of contraception. Every consultation with a man or woman, regardless of age, may be an opportunity to raise the issue of sexual health. The reasons for a woman seeking a consultation with the practice nurse may include:

- pregnancy testing
- emergency contraception
- unplanned pregnancy
- contraception
- menstrual disorders
- fertility advice

- preconception advice
- infertility
- sexual difficulties
- STIs
- breast problems
- menopause
- cervical screening.

Box 1.1 Service specifications for levels 1–3 of sexual health strategy (DoH 2001)

Level 1

- Sexual history taking and risk assessment
- Sexually transmitted infection (STI) testing for women
- HIV testing and counselling
- Pregnancy testing and referral
- Contraceptive information and services
- Assessment and referral of men with STI symptoms
- Cervical cytology screening and referral
- Hepatitis B immunization

Level 2

- Intrauterine device insertion
- Testing and treatment for STIs
- Partner notification
- Invasive STI testing for men (until non-invasive tests are available)
- Vasectomy
- Contraceptive implant insertion

Level 3

- Specialized HIV treatment and care
- Highly specialized contraception
- Specialized infection management, including partner notification
- Outreach contraceptive services
- Outreach for STI prevention
- Special responsibility for service need assessment
- Special responsibility for supporting provider quality and meeting clinical governance requirements

Contraception is the means by which fertility and reproduction are controlled. When discussing contraception with a woman it is important to take an accurate personal, family and sexual history before helping her to make an informed choice about her contraceptive method. It is also important to discuss the risks and benefits of the methods and how the methods work. Information should be given about what to do if a method fails or if its efficacy is compromised and this must include the availability of emergency contraception. All information must be regularly updated and backed up by accurate and updated leaflets. Time spent on accurate teaching of the chosen method is well spent. It is vital to use suitable up-to-date language and be aware of non-verbal communication and body language.

Contraceptive needs can be influenced by age, health, relationships, career stage, financial stability, lifestyle, religion, ethnicity, perceptions, anxieties, embarrassment and decisions about having children.

It is important to recognize that contraception and sexual health are linked and all consultations must reflect this.

Decisions on the choice of contraceptive method may be influenced by:

- effectiveness
- perceived safety
- recognized contraindications
- acceptability
- availability
- ease of use
- reversibility
- partner acceptability
- previous experience
- reasons for avoiding pregnancy
- motivation.

Most women will use more than one method during their reproductive lives and special consideration of the method chosen will be necessary at certain times, such as after a pregnancy and as the woman approaches menopause. Increasing user effectiveness depends on:

- ensuring correct knowledge of use of chosen method
- teaching how to use chosen method
- encouraging disclosure of problems
- being prepared to discuss women's experiences, perceptions and interpretation of side-effects
- advising on the availability and use of emergency contraception and 'back-up' methods.

Contraceptive methods fall into the following categories.

- *Hormonal methods* – combined oral contraceptive pill (COC), progesterone only pill (POP), injectables, implants, intrauterine systems (IUS)
- *Mechanical methods* – intrauterine contraceptive device (IUD)

- *Barrier methods* – diaphragm, caps with spermicides, sponges and male and female condoms
- *Natural methods* – natural family planning, Persona and coitus interruptus
- *Permanent methods* – male and female sterilization
- *Emergency methods* – hormonal and postcoital IUD

Where concerns about STIs are relevant, the use of condoms with another method is desirable. The value of risk assessment at the contraceptive consultation cannot be overemphasized.

HORMONAL CONTRACEPTION

All hormonal methods work in a similar way and provide highly effective and long-lasting choices.

Combined oral contraceptive pill (COC)

This was introduced into the UK in 1961 after many years of research. It is used extensively and despite the concerns and scares which inevitably arise, there are few risks provided that it is prescribed appropriately to well women with no medical contraindications. It is safer than pregnancy and childbirth.

The COC contains two hormones – oestrogen (usually ethinyloestradiol) and a progestogen. It works by:

- inhibiting ovulation
- making the endometrium unsuitable for implantation
- making the cervical mucus impenetrable to sperm.

Research has resulted in low-dose pills and many varieties to ensure safety and choice.

The COC is very effective provided that it is taken correctly but efficacy is lost if:

- pills are missed or a dose is taken more than 12 hours late especially if this extends the pill-free week
- the woman vomits within 3 hours of taking the pill
- there is severe diarrhoea
- she is taking medication which is an enzyme inducer or affects the absorption in the bowel such as broad-spectrum antibiotics.

Types of COC

- Monophasic COCs contain the same doses of oestrogen and progestogen in every pill.
- Biphasic COCs contain two different levels of progestogen.
- Triphasic COCs contain usually two varying amounts of oestrogen and three varying amounts of progestogen.
- Every-day pills have seven inactive or placebo pills equivalent to a pill-free week.

Advantages

- Reliable
- Easily reversible
- No interference with intercourse
- Relief of menorrhagia and dysmenorrhoea
- Reduced risk of iron deficiency anaemia
- Less benign breast disease
- Relief of PMT
- Reduced risk of ectopic pregnancy
- Protection against pelvic inflammatory disease (PID)
- Protection against endometrial and ovarian cancer

Disadvantages

- Needs to be taken consistently
- No protection against STIs
- Increased risk of hypertension, arterial disease and venous thromboembolism
- Increased risk of liver adenoma, cholestatic jaundice and gallstones
- Small increased risk of breast cancer while taking the pill and for 10 years after stopping. The cancers appear to be less advanced and are less likely to have spread
- Unsuitable for smokers over the age of 35
- Unsuitable for those with a BMI of 35 kg/m^2

The COC and liver enzyme-inducing drugs

- Anticonvulsants – barbiturates, primidone, phenytoin, carbamazepine, topiramate
- Antitubercular – rifampicin
- Antifungal – griseofulvin
- Diuretic – spironolactone
- Tranquillizer – meprobamate

If the woman is using a drug that induces liver enzymes an alternative type of contraception is preferred but if she still wishes to take the COC she will need a pill containing at least 50 μg oestrogen. She should take three packets of monophasic pills consecutively without a break (tricycling). To increase efficacy the pill-free period may be cut to 4 days.

If she experiences breakthrough bleeding and STI risk has been excluded, increasing the oestrogen should be considered.

If the woman stops taking the liver enzyme-inducing drug she should wait for 8 weeks before reducing the dose of oestrogen.

The COC and broad-spectrum antibiotics

- Penicillins
- Tetracyclines
- Cephalosporins

If the woman has been on long-term antibiotics for more than 2 weeks she may start taking the pill on day 1 of her cycle as normal. If she is already established on the COC and is about to start long-term antibiotic treatment or switch to a different antibiotic, she will need to use condoms or abstain from sex for 2 weeks. If this runs into her pill-free week she should start her next packet immediately. If she is taking phasic pills she should take the last section of pills in her next packet. She should be on the highest dose of oestrogen for a full 2-week period before taking a 7-day break.

If the pill taker is prescribed a short course of antibiotics she should use condoms during the treatment and for 7 days after finishing the course.

Use of the COC A medical history should be taken to consider:

- cardiovascular disease risk
- risk factors for venous thromboembolism
- liver disease
- migraine with aura
- pregnancy
- undiagnosed vaginal bleeding
- age
- smoking status.

Examination should include blood pressure and BMI. It is not necessary for a woman starting hormonal methods of contraception to undergo a pelvic examination. Nor is it necessary for a woman under the age of 20 to have a cervical smear.

Pill taking Pill taking should be carefully taught and advice given about action to be taken if a pill is missed. Condoms should be advised to protect against STIs. If the pill is started on the first day of a period the woman will be contraceptively safe straight away but if the pill is started on day 2–5 she will not be safe for 7 days. Ideally the pill should be taken at the same time every day but there are 12 hours to spare.

At the end of 21 days there is usually a break of 7 days when no pills are taken and the woman starts her new packet of pills on the 8th day. Every new packet of pills will begin on the same day of the week.

Some women are advised to tricycle their pill regime especially if they experience headaches in their pill-free week.

Choice of COC Usually a second-generation pill containing 30 μg of oestrogen is chosen initially but if a woman is older or has possible cardiovascular risk factors pills containing 20 μg of oestrogen may be preferred.

If a woman has acne third-generation pills will be more appropriate. In severe cases of acne a pill containing cyproterone, which is an antiandrogen, may be recommended. This pill (Dianette) is also used for women suffering from hirsutism, especially when associated with PCOS.

Follow-up Follow-up is usually at 3 months and then every 6 months if all is well. At each appointment blood pressure is recorded and weight if there are concerns about weight gain. Any problems should be discussed and advice on sexual health should be offered and reinforced. Condoms should be offered if these are available. This is also an ideal time to check on cervical smear status.

Side-effects These may be oestrogenic, progestogenic or androgenic.
Oestrogenic:

- nausea
- headache
- dizziness
- breast tenderness
- increased vaginal secretions.

Progestogenic:

- headache
- mood changes
- breast tenderness
- bloating
- weight changes
- vaginal dryness.

Androgenic:

- acne
- hirsutism
- weight gain.

If any of the above symptoms are experienced after 3 months on the pill a change to another type of pill should be considered.

Breakthrough bleeding If this persists after the first 3 months settling in period, it should be investigated. Chlamydia should be excluded and cervical ectropion or neoplasm. Pill taking should be checked and possible drug interactions. If all the above are satisfactory then a change of pill may be indicated.

Progesterone only pill (POP)

The POPs contain only progesterone and they prevent pregnancy by:

- thickening cervical mucus, making a barrier to sperm
- making the endometrium unreceptive to implantation
- reducing Fallopian tube function
- preventing ovulation in some cycles.

The efficacy of the POP relies more on patient ability to remember to take it at the same time every day because it only has a 3-hour window. It is more effective in older women who are less fertile. In women who are over 70 kg in weight it may not be so effective and so two pills a day are recommended.

Advantages
- Does not interfere with breastfeeding
- Useful for women with contraindications to COC (heavy smokers over 35, hypertension, VTE and valvular heart disease)
- Not affected by broad-spectrum antibiotics
- Need not be stopped prior to surgery
- Suitable for diabetics
- Suitable for women with focal migraine
- May relieve PMS
- Reduces dysmenorrhoea

Disadvantages
- Requires consistent use
- Higher risk of pregnancy among younger women
- Menstrual irregularities
- Possible increase in ectopic pregnancies
- May cause functional ovarian cysts
- Same breast cancer risk as COC

Contraindications
Absolute:

- pregnancy
- undiagnosed vaginal bleeding
- severe arterial disease
- severe dyslipidaemia
- recent trophoblastic disease
- severe progestogenic side-effects on COC
- previous ectopic pregnancy
- liver disease.

Relative:

- chronic systemic disease
- recurrent cholestatic jaundice
- sex steroid-dependent cancer
- symptomatic ovarian cysts
- risk factors for arterial disease.

There are three types of POP – norethisterone based, levonorgestrel based and a new type which is desogestrel based. This POP is licensed for ovulation suppression and has only recently been marketed.

Possible side-effects
- Ovarian cysts
- Breast tenderness
- Weight gain
- Depression
- Nausea
- Irregular bleeding
- Amenorrhoea

Method of use The initial consultation should include blood pressure and weight recording. It is important to stress that this pill should be taken at the same time every day. If the POP is taken on the first day of a period no extra precautions are needed. The pills are then taken continuously without any breaks. There should not be a break when changing from different brands of POP or from the COC.

After pregnancy it is advisable to start 21 days post delivery but it may be started immediately after a miscarriage or termination of pregnancy.

It is important to stress to the woman that if she is more than 3 hours late taking her POP she must take the pill when she remembers it but must use condoms or abstain from sex for the next 7 days.

Follow-up consultation should be at 3 months initially and if all is well, 6 monthly.

Injectable contraceptives (long-acting progestogens)

Depo-Provera is the only injectable currently available for long-term contraceptive use and it is highly effective. It inhibits ovulation and also thickens cervical mucus.

Advantages
- Very effective
- Long lasting
- Not related to intercourse
- Reduced bleeding or amenorrhoea
- No cardiovascular complications
- Protects against ovarian and endometrial cancer
- Does not interfere with breastfeeding
- May reduce frequency of sickle cell crisis

Disadvantages
- Irregular bleeding which can be erratic and heavy

- Possible delay in return to fertility
- Amenorrhoea (an advantage to most women)
- Weight gain or loss
- Possible mood changes
- Facial spots
- Bloating
- Cannot be removed

Administration It is administered by deep intramuscular injection into the gluteal muscle. The first dose is given during the first 5 days of a normal menstrual cycle or immediately after a termination of pregnancy or a miscarriage. Subsequent injections are given usually at 11–12 week intervals. Depo-Provera is effective for 89 days. If a woman is late for her injection it is not practical to wait for her next period to restart her injection as she may be amenorrhoeic for some time and so certain guidelines need to be followed to avoid an unplanned pregnancy.

1. *If no unprotected intercourse since last injection expired at 89 days.* Give the next injection immediately and advise condoms for the next 7 days. Pregnancy test in 2 weeks if any doubts about unprotected sexual intercourse (UPSI).
2. *UPSI but only in last 72 hours.* Give emergency hormonal contraception and counsel about possible failure and administer injection if informed consent given. Pregnancy test in 2 weeks to exclude failure of emergency contraception.
3. *UPSI in last 5 days.* Consider emergency IUD insertion. Give the next injection at the same time as the IUD fit if not going to keep the IUD for long-term contraception. Always document informed consent. Do a pregnancy test 2 weeks later to exclude emergency contraception failure.
4. *UPSI and emergency contraception is not appropriate.* Pregnancy must be excluded by doing two pregnancy tests 2 weeks apart before the next injection is given. Abstinence or careful condom use should be advised between the two tests. If both tests are negative Depo-Provera can be given with advice to use condoms for the next 7 days. A further pregnancy test is advisable 2 weeks later.

Implants

Implanon is a single rod etonogestrel-releasing implant. It is inserted subdermally into the medial aspect of the upper arm using a preloaded applicator. Local anaesthetic is administered prior to insertion. In thin women an impression may be noticeable and the capsule can always be felt if it is inserted correctly. It inhibits ovulation and will also thicken cervical mucus and alter endometrium.

It is essential that the health professional fitting and removing Implanon should have received the appropriate training and supervision as specified by the manufacturers.

Implanon is effective for up to 3 years and is contraceptively effective within 24 hours of insertion.

Advantages

- Long lasting, very effective
- Not intercourse related
- Effects are rapidly reversible after removal
- Reduced bleeding or amenorrhoea
- No effect on future fertility
- Easy insertion and removal by appropriately trained healthcare professional
- Does not interfere with breastfeeding

Disadvantages

- Possible irregular bleeding
- Minor operative procedure
- Possible development of ovarian cysts
- Breast tenderness
- Weight gain
- Contraceptive efficacy reduced by enzyme-inducing drugs

Intrauterine system (IUS)

This is a T-shaped device similar to an IUD which releases a small amount of levonorgestrel (progestogen) daily. It is inserted into the uterus and works by a localized effect. The endometrium is suppressed and the cervical mucus is thickened. It is effective for 5 years and the pregnancy rate is 0.2 per 100 woman-years.

Advantages

- Reduction in menstrual blood loss
- Less dysmenorrhoea
- Does not interfere with breastfeeding
- Effective for 5 years
- Easily reversible
- Not intercourse related
- Reduces pelvic inflammatory disease

Disadvantages

- Possibility of expulsion
- Insertion may be difficult
- It may cause irregular bleeding initially
- Possible development of ovarian cysts
- Possible nuisance side-effects such as weight gain, spots and bloatedness
- Possible ectopic pregnancy

INTRAUTERINE DEVICES (IUD)

IUDs are small plastic and copper devices available in a variety of shapes and sizes. They are inserted into the uterus and work by preventing the sperm reaching the egg due to the action of the copper. IUDs containing more than 300 mm copper are more effective. They can be used by all women, whether or not they have had children. They are not suitable for women who are at high risk of infection, e.g. women with multiple sexual partners.

Advantages

- Highly effective 98–99% depending on type
- Long lasting, 5–8 years
- Not intercourse related
- Fully reversible
- No effect on future fertility
- Effective immediately after insertion
- No interference with breastfeeding
- More effective as emergency contraceptive than oral form

Disadvantages

- Menstrual disturbances – longer, heavier
- Dysmenorrhoea
- Small risk of uterine perforation dependent on the skill of fitter
- Risk of infection dependent on lifestyle – highest risk in first 20 days after insertion
- Possible risk of ectopic pregnancy

BARRIER METHODS

These work by preventing the sperm and the egg meeting. Barriers can be diaphragms, cervical caps, male and female condoms and spermicides.

Diaphragm

Diaphragms and caps can be latex or silicone and come in different sizes and types. To be effective they must be used with a spermicide. If fitted correctly and the method taught well and with empathy and patience, this method can be very successful. It is 96% effective when used in conjunction with a spermicide.

Advantages

- Effective with careful use
- Under control of woman
- No established health risks
- May help to protect cervix from STIs and cancer by acting as a barrier
- Possible to use in advance of intercourse
- Can be used when menstruating

Disadvantages

- Requires thinking ahead
- Not as effective as other methods
- May cause increase in cystitis and urinary tract infections by pressure irritating the bladder
- Possible latex or spermicide allergy or irritation
- Oil-based preparations must not be used with latex
- May cause vaginal irritation

Contraindications

- Congenital abnormalities of vagina or cervix
- Allergy to rubber or latex
- Poor muscle tone
- Unacceptability of touching genital area and cervix
- Pelvic or vaginal infection
- Undiagnosed vaginal bleeding
- Lack of personal hygiene
- Vaginal prolapse
- Virgo intacta. Diaphragm may be fitted before intercourse has taken place if the hymen is intact
- Previous toxic shock syndrome

A diaphragm may take up to 30 minutes to successfully fit and teach and this should be done by a trained family planning nurse or doctor.

A vaginal examination needs to be carried out to check the position of the cervix. It is also possible to check muscle tone to exclude vaginal wall prolapse and also position of the retropubic ridge.

There are three types of diaphragm:

- coil spring
- flat spring
- arcing spring.

The arcing spring is used for women whose cervix is very posterior and who find it difficult to feel their cervix. The flat spring is used for women who have an anterior or midplane cervix and the coil spring may be suitable for women with a shallow symphysis pubis.

The diaphragm should be inserted prior to intercourse and left in for a minimum of 6 hours afterwards and no longer than 24 hours. After use it should be washed in warm soapy water and rinsed and dried and bent carefully back into shape. It should be checked regularly for holes or deterioration in quality.

Checks should be repeated if the woman loses or gains more than 3 kg in weight and following pregnancy. A new diaphragm should always be supplied if the woman has a vaginal infection to prevent reinfection after treatment.

Cap

The cap is smaller than the diaphragm and only covers the cervix and is held in place by suction. Like the diaphragm, it is important to use it with a spermicide to improve effectiveness.

The types of cap are the cervical cap, the vault cap (Dumas), the vimule and more recently the Oves cap. The Oves cap is made from silicone and is very thin. It is available in three sizes. It can remain in place for 72 hours and is available to buy over the counter.

It is essential that a woman is taught to insert and remove a cap in the same way as the diaphragm.

Male and female condoms

These can be up to 98% effective and are essential to protect against sexually transmitted infections.

Advantages

- Very effective with careful use
- No health risks
- Woman or man can take responsibility
- Effective protection against STIs, including HIV
- Easily obtained
- Possible protection against cervical neoplasia

Disadvantages

- May break, slip off or come out
- May be perceived to interrupt intercourse
- Can only be used once
- Femidom is expensive
- Latex condoms cannot be used with oil-based lubricants
- Possible loss of sensitivity

Femidom The Femidom is a polyurethane condom with a non-spermicide lubricant. It has two small rings: one helps insertion like a tampon and the outside ring keeps it in place over the genital area. It can be used with any type of lubricant.

Spermicides

Spermicides prevent pregnancy by destroying sperm and by changing the pH of the vagina. Usually spermicides are used in conjunction with another method and increase the efficacy of the diaphragm and condom. They are available as gels, creams, pessaries and foams and usually contain a chemical called nonoxynol 9.

Advantages

- No systemic effects
- Easy to obtain and use
- Provide lubrication
- Possible protection against STIs and HIV

Disadvantages

- Possible local allergic reaction
- Poor efficacy when used alone
- Possibly perceived as messy

NATURAL METHODS

Natural family planning

This is also known as the temperature method, the cervical mucus or Billings method or the symptothermal method. The woman is able to recognize and predict ovulation with these methods and is thus able to identify fertile and infertile phases of her menstrual cycle. Can be up to 98% effective if two or more fertility indicators are used. These indicators are cervical mucus changes, temperature changes and cycle length. Ovulation occurs 12–16 days before the woman's next period.

Advantages

- Can be used to plan a pregnancy as well as prevent pregnancy
- No known health risks
- No hormones or devices used
- Not intercourse related
- May be the only acceptable method for some couples with particular religious or personal beliefs
- Effective when properly taught
- Shared responsibility

Disadvantages

- Requires commitment from both partners
- Should be taught by specialist NFP teacher
- Requires daily observation and record keeping
- Expensive if Persona is used

Persona

Persona is a small handheld computerized monitor. Via a database it monitors luteinizing hormone and oestrone levels. It tells a woman by a series of coloured lights when to test her urine. A green light indicates that it is safe to have sex because she is in her infertile period, a red light means that she is in her fertile period and should use a condom or abstain from sex. A yellow light means that a further test is needed to give more information. It is not suitable for:

- breastfeeding women
- women approaching menopause
- women on hormone treatment
- polycystic ovary syndrome
- women who are within 2 months of having emergency hormonal contraception
- women with kidney or liver disease.

Coitus interruptus

This method, also known as withdrawal, is the oldest and possibly most widely used method of contraception. It involves removing the penis from the vagina before ejaculation occurs. It fails when small amounts of semen leak out before ejaculation occurs.

Advantages

- Allows the couple to choose full intercourse or coitus interruptus
- Free of charge

Disadvantages

- Can be dissatisfying for couple
- Under control of male
- Unsuitable for men with premature ejaculation
- Increased anxiety
- Risk of pregnancy occurring

PERMANENT METHODS

Female sterilization

Female sterilization involves blocking of the Fallopian tubes to prevent the ovum travelling along the tube and thus preventing the sperm and ovum meeting and fertilization taking place. Tubal sterilization is highly effective but it does have a failure rate depending on the type of tube-blocking method used. This can be cutting, sealing or blocking the tube with clips, diathermy and cautery or excising and ligating the Fallopian tube.

Counselling and full information are essential to ensure that the decision is informed and that the woman is aware that the procedure is not reversible and she must be certain that her family is complete.

Advantages

- Permanent
- High efficacy
- Immediately effective
- Removes fears of pregnancy more than other methods

Disadvantages

- Not reversible easily
- Surgical procedure requiring anaesthetic
- Occasional failure
- Possible regret, especially if carried out without proper counselling

Contraindications

- Relationship problems
- Psychiatric illness
- Ill health which could increase operative risk
- Indecisiveness about desire for operation

Male sterilization

Vasectomy involves the removal by excision of part of the vas deferens which is the tube which transports sperm from the testes to the penis. It is 99.9% effective and should be regarded as irreversible. It is carried out usually under local anaesthesia. It takes approximately 3 months for the sperms to clear and two negative sperm counts are advised before a man will be contraceptively safe.

As in female sterilization, careful counselling is essential and the man should be advised that his libido will not be affected and the appearance of the ejaculate will remain the same.

Advantages

- Permanent
- Very effective

Disadvantages

- Minor surgical procedure
- Not easily reversed
- Not immediately effective

Contraindications

- Urological problems
- Psychiatric illness
- Relationship problems
- Indecision by either partner

EMERGENCY CONTRACEPTION

Emergency contraception is a very important method of preventing a pregnancy and is used after unprotected sexual intercourse (UPSI) or when there has been a possible problem with a woman's usual method. This may include:

- forgetting to restart the COC after a 7-day break
- missing four or more COC pills in the middle of a packet and then having sexual intercourse

- condom splitting or coming off during intercourse
- recent use of drugs which might affect a fetus
- rape or sexual assault
- cap or diaphragm not fitted properly.

There are two methods of emergency contraception:

- hormonal method
- copper-releasing IUD.

Emergency contraceptive pills (Levonelle-2)

- Delay or prevent ovulation
- Alter the endometrium to prevent implantation of a fertilized ovum
- Alter the activity of the wall of the uterine tubes to prevent the ovum and sperm meeting

This method must be used within 72 hours of unprotected sex, but is more effective the earlier it is started. It is 95% effective if taken within 24 hours of UPSI and 85% effective if taken within 48 hours.

Emergency copper-releasing IUD

- Used within 5 days of UPSI or up to 5 days after the earliest calculated ovulation day in the cycle
- Highly effective
- Alters the endometrium so that a fertilized ovum does not implant
- Affects sperm motility and so lessens the chance of an ovum being fertilized

Emergency contraception is now much more widely available and some pharmacies are now selling it over the counter or in some areas supplying it free of charge to under-21 s. It can be taken more than once in a cycle should the need arise and there is no limit to how many times it can be taken.

CONTRACEPTION AFTER PREGNANCY

If the woman is breastfeeding she should not take the COC because it inhibits lactation. The POP is safe and does not affect the supply of breast milk. It should be started 28 days after delivery in breastfeeding women.

If the woman is not breastfeeding she should start the POP or COC 21 days after delivery because she will potentially ovulate 28 days after childbirth.

If she is going to use Depo-Provera she should start this 6 weeks post delivery to minimize the risk of irregular bleeding, whether breastfeeding or not.

An IUD can be inserted 6 weeks post delivery but care must be taken to avoid perforating the uterus which can be softer, especially if the woman is breastfeeding.

Diaphragms and caps need refitting 5–6 weeks after delivery because a different size might be needed.

The COC, POP and contraceptive injection can all be started immediately after a miscarriage or after a termination of pregnancy. This is because ovulation can occur as early as 10 days after such an event.

MIDLIFE CONTRACEPTION

It is advisable to use contraception for 2 years after the last menstrual period if a woman is under 50 and for 1 year if a woman is over 50.

Individual needs and general health should be taken into consideration because an unplanned pregnancy at this time in life can be very distressing.

The COC can be continued to menopause provided the woman does not smoke and has no other risk factors. IUDs and implants may be preferred because they remove a lot of the anxiety of unplanned pregnancy.

The perimenopausal woman already on HRT must be advised to continue contraception. IUDs, IUS or barrier methods are ideal. The POP appears to be effective and is taken continuously with the HRT. There are no clinical data to support such use but it does appear to be effective.

THE FUTURE

Research continues into new and improved methods of contraception. There will be different types of oral pills. A contraceptive patch is soon to be released. Biodegradable implants, vaginal hormonal rings, nasal sprays, improved condoms and spermicidally impregnated diaphragms are all possible in the future.

A couple need to have choice and to be as well informed as possible by appropriately trained health professionals.

URINARY INCONTINENCE

This section is reproduced with permission of Elsevier Science from the *Pocket book of general practice* by S Cartwright and C Goodlee.

Incontinence is involuntary leakage of urine and is a common and disabling condition, which can be significantly improved by appropriate intervention.

HISTORY TAKING

General questions should be asked relating to:

- pain on passing urine – suggestive of urinary tract infection, atrophic vaginitis or obstruction
- liquid intake – alcohol and coffee are diuretics
- drugs, e.g. diuretics, antidepressants
- use of pads or towels
- past medical history, e.g. stroke, Parkinson's disease, multiple sclerosis, spinal injury, obstetric history.

Specific questions relating to the type of incontinence include the following.

1. Stress incontinence due to weakness of the urethral sphincter:
   - leakage of urine with exercise, coughing or sneezing
2. Urge incontinence:
   - urinary frequency day or night
   - hurrying to get to the toilet
   - not being able to get to the toilet in time
3. Overflow incontinence (bladder outflow obstruction):
   - difficulty passing urine (hesitancy)
   - dribbling after passing urine
   - poor stream
   - nocturia
   - sensation of incomplete bladder emptying
4. Passive incontinence:
   - passing urine without being aware of it
   - accidents in bed at night

EXAMINATION

The practitioner should look for:

- constipation
- palpable bladder
- overflow incontinence
- pelvic masses, e.g. fibroids
- local lumps, e.g. inguinal hernia
- cystocoele
- local infections, e.g. Candida
- atrophic vaginitis
- assessment of pelvic floor muscles by asking the patient to pull up her pelvic floor during pelvic examination.

INVESTIGATIONS

Investigations could include:

- dipstick urine for blood, sugar, protein and nitrates
- midstream urine for microscopy, culture and antibiotic sensitivities
- urinary diary documenting frequency and volume of urine passed and drinks taken.

MANAGEMENT

Stress incontinence

Encourage reduction of intraabdominal pressure by:

- reducing weight
- stopping smoking
- avoiding constipation
- avoiding heavy lifting.

Regular pelvic floor exercises will help to improve tone and support. Advise women to:

- tighten the muscles of the front (bladder) and back (bowel) passages
- count to four slowly
- release slowly
- repeat several times an hour.

Local oestrogen cream or oral HRT can be useful for atrophic vaginitis.

Consider referral to a physiotherapist for:

- instruction on pelvic floor exercises
- graduated vaginal cones
- electrical stimulation of the pelvic floor

or a urologist for:

- urodynamic investigations and/or surgery if exact diagnosis is in doubt, conservative methods have failed or symptoms reoccur following surgery.

Urge incontinence

Bladder retraining involves encouraging the patient to void increasingly larger volumes of urine at less frequent intervals, thus relearning inhibition of abnormal detrusor muscle contractions. Drugs to stabilize the detrusor muscle can be used in addition to bladder retraining, e.g. oxybutynin, propantheline or isipramine. Once continence has been regained, medication can be reviewed and possibly discontinued.

Living with incontinence

Referral to a continence adviser or to district nursing services may be necessary.

References

Adams J, Polson DW, Franks S 1986 Prevalence of polycystic ovaries in women with anovulation and idiopathic hirsutism. British Medical Journal 293:355–359

Aiken C 2000 The impact of the cyclical symptoms of PMS. Practice Nurse 19(4):148–152

Andrews G 1998 PMS: head or hormones? Women's Health Journal for the Health Professional 3(4):12–15

Andrews G 2001 Women's sexual health, 2nd edn. Baillière Tindall, Edinburgh

Barter J 1999 Premenstrual syndrome. In: Kubba A, Sanfilippo J, Hampton N (eds) Contraception and office gynaecology choices in reproductive healthcare. WB Saunders, London

Belfield T 1999a Patient communication. In: Ferguson J, Upsdell M (eds) Key advances in the effective management of contraception. Royal Society of Medicine, London

Belfield T 1999b The contraceptive decision – information and counselling. In: Kubba A, Hampton N, Sanfilipo J (eds) Contraception and office gynaecology: choices in reproductive healthcare. WB Saunders, London

Bray JJ, Cragg PA, MacKnight ADC, Mills RG 1999 Lecture notes on human physiology, 4th edn. Blackwell Science, Oxford

Buck P 1997 Pelvic pain. In: Luesley DM (ed) Common conditions in gynaecology. Chapman and Hall Medical, London

Chamberlain G (ed) 1995 Gynaecology by ten teachers, 16th edn. Arnold, London

Chandler C 2000 Walk-in clinic endometriosis. Practice Nursing 11(13):19–21

Conway GS, Honour JW, Jacobs HS 1989 Heterogeneity of the polycystic ovary syndrome: clinical, endocrine and ultrasound features in 556 patients. Clinical Endocrinology 30(4):459–470

Coope J 1997 The menopause. In: McPherson A, Waller D (eds) Women's health, 4th edn. Oxford General Practice Series, 39. Oxford University Press, Oxford

Dahlgren E, Jansen PO, Johansen S et al 1992 Polycystic ovary syndrome and risk for myocardial infarction. Evaluated from a risk factor model based on a prospective population study of women. Acta Obstetrica Gynaecologica 71(8):599–604

DoH 2001 Sexual health strategy. Department of Health, London

Doyal L 1998 Women and health services. Open University Press, Buckingham

Edwards M 1999 Know the symptoms and the risks of PCOS. Practice Nurse 18:502–506

Ernst E 1999 Second thoughts about safety of St John's Wort. Lancet 354:2014–2016

Farquhar C 2002 Endometriosis. Clinical Evidence Concise 7:321–322

Grady D, Gebrretsadik T, Kerlikowske K et al 1995 HRT and endometrial cancer risk: a metanalysis. Obstetrics and Gynaecology 85:304–313.

Guillebaud J, Hannaford P 1998 Providing high quality contraceptive services in primary care. In: Carter Y, Moss C, Weyman A (eds) Handbook of sexual health in primary care. RCGP, London

Guyton AC, Hall JE 1997 Human physiology and mechanisms of disease, 6th edn. WB Saunders, Philadelphia

Halbreich U, Rojansky N, Palter S 1991 Elimination of ovulation and menstrual cyclicity (with Danazol) improves dysphoric premenstrual syndrome. Fertility and Sterility 56:1066

Hopkinson ZEC, Sattar N, Fleming R, Greer IA 1998 Polycystic ovarian syndrome: the metabolic syndrome comes to gynaecology. British Medical Journal 317:329–332

Kiddy D, Hamilton-Fairley D, Bush A et al 1992 Improvement in endocrine and ovarian function during dietary treatment of obese women with polycystic ovary syndrome. Clinical Endocrinology 36:105–111

Leather AT, Holland EFN, Andrews GD, Studd JWW 1993 A study of the referral patterns and therapeutic experiences of 100 women attending a specialist premenstrual syndrome clinic. Journal of the Royal Society of Medicine 86(4):199–201

Liu DT, Hitchcock A 1986 Endometriosis: its association with retrograde menstruation, dysmenorrhoea and tubal pathology. British Journal of Obstetrics and Gynaecology 93(8):859–862

Logue CM, Moos RH 1988 Positive perimenstrual changes: towards a new perspective on the menstrual cycle. Journal of Psychosomatic Research 32:31–40

MHRA 2003 Hormone replacement therapy (HRT). Latest safety update. www.mhra.gov.uk

Mira M, McNeil D, Fraser IS, Vizzard J, Abraham S 1986 Mefenamic acid in the treatment of premenstrual syndrome. Obstetrics and Gynaecology 68:395–398

NIH 2000 NIH Consensus statement. Osteoporosis prevention, diagnosis and therapy. 17(1):27–29

NMC 2002 Code of professional conduct. Nursing and Midwifery Council, London

O'Brien PMS 1987 Premenstrual syndrome. Blackwell Scientific, Oxford

O'Brien PMS 1993 Helping women with premenstrual syndrome. British Medical Journal 307:1471–1475

Perry E 1998 Alzheimer's disease, acetylcholine and oestrogen. Journal of the British Menopause Society 4:144–147, 149, 151

RCOG 1998 The management of infertility in secondary care. Evidence-based clinical guidelines no 3. Royal College of Obstetricians and Gynaecologists Press, London

Rees MCP 1999 Physiology of the normal menopause and end-points of treatment. In: Hope S, Rees M, Brockie J (eds) Hormone replacement therapy: a guide for primary care. Oxford University Press, Oxford

Rees M, Purdie DW 2002 Management of the menopause: the handbook of the British Menopause Society, 3rd edn. BMS Publications, Marlow

Steiner M, Steiner S, Stewart D et al 1995 Fluoxetine in the treatment of premenstrual dysphoria. New England Journal of Medicine 332(23):1529–1534

Stevenson JC 1996 Metabolic effects of the menopause and oestrogen replacement. Baillière's Clinical Obstetrics and Gynecology 10(3):449–468

Sutherland C 2001 Women's health: a handbook for nurses. Churchill Livingstone, Edinburgh

Taylor R, Marsden PJ 2000 Insulin sensitivity and fertility. Human Fertility 3:65–69

Utian WH 1999 The International Menopause Society menopause related terminology definitions. Climacteric 2:284–286

Walker AF, De Souza MC, Vickers MF, Abayasekera S, Collins ML, Trinca LA 1998 Magnesium supplementation alleviates premenstrual symptoms of fluid retention. Journal of Women's Health 7(9):1157–1165.

Watson NR, Studd JWW, Savas M, Garnett T, Baber RJ 1989 Treatment of severe premenstrual syndrome with oestradiol patches and cyclical norethisterone. Lancet ii:730–732

Whitehead M, Godfree V 1992 Hormone replacement therapy: your questions answered. Churchill Livingstone, Edinburgh

WHO 1996 Research in the menopause in the 1990s. WHO Technical Report Series 866. World Health Organisation, Geneva

Wilson KJW 1990 Ross and Wilson anatomy and physiology in health and illness, 7th edn. Churchill Livingstone, Edinburgh

Woolf AD, St John Dixon A 1998 Osteoporosis: a clinical guide, 2nd edn. Martin Dunitz, London

Wyatt KM, Dimmock PW, O'Brien PM 1999 Premenstrual syndrome. In: Clinical evidence 99. BMJ Publishing Group, London

Further reading

Belfield T 2000 Walk-in clinic – contraception. Practice Nursing 11(12):19–21

Everett S 2001 Contraception. In: Andrews G (ed) Women's sexual health, 2nd edn. Baillière Tindall in association with RCN, Edinburgh

Guillebaud J 1999 Contraception: your questions answered, 3rd edn. Churchill Livingstone, London

Hawkridge C 1989 Understanding endometriosis. Macdonald Optima, London

Henderson R 1999 Endometriosis. Health in Focus. www.healthinfocus.com

Marsden P 2002 Polycystic ovary syndrome. Gynaecology Update. www.DoctorUpdate.net

Talbott E, Guzick D, Clerici A et al 1995 Coronary heart disease risk factors in women with polycystic ovary syndrome. Arteriosclerosis Thrombosis and Vascular Biology 15:821–826

Walsh J, Lythgoe H, Peckham S 1996 Contraceptive choices: supporting effective contraceptive use of methods. Family Planning Association, London

Chapter 2

Cervical and breast screening and abnormalities

Vicky Padbury

CHAPTER CONTENTS

CERVICAL SCREENING AND ABNORMALITIES

The vast majority of cervical screening takes place in GP surgeries (Table 2.1). It has been shown (Atkin et al 1993) that 75% of practice nurses are undertaking the role of cervical smear-taker. As nurses, we are all accountable for our own actions and therefore should not take on any tasks for which we do not feel competent but should seek out further training. The NMC document *The code of professional conduct* (NMC 2002) is useful to refer to.

Problems within some laboratories have been widely reported by the media, leading to much anxiety for the women concerned. This has led to the compulsory accreditation of all laboratories involved in cervical cytology, with some staff being retrained and small laboratories being merged or closed (Warden 1998).

NATIONAL HEALTH SERVICE CERVICAL SCREENING PROGRAMME

Britain has been screening since 1964, although initially in an ad hoc, uncoordinated way; 15 years ago more efficient organization, computerization and government initiatives made screening more effective. Following Department of Health guidelines, the district health authorities (DHAs) established computerized call/recall systems and in 1988 organized cervical screening really started in England and Wales, as the NHS Cervical Screening Programme (NHSCSP).

The Department of Health guidelines (DoH 1988) updated in 1993 (DoH 1993) gave clear guidance on recall intervals, age groups to be invited and training requirements for cyto-screeners, among its main points.

Table 2.1 Percentage of smears examined by source of smear, England 2002–3

Source	Percentage
General practice	87.4
NHS hospitals	6.2
Community clinics	4.5
GUM clinics	0.8
Private hospitals	0.6
Other	0.5

Adapted from DoH Cervical Cytology Summary, form KC 61 2002–3. Crown copyright material is adapted with permission of the Controller of Her Majesty's Stationery Office

NATIONAL COORDINATING NETWORK

The NCN was originally set up in 1991. It has since become the National Health Service Cancer Screening Programme (NHSCSP) and there is an overall National Director. The NHSCSP is responsible for improving the overall performance of the screening programme with priorities to:

- develop systems and guidelines which will assure a high quality of cervical screening throughout the country
- identify important policy issues and help resolve them and improve communications within the programme and with the public.

To complete the history of our cervical screening programme, two more events need mentioning. The first event was the 1990 GP Contract which brought in target payments as incentives to GPs to screen 50% (lower payment) and 80% (higher payment) of their target population of women (aged 20–64 years) every 5 years. This initiative has proved to be very successful, with the majority of GPs in the country reaching the higher target, but has raised some problems along the way.

- Not all 20-year-olds and onwards will be sexually active so some will be inappropriately screened.
- If a GP has a highly mobile practice population it may be difficult to reach targets; therefore cervical screening might become a low priority within the practice.
- Coercive tactics encouraging women to have their smear test at their GP's surgery have been reported. This creates a conflict, in that it goes against the spirit of enabling women to make informed choices about whether they wish to be screened and where they wish to attend (Austoker & McPherson 1992). The changes to the GP Contract (2003) may have implications for target payments.

The second event was the publication in July 1992 of the DoH's *Health of the nation* document in which targets were set for the reduction of preventable disease. Cancers are the second most common cause of death (25%) in England: four cancers (breast, cervical, lung and skin) were targeted for action.

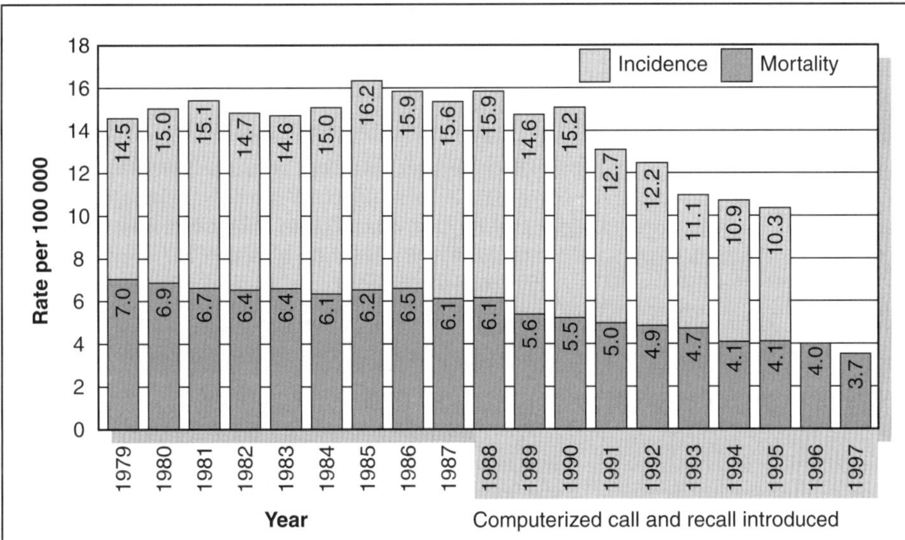

Figure 2.1 Incidence and mortality rates for cervical cancer in England 1979–97. (Reproduced with permission of the NHS Cervical Screening Programme.)

Box 2.1 The principles of screening

The *Principles and practice of screening for disease* was a Public Health Paper formulated in 1968 for the World Health Organization by Wilson & Junger and seems just as appropriate four decades later when we are considering cervical screening. The basic principles are as follows.

- The condition should pose an important health problem.
- The natural history of the disease should be well understood.
- There should be a recognizable early stage.
- Early treatment should be more beneficial than at a later stage.
- There should be a suitable test.
- The test should be acceptable to the population.
- There should be adequate facilities for the diagnosis and treatment of abnormalities detected.
- For disease of insidious onset, screening should be repeated at intervals determined by the natural history of the disease.
- The chance of physical or psychological harm must be less than the benefits.
- Cost of screening should be balanced against the benefits it provides.

With cervical cancer the aim was to reduce the number of women with newly detected invasive cancer by at least 20% by the year 2000 which would equal 12.8 per 100 000 women.

This number was achieved early (NHSCSP 1998a) (Fig. 2.1).

Screening in itself can cause stress and anxiety. It should be remembered that we are dealing with a seemingly healthy population and if a smear has to be repeated for any reason, it can cause great anxiety.

The principles of screening for disease are outlined in Box 2.1. You will see as we go through this chapter how well cervical screening fits in with most of these principles.

WHAT IS CERVICAL SCREENING LOOKING FOR?

Cervical screening is undertaken to detect very early changes in cells from the cervix which, if left untreated, could lead to squamous cell carcinoma. Cervical screening is a way of interrupting the natural history of the disease at an earlier and more treatable stage.

Other abnormalities may be picked up coincidentally on smear. These will be discussed.

CERVICAL SMEAR TEST OR 'PAP' SMEAR

We have the Greek scientist and humanitarian George N Papanicolaou (1883–1962) to thank for the modern smear test. He developed a cytological test for malignant change in the squamous epithelial tissue of the cervix uteri, using a pipette to draw fluid from the posterior fornix of the vagina in which can be found cervical cells which exfoliate like any other epithelial covering.

This test for the early detection of cervical cancer has been widely used since the late 1940s and is known as the 'Pap' test.

EPIDEMIOLOGY OF CERVICAL CANCER

Cervical cancer rates vary greatly throughout the world.

- In developing countries cervical cancer is the most common female cancer.
- Of the estimated 471 000 new cases each year in the world, 80% were in developing countries.
- Taking the world as a whole, cervical cancer is the second most common female cancer after breast cancer.
- The UK has the second highest recorded incidence of cervical cancer in the European Community.
- Cervical cancer is the 11th most common cause of cancer deaths in women in England and Wales.
- Deaths from cervical cancer have fallen by nearly 50%, from 7.1 per 100 000 in 1979 to 3.3 per 100 000 in 2000 (Fig. 2.2).

NATURAL HISTORY OF CERVICAL CANCER

The majority of cancer of the cervix is squamous cell carcinoma.

> *Adenocarcinomas, which originate deep within the glands of the endocervical canal, are very difficult to pick up on a cervical smear. The number of smears reported with a potential glandular abnormality remains a very small proportion of all smears reported, at 0.04% 2002–03.* (NHSCSP 2003)

SQUAMOUS CELL CARCINOMA

Epidemiological evidence has linked squamous cell carcinoma with sexual habits. One of the first people to take an epidemiological approach to cancer was a doctor called Domenico Rigoni-Stern who was born in 1810 in Italy. In 1842 he published his most notable study of 'Statistical data relative to the disease of cancer' (Scotto & Bailar 1969). In this study he noted the higher frequency of breast cancer among unmarried women and nuns, relative to married or widowed women. He also found that uterine and cervical cancer were not common in unmarried women and were very rare in nuns. Over time these findings have been confirmed by other studies.

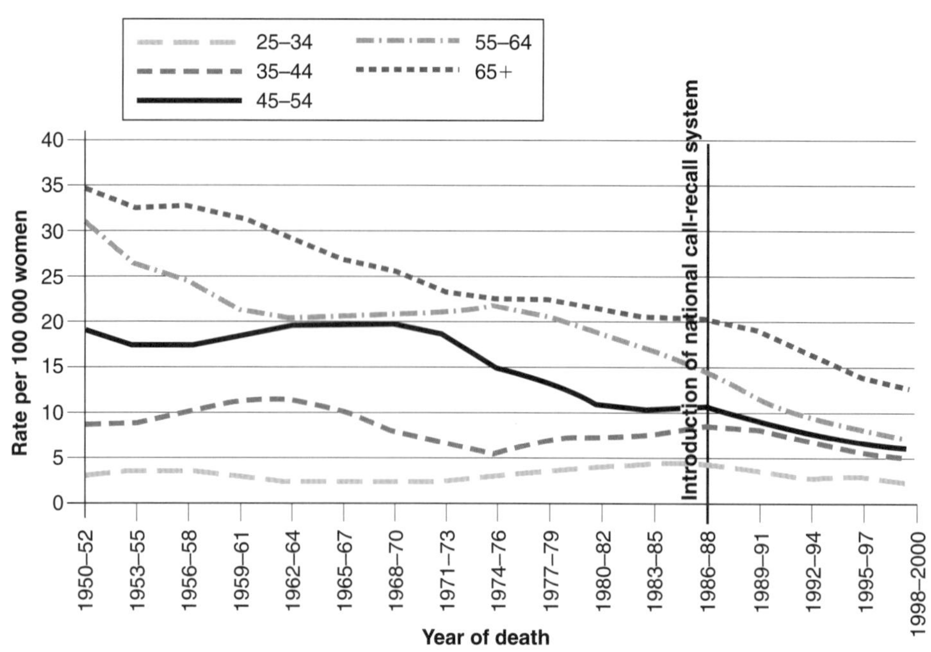

Figure 2.2 Deaths from cervical cancer have fallen by nearly 50% from 7.1 per 100 000 in 1960 to 3.7 per 100 000 in 1997. (Reproduced with permission of Cancer Research UK.)

In the 1960s attention turned to the role of the male in the incidence of cervical cancer and the concept of the 'high-risk' male.

In general the disease is more common in women of lower socio-economic groups (Fig. 2.3). There may be many co-factors within this, such as smoking habits (Simons et al 1993) and early age of sexual intercourse, leading to the likelihood of having more than one partner in a lifetime and increased probability of having more pregnancies.

The sexually transmitted agent that is strongly linked with cervical cancer is the human papillomavirus (HPV), also known as the wart virus. When a cell is invaded by a wart virus, characteristic changes can be seen under the microscope (the nucleus gives the appearance of having a halo round it). The cells invaded are called koilocytes.

There are over 60 different kinds of wart virus, identified by the type of DNA they contain, and they are individually numbered. The association with cervical cancer is verified by the fact that around 90% of women with cervical cancer have antibodies to HPV in blood samples, while antibodies to HPV have also been found in about 95% of people who have genital warts.

There are about 13 so-called 'high-risk' HPV types, for example 16 and 18 are known to be associated with cervical cancer, but unfortunately they cannot be specifically identified from a smear test alone. To distinguish which HPV was present the DNA would have to be examined. Advances in HPV testing are discussed in more detail on p.44.

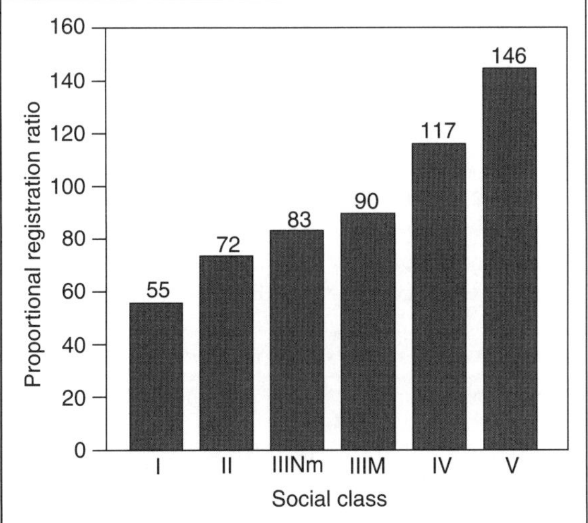

Figure 2.3 In general, cervical cancer is more common in women of lower socio-economic groups.

RISK FACTORS ASSOCIATED WITH CERVICAL CANCER

SEXUAL BEHAVIOUR

It is recognized that certain areas of sexual behaviour are associated with increased risk of cervical cancer. These include the following.

- Age at first sexual intercourse. The transformation zone (see p.35) is very evident and active in puberty, making it more susceptible to possible carcinogens such as HPV.
- Number of sexual partners. Because HPV is transmitted through sexual activity, the numbers of sexual partners of both the woman and her partner are risk factors.
- Number of pregnancies. During pregnancy the transformation zone is very evident and active and therefore more vulnerable to sexually transmitted agents. Pregnancy also suppresses the immune system.

Along with these risk factors associated with sexual behaviour run the previously discussed risk factors of smoking and socio-economic group. Barton et al (1988) showed that in those smoking over 20 cigarettes a day, nicotine found in high concentrations in the cervical cells damages the cells' immune response (Langerhans cells), making them more susceptible to infections such as wart virus.

METHOD OF CONTRACEPTION

The combined oral contraceptive pill has been implicated in cervical cancer, possibly due to the oestrogen in the pill making the ectropion on the cervix more extensive, producing a larger area where metaplasia can be more vulnerable to HPV. The connection with pill use is inconclusive and studies continue (Smith et al 2003).

The co-factor could be that pill users are less likely to use barrier methods in addition to the pill. The message that health professionals should give to clients is that the pill will protect against pregnancy and the use of condoms will protect against sexually transmitted infections and cervical abnormalities.

ALTERNATIVE SEXUAL PRACTICES

So far, we have been discussing risks associated with penetrative sexual intercourse. Not all women are in a heterosexual relationship and lesbian relationships need to be considered.

A lesbian coming for a cervical smear should have her own sexual activities discussed in a sensitive manner. Knowing that the high-risk agent is the wart virus, sexual practices should be addressed, to decide if the woman is at risk and whether a smear is relevant. Ultimately it is the woman's choice.

ANATOMY AND PHYSIOLOGY

THE UTERUS

The uterus is situated in the pelvic cavity between the bladder and the rectum. In 80% of women it is anteverted (tilted forward) and anteflexed (curved forward on itself).

The inner layer of the body of the uterus is lined with endometrial cells which are constantly changing in thickness and vascularity according to the phases of the menstrual cycle. The superficial layers are shed during menstruation; evidence of them can be found up to days 10–12 of the next menstrual cycle if cervical mucus is examined under the microscope.

This underlines the importance of recording the *first* day of the last menstrual period on the laboratory form. If there are endometrial cells present and your client is more than 10–12 days into her menstrual cycle the laboratory may ask for a repeat smear. The importance of informing the laboratory of an intrauterine contraceptive device being in situ is also associated with endometrial cells being present later in the cycle (Hopwood 1995).

THE CERVIX

The outer part of the cervix, the ectocervix, is covered by thick, multilayered, stratified squamous epithelium. In healthy women in their reproductive years, this consists of up to 20 layers of cells which arise at the basement membrane and mature in an orderly way, gaining increased amounts of cytoplasm as they approach the surface of the epithelium. The blood vessels and glands are contained in the basement membrane under the tough squamous epithelium, giving the ectocervix a dusky pink sheen, which can be a helpful guide to you when endeavouring to locate the cervix during smear taking. It is quite different from the darker pink epithelium of the vaginal walls.

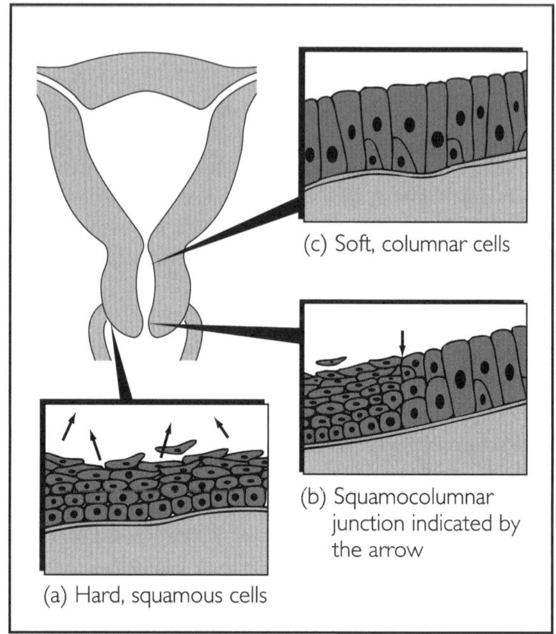

Figure 2.4 Squamocolumnar junction of the cervix.

Under the microscope, the surface of the ectocervix is not smooth but contains many irregular folds. Sometimes these folds become blocked with mucus; when this happens they look like little cysts on the surface of the cervix and are called retention cysts or Nabothian follicles.

The cervical os is the opening into the cervical canal, which is lined by epithelium only one cell thick, arranged in columns called columnar epithelium (Fig. 2.4). Within these cells are found deep branching glands, which secrete alkaline mucus. It is within these glands that the precursor to the (uncommon) glandular carcinoma, adenocarcinoma, can arise.

The cervix is a very dynamic organ and changes throughout the different phases of a woman's life, under the influence of ovarian and pituitary hormones which are very active at puberty and during pregnancy. These start to decline during the climacteric and cease completely after the menopause.

An experienced smear-taker could probably guess the approximate age of a woman just by looking at her cervix.

THE SQUAMOCOLUMNAR JUNCTION (SCJ)

The point at which the squamous cells of the ectocervix meet the columnar cells of the endocervix is known as the SCJ. Depending on the age and

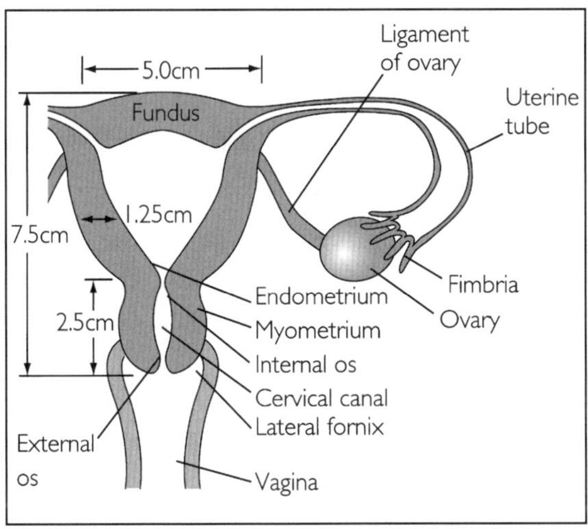

Figure 2.5 The uterus and left fallopian tube and ovary.

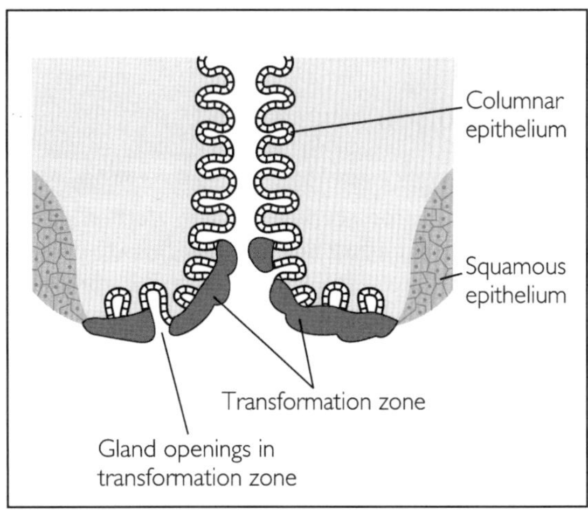

Figure 2.6 The transformation zone.

hormonal state of the woman, this junction could be in the lower third of the endocervical canal or out on the ectocervix.

Within the confines of the alkaline endocervical canal the delicate columnar cells are protected from the acid pH of the vagina and also from the natural friction of the penis pushing against the cervix during sexual intercourse.

It is a natural process for the columnar cells to migrate downwards onto the ectocervix, moving the SCJ to a new position. Ectropion, or ectopy, is the appearance of a red area of columnar epithelium around the cervical os (Hopwood 1990). This is a normal physiological state and the term 'erosion' formerly used should be avoided.

TRANSFORMATION ZONE OR TRANSITIONAL ZONE (TZ)

The migrated columnar cells at the SCJ will start to break down in the acid environment of the vagina; squamous cells begin to grow from beneath the columnar epithelium and gradually replace it.

This normal replacement of one type of cell by another is called squamous metaplasia and where it takes place is called the transformation or transitional zone (TZ) (Fig. 2.6).

The SCJ and the TZ are the most common sites where precancerous changes originate.

It is imperative that the smear-taker understands this concept in order to take the best possible smears.

THE NURSE'S ROLE AS A SMEAR-TAKER

It is important for smear-takers to be up to date and well informed regarding all aspects of cervical cytology and this in turn will allow you to give your client advice and information prior to her smear being taken.

All nurses who take cervical smears should have undertaken an appropriate course.

- The Family Planning Courses (formerly ENB 901 and A08) have now been superseded by courses in Reproductive and Sexual Health that may not necessarily include cervical cytology training. Each course should be carefully checked to ensure that the contents fulfil your specific needs.
- The 8103 and S103 are the present courses and are linked to universities.
- The Marie Curie Cancer Screening for Practice Nurse Course; similar courses are available in Scotland, Wales and Northern Ireland.
- Many primary care organisations are now running basic courses in Cervical Cytology, including theory and practice.
- The NHSCSP has produced an excellent aid to training, 'Resource pack for training smear-takers' (1998b), that has enabled trainers to offer a common core of learning to all smear-takers.

Smear taking should not be task orientated. A sound knowledge of relevant anatomy and physiology; the natural history of the disease; associated risk factors; abnormalities and possible treatment would all be a distinct advantage not only to you but also to your clients.

INFORMATION FOR WOMEN BEFORE THE SMEAR

Before attending for a cervical smear, women should be provided with information about how to prepare for the procedure. This could be in the form of a leaflet given out in your practice or clinic or details given over the telephone when women make their appointments.

The information should include the following recommendations.

- Ideally your smear should be taken halfway between your periods.
- Avoid having a bath on the day of your smear; a shower or stand-up wash would be better.
- For about 48 hours before your smear use a condom or abstain from sexual intercourse.
- If you have recently used a vaginal pessary for treating an infection such as thrush, allow yourself to have a period before your next smear, to make sure all traces of the pessary have gone.
- If you are using an oestrogen cream, do not apply it on the day of your smear.

These are ideals and few women can manage all of them. The most important is that the woman is not too near the time of her period.

TAKING A CERVICAL SMEAR

A smear should be taken in such a way as to provide an adequate sample for assessment with the minimum of distress or discomfort to the client. The client should be fully informed of the reason for the procedure and the implications for her future health and well-being. See the resource section (p.45) for NHSCSP booklet details, which is provided nationally with each invitation for a smear.

The environment is important, so try to provide warmth, privacy, a good adjustable light and no interruptions.

EQUIPMENT NEEDED

1. An autoclave which is regularly serviced and complies with current guidelines (DoH 1994)
2. Vaginal specula (stainless steel or disposable in various sizes)
3. Cytology slides with frosted ends and a sharp pencil
4. Fixative containing alcohol and carbo wax (dropper or spray)
5. Assorted spatulas and cervical brushes currently recommended
6. Swabs for culture
7. Latex examination gloves (protein/powder free). Non-latex gloves should also be available in case of allergy being present
8. Water-based lubricating jelly
9. Smear request forms and boxes for transporting slides
10. Disposable paper roll for the couch and cover if necessary

Points 3, 4, 5 and 9 will change when LBC is rolled out over the next few years (see p.44).

INTERVIEW AND COMPLETION OF THE SMEAR FORM

Record a menstrual/obstetric/contraceptive history in the patient's notes or on the computer. These are relevant to cervical cytology. Key questions are listed in Box 2.2.

Box 2.2 Key questions to ask prior to taking a smear

- Do you understand the purpose of this test?
- Do you have any bleeding after sexual intercourse (postcoital)?
- Are you currently using a method of contraception?
- Do you have any intermenstrual bleeding (if the patient is using oral contraception this may be the reason)?
- Do you have any pain during or after sexual intercourse (dyspareunia)?
- Do you have painful or heavy periods? (This would be important if the pattern and severity had altered without any changes in circumstances or lifestyle.)
- Have you noticed any difference in your vaginal discharge?

WOMEN WHO DO NOT NEED SMEARS

Women are sent a request for a smear by age alone which means that many women who do not need smears at the present time are sent for. Austoker & McPherson (1992) state that 'all women aged 20–64 who are or ever have been sexually active should be screened'.

During the interview with the client you should sensitively find out if the woman has been sexually active (i.e. engaging in sexual intercourse). If a smear is not needed at this time, the woman should be informed that if circumstances change and she becomes sexually active she needs to return for a smear. The primary care agency should be informed by writing on the invitation 'not applicable at this time'. She will then be recalled after a suitable interval.

If a woman chooses not to have a smear, this is her choice. It is now a recommendation that 'disclaimer' forms are kept in each practice for the woman to read and sign.

Women who have had a hysterectomy for benign reasons do not need smears. A hysterectomy undertaken for precancer/cancer is different and the woman would have vault smears at intervals according to the present guidelines. Vault smears are not part of the screening programme.

A woman who has had a subtotal hysterectomy with the cervix remaining will still need to have cervical smears.

Frequency of cervical screening

Recommendations made by Cancer Research UK scientists on the optimal frequency of cervical screening (Sasieni et al 2003) are as follows:

- first invitation: age 25 years
- 3 yearly: ages 25–49 years
- 5 yearly: ages 50–64 years.

> *Screening of teenagers is not recommended as the cervix of a girl in her teens is rapidly developing. These rapid changes often cannot be distinguished on a smear from the changes when there is a low grade abnormality on the smear of a mature woman.*
>
> (NHSCSP 1999a)

Women under 25 who are anxious should be advised to seek further information.

TAKING THE SMEAR

Write in pencil the name and date of birth on the frosted end of the glass slide, ensuring that the slide is free from dust and grease.

Check that the woman gives permission for the smear to be taken.

Warm (or cool) the speculum under running water to reach body temperature. (Nowadays there are good-quality disposable perspex specula available as alternatives.) If necessary, lightly smear the sides but not the end of the speculum with a water-based lubricant, but usually the warm water is sufficient.

Inspect the vulva, looking for any sore areas, genital warts or unusual skin textures or colours. A gentle one-finger examination to locate the cervix can be helpful, but care should be taken that the immediate area surrounding the os is not touched roughly.

Pass the speculum into the vagina gently, with due regard to the woman's reaction. Locate and visualize the cervix, making sure the cervical os is well in view. It is only after the os has been seen that the appropriate spatula can be chosen.

Note the position of the SCJ to ensure that the TZ is sampled. It is the responsibility of the smear-taker to make every effort to sample the whole of the TZ. The cervix must be visualized at the time the smear is taken and the full circumference of the cervix must be sampled.

Primary screening should not be carried out with an endocervical brush alone.

Evidence of TZ sampling is not firm evidence that the cervix has been adequately sampled. It is only evidence that part of the TZ has been sampled (NHSCSP 2000).

Insert the spatula well into the cervical os and rotate it twice (using pencil pressure) through 360°. A cervical brush may be used, if the os is tight. First the blunt end of a spatula should be rotated around the ectocervix, then the brush inserted for sampling the endocervix.

Due to the horizontal position of the bristles there is no need to twist the brush through 360°. Introducing it gently into the cervical canal and twisting through about 40° is sufficient to sample the endocervical canal without causing too much discomfort and bleeding.

A plastic Cervex brush has the advantage of sampling both the endocervix and ectocervix at the same time. Care should be taken, as the Cervex brush should only be rotated clockwise (Waddell 1994) through five turns.

One of the main findings of a systematic review and metaanalysis (Martin-Hirsch et al 1999) was that the blunt-ended Ayre's spatula, when used alone, is the least effective device for cervical sampling and should be superseded by extended-tip spatulas for primary screening (Fig. 2.7).

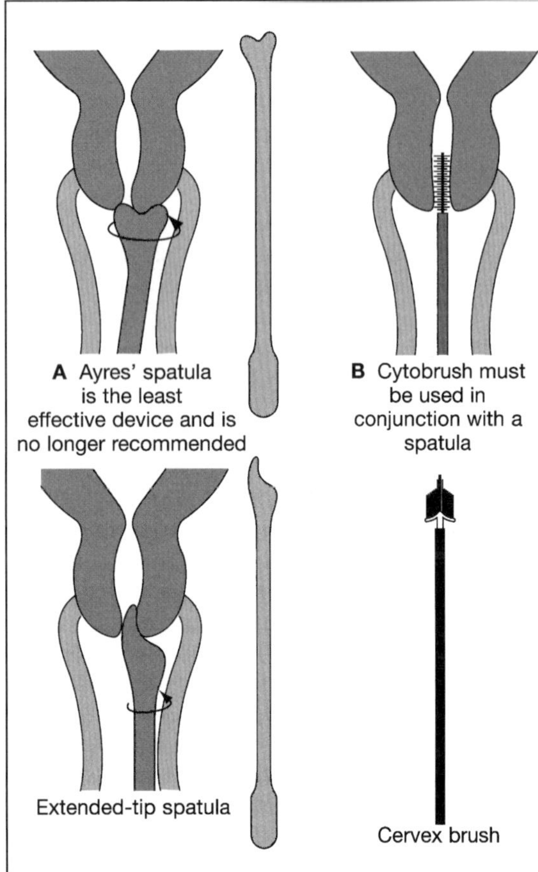

Figure 2.7 Cervical spatulas and their position within the external os. (Redrawn with permission from Szarewski 1994.)

Transfer the cells from the spatula onto the slide, using two lengthways strokes, spreading the specimen evenly. If a brush is used, the specimen should be applied using a rolling action.

Fixative must be applied immediately, gently flooding the slide, and left to dry horizontally for at least 15 minutes.

The experienced smear-taker might remove the speculum at the same time as the sample is taken, having a receptacle at hand to drop the used speculum into. Nurses new to the procedure may find it better to leave the speculum in position until the specimen is fixed.

Bacterial swabs should be taken after the smear if there is a heavy or unusual discharge.

Gently remove the speculum, making sure that it is clear of the cervix before allowing the blades to start closing.

Bimanual examination of the pelvis is not routinely carried out on an asymptomatic woman. However, if the patient has any of the following symptoms an examination should be carried out by a health professional who is qualified and competent (RCN 1995).

- Very painful and/or heavy periods
- Intermenstrual bleeding
- Urinary symptoms
- Abdominal swelling
- Lower abdominal pain or discomfort
- Pain on sexual intercourse (dyspareunia)
- Postcoital bleeding. It may also be worthwhile considering testing for chlamydia if PCB is a problem.

COMPLETING THE LABORATORY REQUEST FORM HMR101

The clinical observations of the cervix should now be recorded on the laboratory request form. You should not diagnose what has been observed on the cervix but just describe exactly what is seen: 'red cervix, bled on contact', 'large ectropion-like area seen', 'greenish vaginal discharge at os'.

Box 2.3 Checklist for filling in the laboratory request form

- Patient's name (correctly spelt) and maiden name if appropriate
- Address with postcode
- Date of birth
- NHS number if known
- Today's date
- The first day of the last menstrual period or bleed if using oral contraception or hormone replacement therapy
- Date of the last smear
- Contraceptive type: oral contraceptive, injectable contraceptive or implant: HRT type with name. State if intrauterine device (IUD) is present
- Call/recall; previous abnormal; indicate which
- If early recall state last test result or if known give the slide serial number from the previous laboratory form

Please note that changes are being made to the form following national guidance.

It is recommended that you record 'cervix and os visualized, transformation zone sampled' (NHSCSP 1998b).

PROBLEMS INSERTING THE VAGINAL SPECULUM

At all times you should be sensitive to the woman's reactions, particularly as you are about to insert the speculum into the vagina. Many things could happen.

- The client clamps her thighs together and informs you she cannot go through with the test. This could possibly be vaginismus and the smear would have to be delayed until the woman felt able to cope with the procedure.
- The entrance to the vagina (introitus) looks small and when a fingertip is inserted an intact hymen is present. The woman has not had sexual intercourse. Inform your client that she does not require a smear at this time, but to return if circumstances change.
- The labia look different, possibly non-existent or made up of scar tissue; the introitus might be just a small opening and the clitoris absent. If these signs are present in a woman who originates from a part of the world where female genital mutilation is still performed, care and sensitivity are even more important (Box 2.4).

Box 2.4 Female genital mutilation

This is a collective term used for different degrees of mutilation of the female external genitals. As more refugees from Africa arrive in the UK, so more nurses working in primary care will come across women who have been genitally mutilated.

The procedure is illegal in Britain under the Prohibition of Female Circumcision Act 1985, though parents determined to have it carried out may take their children abroad.

It has no benefits to the woman and can cause problems such as painful intercourse (dyspareunia), no orgasms (as the clitoris is removed) and urinary and menstrual problems. Often the first time the mutilation is observed is during pregnancy.

Problems commonly occur during labour. There are no easy answers to this problem but when found, you should be sensitive, non-judgemental and supportive to the woman. It may be impossible to take a smear without surgical intervention.

- Women who have undergone caesarean section(s) only may have tight vaginal muscles.
- Peri- and postmenopausal women often present with drying and thinning of the vaginal epithelium. The choice of speculum is important and the careful use of lubricating jelly or warm water will be helpful (RCOG 1987).

DOUBTS WHEN THE CERVIX IS VISUALIZED

- If the cervix is covered with thick mucus, do not clean it off. Cells which might be abnormal may be lost. A first sweep of the cervix with a spatula should be followed by a second sweep with another, spread side by side on the slide, fixed without delay and described on the laboratory form. Two slides could be sent marked 'first' and 'second'. If there is a mucus plug in the cervical os, this can be carefully lifted off with the tip of a spatula.
- If the cervix bleeds on the first circumference do not make a second sweep; spread the specimen immediately and fix; record the bleeding on the laboratory form.
- If the cervix looks sore and very red take a high vaginal and chlamydia swab after the smear is taken, noting this on the form. The patient should be told of the difference between cytology and bacteriology.
- If there is a wide TZ take a first sweep with an Aylesbury spatula within the cervical os and a second sweep with the blunt end of the spatula to sample the wide TZ. Spread the specimens side by side on one slide and fix.
- A cervical polyp may be seen, which is an overgrowth of epithelial tissue often on a stalk and looking like a grape. Polyps are rarely associated with malignancy, but they are worth referring to a gynaecologist for removal.
- If the cervix looks unusual in any way it is appropriate to get a second opinion from a practitioner. It is quite acceptable for a patient to be referred for further investigations and colposcopy on the look of the cervix alone.

COMMON FAULTS WHEN TRYING TO LOCATE THE CERVIX

You can never judge by outward appearances exactly where and in what position your patient's cervix will be. The 'one-finger' examination will be a good guide as to the position and angle of the cervix.

Incorrect position of the speculum

You have inserted the speculum into the vagina, opened up the blades and all you see is a space surrounded by the vaginal walls. Often this is because you are in the posterior fornix.

Solution: gently ease the speculum towards you while watching carefully to see if the cervix drops into view; it is useful to ask your patient to cough.

When inserting the speculum, open it up slightly when half of it is inside the vagina; you may be surprised to see the cervix coming into view already.

Acute position of the cervix (1)

The cervix is pointing into the anterior wall of the vagina, due to a retroverted uterus. You cannot encompass the cervix with your speculum.

Solution: ask your client to half-sit up, resting on her elbows, keeping her informed of why you are asking her to do this, or ask her to put her hands underneath her buttocks to raise her pelvis.

Acute position of the cervix (2)

The cervix is pointing into the posterior wall of the vagina, due to a very anteverted uterus.

Solution: ask your client to press down with her hands over her lower abdomen or bring her knees up against her abdomen, holding them with her arms. Either of these solutions could help flip the cervix forward.

If this fails, ask her to get into the left-lateral position where, by inserting the speculum into the vagina from the back, you should be able to view the cervix.

Prolapsed vaginal walls obscuring the view of the cervix

You insert the speculum and can only see the lateral walls of the vagina.

Solution: instead of turning the speculum through 90° after you have inserted the tip into the introitus, keep it in the lateral position, then continue introducing the speculum further into the vagina. The walls will be against the blades and unable to collapse. This method can only be used if the area around your client's inner thighs allows.

Alternatively, use a condom with the closed end cut off and 'sheath' the speculum with this.

A very deep (posterior) cervix

Solution: use a Winterton speculum, which has extra long blades, or ask your client to press over her lower abdomen or come up into the semi-sitting position, which may push the uterus down.

Remember the very delicate structures, clitoris and labia, that your speculum may be pressed closely against.

As you progress and see more cervices, you will realize that there are many different shapes and sizes, ranging from small flat to long pointed ones.

RESULTS

It is part of your job to inform your client of how and when she will receive her results and what action to take if no results appear. All women should receive their results in writing. Offer advice and interpretation of smear results.

THE OPPORTUNISTIC SMEAR

Beware of the woman who is always menstruating or 'having a bleed' when you see her, as this may indicate some underlying pathology. It may be safer to take the smear despite bleeding, noting such on the laboratory form.

Any woman who presents with abnormal vaginal bleeding should always be investigated and referred for a specialist opinion (NHS Executive 1998).

THE POSTNATAL SMEAR

Before the reforms of 1988 smears were taken at the 6-week postnatal check. Many doctors and nurses are mistakenly continuing this practice. A smear should only be taken if it is due as part of the NHS screening programme and ideally not before 12 weeks postnatal.

SMEAR RESULTS AND CLASSIFICATION

Inadequate smears may be due to insufficient or unsuitable material being present. This could be due to various causes.

- Transformation zone not sampled sufficiently.
- Excessive lubricant used.
- Atrophic cervix. This can be due to low oestrogen levels not allowing exfoliation of cervical cells.
- Cytolysis. This is the normal process of cell disintegration due to the high glycogen content of cells during the second half of the menstrual cycle. If a repeat is requested the smear should be taken before ovulation, when the glycogen content is less.

- Poor spreading of cervical mucus on the slide.
- Inadequate fixation. Is the fixative out of date; shaken before use; all mucus completely covered by fixative; the slide flooded too much, pushing off the cells? Was the slide allowed to dry before putting it in the transport box?
- The smear consists mainly of blood, pus or inflammatory exudate.

If the laboratory sends back a smear result reported as 'inadequate' they will usually give details; contact the laboratory if in doubt.

With the advent of LBC inadequate results will not be such a problem.

HUMAN PAPILLOMAVIRUS, KOILOCYTOSIS

This is a common result and there is no treatment. It is not the same as having warts and this distinction is very important. HPV appearing alone on a smear does not mean a referral for colposcopy is needed.

Great care should be taken when discussing a result of HPV. Your client may wonder how she came to have the virus; emphasize the fact that the natural history of HPV is fairly obscure, that it is common and can lie dormant for many years before it is seen in cervical cells.

The main types (according to the DNA in the cell) of HPV associated with precancer changes are HPV 16 and 18 which do not show up as genital warts in either women or men and there is no way of knowing if a man has it on his penis.

Visible genital warts are HPV 6 and 11 and are not thought to be important as far as cervical cancer is concerned.

INFLAMMATORY SMEAR OR INFLAMMATORY CHANGES

These changes can be caused by a background infection. If there is a suspicion of an infection, bacterial screening should be suggested. A simple reason for an inflammatory smear can be one taken near to menstruation.

Repeated inflammatory changes may need a referral for colposcopy as they can be implicated in advanced cancer.

BORDERLINE CHANGES

This term is used to describe a cellular appearance that cannot definitely be described as normal. There are usually severe inflammatory changes on the borderline with mild dyskaryosis.

The presence of HPV infection is the main reason for recording borderline nuclear changes (Austoker & Davey 1997).

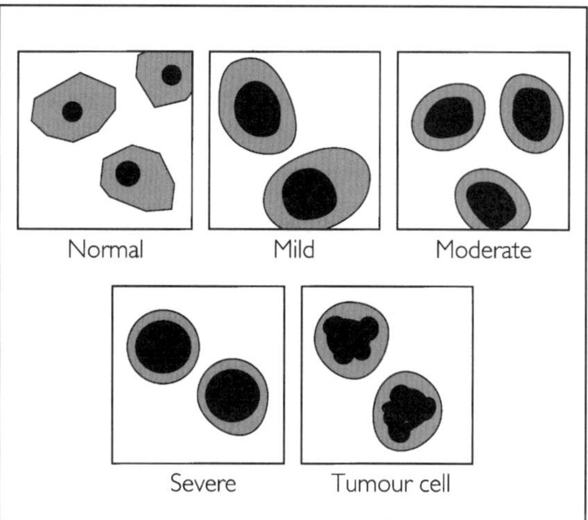

Figure 2.8 Dyskaryotic changes in the cell. (Redrawn with permission from Barker 1987.)

DYSKARYOSIS

Dyskaryosis is a cytological term. Cytology is the study of individual cells focusing on the size and shape of the nucleus within the cytoplasm.

There are three grades of abnormality between a normal cell and a tumour cell (Fig. 2.8).

- Mild dyskaryosis
- Moderate dyskaryosis
- Severe dyskaryosis

HISTOLOGY

Histology is the study of a portion (or biopsy) of epithelium looked at microscopically and obtained at colposcopy. Dysplasia is a histological term describing the abnormal architecture of the epithelium.

In a sample of cervical epithelium looked at under the microscope, the histologist can see how far through the layers of squamous cells the dyskaryotic cells have progressed.

Cervical intraepithelial neoplasia (CIN) (Fig. 2.9)

CIN means 'new change in the outer layer of the cervix'.

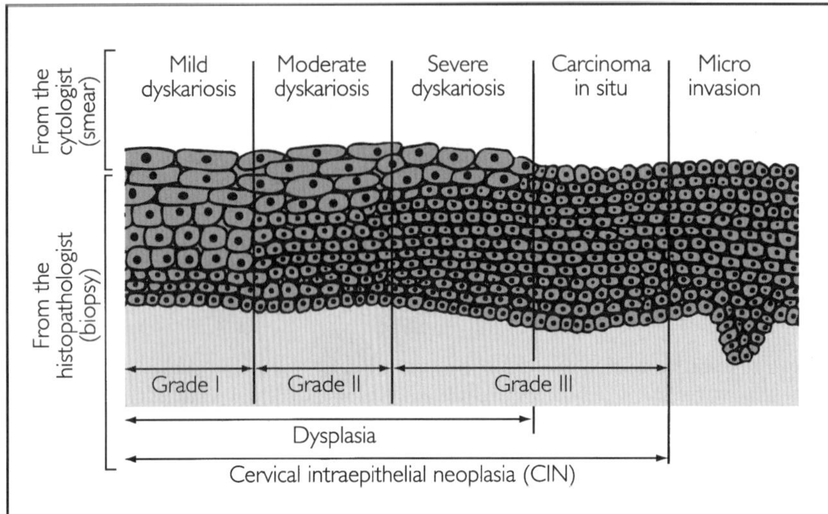

Figure 2.9 The CIN grading system. (Redrawn with permission from Barker 1987.)

- CIN I occurs if the outer third of the epithelium is abnormal (mildly dyskaryotic cells appear in the smear); the epithelium shows 'mild dysplasia'. CIN I may resolve without any intervention but the woman will be monitored (repeat smears) according to guidelines.
- CIN II occurs if a half to two-thirds of the epithelium is involved (moderate dyskaryotic cells appear in the smear); the epithelium shows 'moderate dysplasia'. Referral for colposcopy will be suggested.
- CIN III occurs if the full thickness of the epithelium is involved, with complete architectural chaos between the basement membrane and the surface of the epithelium (severely dyskaryotic cells appear in the smear); the epithelium shows 'severe dysplasia'. This is also called carcinoma in situ. CIN III is still 'skin deep', being confined by the basement membrane.

Microinvasion

If the basement membrane has been breached by the abnormal cancer cells for a distance of 2 or 3 mm microinvasion has occurred. This is the first sign that the abnormal cells on the surface of the cervix are becoming malignant and starting to invade the cervix.

Invasive tumour

If the depth of invasion reaches 5 mm, involvement of the lymphatic channels and blood vessels becomes likely. At this stage your patient would no longer be asymptomatic but may present with a blood-stained vaginal discharge, intermenstrual bleeding, postcoital bleeding or unexpected postmenopausal bleeding.

On examination of the cervix, the tumour may appear as a bleeding ulcer.

Staging of cervical cancer

- Ib The cancer is confined to the cervix and uterus
- IIa The cancer has encroached on to the top of the vagina
- IIb The cancer has invaded the tissue around the cervix (parametrium)
- III There is extensive involvement of the vagina and invasion out to the bones of the side wall of the pelvis
- IV The cancer has invaded beyond the pelvis and adjacent organs such as the bladder or rectum

Incidental findings on smears

The smear, though taken primarily to look for precancer changes, may also identify specific infections present.

- Anaerobes or anaerobic bacteria.
- Organisms such as bacteria or fungi which can live without oxygen may be found in the moist, airless genital tract.
- Bacterial vaginosis or *Gardnerella vaginalis*: laboratories no longer report on this.

• *Candida albicans* is another quite innocent vaginal infection which often shows up on a smear and can give rise to 'many polymorphs or neutrophils'.

• *Trichomonas vaginalis* is a sexually transmitted protozoan. Its presence makes smears very difficult to read, often mimicking precancer in the cells. This infection can give the cervix the appearance of a strawberry.

• Herpes simplex virus (HSV) can be identified on a smear and would be indicated by 'multinucleated giant cells' on the result.

• Gonorrhoea and chlamydia cannot be diagnosed from a cervical smear, but there can be intracellular detail that may suggest that one or the other is a possibility.

• Actinomyces-type organisms are bacteria which live normally in the mouth and intestines in women who have an intrauterine device (IUD) in situ.

All of these 'incidental findings' should be treated and managed according to the woman's clinical symptoms and local policies.

THE NURSE'S ROLE IN GIVING RESULTS

The laboratory will report the result of the smear and recommend the timing for future recall, treatment or referral. If you are in doubt or have a query about this you should contact the laboratory.

As the nurse who took the smear, your client might come and ask you for advice or further information about her result. It is important to be able to undertake this with a thorough knowledge of the subject which highlights the need for keeping up to date with issues around the screening programme. Updating is recommended once in 3 years (NHSCSP 1998b).

COLPOSCOPY

Colposcopy clinics are an important part of the NHSCSP.

Referral for colposcopy has always been via the GP, unless the woman is not registered in which case referral is via the source of the smear. Direct referral from the laboratory to colposcopy is now seen as ideal and is up and running already in Cleveland (NHSCSP 2001). There is an increasing number of nurse colposcopists, contact BSCCP for details (see Resources p.45).

The colposcope is a binocular microscope which allows the whole cervix to be viewed in detail using magnification of up to 10 times life size.

Many colposcopy clinics nowadays send out patient information leaflets giving details of what to expect at the consultation, with clarification of some of the abnormalities that may be found and possible treatments. You should be up to date with knowledge of your own local service.

Box 2.5 Useful information sent out by colposcopy clinics prior to a first consultation

- You should cancel your appointment if you are likely to be menstruating
- Bring a friend with you
- Arrange to have some time off work in case you have any treatment at your appointment; minor abnormalities may be dealt with the same day
- If you are pregnant you can still have colposcopy, but if you require treatment this may be deferred until after the birth of your baby
- Wear loose clothing, ideally in two halves, as you will be asked to remove your underwear
- It will be useful for you to know the first day of your last menstrual period
- Write down any questions that you would like to discuss

THE EXAMINATION

• Dilute acetic acid shows up the degree of aceto-white (protein-rich 'active' areas), indicating the likely severity of underlying CIN.

• Lugol's iodine (Schiller's test) reacts with glycogen, delineating 'active' areas which produce less glycogen, therefore not taking up the stain as much, whereas healthy areas stain dark brown.

• One or more colposcopically directed 'punch' biopsies may be taken from what appear to be the most severely affected areas.

TREATMENT OF CIN

Laser treatment

The laser beam boils the water in the cells, vaporizing the tissue. The lesion is destroyed to a depth of approximately 1 cm. Sufficient depth is important as abnormalities often extend deep into the endocervical glands. The ablation should also extend beyond the margin of the lesion. This procedure has to a large extent been superseded by large loop excision of transformation zone (LLETZ) (see below).

Cold coagulation

Probes are used depending on the contour of the area to be treated. They are heated electrically and are applied to the cervix for up to 30 seconds. This method has mainly been superseded by LLETZ (see below).

Cryocautery

This destroys the abnormal cells by freezing them with a cryoprobe through which nitrous oxide is released. This method has mainly been replaced by LLETZ but is still used for cervical ectopy.

Diathermy

LLETZ has become an increasingly popular method of treatment for CIN and could be used for routine management of CIN or as a quick and acceptable outpatient alternative to other cone biopsy techniques. It has the advantage of providing a specimen of tissue for histology to see if all the affected area has been removed.

The patient is given written information before she leaves the clinic and follow-up will be according to local policy and guidelines.

Surgical cone biopsy

The need for this operation has been largely superseded by LLETZ. If a very deep cone is taken it is usually carried out under general anaesthetic and will be used mainly when the upper limits of the lesion cannot be visualized.

With the advent of LLETZ problems such as cervical incompetence are not as common as they were.

Hysterectomy

A hysterectomy may be indicated when there are recurrent abnormal results following treatment or where there are other additional gynaecological problems such as menorrhagia or symptomatic fibroids.

Invasive disease

If invasive disease has been diagnosed, the patient will be treated surgically and (depending on the stage of the disease) by radiotherapy or chemotherapy.

Wertheim's hysterectomy is the removal of the uterus and the upper third of the vagina with lymph node clearance. The ovaries may be removed if the woman is approaching the menopause or is postmenopausal.

THE FUTURE

LIQUID BASED CYTOLOGY (LBC)

In October 2003 the NHSCSP announced that, following recommendations from the National Institute for Clinical Excellence (NICE), LBC will be rolled out across England over the following 5 years. This new system has implications for training smear-takers; the old style 'spreading and fixing' the sample is replaced by cells being transferred into a vial of liquid to be processed by the laboratory.

HPV TESTING

If the DNA of HPV could be identified, women with high-risk DNA (16 and 18) could be managed accordingly, and it would also reduce the need for repeat smears from women with low-risk DNA.

It is a possibility (with the appropriate machinery in laboratories) that HPV and chlamydia could also be tested for, from the LBC sample sent.

Trials of an HPV vaccine are under way in America, Australia, China and Manchester (NHSCSP 1999c).

CONCLUSION

In becoming a competent, sensitive smear-taker you will be helping not only to spread the positive news about the 'programme' but also to discover this disease in its early, very treatable stages.

References

Atkin K, Lunt N, Parker G, Hirst M 1993 A national census of practice nurses. York University, York

Austoker J, Davey C 1997 Cervical smear results explained: a guide for primary care. Cancer Research Campaign and NHSCSP, London

Austoker J, McPherson A 1992 Cervical screening, 2nd edn. Oxford University Press, Oxford

Barton SE, Maddox PH, Jenkins D, Edwards R, Cuzick J, Singer A 1988 Effects of cigarette smoking on cervical epithelial immunity. Lancet 11:652

DoH 1988 HC(88)1. Department of Health, London

DoH 1992 The health of the nation. Department of Health, London

DoH 1993 HSG(93)41. Department of Health, London

DoH 1994 Instruments and appliances used in the vagina and cervix: recommended methods for decontamination. SAB(94)22. Department of Health, London

Hopwood J 1990 Background to colposcopy and treatment of the cervix. Schering Healthcare, Burgess Hill

Hopwood J 1995 Background to cervical cytology reports, 3rd edn. Schering Healthcare, Burgess Hill

Martin-Hirsch P, Lilford R, Jarvis G, Kitchener HC 1999 Efficacy of cervical smear collection devices: a systematic review and meta-analysis. Lancet 354:1763–1770

NHSCSP 1998a A national priority: review. NHSCSP, Sheffield

NHSCSP 1998b Resource pack for training smear-takers. NHSCSP, Sheffield

NHSCSP 1999a A national priority: review. NHSCSP, Sheffield

NHSCSP 1999b A pocket guide. NHSCSP, Sheffield

NHSCSP 1999c Links newsletter. Issue 28. NHSCSP, Sheffield

NHSCSP 2000 Achievable standards, benchmarks for reporting, and criteria for evaluating cervical cytopathology, 2nd edn. NHSCSP, Sheffield

NHSCSP 2001 Informing choice: annual review. NHSCSP, Sheffield

NHS Executive 1998 Cervical screening action team – the report. NHS Executive, Leeds

NMC 2002 The NMC code of professional conduct. Nursing and Midwifery Council, London

RCN 1995 Bimanual pelvic examination – guidance for nurses. Royal College of Nurses, London

RCOG, RCP, RCGP, FCM 1987 Report of the Intercollegiate Working Party on Cervical Cytology Screening. Royal College of Obstetricians and Gynaecologists, Royal College of Pathologists, Royal College of General Practitioners, Faculty of Community Medicine, London

Sasieni P, Adams J, Cuzick J 2003 Benefit of cervical screening at different ages: evidence from the UK audit of screening histories. British Journal of Cancer 89:88–93

Scotto J, Bailar JC III 1969 Domenico Rigoni-Stern and medical statistics (a nineteenth century approach to cancer research). Journal of the History of Medicine and Allied Sciences 24:65–75

Simons AM, Phillips DH, Coleman DV 1993 Damage to DNA in cervical epithelium related to smoking tobacco. British Medical Journal 306:1444–1448

Smith JE, Green J, Berrington De Gonzales A et al 2003 Cervical cancer and use of oral contraceptives: a systematic review. Lancet 361(9364):1159–1167

Waddell C 1994 Update in cytology with a focus on smear adequacy. Journal of the National Association of Family Planning Nurses 27:43–48

Warden J 1998 Moves to end cervical screening failures in England. British Medical Journal 317:558

Resources

British Society for Clinical Cytology (BSCC). New video/CD with booklet/workbook *Taking cervical smears*. £75 including p&p from BSCC Office, PO Box 352, Uxbridge UB10 9TX. Cheque payable to 'Cansearch Limited'.

NHSCSP leaflets *What your abnormal result means, The colposcopy examination* and *Cervical screening – the facts*. www.hpe.org.uk

To order any of the following contact the NHS response line on 08701 555 455 or email doh@prolog.uk.com
NHSCSP (updated 2003) *A pocket guide to cervical screening*; NHSCSP (updated 2003) *Cervical smear results explained* (booklet): a guide for primary care; NHSCSP (updated 2002) *Cervical screening – the facts* (booklet): good practice in cervical screening for women with learning difficulties

Useful addresses and websites

British Society for Colposcopy and Cervical Pathology (BSCCP). Mrs E Dollery, The Women's Hospital, Edgbaston, Birmingham B15 2TG. Tel: 0121 607 4716. email: lizdollery@orbite.co.uk

Cancer Research UK. PO Box 123, London WC2A 3PX. Tel: 020 7242 0200. www.cancerresearchuk.org

Marie Curie Cancer Care. 28 Belgrave Square, London SW1X 8QG. Tel: 020 7599 7777. www.mariecurie.org.uk

NHSCSP. 260 Ecclesall Road South, Sheffield S11 9PS. Tel: 0114 271 1060. www.cancerscreening.nhs.uk/ce

Women's National Cancer Control Campaign (WNCCC). www.wnccc.org.uk

Further reading

Andrews G (ed) 2001 Women's sexual health, 3rd edn. Baillière Tindall, London

National Coordinating Network 1994 Report of the first five years of the NHS cervical screening programme. NCN, London

Royal College of Nursing 1994 Female genital mutilation. RCN, London

Szarewski A 1994 A woman's guide to the cervical smear test. Optima, London

Wilson JMC, Junger OGH 1968 Principles and practice of screening for disease. Paper 34. WHO, Geneva

BREAST SCREENING AND ABNORMALITIES

Breast problems account for a large number of consultations in general practice and other primary care locations. Generally nurses are seen as approachable and possibly more accessible than doctors; it is important therefore to have up-to-date information about all aspects of:

- anatomy and physiology of the breasts
- epidemiology and risk factors for breast cancer
- common breast problems with possible signs and symptoms
- importance of breast self-awareness (BSA)
- the NHS Breast Screening Programme (NHSBSP).

ANATOMY AND PHYSIOLOGY

The breasts or mammary glands are intended for lactation but in Western societies they are associated with sexual attractiveness and can be the cause of great anxiety in all the age ranges.

The breast lies over the rib cage and is made up of fatty tissue and 15–20 ducts which extend from the nipple to lobules which in turn end in 100 or so tiny bulbs called acini, where milk is produced.

Looking at the outer breast, the nipple contains lactiferous sinuses which are the enlarged terminals of the ducts; it is from these that milk is secreted. The nipple is surrounded by the areola on which is found small pimple-like elevations known as the tubercles of Montgomery, which help to lubricate the area during breastfeeding.

The breasts' major lymphatic drainage is to the axilla and internal mammary chain which has implications when the spread of malignant disease is considered. The breast tissue is held in position by Cooper's ligaments, fibrous bands which run between the lobes to the skin, extending upwards to the armpit, forming the axillary tail.

The breasts are under the influence of oestrogen and progesterone and each month when a woman approaches menstruation, the size of the breasts may fluctuate in response to these sex hormones.

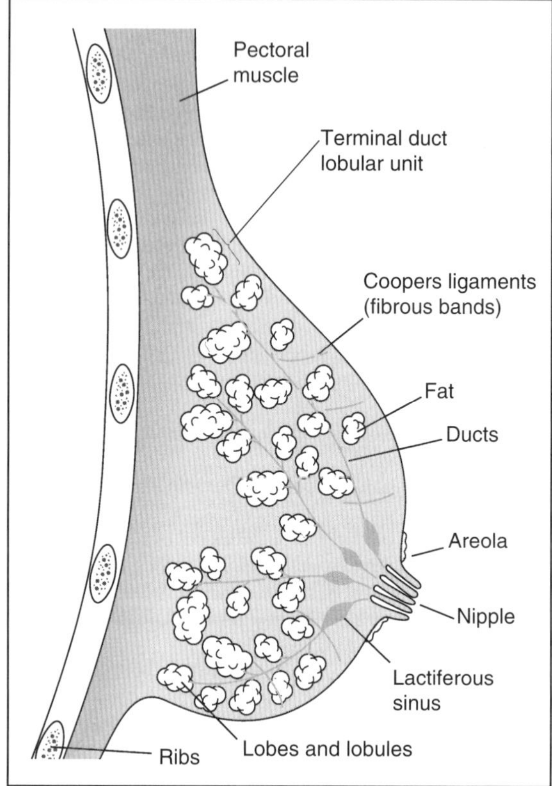

Figure 2.10 Sagittal section of the breast.

EPIDEMIOLOGY OF BREAST CANCER

Breast cancer is the most common malignancy in the female population worldwide (Parkin et al 1984) and is the most common cause of death in women between the ages of 44 and 50. In the UK 1 in 9 women develop breast cancer.

RISK FACTORS

- *Family history*. History of breast cancer in a first-degree relative on the maternal side. Risk increases if the relative was premenopausal.
- *Genetic predisposition*. All breast cancer can be termed 'genetic' as cancer is caused by genetic mutations resulting in abnormal cellular growth, but only 5–10% of breast cancers are due to inheriting a mutated gene. Two genes have been isolated in which mutations are associated with an increased risk of breast and ovarian cancer: *BRCA1* and *BRCA2*.
- *Menstrual history*. An early menarche before age 12 years and a late menopause after age 55 years increases a woman's risk factors.
- *Age*. Risk rises steadily from the age of 40.
- *Reproductive history*. Nulliparity increases the risk as does the age at first full-term pregnancy (after the age of 35) (Dixon & Sainsbury 1993).
- *Breastfeeding* appears to be protective against breast cancer, with the risk decreasing further

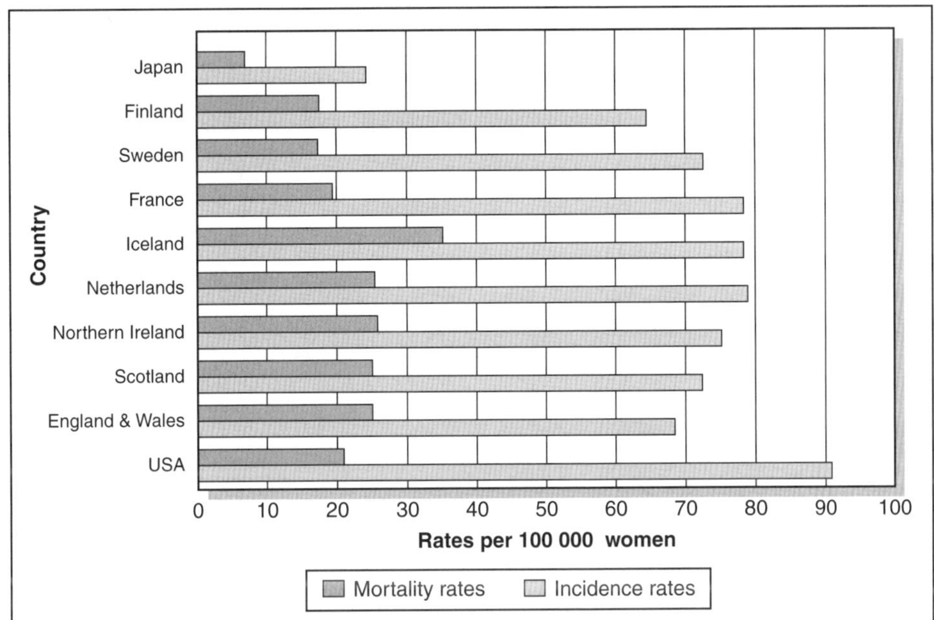

Figure 2.11 International incidence and mortality rates for breast cancer. Data on mortality from WHO database which can be accessed via www.dep.iarc.fr

with increasing duration of feeding (Chilvers et al 1993).

- *Oral contraceptive pill.* There is a small increased risk of breast cancer in current users of the combined oral contraceptive pill compared to non-users, but this decreases after stopping the pill and disappears after 10 years.
- *Hormone replacement therapy* (HRT). There is a slight increased risk in long duration of use (an additional 2 in 1000 women after 5 years' use; 6 in 1000 women after 10 years' use; 12 in 1000 women after 15 years' use, all having started HRT at age 50).
- *Exposure to radiation.* Women who have received large doses of ionizing radiation for medical reasons (also women who survived the nuclear bombings in Japan demonstrated an increased risk to breast cancer).
- *Obesity.* It has been shown that obese women have a greater risk than slim women.
- *Alcohol* has been associated with a moderate increased risk (IARC 1988).
- *Geographic variations* (Fig. 2.11).

Cigarette smoking is not related to an increased risk of developing breast cancer.

COMMON BREAST PROBLEMS WITH POSSIBLE SIGNS AND SYMPTOMS

- Fibroadenomas are the most common benign lumps in women between the ages of 20 and 30 years. These are fibrous nodules which are usually firm and mobile, often referred to as a 'breast mouse' because of its mobility. They will commonly be found by the woman, causing anxiety if not investigated. A referral to a breast care specialist may be advisable.
- Cysts are fluid-filled sacs found most commonly in women in the 40–60 age group. They can vary in size and feel either soft ('lax') or hard, in which case they may resemble a carcinoma. Investigations may include a mammogram to rule out cancer or ultrasound. They can be aspirated by fine needle, especially if they are causing discomfort, but some persistent cysts may have to be removed surgically.
- Breast discomfort (mastalgia), in which the breasts are generally lumpy, causes great anxiety to women. There is a great need for education here and a sound knowledge of the normal physiology of breast tissue and the influence of cyclical hormones will be of enormous benefit. This could include keeping a chart of dates and symptoms to see a pattern evolve, which is always reassuring. Advice regarding the importance of a well-fitting bra and reducing the consumption of caffeine and salt in the diet can be helpful. Evening primrose oil or starflower oil can be helpful at the recommended dose. *Reassuringly, breast pain is a rare symptom of breast cancer.*
- Duct papillomas are very common, caused by solitary benign lesions growing in one of the main ducts close to the nipple. Nipple discharge will be a sign. Treatment is usually excision of the duct.

- Duct ectasia is due to dilatation of major or minor ducts within the breast leading to retention of secretions within them. Symptoms can be nipple discharge/retraction and/or a palpable mass.
- Intertrigo is a rash in the fold of skin under (large) breasts, usually caused by not drying the area thoroughly or after excessive perspiration. Advice on wearing cotton next to the skin, the use of calamine cream and non-use of talcum powder will be useful.
- Hairs around the areola are common and can be removed with tweezers or with electrolysis by a trained professional.

BREAST AWARENESS

The government advisory committee on breast cancer screening revised its advice in 1998, stating there was no evidence to support the efficacy of breast examination as a routine part of health promotion on asymptomatic women. It was 'inappropriate' in the primary care setting to be offering this service, as it could give false reassurance.

Nowadays the concept of 'breast awareness' is what all health professionals should be promoting. The difference between the two is subtle as women are still being asked to look at and feel their breasts but not in such a ritualistic way as previously.

Women should be encouraged to become familiar with how their breasts normally look and feel and how this can vary throughout the month. There is still controversy around this advice but it could be argued that even if BSA does not alter the course of the disease, perhaps initial treatment need not be so aggressive.

Box 2.6 Breast awareness: a summary

Women should be aware of:
- change in breast shape or size
- any dimpling/puckering or creases in the skin
- any lump or thickening in the breast
- any alteration in the nipple, whether it starts to go in or starts pointing in a different direction
- any discharge from the nipple

The Marie Curie Cancer Screening Course has a breast awareness component within it (see p.45 for address).

There are some useful booklets to give out to women to back up information. See resource section for details (p.49).

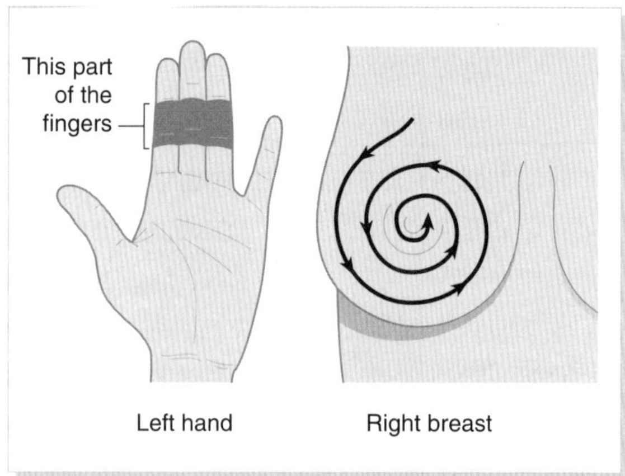

Figure 2.12 Area of fingers to be used in breast awareness and circular method of self-examination.

NATIONAL HEALTH SERVICE BREAST SCREENING PROGRAMME

Mammography uses an X-ray technique to visualize the internal structures of the breast. Following the Forrest Report (DHSS 1986), a national breast screening programme was set up, offering mammography to asymptomatic women aged 50–64 years every 3 years (though the age range is being changed to include those up to age 70). There has also been a study looking at screening women from age 40. The aim of the NHSBSC is to reduce mortality from breast cancer by 25% in the population of women invited to be screened.

Information on women in the screening age range is based on primary care agency computer records, which in turn rely on all women being registered with a GP.

Screening can generate much anxiety and nurses have a significant role in informing and encouraging women to make use of the service.

The most common question asked is 'does breast screening prevent breast cancer'. The answer is no; breast screening only helps find breast cancer if it is already there at an earlier more treatable stage. Some women will develop cancer before their first mammogram or between mammograms. This highlights the importance of encouraging BSA.

The NHS Cancer Screening Programme have published a free booklet on *'Breast screening – the facts'* which will be sent out to all women with their invitation.

Breast care and screening is a huge area which cannot be discussed fully here. Treatments for breast cancer are moving on apace so it is recommended that further reading around the topic is undertaken.

References

Chilvers C, McPherson K, Peto J, Pike M, Vessey M 1993 Breast feeding and risk of breast cancer in young women. British Medical Journal 307:17–20

DHSS 1986 The Forrest Report. HMSO, London

Dixon M, Sainsbury R 1993 Diseases of the breast. Churchill Livingstone, Edinburgh

IARC Monographs on the evaluation of carcinogenic risks to humans: alcohol drinking. International Agency for Research on Cancer, Lyon

Parkin D, Srjeinswaard J, Muir C 1984 Estimates of the worldwide frequency of twelve major cancers. Bulletin of the World Health Organization 62:162–163

Resources

NHSBSP. *Be breast aware* (1998). Leaflet produced by the DoH. The Manor House, 260 Ecclesall Road South, Sheffield S11 9PS. Tel: 0114 271 1060

NHS Cancer Screening Programme. *Breast screening – the facts*. Booklet published by Health Promotion England. www.cancerscreening.nhs.uk/breastscreen

Breast Cancer Care. *Breast awareness* and many other booklets. Kiln House, 210 New Kings Road, London SW6 4NZ. Tel: 020 7867 1101. National free phone: 0808 800 6000. www.breastcancercare.org.uk. Fax: 0870 191 1219

Male breast cancer. interact.withus.com/interact/mbc

Further reading

Baum M, Saunders C, Meredith S 1994 Breast cancer: a guide for every woman. Oxford University Press, Oxford

Curling G, Burnet K 2001 Breast screening and breast disorders. In: Andrews G (ed) Women's sexual health. Baillière Tindall, London

Collaborative Group on Hormonal Factors in Breast Cancer 1996 Breast cancer and hormonal contraceptives. Lancet 347:1713–1727

Million Women Study Collaborators. The British Million Women Study 2003. Lancet 362:414–415, 419–427

Chapter 3

Men's health

Andy Shave

CHAPTER CONTENTS

INTRODUCTION

The aim of this chapter is to highlight issues that are specific to men. It will look at how men view their health and some of the difficulties they experience when accessing healthcare. It will also look at perceptions of men and their health by healthcare providers, particularly in primary healthcare.

The majority of the chapter will focus on the two issues facing many men today:

1. prostate cancer and the role of prostate-specific antigen (PSA) screening
2. erectile dysfunction and new treatments available.

The chapter will also give useful addresses and website information for health professionals to help them with assessment and aftercare provided for men presenting with the above conditions.

MEN'S APPROACH TO HEALTHCARE

It is a universally acknowledged fact that being a man is a dangerous occupation!

- In every age group male death rates are higher than female death rates, from birth to adulthood (Whitehead 1988).
- Men are more at risk of life-threatening conditions such as circulatory disease (Callman 1992).
- Suicide rates for men are twice as high as those for women – 13.1% male to 6.8% female (Callman 1992).
- There are a number of male-specific diseases, such as prostate and testicular cancers.
- Twice as many men die from skin cancer as do women.

Despite these figures and increasing health promotion targeting men, little seems to have changed to improve men's mortality. There are a number of reasons for this, most centring on belief systems. Robertson (1995) believes that women are healthier due to the fact that their healthcare is not just centred on a medical model but takes account of a second model, which is focused on a holistic approach and self-help. This is in direct contrast to men who concentrate on the medical model and completely ignore the psychological aspects of their health. Robertson (1995) states his belief that this may stem from the patriarchal nature of medicine, which causes a paradox by preventing men from expressing their healthcare needs and thus contributing to higher levels of morbidity and mortality. Richman summed this up perfectly when he stated that:

> *Thou shalt not cry or expose feelings of emotion, fear, weakness, symptoms, empathy or involvement before thy neighbour.* (Richman & Holland 1983)

Although Richman was specifically talking of men's experience of childbirth, this 'first commandment of masculinity' adequately conjures up the traditional image of the macho man who is dominant, competitive, strong, fit, healthy and the family provider, as identified by Platzer (1988). Unfortunately these images have remained at the forefront of cultural stereotyping, creating ideals and expectations to be met. Women have been able to cast off their soft, weak, housekeeper stereotype with the emergence of the women's movement; however, men still have the need to appear strong and independent, which is continually reinforced by expectations from the media and others.

Platzer recognized that if these ideals go unrecognized or are challenged, such as happens in unemployment, then both physical and mental health may suffer as a consequence of the blow to this macho role. This could be the start of a vicious cycle of events, which may prove difficult to break. If we again use the example of unemployment, we can see from several studies that men who are unemployed are more prone to severe psychological strain and mental illness. This stems from anxiety and depression, which in some instances may manifest in a higher incidence of divorce and violence (Fareed 1994). This may be attributed to the fact that men perceive themselves as the breadwinner and when they see this role taken away they may feel emasculated.

The cycle continues as these men will be more reluctant to seek advice as they see this as a further threat because they have been socialized not to express emotional concerns (Richman & Holland 1983), even though they are much more susceptible to stress than women (Fareed 1994, Matthews 1988). Stafford et al (1994) felt that stress was further compounded in the unemployed male, as the workplace was often where men gained psychological support. This in itself may lead to further 'compensatory risk-taking behaviours' as outlined by Forrester (1986).

Men's approach to their own healthcare is often interwoven with their ideas of macho identity, which inevitably brings them into conflict with themselves. They identify with the expectations placed on men and perceive a need for maintaining the masculine image. One only has to look at the rising trend of glossy men's health magazines which do not offer adequate health promotion but often capitalize on perceived healthy, masculine activities such as rock climbing, sailing, etc. They often promote the body culture with the assumption that the sign of being healthy and fit is to have a six-pack and perfect pectorals. The reasons men are willing to buy into this culture are often cited as appearing more physically attractive to women, yet the emergence of this 'body culture' has its roots in wanting to give the appearance of well-being and masculinity.

Gay men originally adopted body culture with the advent of the HIV/AIDS epidemic in the early 1980s when they were singled out as the cause of AIDS. There was general panic within the gay population as to who was infected and who was not (HIV testing had not been developed at that stage). The way to 'prove' that one was uninfected was to present a picture of health and fitness. Even when HIV testing was introduced the body culture continued to flourish, as it still remained an unspoken testimony of wellness. This, however, has taken its toll with many gay men being unable to meet the demands of 'physical perfection', often leading to psychological distress and in some cases suicide. Whether these negative effects translate to the heterosexual male remains to be seen but there is much media manipulation, promoting high expectations.

To summarize, many men are reluctant to access healthcare, usually because they identify with the expectations placed upon men and their perceived need for maintaining the masculine image. Ultimately they do not wish to be seen as weak or dependent or to be assuming a feminine role, based on the belief that sickness or ill health is the domain of women.

PERCEPTIONS OF A HOSTILE ENVIRONMENT

Men are reported as much less likely to utilize their GPs, again partly due to a refusal to acknowledge symptoms, thereby maintaining the macho image, but this is implicitly reinforced by health professionals who tend to view men's health problems as less severe (Macintyre et al 1996). One has only to look at male registrations in GP surgeries to appreciate this. The very act of registration is difficult for men who are often working during surgery hours, combined with taking more time off for a health screen by the nurse. There are often no 'fast-track' facilities for men who attend. There are very few surgeries which provide men-only spaces or allocated times for men only and even fewer which provide these facilities run by male staff. This will have the knock-on effect that males will find it very difficult to discuss sexual dysfunction or other sexual health needs in this environment, just as female patients will not want to discuss contraception and reproductive health in a male-dominated environment. Many surgeries need to evaluate the service they offer if they are to comply with access to care outlined in the DoH *Sexual health strategy* (DoH 2001).

SINGLE MEN

Unmarried men, particularly widowed, divorced or separated, have a higher mortality rate than men who live with partners (Gove 1979). Statistics show that this group are more likely to smoke and drink to excess. This partly explains the number of car, cycling and motorcycling accidents that involve younger men, usually under the influence of alcohol (Fareed 1994). Diet may also be a contributing factor. Single men are much more likely to have an unhealthy diet. This may be due to working hours, lack of motivation or the simple inability to take on a role seen as the preserve of women. Men also have limited access to information on healthy eating; one only has to look at the amount of literature found in women's magazines to appreciate this. If men are also consuming large amounts of alcohol then food becomes of secondary importance.

Bereavement has been shown to increase the risk of death in men, with men being 40% more likely to die in the year following the death of a spouse (Fareed 1994). This is attributed to the level of support that society gives to a female survivor, which it withholds from men, suggesting that social support is a protector of health. This may be due to the fact that men have become dependent on their spouse and are therefore unable to care for their own needs or that they are unable to seek support because of maintenance of the macho image.

HEALTH PROMOTION TARGETED AT MEN AND THEIR NEEDS

In 1995 the UK National Men's Awareness Campaign undertook a survey of 5000 men, the largest ever performed in the UK. From this survey the following data were collated:

- 96% believed there wasn't enough information about healthcare for men
- 88% thought that society placed a higher value on women's health
- 79% wanted more information about diet; 62% about stress; 19% about alcohol and 14% about smoking
- a staggering 91% didn't share their health concerns with their GP and only made an appointment when they were ill
- 20% didn't talk to anyone about their health concerns
- 60% said they suffered from depression, of which two thirds had not requested any help
- 92% said they would attend a well-man clinic.

Most of these findings correlate with the research already outlined; however, a startling number of men felt that their healthcare needs were not taken seriously and that they were concerned about their healthcare needs. This assertion seems to be supported by the literature available. Fareed (1994) states that:

> *A search for information on men's health between 1983 and 1993 using the nursing index, CINAHL, and the key words 'men's health' revealed only 10 articles.*

Little appears to have changed in the interim for when I recently did a similar search I was rewarded with only a few more articles. There is much complacency about men's health needs. This ranges from one health trust admitting 'We are neglecting men's health needs' to accusations that the Department of Health refuses to take any responsibility, although it recognizes the disparity between women's and men's health. This has been clearly illustrated in Callman's tacit agreement that:

> *The health profiles of men and women clearly differ. Greater knowledge about the reasons for sex*

> *differences in susceptibility to common diseases might give a better understanding of the disease mechanisms, to the benefit of men and women alike*
>
> (Callman 1992)

Although there is a clear recognition of the differences in health needs there appears to be little commitment to improving men's healthcare. An example of how little has changed is provided by Fareed (1994). He argued that although 8000 men were dying of prostate cancer (the third biggest killer of men at the time), with 12 500 new diagnoses in 1989 alone and figures rising yearly, there was no money set aside to target screening. This was in contrast to the £54 million set aside to screen women for breast and cervical cancer. Little has changed since then although cancer is now the second biggest killer of men. In 1997–8 government funding for research into prostate cancer was just £47 000 compared with £4.3 million spent on breast cancer research. An extra £1 million was given by the government in March 2000 (Templeton 2003). There are, of course, a number of reasons why the government may choose not to target prostate cancer, due to the controversy surrounding the effectiveness of screening and treatment. This is something which the practice nurse will encounter and therefore it is discussed in more depth later in the chapter.

Three approaches to men's health promotion have been identified:

1. the medical screening approach
2. the sporadic approach
3. the holistic approach (Robertson 1995).

Although there is some value in the sporadic approach it is hit and miss, whereas the medical screening approach, which is usually adopted, is ineffective. One way to explain this is that the men often most in need of information are manual workers who tend to view health checks as less valid than professionals (Fareed 1994). Other reasons suggested for failure are that, because healthcare professionals adopt the medical approach, they do not look at the social and behavioural issues which would be addressed by a holistic approach, such as that which has proved successful in women's health screening. Unfortunately, with the advent of GP purchasing, the holistic approach is often dropped in favour of the medical approach; this may be because task screening attracts additional government funding.

To assess the level of health promotion that is tailored to men it would be useful to analyse the targets set for the *Health of the Nation* (DoH 1992) and how they have been applied to men's health issues.

MENTAL HEALTH

Mental health issues are relatively common in men but are often underestimated. This is partly because men often feel unable to express their feelings or they have 'masculine' expectations which do not allow them to acknowledge their feelings, leading to gender role conflict. The RCN (1996) stated in its review that:

> *Men who take on behaviour thought to be 'feminine' are thought to be 'less than men' ... This can lead to lower self-esteem and gender role conflict and strain.*

If this is the case for all men then it must follow that gay men must be especially vulnerable. There are a number of studies that identify the risks of mental ill health (Stanford 1988) and parasuicide (Paul et al 2002) for gay adolescents, thought to be due to lack of support when coming to terms with their sexuality. In the UK there has been a steady increase in the number of men committing suicide (four times the rate of increase among women), particularly in the young population. Up to half of these men were divorced or single (Charlton 1993).

CORONARY HEART DISEASE

In the UK coronary heart disease is the biggest killer, being responsible for nearly 150 000 deaths per annum, with a ratio of one in four deaths in men to one in five in women. It is also the most common cause of premature death: 28% in men and 17% in women. There is debate as to the cause of this, with most studies citing risk factors and risk groups, with much controversy as to how these are identified and how effective preventive campaigns were. We have identified that because of behaviour, attitude and beliefs, men are risk takers so it should come as no surprise that most heart attacks are caused by excessive smoking, with alcohol consumption and poor diet adding to the risk.

There are numerous campaigns targeting preventive measures, such as smoking and healthy eating, but this could be seen as treating the symptoms without treating the cause. Only when we start challenging the beliefs and value systems of men will health campaigns like this have some impact. After all, we know that most pregnant women will only stop smoking if they feel that it will affect the health of their unborn child.

ACCIDENTS

Forty-nine percent of male accidental deaths are caused by road traffic accidents, usually with exacerbating factors such as alcohol and sometimes drugs (RCN 1996). Most of these tend to be in younger age groups and there has been a rising trend since 1990.

CANCERS

Lung cancer is still the most common in England, with men twice as likely to die from it as women (even though the incidence in women is increasing) (RCN 1996). Reducing lung cancer deaths in men under 75 was the stated target. It is well recognized that smoking plays an active part in the development of the disease so it is reasonable to expect that health promotion would focus around this. Most of the promotion was not gender specific. However, the Health Education Report for 1994–5 highlighted that some campaigns were targeted at women, particularly around pregnancy, encouraging partners of pregnant women to give up smoking, not for their own sake but for the woman and unborn baby. There were no specific campaigns aimed at men, totally ignoring the identified target group.

Testicular cancer is also a concern for men. There are approximately 4900 new cases a year, mainly in the 20–34 age group, with a 90% chance of recovery if caught early. Unfortunately, in the Men's Health Awareness Survey (1995) only one third of respondents had ever heard of this and only 5% undertook regular self-examination. The number of new cases are only 500 less than women who are diagnosed as having cervical cancer, yet the health promotion is poles apart, with targeting often relegated to leaflets in the GP surgery. This is an important role that the practice nurse must put on the agenda, if we are not to waste the opportunities provided by the rare visits of men to the GP surgery.

PROSTATE CANCER

Prostate cancer is the second most common cancer in men in the UK and it is estimated that around 20 000 men are diagnosed and approximately 10 000 men die of the disease each year (NHS 2003). Prostate cancer is more common in older men with the rate of disease increasing with age. The incidence of prostate cancer increased sharply in the 1990s, partly caused by the introduction of a rapid and sensitive test for PSA and an ageing population. There is much debate as to whether a national screening programme using PSA will reduce prostate cancer-related mortality, with several studies giving conflicting results. The facts that high levels of PSA are not indicative of prostate cancer and that many men who have prostate cancer have normal levels of PSA further complicate this already complex and contentious issue.

Several studies indicate the benefits of PSA screening in reducing prostate cancer mortality whilst others indicate that PSA screening does not fulfil the required conditions to be introduced as a national screening programme (Ransohoff et al 2002). Confusion over the perceived benefits of PSA screening does not help the patient. The practice nurse needs to be informed of the benefits and negative aspects of PSA screening. The patient needs to be aware that high levels of PSA may not mean that he has prostate cancer and, conversely, low levels may not mean that he does not have prostate cancer although, in conjunction with digital rectal examination (DRE), PSA levels may give a clearer picture. The practice nurse needs also to be aware of the psychosocial aspects of PSA screening – increased worry and distress following a high PSA test for a healthy male, for example – and help the patient come to a decision over whether to submit to testing.

AGE AND INCIDENCE: SOME FACTS AND FIGURES

The *NHS Prostate Cancer Risk Management Statistics* (NHS 2003) give the following figures for the UK incidence and mortality of prostate cancer (Fig. 3.1).

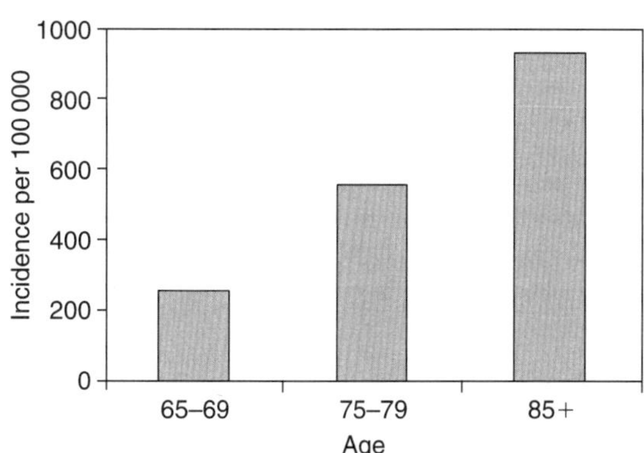

Figure 3.1 Prostate cancer incidence increases with age but is rare in men under 50. Average age of diagnosis is 75.

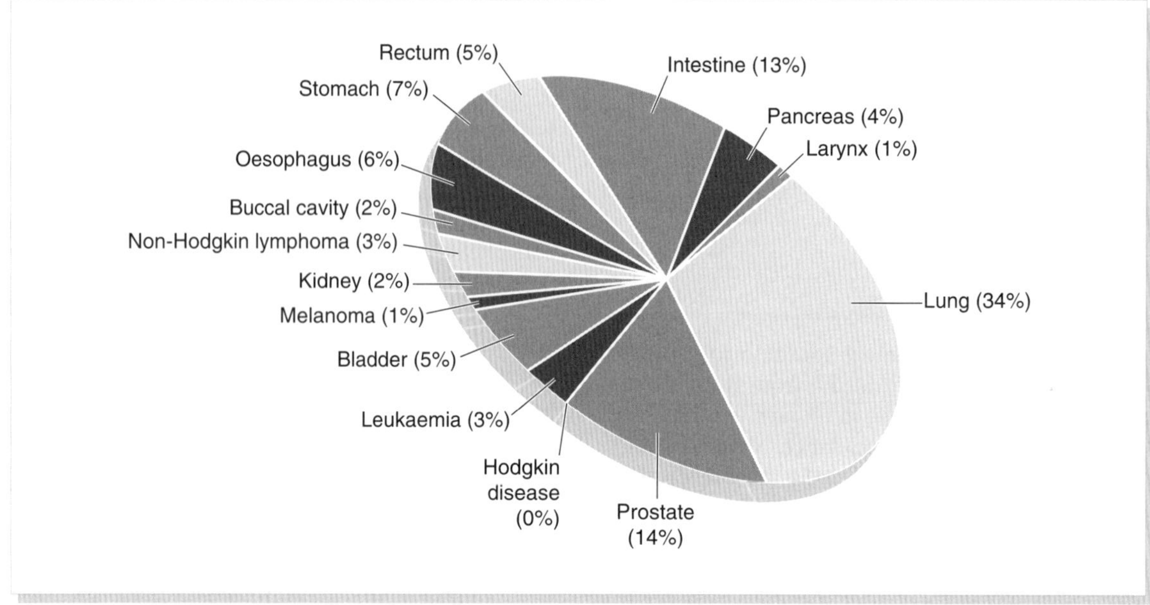

Figure 3.2 Cancer deaths in the UK from 1990 to 1999 in males aged 50+ (data from WHO).

Prostate cancer is mainly a disease of the elderly and increased disease correlates with age. In 1997 there were 21 748 new cases of prostate cancer registered in the UK, giving an approximate incidence of 75 cases per 100 000 men. The average age at diagnosis is 75. Overall, prostate cancer is the second largest cause of cancer deaths in the UK (Fig. 3.2), a trend repeated in many countries around the world. However, despite significant increases in the incidence of prostate cancer in many countries there has been a concurrent decrease in mortality in some age groups. In the UK, however, using statistics from 1970 to 1999, only the beginning of a decrease in mortality is apparent (Fig. 3.3); this is much more marked in the USA over the same time period (data not shown).

The cause of prostate cancer is not known and several factors are thought to play a role in causation. Factors such as age, hormones, dietary fat and genetics could potentially be involved. As with many cancers, it is very difficult to suggest a causative agent or one particular factor that leads to disease.

Hormones

Some hormones have been thought to play a role in prostate cancer and oestrogens have been used therapeutically to treat disease.

Sexual activity

Another factor implicated in prostate disease is sexual activity. Some studies have found links with the number of sexual partners and also the age at the time of first intercourse. In addition, sexually transmitted diseases have been implicated in prostate cancer. Several studies show that previous infections increase the risk of prostate cancer. However, these increases in incidence are slight and not all studies agree (Dennis & Dawson 2002, Key 1995).

Family history

Prostate cancer can also have a strong family association. Simply put, if one family member has prostate cancer, the risk of another male family member having prostate cancer is increased. It has been estimated that around 5–10% of all prostate cancer cases are caused by susceptibility genes (Bratt 2002). Interestingly, the predictive value of a PSA screen increases if a family member has prostate cancer. Environment may also play a part in prostate cancer incidence in families.

Ethnicity is also a factor in prostate cancer incidence. African American men have a much increased risk compared to white American men; in fact, the risk is almost double (Moul 2000). The lowest risk of prostate cancer is in Asian men.

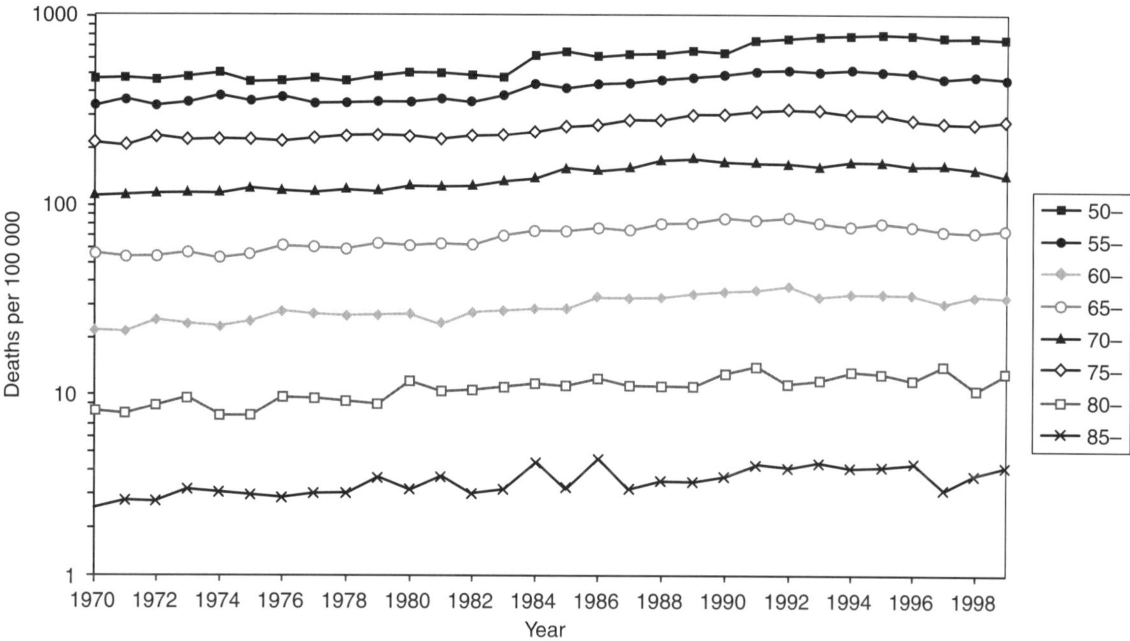

Figure 3.3 Trends in mortality from prostate cancer in the UK from 1990 to 1999 (data from WHO).

Environmental factors

Prostate cancer incidence is greater in the West and one of the contributory factors for this has been thought to be dietary fats. Increased intake of dietary fat has been associated with an increase in prostate cancer. It has been suggested that different types of fats may be protective or increase prostate cancer.

Several other factors have been suggested to alter prostate cancer incidence, including smoking and exposure to chemicals, but the evidence for these and other factors influencing prostate cancer is limited (Key 1995).

Finally, there has been much controversy relating to vasectomy and prostate cancer. Some studies have suggested that vasectomy increases the risk of prostate cancer. However, other studies have shown no link (Weiske 2001).

It is well worth noting that more men die *with* prostate cancer than *of* prostate cancer. This is the main reason for the controversy over implementation of a national screening programme.

PSA SCREENING

What is PSA?

PSA is a protein made in the prostate by both normal and cancerous cells. Technically, PSA is a serine protease. Its function is to cut up proteins present in semen; more specifically, it cleaves semenogelins. During PSA synthesis in the prostate, PSA enters the circulation and its levels can be detected in the blood. The amount of PSA in the blood can indicate the presence of prostate cancer.

As already mentioned above, normal prostate cells make PSA. That cancerous cells also make PSA is one of the reasons for using it for prostate cancer screening, the larger number of tumour cells making more and more PSA. However, this is the crux of the PSA testing problem. High levels of PSA do not necessarily mean prostate cancer – and many men who have prostate cancer have normal levels of PSA. Put another way, high levels of PSA (deemed >4 ng/ml) are not disease specific. This can cause difficulty when informing patients of the advantages and disadvantages of PSA screening.

A national PSA screening programme

As already mentioned, there are many complexities in deciding if a national PSA screening programme should be implemented in the UK. The efficacy of a screening programme must be clearly demonstrated and Wilson and Junger of the WHO published a list of criteria to be met and these were reproduced on the NHS Cancer Screening Programmes website (NHS 2003).

1. The condition is an important health problem.
2. Its natural history is well understood.
3. It is recognizable at an early stage.
4. Treatment is better at an early stage.
5. A suitable test exists.
6. An acceptable test exists.
7. Adequate facilities exist to cope with abnormalities detected.
8. Screening is done at repeated intervals when the onset is insidious.
9. The chance of harm is less than the chance of benefit.
10. The cost is balanced against benefit.

It is generally agreed that prostate cancer and PSA screening do not fulfil all of these criteria and it is for this reason that the government has not recommended a national PSA screening.

These characteristics apply to national screening programmes, but not to the screening of symptomatic men. A PSA test may be advised by the patient's GP if appropriate symptoms are described at consultation.

What are the benefits of a national screening programme? Should all men over 50 be offered an annual PSA test?

There are conflicting reports over the efficacy and benefit of PSA screening for prostate cancer. At first glance, it may seem that PSA screening is definitely a good thing. In the USA, where PSA screening is more prevalent, there has been a drop in prostate cancer-related mortality in the last 10 years. In the UK, where PSA screening is still uncommon, there has been only a slight decrease in mortality in certain age groups. Does this mean that PSA screening is beneficial? At first glance it may seem that way but there are other factors to be aware of.

It is important to weigh up the benefit gained from a PSA test. Obviously, PSA screening could detect asymptomatic men with prostate cancer, perhaps at an early stage of disease. However, how many men who are tested will have prostate cancer? What are the psychological effects of annual testing from the age of 50 plus? Given that the average age of prostate cancer diagnosis is 75, does the annual test, with the attendant anxiety, justify PSA screening?

Another serious problem is the number of false-positive results. As mentioned several times before in this chapter, high levels of PSA do not indicate prostate cancer. In fact, around two thirds of men who have elevated PSA do not have prostate cancer. Equally seriously, if a tested man had high levels of PSA, what happens next? It is difficult to ignore an elevated PSA level and the GP may suggest referral to a urologist who may then decide to perform a prostate biopsy. So the report of a high PSA level may lead to medical intervention in the form of a biopsy, with all the anxiety that this may bring.

In addition, there is always the risk of alarming men with clinically unimportant prostate cancer. More men die *with* prostate cancer than *of* it. In screening for PSA, asymptomatic men who may never develop clinically important disease will have to decide whether or not to have a biopsy and further treatment.

All these factors must be taken into account when looking at the figures for the efficacy of PSA screening.

There are several major studies under way in several countries to test the efficacy of PSA testing in reducing prostate cancer-related mortality. Until those results have been collated and examined (in several years' time), the UK government will not recommend a national PSA screening programme.

However, what does all this mean to the practice nurse who is advising a patient of the risks and benefits of a PSA screen? Ito & Schrder (2003) offer the following suggestions for giving information to men who are at risk of prostate cancer.

1. Information on risk factors, including age, race, family history, diet and lifestyle.
2. The risk of diagnosis in the patient's lifetime with and without screening. How the risk of prostate cancer would change if there is a family history of disease.
3. The chances of having an abnormal test and biopsy.
4. Biopsies and the risks attached.
5. The risk of prostate cancer following a positive result.
6. The effects of treatment and its efficacy.
7. Complications following treatment.
8. Risks of overdiagnosis and unnecessary treatment.

So the patient must be advised of the limitations of a PSA screen, particularly men who are asymptomatic. In men who have symptoms the role of PSA is perhaps clearer and after discussion with the practice nurse and the GP, the patient may be referred to a urologist who will be able to advise further.

PROSTATE CANCER TREATMENTS

There are three main treatments offered in the UK: monitoring, radical prostatectomy and radiotherapy. The life expectancy of the patient will affect the option chosen. Active monitoring involves regular urology follow-ups. It is particularly suitable for men who have slow-growing tumours or are perhaps older or for those who find the risks of alternative therapies unacceptable. Of course, the risk of monitoring is that some men may develop metastatic disease.

Prostatectomy involves removal of the prostate gland and has a significant risk of impotence and incontinence. Some studies have reported impotence levels as high as 80%. In younger, sexually active men, this could lead to considerable emotional and psychological distress. In addition, complete removal of the tumour cannot be guaranteed.

Radiotherapy also carries with it considerable risks of impotence and incontinence although not as high as those reported for prostatectomy. Impotence has been shown to be as high as 60% following treatment. Bowel problems and rectal bleeding are also side-effects of treatment.

SUMMARY

The role of the practice nurse in prostate cancer and screening is manifold. The practice nurse may explain the pros and cons of PSA screening to at-risk men, giving a detailed account of the difficulties involved in measuring PSA levels and also understanding what those results may mean. The issues at the heart of prostate cancer and PSA screening are complex and the patient needs as much information as possible to make the decision on whether to go ahead with a PSA test.

ERECTILE DYSFUNCTION

Erectile dysfunction is the umbrella term for the inability to achieve and/or maintain an erection which is sufficient for sexual intercourse. It is the currently preferred term, replacing impotence. It is said that nearly all men at one time or another will experience erectile dysfunction.

Erectile dysfunction is characterized by a persistent and continuing inability to achieve or maintain an erection. Erectile dysfunction is often short term or limited to a few episodes, but for some erectile dysfunction blights their lives, affects self-esteem and how they view their masculinity. Partners may believe that they are no longer attractive or wanted. Obviously all of these things can have a major effect on men's lives.

Incredibly, it is said that around 75% of men do not seek advice for this problem. Some men feel that erectile dysfunction is just another part of ageing and do not want to seek advice or perhaps do not think that their problem merits help or advice. There is a link between age and erectile dysfunction as the incidence of erectile dysfunction does increase with age. However, age is not important when it comes to treatment. All men of any age should feel free to discuss this issue with a health professional (Dinsmore & Kell 2002).

NORMAL ERECTILE FUNCTION

So how does an erection happen? Quite simply, an erection occurs when the penis is filled with blood. In the normal, flaccid state, blood vessels in the penis limit the flow of blood but during arousal these vessels open and the penis fills with blood. Columns in the penis called the corpus cavernosum and the corpus spongiosum fill with blood and harden. Firm tissues surrounding these columns prevent blood leaking out, maintaining the erection. After ejaculation the blood vessels return to their state of restricted blood flow and the penis returns to its flaccid state.

COMMON CAUSES OF ERECTILE DYSFUNCTION

Psychological

Around 20% of erectile dysfunction has a psychological cause, including sexual inexperience, stress, depression, bereavement, new partner and anxiety. However, the important thing to remember is that these men will still have erections at night and in the morning, when they are not placed in a sexual situation. This of course means that the penis is working and that there is no physical bar to sex. It is more common in younger men.

Physical/organic

There are several physical reasons why men have erectile dysfunction. These can broadly be divided into four areas:

1. vascular
2. neurogenic
3. endocrinological
4. drug side-effects.

Vascular Erectile function needs healthy veins to work properly. If a man has vascular disease this may cause a decrease in blood flow and a loss of erection. Typical vascular problems are atherosclerosis, hyperlipidaemia, smoking, diabetes and hypertension. Atherosclerosis accounts for around half of all erectile dysfunction in men over 50.

Neurogenic Neurogenic reasons for erectile dysfunction include multiple sclerosis, surgery, diabetes, trauma and alcohol. Prostatectomy is a major cause of erectile dysfunction.

Endocrinological Androgen deficiency and thyroid disorders can cause erectile dysfunction.

Drug side-effects Men who take antidepressants or antihypertensives often report erectile dysfunction. Of course, men should not stop taking these drugs without discussion with their GP.

TREATMENTS FOR ERECTILE DYSFUNCTION

When a man comes to a surgery with erectile dysfunction he will have an examination, both genital and physical. Diabetes may be tested for as well as testosterone measurement (especially for loss of libido). Men may be referred if the erectile dysfunction cannot be treated by the GP.

There are several treatments available for erectile dysfunction. First, a discussion on smoking, drinking and lifestyle may be of benefit. Diabetes should be under control and psychological factors examined. Sexual counselling may be offered and partner involvement is welcomed. However, there are other methods of treatment for erectile dysfunction.

Vacuum devices

A vacuum pump can be used to draw blood into the penis and the blood flow from the penis limited by a band around its base. Pumps have benefit in that they are non-invasive and work in the majority of men. However, they can cause discomfort and the penis can feel cold. Ejaculation is also often blocked.

Intracavernosal injection therapy

Alprostadil is the most widely used injection therapy. The drug is injected into the penis (the patient can be trained to do this) and an erection occurs around 10 minutes later. However, side-effects include fibrosis and priapism.

Transurethral administration

Alprostadil can be given intraurethrally with a pellet. The patient at home will administer the pellet into the urethra after careful instruction. However, this treatment is not suitable if the partner is trying to conceive or is pregnant.

Oral therapy

Oral therapies for erectile dysfunction have been given much attention in the media over the last few years. It is the treatment of choice for many men. Sildenafil, a phosphodiesterase inhibitor (Viagra®), is the most widely known treatment. It is usually taken around 1 hour before intercourse and it will remain active for 3 or 4 hours. Some men feel that this pressure to have sex quickly after taking sildenafil is problematic and there are other drugs that may be available in the near future that may last for around 24 hours. The important thing to remember is that sildenafil will not work without sexual stimulation and is therefore not suitable for men with a loss of libido. Side-effects include headache, flushing of the face, indigestion and nasal congestion. Patients with heart problems must discuss the possibility of taking sildenafil with their GP.

Another phosphodiesterase inhibitor is tadalafil (Cialis®). This is not yet available in the UK. Similar to sildenafil in function, it will last for longer and can be taken with food and alcohol. Its longer action also means that couples do not have to plan when they have sex.

Erectile dysfunction is a subject that men find very difficult to discuss and are reluctant to seek help for. Most men can be helped to overcome their erectile dysfunction and there is a range of treatment options available. Frank discussion with their GP and other health professionals is important to give the maximum health benefit to the patient.

References

Bratt O 2002 Hereditary prostate cancer: clinical aspects. Journal of Neurology 168(3):906–913

Callman K 1992 On the state of the public health. HMSO, London

Charlton J 1993 Suicide deaths in England and Wales: trends in factors associated with suicide deaths. Population Trends 71:34–43

Dennis LK, Dawson DV 2002 Meta-analysis of measures of sexual activity and prostate cancer. Epidemiology 13(1):72–79

Dinsmore P, Kell W 2002 Impotence: a guide for men of all ages. Royal Society of Medicine Press, London

DoH 1992 Health of the nation. HMSO, London

DoH 2001 Sexual health strategy. Department of Health, London

Fareed A 1994 Equal rights for men. Nursing Times 90:26–29

Forrester DA 1986 Myths of masculinity. Impact upon men's health. Nursing Clinics of North America 21(1):15–23

Gove WR 1979 Sex, marital status and mortality. American Journal of Sociology 79(1):45–67

Ito K, Schrder FH 2003 Informed consent for prostate-specific antigen-based screening – European view. Urology 61(1):20–22

Jacobson B, Smith A, Whitehead M (eds) 1990 The nation's health: a strategy for the 1990s. King's Fund Centre, London

Key T 1995 Risk factors for prostate cancer. Cancer Surgery 23:63–77

Macintyre S, Hunt K, Sweeting H 1996 Gender differences in health: are things really as simple as they seem? Social Science and Medicine 42(4):617–624

Matthews SJ 1988 Men and stress. Nursing 3(26):972–974

Moul JW 2000 Screening for prostate cancer in African Americans. Current Urology Report 1(1):57–64

NHS 2003 www.cancerscreening.nhs.uk/prostate/index.html

Paul JP, Catania J, Pollack L et al 2002 Suicide attempts among gay and bisexual men: lifetime prevalence and antecedents. American Journal of Public Health 92(8):1338–1345

Platzer H 1988 Ageing in men and the crisis of middle age. Nursing 3(26):963–965

Ransohoff DF, McNaughton Collins M, Fowler FJ 2002 Why is prostate cancer screening so common when the evidence is so uncertain? A system without negative feedback. American Journal of Medicine 113(8):663–667

RCN 1996 Men's health review. Royal College of Nursing, London

Richman J, Holland J 1983 Counselling of fathers during a pregnancy. Occupational Health 35(7):300–305

Robertson S 1995 Men's health promotion in the UK: a hidden problem. British Journal of Nursing 4(7):382, 399–401

Stafford EM, Jackson PE, Bank MH 1990 Employment, work involvement and mental health in less qualified young people. Journal of Occupational Psychology 53(4):291–304

Stanford J 1988 Knowledge and attitudes to AIDS. Nursing Times 84(24):47–50

Templeton H 2003 The management of prostate cancer. Nursing Standard 17(21):45–53

United Kingdom National Men's Health Awareness Campaign 1995 Surrey, UK. www.nhsinherts.nhs.uk/hp/healthtopics/menshealth.htm

Weiske WH 2001 Vasectomy. Andrologia 33(3):125–134

Whitehead M 1988 Inequalities in health. The Black Report and the health divide. Penguin, London

Resources

Prostate cancer

The Prostate Cancer Charity
Offers support and information to anyone concerned with prostate cancer.
www.prostate-cancer.org.uk

Prostate Cancer Research Institute
www.prostate-cancer.org

CancerHelp UK
Offers news and information about the prevention, treatment and cure of prostate cancer.
www.cancerhelp.org.uk

Scottish Association of Prostate Cancer Support
Details support groups in Scotland. Information and links to treatments, sites, drugs, books and diet.
www.pcansupportscot.f9.co.uk

Erectile dysfunction

Jayne Wadsworth Clinic
Jefferiss Wing
St Mary's NHS Trust
Praed St
London W2 1NY

Impotence Association
PO Box 10296
London SW17 9WH

British Association for Sexual and Relationship Therapy (BARST)
PO Box 13686
London SW20 9ZH

Chapter 4

Lifestyle advice

Lesley Hand

CHAPTER CONTENTS

INTRODUCTION

The publication of *Health of the nation* in 1992 made it clear that much of the responsibility for the primary prevention of disease lay with general practitioners and their teams. Health was to be actively promoted with the introduction of clinics specifically designed to identify and treat those patients with risk factors for mortality and morbidity. Cervical screening, mammography, antenatal care and immunizations programmes were already well established but the new health promotion clinics had a holistic approach to patient well-being.

It was hoped that there would be a demonstrable health gain from these activities, described as 'A measurable improvement in the status of health and well-being, in an individual or population, which is attributable to an earlier intervention' (DoH 1992).

Primary care was required to screen all patients for risk markers such as obesity, hypertension, smoking, drug and alcohol misuse. Other markers, family history, mental health and stress were also identified. If any of these were outside the normal range they were addressed and help offered. Practice nurses were deemed to be the most suitable people for the job of health advisor and their role has evolved subsequently. The public accepted this extension to the practice nurse's role and over the years have grown used to seeking nurses' advice for help with lifestyle changes.

The evidence for the efficacy of these clinics, in terms of actual weight reduction or smoking cessation, remains doubtful (Kinmonth et al 1998) so it is important that the nurse has some insight into the patient's health beliefs and their commitment to change.

HEALTH PSYCHOLOGY

What people believe about their lifestyle, and how this influences their decision to alter it, seems as much to do with psychosocial factors as biomedical ones. It follows that psychosocial factors should be reviewed to see if there are any specific patient characteristics that predict effective changes in lifestyle. The internal influences to change have been examined in depth from a behavioural scientific perspective (Rosenstock et al 1988) and by the nursing profession (Schain 1994, Schroer & Wilcox 1996). The three models favoured as being conceptually and theoretically representative are the Health Belief Model (HBM) (Rosenstock et al 1988), social cognitive theory (SCT) (Bandura 1982) and the theory of reasoned action (TRA) (Ajzen 1985). The models have already made a significant contribution towards our understanding of ways to predict health-related behaviours.

HEALTH BELIEF MODEL

Rosenstock, who sought to develop ways of predicting health-related behaviours such as smoking, alcohol consumption and attending screening programmes, first defined the HBM in 1966. He based his theory on four cues to action:

- susceptibility
- severity
- benefit
- costs.

The cues to action may focus internally or externally and it is these cues which influence decisions to change. They are referred to as the locus of control (Table 4.1).

Table 4.1 Locus of control

Internal	External
Believe that they are responsible for their own life and health	Believe that their lives/health are influenced by powerful others, chance or luck
Believe that they have the power to make choices which will affect their life	Believe that they are relatively powerless to make changes that affect their life
Can be motivated to make recommended changes to improve health	More likely to be fatalistic about the future and are difficult to motivate

In the case of deciding whether or not to reduce weight, the internal cue might be a fear of developing a condition linked with obesity such as diabetes and the external cue information about the prevention of the condition in the research documentation or lay press. If individuals perceive themselves to be susceptible to the condition (because of a strong family history) and rate its severity as high (serious illness, impaired vision) they would then weigh up the benefits and costs of going on a diet. The benefits (reducing the risk of developing diabetes) would be balanced against the costs (not eating the foods they most enjoy).

The model was criticized initially for being too rigid, relying heavily on a rational process that did not alter with time. There was no room for the influence of economic or social variables, focusing as it did on the individual, nor were emotional factors, such as fear or denial, included. These shortcomings made the model a poor predictor and it was revised in 1988 to include self-efficacy (Bandura 1982).

SOCIAL COGNITIVE THEORY

Self-efficacy is a product of Bandura's social cognitive theory which has as its foundation the concept that all behaviour is determined by personal expectations and incentives. The expectations are categorised as environmental (how events are connected), consequential (what will the outcomes be) and competence (ability to perform the behaviour).

Incentives relate to the value of the outcome, which in the case of weight reduction might be improved health or the approval of others. However, any change in health-related behaviour cannot be carried out unless individuals believe that they will be successful in achieving it (self-efficacy).

THEORY OF REASONED ACTION

Ajzen and Fishbein's TRA (Ajzen 1985) emphasizes the importance that people attach to others' (important others) attitudes to their planned behaviour. If they trust and respect their important others they are more motivated to comply with what is being asked of them by these people. The theory allows for the social context of the patient in that if the behaviour is important to others whose opinion they respect within their environment (the GP, nurse, family or community), then they are more likely to adopt that behaviour which is most acceptable.

These important others may include:

- social influences: family, friends
- relationship with the nurse or general practitioner
- inducements
- social capital.

RISK ASSESSMENT

People may have to make a personal risk assessment when deciding whether to change their behaviour. They may have an idea about whether or not they are susceptible to particular conditions but it will be the task of the nurse to identify risk factors and explain them to patients so they understand the relevance to them. Sir Kenneth Calman (1996) proposed a standardized 'language of risk' as an instrument to aid communication between health professionals and patients. The Calman scale ranks risk as high, moderate or low but these terms have a very subjective interpretation. One person might find a moderate risk of no concern, whereas a more anxious person would find a moderate risk unacceptable. Similarly low risk might be interpreted as of no importance and not worth addressing. The risk might be clarified by written information, but also by visual aids such as graphs and charts. Charts can show the risk associated with a specific condition (e.g. heart disease) compared to something within everyone's experience (e.g. driving a car). The individual's perception of risk has been shown to influence the decision to change behaviour and should be explored.

CULTURAL AND AGE DIFFERENCES

Britain is now a multiethnic population and as such the practice nurse has to recognize and acknowledge the differences in health beliefs. Qualitative research has shown how different cultures influence health beliefs. A study of working-class mothers demonstrated how they considered their poor health to be linked to germs and hereditary factors rather than elements from their own lifestyle such as smoking or poor housing (Pill & Stott 1982).

Another study examining Bangladeshi beliefs showed how attitudes to eating and exercise are strongly influenced by religious and cultural mores which make the standard British advice for a healthy lifestyle unacceptable (Greenhalgh et al 1998). For Bangladeshi women sport and physical exercise have no cultural meaning, the wearing of sports clothing is considered inappropriate and women should generally remain within the home. This ethnic group believed that the British climate and damp housing were to blame for their poor health.

Different generations have different concepts of what is healthy. Young people associate health with fitness and energy, the old with inner strength and the ability to cope. Social classes I and II link good health with enjoying life whilst classes IV and V see it as functional, a means to avoid illness and get through the day (Blaxter 1993). Practice nurses need to understand the various cultures in their community and be able to communicate effectively (Gerrish 2001).

SOCIAL INEQUALITIES AND HEALTH

Differences in living standards may be a bar or incentive to health behaviour changes. These social inequalities in health were first recognized in reports published in the mid-19th century, revealing that the poor suffered more illness than the rich (Nettleton 1995). Little has changed in the 21st century; social classes IV and V are still more likely to be parents of stillbirths or neonatal deaths and death rates have widened between deprived and affluent areas, particularly in northern England. Using data from the Office of Population Censuses and Surveys, White et al (1993) drew up Table 4.2 which shows self-reported health by sex and social class of head of household.

Table 4.2 Self-reported health by sex and social class of head of household

Social class of head of household	Health				
	Very good	Good	Fair	Bad	Very bad
Men					
I and II	585	43	44	10	2
IIIN	139	40	41	16	2
IIIM	456	30	42	23	5
IV and V	274	29	38	25	8
Women					
I and II	598	43	40	15	2
IIIN	256	35	43	17	5
IIIM	442	25	41	26	8
IV and V	382	25	41	26	8

These data show that the lower social classes have an awareness that their health is fair or bad. This perception is borne out by morbidity and mortality statistics; the mortality rates in social class V are approximately twice as high as those in social class I (OPCS 1986). It is difficult to see how the practice nurse can have any impact on these social inequalities other than to be aware of them and seek additional funding via the primary care trust (PCT). Certainly nothing has changed since Tudor Hart's comments three decades ago when he noted 'the availability of good medical care tends to vary inversely with the need of the population served' (Tudor Hart 1971). In other words those people who are most deprived materially and educationally tend to live in areas that are near to the bottom in terms of health service provision.

MOTIVATION

The majority of people who have changed their health behaviour have done so without any professional help and many will comment that they just decided to change, demonstrating belief in their confidence and efficacy. Certainly timing is crucial when discussing lifestyle changes and resistance may arise if patients feel judged or are offered advice when they are not receptive. The concept of motivational interviewing to assess the patient's level of commitment and motivation was first defined by Miller & Rollnick in 1991 (Rollnick et al 2000). Using previous psychological models they sought ways to motivate those with addictive behaviours to change. Whether a patient was really motivated to change could be assessed by the importance he attached to the change (why it is important to change) and his confidence (how will I achieve the change?). The authors deduced that patients showing high importance and high confidence were displaying a willingness to change. Furthermore, anything the patients did to increase either the importance or their confidence in their ability to achieve the change would enhance their chance of success.

CYCLE OF CHANGE

Prochaska & DiClimente introduced the cycle of change in 1982 (Fig. 4.1). It is a useful tool for discovering if the patient is motivated to change and it can be applied to any behaviour.

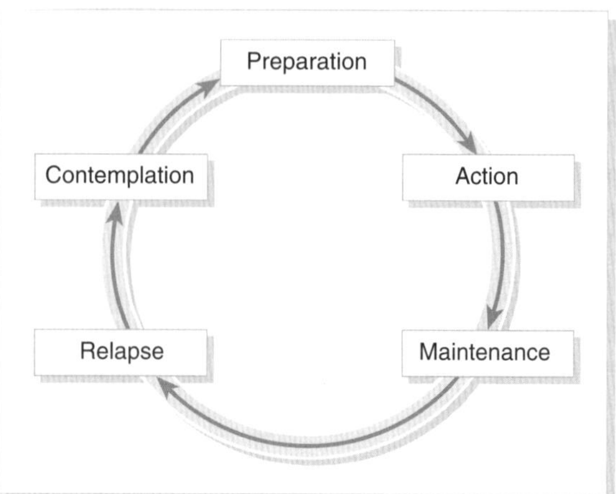

Figure 4.1 The cycle of change.

The cycle revolves round a wheel of change and can have four, five or six stages. The stages include thinking about, planning and acting on the behavioural change. The final stage is usually maintenance and the prevention of relapse. The cycle can be joined at any point depending on the patient's readiness to change, but it is particularly useful in the precontemplation phase. Here the patient may be resisting any thought that the health behaviour might be risky. This may be because of reluctance, rebellion, resignation or rationalization (DiClemente 1991). These are known as the four Rs.

The reluctant precontemplator will have refused to acknowledge the impact of the information offered or chooses to ignore it. The rebellious contemplator is one who denies there is a problem, disputes the facts and is hostile to change. The resigned precontemplator may have tried to change his behaviour in the past with no success, so he accepts that he is a hopeless case and needs the opportunity to push down the barriers that stop him from being hopeful. The rationalizing precontemplator may have made her own risk assessment and concluded that her relative risk is not sufficiently great to merit a behavioural change. Patients in the precontemplation phase are not ready to change, but may be offered the opportunity to come back if they have a change of heart.

SUPPORT

The practice nurse can best help the patient by using skills and knowledge drawn from the above that she is most comfortable with and by offering ongoing support. She can provide information relevant to the patients' wants and work with them to structure and direct the planned change.

Even a brief intervention in a busy clinic can be effective. Strategies to assess readiness to change might include scaling. This is when patients are asked to give a score of 1–10 to show how important they feel the proposed change is and their confidence in their ability to perform it. For example, if someone scores 9 for recognizing the importance of losing weight but only 2 for having the confidence to accomplish weight loss, she is probably in the precontemplation phase and not ready to move forward.

RESOURCES

Before embarking on any type of lifestyle advice the practice nurse needs to identify and evaluate the resources available. The local health education department should be able to help with leaflets, videos, posters or audiocassettes. There may be self-help groups within the area such as Weight Watchers or Alcoholics Anonymous. Most practice computers have a patient information programme, which can provide additional information. Whatever information is chosen all the members of the practice team and ideally the primary care team (PCT) should be aware of their use. This way the information can be standardized and a degree of consistency maintained.

DIET

Food is one of life's necessities and so much is at stake that it is hardly surprising that the media and advertising industry continue to publish a plethora of advice on diets, good/bad foods, slimming products and food scares. The agenda changes daily: eggs, high-fat cheese, beef, nuts, honey and paté have all been vilified at some point whereas olive oil, oily fish, fresh fruit and vegetables remain stalwarts of a safe diet. The practice nurse is often asked about conflicting messages and has to try to put the whole diet question in perspective.

GENERAL RULES

The Food Standards Agency (2001) published eight guidelines for a healthy diet which are good bases for dietary advice.

- Enjoy your food.
- Eat a variety of different foods.
- Eat the right amount to be a healthy weight.
- Eat plenty of foods rich in starch and fibre.
- Eat plenty of fruit and vegetables.
- Don't eat too many foods that contain fat.
- Don't have sugary foods and drinks too often.
- If you drink alcohol, drink sensibly.

These guidelines, whilst not being too prescriptive, point out the fact that the key to a successful diet lies in the balance between types of food.

As mentioned earlier, one of the formats used for providing lifestyle advice is a chart. The coloured pie chart showing optimal proportions of different foods published by the Food Standards Agency has been shown to be particularly effective and well accepted.

WEIGHT CONTROL

The 1999 *Health survey for England* (DoH 1999) showed that 19% of men and 21% of women were clinically obese compared with 6% men and 8% women in 1980. A further 44% of men and 33% of women were overweight. Clearly if current trends continue 1 in 4 adults will be obese in 2010. This trend is not confined to adults, as there is also an increase in obese children. Being overweight matters; it places patients at greater risk of certain conditions, which include:

- coronary artery disease
- cerebral vascular events
- diabetes
- hypertension
- gallstones
- osteoarthritis of weight-bearing joints
- respiratory problems
- back pain.

It is also associated with psychosocial problems arising from poor self-esteem, such as depression, phobic behaviour and eating disorders. By way of encouragement, it should be noted that a 5–10% reduction in weight would have significant benefits. The benefits of a 10 kg weight loss include the following.

Fall of:

- 20 mmHg systolic and 10 mmHg diastolic BP
- 50% in fasting blood glucose
- 10% total cholesterol

- 15% LDL
- 30% triglycerides.

Rise of:

- 8% HDL.

What is overweight?

The body mass index (BMI) or Quetlet index is the best known and most reliable measurement of a patient's weight status. It is calculated using the formula:

$$\frac{\text{Weight (kilos)}}{\text{Height (metres}^2\text{)}}$$

Most practice computer programs will calculate the BMI given the height and weight and there are coloured ready reckoner charts available. The chart has five bands indicating the level of risk.

	Less than 19	Underweight
Grade 0	19–24.9	Acceptable
Grade I	25–29.9	Overweight
Grade II	30–39.9	Obese
Grade III	Over 40	Gross obesity

Trying to help a patient to lose weight can be one of the most rewarding or frustrating tasks the practice nurse has to face. There are a very few patients whose weight problem is caused by morbidity such as hypothyroidism, genetic or endocrine dysfunction. Usually it is an imbalance between the energy intake (too much) and the energy output (too little).

MANAGEMENT

The initial assessment will allow the practice nurse to investigate motivation and plan the proposed change. It is useful to negotiate some form of contract so both patient and nurse understand the commitment each is going to give to the project. A realistic target weight and timescale should be set at the beginning of a weight reduction programme and the frequency of follow-up visits stated. Successful weight loss is usually achieved in the first 3–6 months of dieting so the contract should not exceed that time. It should be explicit that follow-up will only continue if there is demonstrable weight loss. Ideally the appointments should be at the same time of day, the scales regularly calibrated and any written information standardized.

Questions about lifestyle and work patterns will help to gauge the timing of meals so that the advice can be relevant to the individual. It is also helpful to ascertain who does the cooking in the household, who is charge of the budget and shopping and whether there are any conflicting dietary needs. Many patients will have other household members to consider and will need to enlist the support of family members to help in gradually changing eating patterns.

Strategies for coping with differing situations can be discussed. The most common problems like missing breakfast, not planning meals ahead and skipping meals only result in grazing on inappropriate quick fix foods such as crisps or chocolate. Getting into the habit of carrying an apple and a bottle of water may prevent eating something high in sugar and fat to stave off a food craving.

When shopping for food patients can be advised to always shop after, not before a meal, to shop with a list with the meals planned for the week and not to buy crisps, biscuits or snacks so they are not in the house. Where possible, patients should avoid tempting situations which trigger food cravings, watching food programmes on the television, smelling cooking or comfort eating. Any of these which are a potential threat to break from the diet should be discussed.

Simple tips to suggest to patients

- Eat small regular meals. Avoid eating between meals, seconds and leftovers.
- Keep fat intake to a minimum. Use low-fat spreads sparingly, measure out oil, grill instead of fry and trim excess fat from meat.
- Eat five portions of fruit and vegetables a day. These need not be raw but can be fresh or frozen.
- Eat oily fish twice a week. Choose white meat (chicken) rather than red meat (steak).
- Avoid all high-calorie, high-fat foods such as cakes, biscuits, chips, pies, pasties.
- Drink plenty of water, avoid sugary drinks and have no more than half a pint of skimmed milk a day.
- Starchy foods such as bread, pasta, rice and cereals should form the main part of the meal.
- Exercise for at least 20 minutes four times a week.
- Keep alcohol intake to a minimum.
- Eat the same meals as the family but in smaller portions and on a smaller plate.

DRUG THERAPIES

There will always be some patients who have yo-yoed on diets for most of their adult life and each time they have lost weight it has been regained with a few extra pounds. This group may include those who have used crash diets or drugs in the past and need special encouragement if they are to succeed.

The GP may be reluctant to prescribe anorectic drugs, as they are addictive and cause numerous side-effects. Diuretics used to treat water retention can precipitate gout or diabetes and giving thyroxine to patients with normal thyroid function is potentially dangerous. Orlistat, a pancreatic lipase inhibitor which reduces fat absorption, is used for patients with a BMI >30 who have demonstrated a weight loss of 2.5 kg in the previous 4 weeks with diet alone. It can be used for up to 2 years and does seem to help weight reduction. Other drug therapies are supported by limited evidence of effectiveness and the long-term outcomes are unclear (Arterburn & Hitchcock 2001).

RELAPSE

Many people who have successfully lost weight put it back on when they have achieved their target. This is usually because of a reversal back to the old ways of eating. The practice nurse needs to continue to offer support and advice if the weight reduction is to be permanent. Once the weight has been lost the daily calorie consumption will be up to 300 less than before the diet started, so it is important to emphasize the need to continue the habits of exercise and healthy eating for a lifetime.

DIET IN DISEASE

Hyperlipidaemia

The Western diet, which is high in fat, plays a significant role in the development of heart disease. Generally everyone should eat less fat but for patients with raised blood lipids it is essential. Whereas some fat in the diet is necessary, patients need to be aware of the different types of fat.

- The *unsaturated* fats can help to lower blood cholesterol. These are present in olive and rapeseed oil (monounsaturates) and in nuts, vegetable oil and oily fish (polyunsaturates).
- The *saturated* fats can raise blood cholesterol. These are present in cooking fats and spreads, fatty meats, full-fat dairy products, chips, cakes, biscuits and confectionery.

A popular and easy to follow low-fat diet is described in the Mediterranean diet which endorses the weekly consumption of three 4 oz portions of oily fish and the use of olive oil for cooking. The Mediterranean diet advises the following.

Eat more fish The Diet and Reinfarction Trial (DART) (Burr et al 1989) showed that increasing the portions of oily fish (mackerel, herring, kipper, sardine, salmon and trout) to two or three per week brought about a 29% reduction in all-cause mortality over a 2-year period.

Eat more fruit and vegetables There is a consensus which suggests that eating more fruit and vegetables is correlated with lower rates of fatal and non-fatal coronary events. This may be causal in that those who do eat more fruit and vegetables may have higher levels of nutritional knowledge and come from a higher social class. Nevertheless, the recommendations from the Food Standards Agency (2001) suggest five portions of fruit and vegetables per day. The beneficial effects of consumption at this rate are said to be as high as 34% reduction in coronary death for a difference of 60 g/day vegetable intake.

Eat a more Mediterranean diet The traditional Mediterranean diet, which leans towards more bread, more green and root vegetables, less red meat and more poultry and replacement of butter and cream with monounsaturated fats, tends to protect against coronary disease with a reduction in mortality.

Hypertension

There is good evidence that a diet high in salt can cause raised blood pressure (Elliot et al 1996). This is partly as a result of sodium retaining more body fluid.

Fresh food contains very little salt but processed foods such as tinned or packet soups, cereals, crisps, nuts and ready meals all have added salt. Foods high in salt include bacon, hard cheese, sausages and corned beef. Salt can be added sparingly in cooking but should not be added at the table. Salt substitutes can be used but it is generally better to omit added salt altogether.

Arthritis

The symptoms of both osteo- and rheumatoid arthritis seem to be helped by a diet biased towards vegetarian foods with oily fish, eggs and low-fat cheese as protein sources. Red meat can aggravate inflammation and lactic acid products are best avoided.

Irritable bowel syndrome (IBS)

There are many causes of IBS, including food intolerance. It is therefore always worth trying a food exclusion diet to identify any triggers. Alcohol, spicy foods and coffee should be avoided as they stimulate bowel contractions. A diet high in fibre is recommended with plenty of fluids (1–1.5 l per day).

ALTERNATIVE THERAPIES

The use of alternative and complementary therapies is increasing and has been recognized by the recent report from the House of Lords Select Committee. Some of the therapies are available within the NHS but others are only available to those who can afford them. The cost of a consultation is upwards of £30 an hour so patients may well ask the practice nurse about the efficacy of complementary treatments and whether it would be appropriate to use them.

It is difficult for the practice nurse to advise on some of these therapies as very little research has been done in this area. Indeed, HRH Prince Charles, a proponent of alternative medicine, noted that the Medical Research Council spent no money in 1998–9 researching complementary medicines (Lantin 2001). However, other research has shown that patients appreciate the holistic approach that practitioners of complementary therapy adopt and subsequently feel more in control of their illness (Rees 2001).

Apart from lack of scientific evidence for their use, many of the therapies are not regulated which is a concern for practice nurses offering advice.

The Select Committee divided the therapies into three groups.

1. Acupuncture, chiropractic, herbal medicine, homeopathy and osteopathy. These do have a research base and are available in the NHS.
2. Aromatherapy, hypnotherapy. These are sometimes available in the NHS as an adjunct to conventional medicine.
3. Crystal therapy, dowsing. These are examples of therapies that are part of certain cultures and have been used for a long time. There is no scientific evidence for their efficacy.

Table 4.3 Examples of conditions and herbal remedies commonly used

Condition	Herbal treatment
To boost the immune system and promote healing	Vitamin A
Iron deficiency anaemia	Iron 24 mg daily with vitamin C
Arthritis	Glucosamine
Atherosclerosis	Fish oil 1–3 g daily
Candida	High-potency garlic tablets
Chilblains, restless legs, tinnitus	Ginkgo biloba 120 mg daily
Colds	*Echinacea purpurea* 200–400 mg for 3 weeks
Cystitis	Concentrated cranberry extract
Depression	St John's wort 1000 μg daily
Endometriosis, premenstrual syndrome	Evening primrose oil 1–2 g daily
Irritable bowel syndrome	Artichoke 320 mg daily
Prevention of Alzheimer's disease	Folic acid (Gottlieb 2002)

Access to complementary therapies is improving and more than 40% of general medical practices offer some of these services.

HERBAL REMEDIES

The use of herbal remedies has increased dramatically over the last decade but as with other complementary medicine advice, it has to be tempered with caution as there can be side-effects. Scientific evidence for herbal, mineral and vitamin supplements has been demonstrated with some substances such as St John's wort (hypericum). In a metaanalysis of randomized controlled trials (RCT) hypericum extracts were found to be as effective as standard antidepressants in the treatment of mild to moderate depression and better tolerated (Linde et al 1996). The levels of selenium in the diet have been falling in Europe over the last 26 years which may have made individuals more susceptible to malignant and other disease (Diplock 1994, Rayman 1997). Hence the increased use of selenium supplements.

ALCOHOL

Alcohol has been an integral part of human life for as long as mankind has been in existence. Currently there is an increase in alcohol consumption, teenagers and young women being particularly affected. A recent report indicated that the cost to the NHS of treating alcohol-related accidents and disease is rising at a rate that marginalizes resources available for other health needs. Excessive drinking can precipitate:

- liver damage
- oesophageal varices
- anaemia
- duodenal ulcer
- gastritis and oesophagitis
- pancreatitis
- vomiting and diarrhoea
- malnutrition
- amnesia
- tremors
- raised blood lipids
- carcinoma of the mouth and oesophagus
- insomnia
- psychological changes, i.e. mood swings
- peripheral neuritis
- male impotence
- miscarriage.

Prolonged heavy drinking can lead to social problems as it impacts on family and career. Days off work through hangovers can result in job loss and the subsequent reductions of income to financial ruin. The family may suffer through physical abuse, the breakdown of relationships and isolation from friends.

On the positive side there are some beneficial effects of alcohol. A small amount of alcohol (one glass of red wine per day) has beneficial reductive effects on HDL blood cholesterol, leading to fewer deaths from coronary artery disease (McElduff & Dobson 1997). Medicinal uses include sherry as a useful appetite stimulant in those with nutritional needs, beer as an effective laxative and whisky as a hypnotic.

The practice nurse may be the first person to enquire about alcohol consumption during a routine screening appointment and should be able to advise on sensible limits. These are 21 units per week for men and 14 units per week for women. There should be alcohol-free days within the week and binge drinking should be avoided.

The number of units per standard measure of alcohol is shown in Table 4.4. It should be remembered that these figures are based on ordinary strength table wine (11%) and the alcohol content of beers, lagers and ciders varies widely from <0.5% low alcohol to >5.6% extra strength.

Table 4.4 Units of alcohol

	Units
Beer or lager	
1 pint	2
1 can	1½
Export beer	
1 pint	2½
1 can	2
Strong ale or lager	
1 pint	4
1 can	3
Extra strong beer or lager	
1 pint	5
1 can	4
Cider	
1 pint	2
Strong cider	
1 pint	4
Spirits	
Standard measure	1
75 cl bottle	30
Wine	
Standard glass 125 ml	1
75 cl bottle	7
Sherry	
1 glass	1
75 cl bottle	15

Alcohol is metabolized in the liver having been absorbed from the stomach and small intestine. The rate of absorption varies according to certain conditions. It is absorbed more quickly on an empty stomach in the absence of food, particularly carbohydrates. Women drinking the same amount as men will achieve a higher level of blood alcohol as they have less blood volume and more subcutaneous fat.

Apart from self-reporting of alcohol use, two blood tests can be indicative of the alcohol consumption level. The mean corpuscular volume (MCV) and the gamma glutamyl transpeptidase (GGT) will both be raised in moderate to heavy drinkers.

Once the problem has been identified the patient may need help to address it. Local organizations such as Alcoholics Anonymous may be approached or the patient encouraged to take responsibility for change themselves.

Simple strategies relevant to other addictive behaviours can be used.

- Assessing readiness to change.
- Assessing confidence in ability to change.
- Keeping a diary of alcohol consumption and drinking patterns.
- Suggesting alternatives to drinking only alcohol, such as interspersing soft drinks with alcohol.
- Avoiding situations where drinking is the norm.

DRUG THERAPIES AND REHABILITATION

Alcohol abuse can be treated with disulfiram, an aldehyde dehydrogenase inhibitor, to control alcohol cravings. It will produce symptoms of severe nausea and flushing if taken with alcohol. Beta-blockers and benzodiazepines may be used for withdrawal symptoms, such as tremor and tachycardia. There are a limited number of rehabilitation beds within the NHS for alcohol detoxification and generally it is the private sector that provides this care.

DRUG DEPENDENCY

The management of opiate dependence requires specialist knowledge and should be undertaken by practitioners who have appropriate training. Health professionals can refer patients to drug dependency units in most areas and put patients in touch with local self-help groups.

SMOKING

Of all the health-related behaviours listed in this chapter, smoking is the most harmful. 'It is the greatest single cause of preventable illness and premature death in the UK' (Secretary of State for Health 1998).

- One in two smokers will die of smoking-related diseases.
- Smoking is implicated in 50% of coronary heart disease (CHD).
- Smokers under 65 are twice as likely to die from CHD as non-smokers.
- Women are especially vulnerable (2–8 times the risk).

In addition to the risk of CHD, smokers are more likely to suffer respiratory disease such as bronchitis and emphysema. Chronic obstructive airways disease is almost entirely related to smoking. The risk of developing cancers, particularly of the lung but also the mouth, throat, bladder, kidneys and cervix, is increased and smoking contributes to the development of gastric and duodenal ulcers. Research has shown how smoking can be injurious to the fetus (ASH 2000) and to those exposed to passive smoking (ASH 2000).

Other consequences of smoking include:

- worsening of existing disease such as asthma, diabetes
- Crohn's disease
- male impotence, sperm abnormalities, early menopause
- facial wrinkles, grey hair, husky voice.

The cost to the NHS of caring for those suffering smoking-related diseases is £1.7 billion per year (Secretary of State for Health 1998) and the present government has allocated £100 million over the next 3 years to reduce the number of smokers, specifically among the under-16s, disadvantaged adults and pregnant women. These groups reflect the government's concern with the 24% of women who smoke during pregnancy causing increased risk of miscarriage, reduced birth weight and perinatal death. The most recent statistics on teenagers show that about 450 children start smoking every day in Great Britain and almost a quarter of 15 year olds are regular smokers (DoH 1998, RCP 1992).

As part of the CHD National Service Framework (DoH 2000), Standard Two states that the NHS and partner agencies should contribute to a reduction in the prevalence of smoking in the local population. Government strategies include the training of smoking advisors and the availability of nicotine replacement therapy on prescription. General practices are encouraged to have a Level Two facilitator trained. The scheme has been successful; 12 700 people have used the service and 48% achieved short-term abstinence (more than 4 weeks) (Raw et al 2001).

There are three levels of intervention.

- *Level 1, brief intervention*. This can be done by any healthcare professional once it has been established that the patient is a smoker. A simple enquiry into how the patient feels about his or her smoking will probably clarify where he or she is in the cycle of change (see p.66). If the patient answers that he or she is thinking about changing behaviour, they can be referred to a Level Two or Three advisor.

• *Level 2.* Advisors facilitate smoking cessation on a one-to-one basis. The advisor will assess readiness to act and facilitate the client in stopping smoking.

• *Level 3.* Advisors working in primary and secondary care facilitate group meetings for those with higher levels of dependency. These advisors facilitate groups of 8–15 smokers and follow the same guidelines as Level Two advisors.

The targets set by the White Paper are:

- to reduce smoking amongst children from 13% to 9% by 2010
- to reduce adult smoking from 28% to 24% by 2010
- to reduce the number of pregnant women smoking from 23% to 15% by 2010.

WHY PEOPLE SMOKE

- Behavioural reasons – habit
- Psychological reasons – confidence
- Physical reasons – weight control
- Because they are addicted to nicotine

WHAT IS NICOTINE?

Nicotine is a highly addictive substance that stimulates the central nervous system. It releases adrenaline to raise the pulse and blood pressure. Nicotine also narrows the arteries, which is made worse by the development of atheroma.

What else is in a cigarette?

Tar, a brown treacly substance which is deposited in the lungs, is present in cigarettes. Tar is a general name for the mixture of over 4000 chemicals that include formaldehyde, cyanide, arsenic, benzene and toluene. All these are known carcinogens.

What effect does it have?

The exact effect of nicotine is unknown but for most smokers it has a calming effect and is used at times of stress as a coping mechanism or when socializing to boost confidence. When smokers inhale deeply, nicotine reaches the brain in 7 seconds and peak plasma levels are reached after 5 minutes, producing a feeling of relaxation. Smokers who inhale less deeply and who consequently have lower levels of plasma concentration seem to be more alert and able to concentrate better. Smoking raises the blood levels of carbon monoxide, which binds to haemoglobin more readily than oxygen, thereby reducing the amount of oxygen in the blood.

Nicotine is sometimes used as an appetite suppressant. The stomach empties more slowly in the presence of nicotine so when smokers stop the rate is returned to normal and they get hungry more quickly. Many smokers will link caffeine and alcohol with nicotine and it seems that smoking enhances the effect of both.

HOW TO HELP PATIENTS STOP SMOKING

The four As are a good starting point to assess the smoker's readiness to change and are integral to the Level One brief intervention.

- Ask about smoking
- Advise them to stop
- Assist them to stop
- Arrange follow-up

Willpower is important for smoking cessation but not always enough on its own (Hughes et al 1992). The Level Two advisor will need an initial 20-minute appointment with the patient to discuss smoking patterns, previous attempts to quit, treatments available, any barriers to quitting and the support he will receive in his usual surroundings. If the patient is ready to stop he will need to set a quit date and have a follow-up appointment arranged. The benefits of stopping smoking should be emphasized as the health risks decline immediately the smoker quits.

Physical benefits of stopping smoking

• 20 minutes Blood pressure and pulse rate return to normal. Circulation improves in hands and feet.

• 8 hours Oxygen levels in the blood return to normal; chance of heart attack starts to fall.

• 24 hours Carbon monoxide is eliminated from the body. Lungs start to clear out the debris.

• 48 hours Sense of taste and smell are improved. The stale smell of smoke on the breath and clothes starts to disappear.

• 3 months Lung function improves, breathing is easier. Tooth staining begins to disappear.

• 5 years The risk of developing mouth, throat or oesophageal cancer is reduced by 50%.

• 10 years The risk of CHD falls to the same level as a non-smoker. The risk of lung cancer falls to about half that of a smoker.

Financial benefits

Smoking 20 manufactured cigarettes a day will cost £30 a week or £1565 a year.

THERAPIES

Nicotine replacement therapy (NRT)

NRT works by reducing the severity of symptoms and the urge to smoke. It delays weight gain and provides a prop to help the smoker cope without cigarettes. It is available in six forms: patches, chewing gum, nasal spray, lozenges, sublingual tablets and inhalator. The patches are the treatment of choice because they are easy to use and there is no technique to learn. NRT is not suitable for everyone, particularly children under 18, pregnant or breast-feeding mothers (only sublingual tablets should be used). Patients on adjunct therapies, theophyllines, beta-blockers, benzodiazepines, lithium carbonates, warfarin, tricyclic antidepressants, antipsychotics and insulin, should be monitored to ensure the serum level of these drugs has not been altered by smoking cessation.

Most NRTs come in different strengths to allow for a gradual decrease over a 10–12 week period. The initial dose is calculated by the level of dependence so that the heavy smoker (>20/day) will start on the highest dose and the moderate smoker (<20/day) on the next step dose.

Current preparations available on prescription include the following:

Patches

- Niquitin CQ 24 hours containing 21 mg, 14 mg, 7 mg
- Nicotinell 24 hours containing 21 mg, 14 mg, 7 mg
- Nicorette patch 16 hours 15 mg, 10 mg, 5 mg

Gum

- Nicorette gum 2 mg, 4 mg. Use 10–15 pieces maximum per day
- Nicotinell gum 2 mg, 4 mg. Use 8–12 pieces per day. Maximum usage of 15 pieces per day for both strengths

Inhalator

- Nicorette inhalator 10 mg per cartridge. Use 6–12 cartridges maximum per day

Lozenge

- Niquitin lozenge 2 mg, 4 mg. Use one every 1–2 hours to a maximum of 15 per day, increasing interval between lozenges to 4–8 hours over a 3-month period

Bupropion

Bupropion was developed as an antidepressant when it was noted that it seemed to suppress the urge to smoke. Bupropion increases the levels of dopamine and noradrenaline transmitters in the area of the brain associated with withdrawal symptoms and the development of dependence. It seems to block pathways that lead to addictive behaviour. The therapy is given for no more than a 2-month period and needs good motivation on the patient's part. It is not suitable during pregnancy, for patients with a history of seizures or psychiatric illness or cirrhosis. Additionally those taking any of the following may have a reduced seizure threshold: antihistamines, theophyllines, antipsychotics, antidepressants, MAOIs, corticosteroids, quinolones.

Common side-effects of bupropion include dry mouth, insomnia and headache. Less common are seizures, confusion, raised blood pressure and allergic reaction.

The patient should be advised about nicotine withdrawal and how long it is likely to last. The symptoms of light-headedness and sleep disturbance last less than a week but irritability, aggressiveness, restlessness and depression can last for up to 4 weeks. Increased appetite lasts more than 10 weeks and the average weight gain (2 kg) is acquired in the first 3 months. Patients still having cravings after 2 weeks of not smoking are more likely to have a relapse but it is worth remembering that many smokers will have more than one attempt to give up smoking before they finally quit.

EXERCISE

Regular exercise increases cardiovascular and musculoskeletal fitness. It also promotes psychological well-being, reduces stress and helps with weight control. The evidence for health gains associated with exercise has been demonstrated by Paffenberger et al (1986) who found that exercise reduced the chance of developing CHD by 40%. The Multiple Risk Factor Intervention Trial (Leon et al 1987) showed the positive effects of regular exercise even extended to those at high risk of developing CHD. However, despite the strong evidence to show the benefits of exercise, levels of physical activity in the population are low, with only 24% of men and 32% of women maintaining their optimal level of exercise (Sports Council 1992). The habits of regular exercise integral in childhood and adolescence need to be carried into adult life as the positive exercise effect only relates to current exercise (Brill 1989).

Effects of exercise include:

- decrease in heart rate and blood pressure
- increase in maximal oxygen uptake
- increase in musculoskeletal efficiency
- increase in bone density and prevention of osteoporosis
- increased level of HDL cholesterol
- decreased level of triglycerides
- stress reduction through lower levels of adrenaline being released
- maintenance of ideal weight.

WHAT IS EXERCISE?

Every human movement, from breathing to running marathons, requires energy. The body's source of energy comes from adenosine triphosphate (ATP). During exercise the stores of ATP in the muscles are depleted and can only be replaced by the process of resynthesis. Aerobic exercise (in the presence of oxygen) is the most effective way of producing ATP whereas anaerobic exercise (without oxygen) can only produce ATP in short bursts.

Aerobic exercise

Regular aerobic exercise, sometimes referred to as isotonic exercise, will increase performance and stamina by increasing the amount of oxygen the cardiorespiratory system can direct to the muscles. This oxygen is calculated as the maximum oxygen uptake (VO_{2max}). A sedentary adult will have an average VO_{2max} of 35 ml per kilogram of bodyweight per minute. In an athlete it may be 60 ml/kg/min. Accurate measurement of a person's VO_{2max} can only be done using sophisticated respiratory equipment but a value can be gauged from the length of time a subject manages on a graded exercise test. The other calculation of aerobic capacity, which originated in the USA but is also used in the UK, is the metabolic equivalent (MET). The MET score can be calculated by dividing the known VO_{2max} by 3.5. Thus the sedentary adult with a VO_{2max} of 35 ml/kg/min will have a MET score of 10.

Anaerobic exercise

Anaerobic or isometric exercise is when the muscles are contracting without any joint involvement. This could be weight lifting or digging. While this form of exercise is useful for developing strength in particular muscle groups, it is not so protective against cardiovascular disease as aerobic exercise.

PLANNING AN EXERCISE PROGRAMME

The planning of a graded exercise programme for individual patients is usually done by a rehabilitation nurse or fitness instructor. However, there are general guidelines that can be applied to most patients. First, the level of exercise needs to be classified. This may be light, which means it is within the patient's present ability. Moderate exercise will raise the pace of the present activity to increase the heart and respiratory rate. Vigorous exercise will provide a challenge to the cardiorespiratory system, resulting in tachycardia, shortness of breath and sweating. The heart rate should return to normal within 90 seconds. The aim is to enable patients to undertake moderate levels of activity on a regular 3–4 times a week basis.

In order to minimize the risk of musculoskeletal injury it is important to emphasize the need for a 15-minute warm-up, involving stretching exercises and limbering up the main joints. Similarly, at the end of the exercise the activity should be gradually reduced and not stopped abruptly to prevent postural hypotension and to allow the muscles to replenish their ATP.

Box 4.1 Types of exercise

Light	*Moderate*	*Vigorous*
Canoeing	Cycling	Climbing hills
Ballroom dancing	Sailing	Dancing, aerobic or square
Golf with a cart	Golf without a cart	Squash
Walking 2 mph	Walking 3–4 mph	Jogging 10 mph

Many forms of exercise involve some initial cost and patients may not be able to afford the membership costs of health clubs and sporting facilities. Local authorities usually have a concessionary fee for pensioners and the disabled, which is sometimes extended to the unemployed or those on a low income. The idea of a prescription for health has been mooted but not pursued.

Walking

The natural and free form of exercise is walking. It can be done at any time and does not require expensive equipment or other players. The Allied Dunbar Fitness Survey (Sports Council 1992) showed that because of the low levels of exercise in the population, a modest half-hour walk every day was enough to produce demonstrable changes in fitness. A graduated walking programme can be easily designed to increase the speed and duration of the daily walk from a quarter of a mile twice a day at a moderate pace to 4 miles three or four times a week walking briskly.

Jogging

Jogging is really only suitable for the younger age group (under 50) who are used to physical activity. Joggers must wear the proper shoes and remember that because jogging on hard surfaces is a high-impact activity it can lead to musculoskeletal injuries. Running on even ground or running tracks is a better alternative but in all cases the patient should spend time warming up and cooling down.

Dancing

Dancing is a very sociable form of exercise and increasing in popularity. The level of exercise will vary with the style of dance and the pace of the music: line or disco dancing can be vigorous whereas waltzing counts only as light exercise.

Swimming

Swimming is an excellent means of attaining fitness for those who are unable to perform weight-bearing exercises. The buoyancy of water helps those with joint or back problems, particularly if obese, to use the upper and lower body aerobically.

Cycling

Cycling is another non-weight bearing exercise that can be used to improve leg muscles. It has limited use in improving upper body strength but will help cardiorespiratory fitness if incorporated into a graduated exercise plan.

Rowing

Rowing machines are expensive but adaptable exercise vehicles. Both the upper and lower body can be used or just one set of muscles; this makes them very useful for patients with amputations or other disabilities. The exercise can be graded by increasing the resistance of each stroke.

As with all changes in lifestyle it is important to be realistic when setting targets for exercise. People having a previously sedentary life will not suddenly see dramatic changes in body shape, but will benefit in the long term from improved health gains. The safety issue also needs to be addressed; any new exercise should be appropriate for the age and build of the individual and the proper clothing and shoes obtained.

TRAINING

The requirements of the Post Registration Education and Practice Project (PREPP), personal and practice development plans mean that all registered nurses are encouraged to pursue lifelong learning. The style and content of training have changed markedly from the didactic approach used in the nursing schools of the 1970s to the adult learning methods used by today's universities. No single body has ownership over nurse education and increasingly, courses are multidisciplinary. The responsibility for providing education for practice nurses has shifted from the health authorities to PCTs. This new initiative provides the opportunity for practices within a PCT to consider the health priorities of their community and then assess the training that they need to meet them. The PCTs are setting up their own courses using in-house and outside expertise. In the context of this chapter the following agencies may be useful for further training.

- NHS helpline for information and support
- BSc/MSc modules on health education
- National seminars/conferences as advertised in the nursing press
- Day release courses run by local universities
- Community dietitians
- PCT members
- Other practice team members

CONCLUSION

Lifestyle advice has become an integral part of the practice nurse's work; patients recognize this and consult them about personal health behaviours that concern them. As has been demonstrated in several research projects, the outcomes of health interventions are not always efficient in terms of time and resources (ICRF 1995, 1996). The most effective way to alter lifestyle or change health behaviour seems to hinge on getting the balance between education and health beliefs right. Education on its own has been shown to be ineffective (Ruddock & Hunt 1997). To be successful there needs to be a rapport between the practice nurse and her patient which allows for the exploration of the patient's health beliefs and his readiness to change.

References

Ajzen J 1985 From intentions to action: a theory of planned behaviour. In: Kuhl J, Beckman J (eds) Action control from cognition to behaviour. Springer Verlag, Berlin

Arterburn D, Hitchcock NP 2001 Obesity. Issue 5, Clinical Evidence Series. BMJ Books, London

ASH 2000 Basic facts no 2. Smoking and disease. Action on Smoking and Health, London

Bandura A 1982 Self-efficacy mechanism in human agency. American Psychologist 84:122–147

Blaxter M 1993 The cause of disease: women talking. Social Science and Medicine 17:59–69

Brill PA 1989 The impact of previous athleticism, exercise habits, physical activity and coronary heart disease risk factors in middle aged men. Research Quarterly for Exercise and Sport 60:209–215

Burr ML, Fehily AM, Gilbert JF et al 1989 Effects of changes in fat, fish and fibre intakes on death and myocardial reinfarction: Diet and Reinfarction Trial (DART). Lancet ii:757–761

Calman KC 1996 Cancer: science and society and the communication of risk. British Medical Journal 313:793–802

Department of Health 1992 Health of the nation: a strategy for health in England. HMSO, London

DiClemente C 1991 Precontemplation: resistance and the 4Rs. In: Motivational interviewing. Guilford Press, New York

Diplock AT 1994 Antioxidants and disease prevention. Molecular Aspects of Medicine 15:295–376

DoH 1998 Statistics on smoking: England 1976–1996. Bulletin 1998/25. Department of Health, London

DoH 1999 Health survey for England 1999. Department of Health, London

DoH 2000 National Service Framework: coronary heart disease. Department of Health, London

Elliot P, Stamler J, Nichols R et al 1996 Intersalt revisited: a further analysis of 24 hour sodium excretion and blood pressure within and across populations. British Medical Journal 312:1249–1253

Food Standards Agency 2001 The balance of good health. FSA, London

Gerrish K 2001 Meeting healthcare needs of ethnic minorities. Nursing in Practice 3:107–108

Gottlieb S 2002 Higher folic acid levels could reduce risk of Alzheimer's disease. British Medical Journal 324:441

Greenhalgh T, Helman C, Chowdhury A 1998 Health beliefs and folk models of diabetes in British Bangladeshis: a qualitative study. British Medical Journal 316:978–983

Hughes JR, Gulliver SB, Fenwick JW et al 1992 Smoking cessation among self-quitters. Health Psychology 11:331–334

ICRF OXCHECK Study Group 1995 Effectiveness of health checks conducted by nurses in primary care: final results of the OXCHECK Study. British Medical Journal 310:1099–1104

ICRF OXCHECK Study Group 1996 Costs and cost effectiveness of health checks conducted by nurses in primary care: the OXCHECK Study. British Medical Journal 312:1265–1268

Kinmonth A, Woodcock A, Griffin S et al 1998 Randomised controlled trial of patient centred care of diabetes in general practice: impact on current wellbeing and future disease risk. British Medical Journal 317:1202–1208

Lantin B 2001 Health and wellbeing. Daily Telegraph 23/11

Leon A, Connett J, Jacobs D et al 1987 Leisure time physical activity levels and risk of coronary heart disease and death. The multiple risk factor intervention trial. Journal of the American Medical Association 258:2388–2395

Linde K, Ramirez G, Mulrow C et al 1996 St John's wort for depression – an overview and metaanalysis of randomised clinical trials. British Medical Journal 313:253–258

McElduff P, Dobson A 1997 How much alcohol and how often? Population based case-control study of alcohol consumption and risk of a major coronary event. British Medical Journal 314:1159

Nettleton S 1995 The sociology of health and illness. Polity Press, Oxford

OPCS 1986 Occupational mortality: decennial supplement 1979–80, 1982–3. HMSO, London

Paffenberger RS, Hyde R, Wing A et al 1986 Physical activity, all cause mortality and longevity of college alumni. New England Journal of Medicine 314:605–613 and 315:399–401

Pill R, Stott NCH 1982 Concepts of illness, causation and responsibility; some preliminary data from a sample of working class mothers. Social Science and Medicine 16:43–52

Prochaska J, DiClemente C 1982 Transtheoretical therapy: toward a more integrative model of change.

In: Psychotherapy: theory, research and practice. Dow Jones/Irwin, Homewood, Illinois
Raw M, McNeill A, Watt J et al 2001 National smoking cessation services at risk. British Medical Journal 323:1140–1141
Rayman M 1997 Dietary selenium: time to act. British Medical Journal 314:387
RCP 1992 Smoking and the young: a report of a working party. Royal College of Physicians, London
Rees L 2001 Integrated medicine. British Medical Journal 322:119–120
Rollnick S, Mason P, Butler C 2000 Importance and confidence. In: Health behaviour change. Harcourt, Edinburgh
Rosenstock IM, Strecher VJ, Becker HB 1988 Social learning and the Health Belief Model. Health Education Quarterly 15:175–183
Ruddock V, Hunt P 1997 A randomised trial to evaluate the effectiveness of dietary advice by practice nurses in lowering diet-related coronary heart disease risk. British Journal of General Practice 47:7–11
Schain WS 1994 Barriers to clinical trials part II: knowledge and attitudes of potential participants. Cancer 74:2266–2271
Schroer S, Wilcox M 1996 Relationship of study participation to health related behaviours. Journal of Vascular Nursing 6:156–167
Secretary of State for Health and Secretaries of State for Scotland, Wales and Northern Ireland 1998 Smoking kills: a White Paper on tobacco. HMSO, London
Sports Council 1992 Allied Dunbar, Health Education Authority, Sports Council National Fitness Survey: a report on activity patterns and fitness levels. Main findings and summary document. Health Education Authority, London
Tudor Hart J 1971 The inverse care law. Lancet 1:405–412
White A, Nicolaas G, Foster K et al 1993 Health survey for England 1991. HMSO, London

Resources

Helplines on smoking

ASH: 020 7739 5902
NHS helpline for information and support: 0800 169 0 169
The Quitline: 0800 00 22 00

Websites

Department of Health: www.givingupsmoking.co.uk
No smoking day: www.no-smoking-day.org.uk
ASH England: www.ash.org.uk
Health Education Authority: www.hea.org.uk

Further reading

Cochrane AC 1972 Effectiveness and efficiency. Random reflections on health services. Nuffield Provincial Hospital Trust, Oxford
Miller W, Rollnick S 1991 Motivational interviewing. Preparing people to change addictive behavior. Guilford Press, New York
Rollnick S, Mason P, Butler C 1999 Health behaviour change. A guide for practitioners. Churchill Livingstone, Edinburgh

Chapter 5

Vaccination

Jeannett Martin

CHAPTER CONTENTS

IMMUNOLOGY

Immunology is the scientific study of the organs, cells and molecules that are able to recognize and respond to foreign non-self substances, known as *antigens*, in order to protect the self from harm. An understanding of the immune system has allowed us to intervene advantageously by encouraging or preventing a response.

The term 'immune response' is used to describe the physiological chain of events induced by exposure to an antigen, which eventually leads to the production of *immune response products*. These products are white cells, which are able to combat antigens (cell-mediated immunity), and humoral (free in the blood) antibodies.

White cells are classified as *granulocytes* or *agranulocytes* simply because of the way they appear under a microscope when stained. The granulocytes, including neutrophils, basophils and eosinophils, are able to release histamine and have a major role in the inflammatory response.

Lymphocytes are agranular white cells which circulate in the blood, policing the self for any non-self material. These are the cells which produce the immune response products after contact with an antigen. There are two lymphocyte populations – *B cells* from the bone marrow and *T cells* from the thymus – which work together to produce an immune response to an invading antigen.

T lymphocyte cells are divided into three main groups depending on their function. Cytotoxic (Tc) cells deposit harmful substances on an 'enemy' cell and thus destroy the cell wall. Transplanted organs can be attacked in this way. Helper (Th) cells stimulate B cells to produce antibodies and are

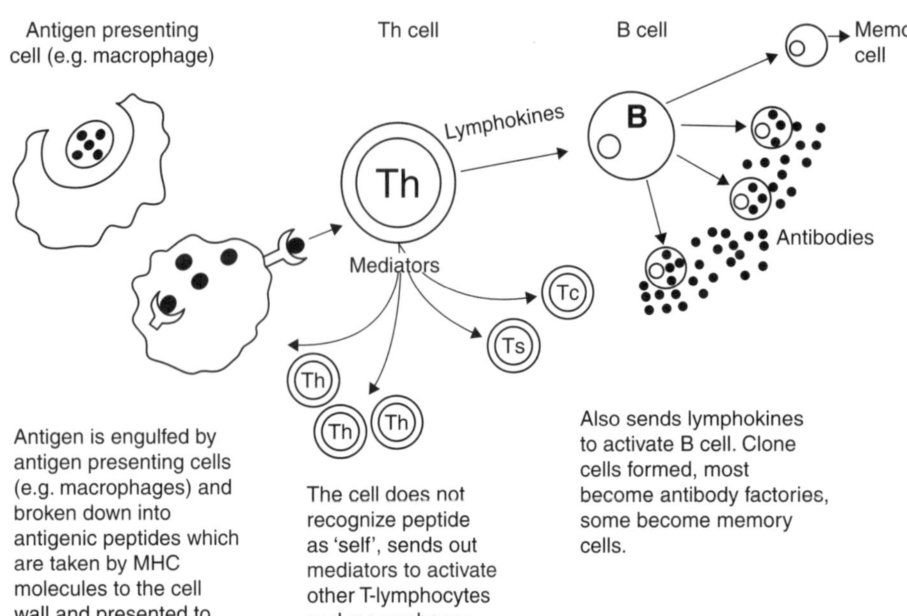

Figure 5.1 Cell-mediated immune response. (Reproduced with kind permission from Joan Sawyer.)

essential for an effective immune response. The human immunodeficiency virus (HIV) can invade these cells and paralyse them. Suppressor (Ts) cells reduce the response of B cells once the situation has been controlled, probably by inhibiting the T helper cells.

CELL-MEDIATED IMMUNITY (T CELLS)

Macrophages, formed from monocytes in the bone marrow, move freely in the blood. They identify a non-self antigen, engulf it and break it down into antigenic peptides. These particles are picked up within a molecule in the cell known as the major histocompatibility complex (MHC) molecule. This then carries the peptide to the surface of the macrophage where it is presented to passing Th cells. If the Th cell identifies this as non-self material it secretes lymphokines to stimulate B cells to produce and secrete specific antibodies. It will also send out mediators which attract other lymphocytes and monocytes, leading to inflammation.

HUMORAL IMMUNITY (B CELLS)

B cells respond to stimulation by T cells or by contact with an antigen. Once activated, B cells secrete millions of specific antibodies to that antigen. These antibodies, also known as *immunoglobulins* (Ig), are free in the blood and are able to bind to the surface and neutralize the antigens that they recognize. The non-self material is then flagged up to be devoured by passing phagocytic white cells such as agranular monocytes or granular neutrophils.

Although B cells can be programmed by T cells to produce antibodies very quickly, they can only recognize the whole antigen when they come across it. Although they can mount an effective challenge to antigens they have previously dealt with, mutating antigens are able to change their outer shell and this will fool circulating B cells. However, the basic protein fragments (peptides) of the antigen do not change and it is these peptides presented by macrophages that the T cells will respond to and then stimulate B cells to produce specific antibodies. This effective partnership between the two lymphocyte populations enables the self to challenge both new and familiar invading antigens.

ACQUIRED IMMUNITY

Once a person possesses antibodies to a specific antigen, he or she can be considered to have 'acquired specific immunity'. Acquired immunity can be active or passive.

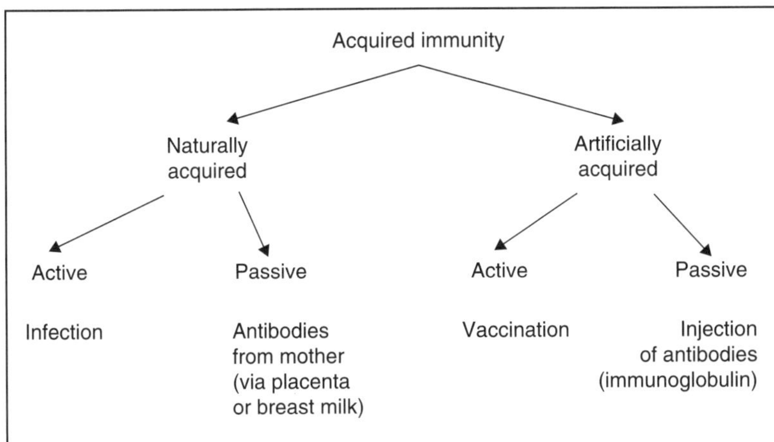

Figure 5.2 Acquired immunity.

Passive immunity

Passive immunity occurs when antibodies are acquired from someone else. Examples of this are:

- antibodies acquired by a newborn baby from the mother via the placenta, colostrum and breast milk
- specific immunoglobulin, which is given by injection to provide immediate immunity to people who have been exposed to a particular disease such as hepatitis B or rabies. These antibodies are taken from the pooled human serum of people known to be immune. Serum is tested to ensure that it is not HIV antibody positive.

Passive immunity is always short-lived. Antibodies are gradually reduced over a period of weeks and are not replaced unless active immunity is developed at the same time.

Active immunity

It has been known for many centuries that active immunity can be naturally acquired after contact with a disease. This was described in ancient Greece, where the observation that recovery from smallpox resulted in future protection was recorded. From then on many attempts were made to develop a method of artificially acquiring the same level of protection from this horrifying disease (Reid & Grist 1988).

The ancient Chinese favoured the inhalation of dried crusts of smallpox pustules. The Turks developed variolation, whereby material from the smallpox pustule was inoculated into the arms of healthy individuals. In fact, rather than protecting people, variolation caused widespread outbreaks of smallpox.

In 1798 Edward Jenner published the results of his research in 1796 into smallpox and described how inoculation of vaccinia (cowpox) would enable people to be immunized effectively and safely against smallpox. Many years later, Louis Pasteur suggested that all inoculations aimed at protecting people against diseases should be called vaccinations in honour of Jenner's work.

VACCINES

Active immunity to many diseases has been established by means of vaccination. Vaccines have been designed to be antigenic; that is, to supply enough antigen to stimulate an immune response.

The result should be an individual who has been immunized against a disease without having to experience morbidity. Vaccination is of particular benefit when the disease has a high mortality rate, for example diphtheria, or severe morbidity such as polio.

TYPES OF VACCINE

Live attenuated vaccine

A live organism replicated to produce a less virulent progeny. It needs a stable level of attenuation to achieve the required response without becoming virulent enough to cause infection.

Inactivated vaccines

Killed or inactivated organisms possessing surface proteins which will stimulate antibody production.

They are often treated with formaldehyde and may have an adjuvant such as thiomersal added to boost the response.

Recombinant bio-engineered vaccines

These use viral surface proteins genetically replicated in other harmless organisms. These will be identified by T cells and stimulate the required immune response.

Toxoid vaccines

Sometimes, for example with tetanus, it is not the organism which causes the symptoms but the toxins it produces. Toxoids stimulate a response to combat these.

Whole-cell, capsular polysaccharide and capsular conjugated vaccines

A useful analogy here is to compare the organism used for a vaccine with an instantly recognizable sweet – a Smartie.

Table 5.1 Types of vaccines

	Viral	Bacterial
Live	Measles Mumps Rubella Oral polio Yellow fever	BCG Oral typhoid
Inactivated	Influenza Hepatitis A Injectable polio Rabies Tick-borne encephalitis Japanese encephalitis	Pertussis Cholera Plague
Toxoids		Diphtheria Tetanus
Bio-engineered	Hepatitis B	
Capsular polysaccharide		Pneumococcal *Haemophilus influenzae* b (Hib) Meningococcal A&C Typhim Vi
Conjugated		Meningitis C Pneumococcal

A Smartie has an outside sugar coat with the centre full of chocolate – this correlates with the whole organism and would be used for whole-cell vaccines.

Remove the chocolate from the middle of the Smartie and leave the outside sugar coat intact; this is a capsular polysaccharide vaccine that would produce an immune response but have fewer side effects than the whole-cell vaccine.

Children under 2 years of age do not respond to capsular polysaccharide vaccines but if this capsular polysaccharide coat is joined (conjugated) to another, harmless protein you have a conjugated capsular polysaccharide vaccine which will create an immune response in children under 2 years.

IMMUNE RESPONSE TO VACCINATION

More than one exposure to the antigen may be required to ensure that a person develops immunity. The immune response at first exposure to an antigen is known as the *primary response*. This may require more than one injection, depending on the potency of the product.

After the primary response, immunoglobulin M (which has no memory cells) is predominant, with only a subsidiary immunoglobulin G level. The memory cells contained within the small amount of immunoglobulin G act like a booster rocket to enable the self to recognize the antigen contained in the vaccine very quickly at the next meeting. This results in a *secondary response* and an increased immunoglobulin G level.

The secondary response takes 2–4 days, but the antibodies produced last for years. Once a person has received a full primary course resulting in both the primary and secondary immune response, it never needs to be repeated but further single boosters may be required if immunity needs to be reinforced.

If a person interrupts a primary course of vaccination but then presents for the next injection, even years later, the immunological memory will mean that the course does not need to be restarted from the beginning, only continued from the point reached and completed according to the recommended schedule. The only exception to this is rabies vaccination where, depending on the interval, the manufacturers provide a sliding scale on what number of doses need to be given.

Routine vaccination in childhood against a range of serious diseases results not only in effective individual protection but also in *herd immunity*.

The main benefit of herd immunity to society is that those not yet vaccinated or those unable to be vaccinated because of genuine contraindications are less likely to come into contact and be infected with the disease. However, 90–95% of the population need to be vaccinated to ensure that herd immunity develops (Kassianos 2001).

THE DISEASES AND EXPANDED PROGRAMME OF VACCINATION

CHILDREN

Table 5.2 shows the DoH (2002) recommendations for children's vaccinations.

Vaccinations should **not** be given into the buttock. The recommended sites are the anterolateral aspect of the thigh for babies and the deltoid for adults and children receiving their preschool booster. See Chapter 20 for information on injection sites and technique.

The DoH (1996) emphasizes the importance of the schedule and states in the Green Book: 'Every effort should be made to ensure that all children are immunized even if they are older than the recommended age range; no opportunity to immunize should be missed'. When new vaccines are introduced into the national schedule a recommended catch-up programme is also incorporated.

ADULTS

The Department of Health recommends that adults should receive the following vaccinations.

- Tetanus/diphtheria and polio (DTP) – previously unimmunized
- Rubella – in women who are seronegative
- Meningitis A&C/*Haemophilus influenzae* b – asplenic individuals
- Hepatitis A – high-risk groups
- Hepatitis B – high-risk groups
- Influenza – high-risk groups
- Pneumococcal – high-risk groups

TRAVEL ABROAD

The Department of Health recommends that all travellers should have completed routine tetanus and polio vaccination schedules and be offered further vaccination depending on the following.

- The country and area to be visited
- The type of holiday
- Season
- Length of stay
- Previous vaccination history

However, it is important to recognize that illness acquired abroad, such as malaria, is not preventable by vaccines (see Chapter 6). Travel health advice is therefore vital. Further information can be obtained from the Department of Health guidance outlined in the Yellow Book *Health information for overseas travel* (2001a).

TETANUS

Tetanus is not spread from person to person; the most common method of transmission is for tetanus

Table 5.2 Children's immunization schedule

Vaccine	Age	Notes
DTP-Hib Meningitis C Polio	2 months 3 months 4 months	Primary course
Measles/mumps/rubella (MMR)	12–15 months	MMR can be given at any age over 12 months. A booster Hib may be added to the childhood schedule in 2004
DTaP, polio, MMR second dose	3–5 years	3 years after completion of primary course. Acellular pertussis is used for preschool booster
BCG	10–14 years or infancy	
Booster tetanus, diphtheria (Td) and polio	13–18 years	

spores present in soil to enter the body as a result of injury. However, neonatal tetanus, where the baby's umbilical stump becomes infected, is still an important cause of neonatal death in developing countries such as Asia and Africa.

The disease is caused by a toxin produced by the tetanus bacilli at the site of injury. The incubation period is 4–21 days and growth is anaerobic so puncture wounds will provide the ideal environment.

Tetanus spores can never be eradicated so herd immunity is not an option; immunization is the only means of ensuring individual protection.

Td vaccine replaced single-antigen tetanus vaccine for the routine booster immunization given to school-leavers in 1994. The CMO's Update 5, issued in March 1995, clarified that Td should now always be given rather than tetanus (T) alone, on the advice of the Joint Committee on Vaccination and Immunization (JCVI), generated by concern at the low levels of immunity to diphtheria in older people in the UK. It brings us into line with recommendations from the World Health Organization. The DoH (2002) issued the advice below for tetanus immunization to replace that in the then current Green Book: *Immunisation against infectious diseases* (1996).

Routine tetanus and diphtheria immunization schedules (DoH 2002)

1. Adults and adolescents requiring tetanus immunization should now receive combined adsorbed tetanus/low-dose diphtheria vaccine for adults and adolescents (Td).

2. A full course of tetanus and diphtheria vaccines consists of five doses as shown in Table 5.3.

3. Older adults may be unimmunized and at particular risk. Opportunities should be taken to check their immunization status when attending surgery, for example for their influenza immunization, and complete the recommended five-dose schedule. Td can be given at the same time as influenza vaccine in a different arm.

4. For travellers to areas where medical attention may not be accessible should a tetanus-prone injury occur and whose last dose of a tetanus-containing vaccine was more than 10 years previously, a booster dose of Td should be given, even if the individual has received five doses of vaccine previously. This is a precautionary measure in case immunoglobulin is not available to the individual should a tetanus-prone injury occur.

Tetanus immunization following injuries

A tetanus-prone wound is:

1. any wound or burn sustained more than 6 hours before surgical treatment of the wound or burn
2. any wound or burn at any interval after injury that shows one or more of the following characteristics:
   - a significant degree of devitalized tissue
   - puncture-type wound
   - contact with soil or manure likely to harbour tetanus organisms
   - clinical evidence of sepsis.

For prevention, the dose of human tetanus immunoglobulin (DoH 1966) is:

- for most uses: 250 iu by intramuscular injection
- if more than 24 hours have elapsed since injury or there is a risk of heavy contamination or following burns: 500 iu by intramuscular injection.

DIPHTHERIA

Diphtheria is an acute infectious disease of the upper respiratory tract that is spread by droplet

Table 5.3 Full course of tetanus and diphtheria vaccination

Schedule	Children	Adults
Primary course	3 doses of vaccine (usually as DTP) at 2, 3 and 4 months of age	3 doses of vaccine (as Td), each 1 month apart
4th dose	At least 3 years after the primary course, usually preschool entry (as DTaP)	10 years after primary course (as Td)
5th dose	Aged 13–18 years before leaving school (as Td)	10 years after 4th dose (as Td)

infection or contact with soiled articles used by an infected person, e.g. handkerchiefs, bedlinen. The incubation period is 2–5 days and a carrier state is possible. Presentation is usually a sore throat without signs of toxicity.

The diphtheria bacillus produces a toxin which causes an inflammatory exudate which forms a greyish membrane in the respiratory tract and can lead to obstruction.

Our successful vaccination programme has resulted in very few cases of diphtheria presenting now in the UK, but there have been large-scale outbreaks elsewhere in the world, e.g. Russia. This can represent a real risk to travellers and then to the community on return, particularly as we know from a study of UK blood donors that there is a trend of decreasing immunity with increasing age (Maple et al 1995).

Immunization protects by stimulating the production of antitoxin which can then protect against the toxin produced by the bacilli. The dose is 0.5 ml given by intramuscular or deep subcutaneous injection. High-dose diphtheria (D) vaccine is used within the triple vaccine given to babies and children under 10 years of age but after this age low-dose diphtheria (d) vaccine must be used, because local or general reactions are possible if the individual is already immune.

Prophylaxis for close contacts

Depending on their age and previous vaccination history, individuals exposed to risk because of contact with a diphtheria case or carrier should be vaccinated (DoH 1996), either with a complete course of three doses at monthly intervals or a single reinforcing dose (high dose if under 10; low dose if over 10). In addition, unimmunized contacts should be given a prophylactic course of erythromycin or penicillin.

Diphtheria antitoxin is no longer used for prophylaxis in unimmunized contacts, because there is an associated risk of a hypersensitivity reaction to

Table 5.4 Tetanus vaccination following injury (Kassianos 2001)

Immunization status	Clean wound	Tetanus-prone wound (see definition p.84)	
	Vaccine	Vaccine	Human tetanus immunoglobulin
Fully immunized, i.e. has received a total of 5 doses of tetanus vaccine at appropriate intervals as single antigen or in a combined vaccine	None required	None required	Only if risk especially high (e.g. contaminated with stable manure)
Primary immunization complete, boosters incomplete but up to date	None required (unless next dose due soon and convenient to give now)	None required (unless next dose due soon and convenient to give now)	Only if risk especially high (see above)
Primary immunization incomplete or boosters not up to date	A reinforcing dose of combined tetanus/diphtheria vaccine and further doses as required to complete the recommended schedule (to ensure future immunity)	A reinforcing dose of combined tetanus/diphtheria vaccine and further doses as required to complete the recommended schedule (to ensure future immunity)	Yes: one dose of human tetanus immunoglobulin in a different site
Not immunized or immunization status not known or uncertain	An immediate dose of vaccine followed, if records confirm this is needed, by completion of a full 3-dose course of combined tetanus/diphtheria vaccine to ensure future immunity	An immediate dose of vaccine followed, if records confirm this is needed, by completion of a full 3-dose course of combined tetanus/diphtheria vaccine to ensure future immunity	Yes: one dose of human tetanus immunoglobulin in a different site

the horse serum from which it is derived. It is now used only in suspected cases of diphtheria and a trial dose should be given first.

PERTUSSIS

Bordetella pertussis, whooping cough, is a bacterial infection of the mucosal layers of the human respiratory tract. There is no carrier state but it is a highly infectious disease with serious complications; these can include pneumonia (1:8 cases), encephalopathy (1:20 cases), brain damage and death (1:200 cases) (Kassianos 2001).

Whole-cell pertussis (wP) vaccines

Derived from whole pertussis organisms that have been inactivated, they also contain endotoxin; higher endotoxin content correlates with increased rates of local reactions (Barakk et al 1989). Possible adverse reactions include:

- local redness
- swelling
- fever and agitation – this can be reduced by paracetamol and is often routinely recommended post vaccination (HEA 1997)
- prolonged crying and febrile convulsions occur in <1:100
- acute encephalopathy occurs very rarely, <1:10.5 million (WHO 1999a).

No causal link has been demonstrated between wP vaccination and permanent brain damage, epilepsy or death (WHO 1999a). However, in the 1970s parental concern relating to this vaccine led to poor uptake and worldwide epidemics of pertussis followed (WHO 1999a).

Acellular pertussis (aP) vaccines

Acellular pertussis vaccines contain inactivated pertussis toxin, which in most cases is combined with filamentous haemagglutinin and sometimes additional pertussis components such as fimbrial antigens and pertactin. A number of different aP vaccines are available; all have a lower endotoxin content and decreased reactogenicity compared to whole-cell vaccines (Conrad & Jenson 1999). These are part of the routine childhood vaccination programme in Japan, USA and some European countries (Finn & Bell 2000).

In the UK whole-cell pertussis vaccination is currently routinely recommended for infants aged 2, 3 and 4 months. However, for a variety of reasons infants may not always begin vaccination at 2 months.

Vaccine-derived immunity from the whole-cell vaccine wanes after 5 years (Lopez & Blumberg 1997). Subclinical pertussis can occur in adults with reduced immunity and Lopez & Blumberg (1997) estimated that 21–26% of adults with a cough lasting 6–14 days have pertussis. Long et al (1990) suggested that young children with pertussis were usually secondary cases in an affected household with one member of the family serving as the index case. In England and Wales there are an estimated 35 000 GP consultations, 5 500 inpatient days and around nine deaths annually from pertussis (DoH 2001b).

Following recommendations from the Joint Committee on Vaccination and Immunization (JCVI), the Department of Health added a preschool booster of acellular pertussis to the routine vaccination schedule in 2001 (DoH 2001b). It is expected that this additional booster will reduce the present morbidity and mortality associated with pertussis and the risk of transmission from older siblings and parents to very young unvaccinated babies.

As whole-cell vaccines can result in increased reactions in older children or adults, this fourth dose of pertussis will need to be the acellular vaccine. Miller & Waight's study (2001) identified that there were no new safety concerns associated with this additional acellular pertussis booster at preschool age and that there was no increase in reactions due to the administration of MMR at the same time.

MENINGITIS

The central nervous system (CNS) is covered by three layers – the meninges. The cerebrospinal fluid (CSF) is an immunologically naive site and any infection can readily thrive and cause inflammation of the meninges (meningitis) and then spread across into the ventricles of the brain.

Causes

Viral Many different viruses can cause meningitis, including polio, rubella and mumps. Viral meningitis will present with the same signs and symptoms as bacterial meningitis. Viral meningitis is more common, but can be less serious and of shorter duration.

Bacterial The pathogen usually colonizes the nasopharynx and then invades the bloodstream, crossing the blood–brain barrier into the CSF.

There are three major pathogens responsible for meningitis: *Neisseria meningitidis* (the meningococcus), *Haemophilus influenzae* type b (Hib) and *Streptococcus pneumoniae* (the pneumococcus). Until the 1980s meningococcus was the commonest cause of meningitis, but then it was subsequently overtaken by Hib. This trend was reversed by the introduction of Hib vaccination.

***Haemophilus influenzae* type b (Hib)** Hib is a small Gram-negative bacterium that may exist with or without a capsule. Most forms of invasive disease are caused by the strains of the organism with a polysaccharide capsule known as type b. It was estimated that before vaccination was available, 1:600 children developed invasive *Haemophilus influenzae* type b disease before they reached 5 years of age (DoH 1996) and that 60% of cases resulted in Hib meningitis with 4–5% fatality. It was the most common cause of bacterial meningitis in children and it was thought that the nasopharynx of approximately 1% of children under 6 years was colonized with Hib (Howard et al 1998).

Pneumococcal *Streptococcus pneumoniae* (the pneumococcus) is an encapsulated Gram-positive organism. Children under 2 years of age and the very old are at the greatest risk of invasive infection (Kassianos 2001). It will cause pneumococcal pneumonia in 1:1000 adults every year and 400 of those will develop meningitis with a mortality of 5–30% (Kassianos 2001). It is also an important cause of meningitis (Aszkensay et al 1995) and of acute otitis media in children, some of who will have multiple recurrences.

There are 84 known capsular types but 8–10 of these cause the majority of the serious infections. Antibiotic resistance against *Strep. pneumoniae* is increasing worldwide and the organism's susceptibility to penicillin, cephalosporin and macrolide antimicrobials is significantly reduced, making treatment more difficult (DoH 1996).

Meningococcal The organism *Neisseria meningitidis* (the meningococcus) is a Gram-negative diplococcus. It has only one host, man, and cannot survive outside the body. It is carried asymptomatically in the nasopharynx by around 10% of the general population and 25% of young adults in closed communities, such as educational institutions, are carriers (PHLS 1999). Transmission to others is by droplet infection or direct contact with respiratory secretions; the risk is increased by close contact such as kissing. There is usually a rapid onset of symptoms and mortality is around 5–10%.

There are several types of meningococci, which have been categorized into groups A, B, C, Y, W135 and others (Vedros 1987) by the structure of the polysaccharide capsule of the antigen. Group A is the commonest cause of meningitis in developing countries such as Africa. Travellers abroad will be at increased risk of infection during travel and may then transmit the disease to others on their return to the UK. In the UK groups B and C predominate; group B is responsible for the majority of meningococcal meningitis followed by group C (see Table 5.5).

Signs and symptoms of meningitis

- Headache
- Vomiting
- Photophobia
- Spasm of spinal muscles which causes neck stiffness
- Fever
- Petechial rash which does not blanch under pressure
- Kernig's sign – can be demonstrated by bending leg up towards abdomen to flex hip to 90° then, while hip is flexed, slowly extending the knee to 45° horizontal. If this causes hamstring spasm and pain it may suggest meningitis

Table 5.5 Meningococcal disease confirmed by group (PHLS Meningococcal Reference Unit; www.phls.co.uk/facts/meni-t03.htm)

Date	Group B	Group C	Other group	Ungrouped	Total
1995–6	872	618	65	0	1555
1996–7	1060	753	86	422	2321
1997–8	1099	775	112	308	2294
1998–9	1405	953	111	328	2797

- In infants and babies:
  - drowsiness
  - irritability and high-pitched cry
  - off feeds
  - tense or bulging fontanelle
  - pale listless floppy body

Complications

Long-term sequelae of the disease can be serious and wide ranging (Erikson 1998) and include:

- general tiredness
- recurring headaches
- aggressive behaviour
- epilepsy
- limb amputation
- brain damage
- skin necrosis requiring grafts.

Meningitis is a notifiable disease and all cases should be reported to the consultant in communicable disease control at the local health authority.

Prophylaxis for close contacts

For close contacts of confirmed cases, antibiotic prophylaxis will be advised, usually either a single dose of ciprofloxacin 500 mg or rifampicin 600 mg bd for 2 days (Kassianos 2001); see Table 5.6 for recommendations for children under 12. Alcohol should be avoided while taking rifampicin and recipients should be informed that it will cause orange-coloured urine.

Unvaccinated close contacts of groups A and C should be offered vaccination, but not group B as there is no vaccine yet available (DoH 1996). Unvaccinated contacts of *Haemophilus influenzae* type b that are under the age of 4 should be offered vaccination.

***Haemophilus influenzae* type b (Hib)** Since the introduction of Hib vaccination into the childhood vaccination schedule, incidence fell dramatically.

Table 5.6 Antibiotic prophylaxis for children under 12 years

Antibiotic	3 months–1 year	1–12 years
Ciprofloxacin	Not recommended	Not recommended
Rifampicin	5 mg/kg bd for 2 days	10 mg/kg bd for 2 days

In 1995 notifications of Hib meningitis declined from 484 to 60, a fall of 88% with only one death (DoH 1996). However, in 2003 there was an increase in cases. Therefore in 2003, children under 4 years of age were offerred a fourth (booster) dose of single Hib vaccine from 6 months of age. The Department of Health is reviewing the need to add a fourth dose to the routine childhood schedule.

Hib is an inactivated conjugated vaccine given by deep subcutaneous or intramuscular injection. Children under the age of 1 year are at high risk of the disease and parents should be offered vaccination for their child at 2, 3 and 4 months. ActHib can be combined with Aventis Pasteur MSD's DTP, Hiberix can be combined with Medeva's DTP.

Children who start a course of Hib vaccine on one product can have the course completed with another product if necessary (DoH 1996).

If the course is interrupted there is no need to restart the course; it can be recommenced and completed with monthly intervals between the remaining doses (DoH 1996).

Unvaccinated children between 13 and 48 months should be offered a single vaccination of Hib (DoH 1996). Routine vaccination or reinforcing doses for children over the age of 4 years and adults is not recommended. However, all asplenic individuals over the age of 1 year should be offered a single dose of Hib vaccine (DoH 1996) and those under 1 year should be offered three doses as part of the routine childhood vaccination schedule (DoH 1996).

Contraindications

- Severe reaction to a previous dose, but see section on adverse reactions below.
- Delay vaccination if the child has an acute illness, but this is not necessary for minor infections without fever or systemic upset.
- Pregnancy, unless there is a significant risk of infection.

Adverse reactions Swelling and redness at the site of injection which usually appear within 3–4 hours and resolve completely within 24 hours.

Introduction of Hib has not resulted in an increase in the number of severe reactions other than those that would be expected to be reported after DTP vaccinations. Therefore the DoH (1996) recommends that:

- if a severe *local* reaction occurs following combined DTP/Hib the course can be continued with DTP and Hib given separately at different sites

- if a severe *generalized* reaction occurs following combined DTP/Hib then the course can be completed with DT (instead of DTP) at one site and Hib at another.

Pneumococcal The inactivated 23-valent capsular polysaccharide vaccine presently available in the UK is effective in preventing severe pneumococcal infections such as pneumonia or meningitis, but does not protect against more common infections where pneumococcus can be implicated, such as otitis media.

The plain polysaccharide vaccine is recommended by the DoH (1996) for patients:

- without a spleen or severe dysfunction of the spleen
- with chronic renal disease or nephrotic syndrome
- with chronic heart or lung disease
- with diabetes.

Contraindications

- Acute febrile illness
- Severe reaction to a previous dose
- Hypersensitivity to any component of the vaccine such as thiomersal
- Children under 2 years as it is a plain polysaccharide vaccine and response is poor
- Pregnancy and breastfeeding
- Previous pneumococcal vaccination within past 3 years

Adverse reactions

- Swelling and redness at the injection site
- Fever, headaches and myalgia in less than 1%

More severe general reactions are possible in those who are reimmunized within 3 years.

The clinical sequelae in survivors of pneumococcal meningitis can be significantly more severe than those after meningitis due to Hib or meningococcus and would be the rationale for the prevention of pneumococcal infections in all children. However, this would require a conjugated pneumococcal vaccine as young children respond poorly to plain polysaccharide vaccines.

Use of pneumococcal conjugate vaccine (Prevenar) in 'at-risk' children under 2 Advice on the use of the pneumococcal conjugate vaccine (Prevenar) in 'at-risk' children under 2 years of age was outlined by the Department of Health in the CMO letter PL/CMO/2002/4 dated August 2002 and is as detailed in Box 5.1.

Box 5.1 Previously unvaccinated older infants and children

- Infants under the age of 6 months: three doses, each of 0.5 ml, the first dose usually given at 2 months of age and with an interval of at least 1 month between doses. A fourth dose is recommended in the second year of life.
- Infants aged 7–11 months: two doses, each of 0.5 ml, with an interval of at least 1 month between doses. A third dose is recommended in the second year of life.
- Children aged 12–23 months: two doses, each of 0.5 ml, with an interval of at least 2 months between doses.

The Department of Health's recommendation that a single dose of 23-valent pneumococcal polysaccharide vaccine should be given to all 'at-risk' children after their second birthday remains the same. This is to provide protection against a number of other serotypes of *Strep. pneumoniae* not covered by the conjugate vaccine. If the conjugate vaccine is given shortly before the child's second birthday, an interval of at least 1 month should be left between the conjugate vaccine and polysaccharide vaccine.

Meningococcal There are four vaccines currently available for protection against some groups of meningococcal meningitis in the UK. There are two A+C polysaccharide vaccines: Meningivac (A+C) produced by Aventis Pasteur MSD and AC Vax by SmithKline Beecham. There are three conjugated C vaccines. Meningitec, produced by Wyeth, Menjugate from Aventis Pasteur MSD, Neisvac-C from Baxter.

No vaccine is as yet licensed for use against meningitis B.

Meningococcal polysaccharide A+C vaccine This is an inactivated plain polysaccharide vaccine. A single dose of 0.5 ml is given by deep subcutaneous or intramuscular injection. It was administered to first-year university students during the meningitis C campaign in 1999, before the new conjugated vaccine was available, and has been used in the past to vaccinate close contacts of confirmed group C cases. However, as it is a polysaccharide vaccine the immune response in very young children can be poor.

The main indication for A+C or ACWY is as recommended by the World Health Organization

(WHO 2000) for travellers to endemic areas; this would include the 'meningitis belt' of Africa. Muslims travelling to the city of Mecca to attend the Hajj will be denied entry to Saudi Arabia if they do not have a valid certificate of vaccination for meningitis ACWY.

Contraindications

- Acute febrile illness
- Severe reaction to a previous dose of the vaccine
- Pregnancy, unless there is a significant risk of infection

Adverse reactions

- Swelling and redness at injection site for 1–2 days in approximately 10%
- Irritability, fever and rigor within 24–48 hours

Meningococcal C conjugate vaccine This inactivated conjugated vaccine is newly licensed in the UK for protection against meningitis C for adults and adolescents; the Wyeth and Chiron vaccines are being supplied by Farillon for use in the routine childhood vaccination schedule. These conjugated vaccines are group specific and do not provide protection against meningitis groups A or B.

Schedule

- Babies under 1 year should receive three doses of 0.5 ml by intramuscular injection at 2, 3 and 4 months; this can be given at the same time as other childhood vaccines.
- Unvaccinated children between 5 and 12 months should receive two doses.
- Those over 1 year, adults and adolescents require a single dose of vaccine.

Contraindications

- Acute febrile illness
- Hypersensitivity to any component of the vaccine, including tetanus or diphtheria toxoid, meningococcal C polysaccharide or CRM 197 carrier protein.
- Pregnancy unless there is a significant risk of infection.

Adverse reactions

- Local swelling and redness at the injection site
- Fever
- Crying, irritability
- Headache and myalgia in adults

There have been 4764 reports of reactions to the vaccine, but as over 13 million doses have been given since its introduction in November 1999, the number of reactions is in line with what would be expected (DoH 2000).

If the A+C vaccine is required for travel in an individual who has previously been vaccinated with the monovalent meningococcal C conjugate vaccine, then there must be a 2-week interval but 6 months is recommended between polysaccharide and conjugated vaccines (see Table 5.7).

Table 5.7 Time interval required after prior vaccination with polysaccharide and conjugated vaccines (Conaty 2000)

Vaccine	Time interval
Meningococcal C conjugate	Minimum 2 weeks before giving A+C or ACWY for travel
Meningococcal plain polysaccharide A+C	Wait 6 months before giving meningococcal C conjugate

Conclusion

It is possible that the future development of conjugated vaccines for pneumococcal and meningitis B may enable a combined vaccine to be produced, providing protection against all the main causes of meningitis – Hib, meningococcal and pneumococcal – in the form of one meningitis vaccine. With the rapid emergence of antibiotic-resistant organisms, vaccine prevention of bacterial meningitis will not only protect very young children from the disease but will also reduce the need for antibiotic treatment and thus the continued emergence of antibiotic-resistant strains.

MEASLES

Measles is a viral infection present worldwide with epidemics every 2–4 years. In temperate climates the peak incidence is between February and April. The WHO (1999b) estimated that in 1998 measles affected 30 million and killed 888 000 children worldwide.

Before routine vaccination was introduced in the UK, measles was common; the majority would be affected at some stage in their childhood. In the UK measles is a notifiable disease – the consultant in communicable diseases should be informed of all cases diagnosed. Notified cases will be confirmed with a salivary test sent from the Public Health Laboratory Service (PHLS), now part of the Health Protection Agency (HPA).

The incubation period of the disease is 9–11 days before signs and symptoms appear. Illness usually starts as a bad cold (coryza), conjunctivitis and fever. Then a blotchy slightly elevated pink rash appears on the neck behind the ears and spreads to face, body and extremities over 2–3 days. The second phase of fever is 48–72 hours after the rash and then subsides. The rash fades after 5–7 days, often leaving a brown staining of the skin. A third phase of fever suggests that there will be complications to the disease (Box 5.2).

Box 5.2 Complications of measles (Kassianos 2001)

Diarrhoea	1:6
Otitis media	1:20
Respiratory • Pneumonitis (inflammation confined to alveoli) can be acute and transient or chronic, leading to increasing respiratory disability • Pneumonia caused by the virus or a secondary bacterial infection	1:25
Febrile convulsions	2:100
Encephalitis occurs 4–7 days after the rash. Of the cases that occur: • 15% fatality rate • 20–40% will have permanent neurological damage	1:5000
Subacute sclerosing panencephalitis • Occurs years after measles infection • Causes deterioration in intellectual and motor abilities • In most cases is fatal	1:100 000

Measles is transmitted by droplet infection. The disease is highly contagious; 95% of unvaccinated people who come into contact with the disease would be expected to contract it.

Parents should be advised to keep an affected child away from other children during the prodromal (before rash) stage and until after the first 4 days of the rash (Southgate et al 1997). Vaccination should be recommended for any unvaccinated contacts over 6 months of age and specific immunoglobulin for unvaccinated contacts less than 6 months old.

The practice of holding 'measles parties' in order to expose healthy children to the measles virus was common before vaccination was introduced and is rising in popularity again amongst those who consider that immunity gained via natural infection will be better or safer than vaccination. However, approval or recommendation of this practice by a healthcare professional could potentially be interpreted as negligence by a parent should their child go on to develop complications of the disease.

MUMPS

Infectious parotitis (mumps) is a viral infection that exists worldwide and with epidemics presenting every 3 years. In 1989 an estimated 20713 children in the UK were affected, with 16 500 under 10 years of age; mumps was the commonest cause of viral meningitis in children. Cases dropped to 1587 in 1998 following the introduction of routine vaccination in 1988. The incubation period of the disease is 14–21 days. Mumps is a notifiable disease in the UK.

Symptoms

- Fever, headache and vomiting
- Swelling of parotid gland – can be unilateral or bilateral. Swelling spreads up from the jaw into the cheek
- Salivary duct openings in mouth can be red and swollen

Box 5.3 Complications of mumps (Kassianos 2001)

Epididymo-orchitis in males post puberty – rarely causes sterility	1:4
Meningoencephalitis	1:300–400
Deafness	1:25
Miscarriage in first trimester	1:4

Mumps is spread by droplet infection. Parents should be advised to keep an affected child away from other children during the infectious stage – 7 days before and 9 days after parotid swelling.

RUBELLA

Rubella, or German measles, is a mild but highly contagious viral illness with a worldwide distribution. In the past epidemics have occurred every 6–9 years.

The highest risk associated with this disease relates to fetal damage if a pregnant woman becomes infected, particularly during the first trimester of pregnancy. The incubation period is 2–3 weeks. Rubella is a notifiable disease in the UK.

Symptoms

- Headache, sore throat, fever
- Swelling and soreness of the neck due to enlargement of lymph glands
- Widespread rash of minute pink spots which spreads from the face to the rest of the body and lasts for about a week
- Transient polyarthralgia

Box 5.4 Complications of rubella (Kassianos 2001)

Thrombocytopenia	7:3000
Encephalitis	1:6000
Congenital rubella syndrome (CRS) – infection during first 4 months of pregnancy is associated with fetal damage:	90% risk of CRS if rubella contracted during first 10 weeks of pregnancy
• Cardiac abnormalities – septal defects, pulmonary artery stenosis • Meningoencephalitis, microcephaly • Deafness	10–20% risk of CRS if rubella contracted in 10th–16th week of pregnancy
• Cataract • Limb abnormality • Learning disabilities	Low risk of CRS if rubella contracted in second half of pregnancy

All women with rubella-like illness during pregnancy, even those previously vaccinated, should be investigated and referred to an obstetrician to discuss risk to the fetus.

Rubella is spread by droplet infection. An individual will be infectious for 1 week before and up to 1 week after the rash appears.

PREVENTION OF MEASLES, MUMPS AND RUBELLA BY VACCINATION

Since 1988 MMR vaccine has been available in the UK as part of the routine childhood vaccination schedule. The vaccine is live attenuated and offered at 12–18 months. A preschool booster was added to the recommended UK schedule in 1996 but this two-dose schedule has been common practice in countries such as the USA, Canada and Finland for many years.

Benefits of vaccination with MMR

The MMR vaccine has significantly reduced the cases of measles, mumps and rubella.

Risks of vaccination with MMR

As with all vaccines there are small risks of side-effects. Most of these will be minor, local reactions such as redness and swelling at the site of injection.

About a week after MMR some children will become feverish and develop a slight rash. Mild mump-like swelling of the glands can occur about 3 weeks after the injection (HEA 1997). If these do occur children will not be infectious. Side-effects from the second dose are rarer than from the first; those that do occur are most likely in non-responders to the first vaccine so these are the children who most need the protection (HEA 1997).

Occasionally children can have more severe reactions to the MMR vaccine, but the risks of these are much less after vaccination than with the natural disease and the conditions are milder, i.e. not fatal (HEA 1997).

Box 5.5 Risks of MMR vaccination

Febrile convulsions	1:1000
Encephalitis	1:3 000 000
Death	0

MMR vaccine controversies

Recently there has been considerable media coverage of MMR vaccination with suggestions made that it may be linked to irritable bowel syndrome/autism. This has caused understandable parental

Table 5.8 Reduction in cases

Disease	1989	1998
Measles	26 222	3728
Mumps	20 713	1587
Rubella	24 570	3208

concern and resulted in a drop in vaccination uptake in many areas. Some parents have begun to access single-antigen vaccination via private clinics. Due to the time interval between vaccines, children are left unprotected against diseases for longer and can then contract the diseases, particularly in cases where parents leave a year between each vaccination. Also single-antigen vaccines used by these clinics are not necessarily as effective or as safe as the strains contained within the combined MMR.

If this trend continues, these diseases will reemerge in the UK, as has happened recently in both the Netherlands and the Republic of Ireland (Ryan 2000). Tragically the effects on the health and well-being of the children affected are severe; in Dublin, for example, two children died from measles.

Evidence supporting possible links between MMR vaccine and irritable bowel disease/autism A study from the Royal Free (Montgomery et al 1999) suggested that children who contracted measles infection and mumps infection in the same year were more likely to develop Crohn's disease than those who did not contract these diseases. The researchers clearly stated in the paper that they had not established an association between inflammatory bowel disease and MMR vaccination.

A previous study by Wakefield et al (1998) described the clinical features of 12 children referred to a gastroenterology unit at the Royal Free.

- All appeared to be developing normally before the parents noticed the disorder.
- All had both intestinal and behavioural disorders on referral to the study team.
- Parents considered that behavioural symptoms appeared shortly after MMR vaccination in eight of the 12 cases.

The sample size of 12 children was so small that no reliable conclusions could be made. The researchers noted that they were unable to establish an association, but suggested that if there was a causal link then further research would identify whether the incidence of autism increased after the introduction of MMR in 1988. When this work was done (Taylor et al 1999) no causal link was identified.

Evidence against possible links Taylor et al (1999) undertook a large population-based study in North East Thames to investigate whether MMR could be causally linked with autism. They identified 498 children with autism born since 1979 and then looked at trends in the incidence of autism before and after the introduction of the MMR vaccine in 1988.

The main findings were:

- incidence of autism began to increase from 1979 (10 years before the introduction of MMR), possibly related to improved diagnostic methods
- there was no sharp change in the trend coinciding with the introduction of MMR
- there was no difference in age of diagnosis of autism in children who received MMR and those who did not; nor was there any clustering of autism diagnosis in the months following vaccination in those children who had received MMR.

At a meeting in March 1998 organized by the Medical Research Council to review the current evidence, a worldwide panel of independent experts concluded that there was no association between MMR vaccine and the development of irritable bowel disease or autism. Their full report can be accessed at: www.mrc.ac.uk/Autism_report.html.

Guidance from the Deputy Chief Medical Officer and the Chairman of the Committee on Safety of Medicines in June 1999 stated that the combined MMR vaccine does not cause autism or Crohn's disease. This guidance was based on the large population study by Taylor et al (1999) and the CSM report from the Working Party on MMR vaccine 'Current Problems in Pharmacovigilance', available at: www.open.gov.uk/mca/cuprblms.htm.

INFLUENZA

Influenza is a highly infectious acute viral infection of the respiratory tract transmitted by droplet. The incubation period is only 1–3 days and so epidemics can occur rapidly, particularly amongst those living in close proximity with others, e.g. in nursing homes, cruise ships.

Presentation is usually with a sudden onset of fever, chills, headache and dry cough. The greatest morbidity and mortality will be amongst those with underlying disease such as cardiac or respiratory conditions, and the elderly.

There are three types of influenza virus: A, B and C. Influenza A is responsible for most cases, but influenza B when it occurs is likely to be more severe. Influenza C is usually mild. The influenza A virus has the ability to gradually and slightly change its structure. This is known as 'drift' and because of this drift the composition of the influenza vaccine may need to be altered from year to year. The WHO therefore issues recommendations on an annual basis on the optimal composition of the vaccine.

As well as the ability to 'drift', it is possible for the influenza A virus to occasionally undergo a sudden and dramatic change. This is known as 'shift' and will result in a new or novel strain of influenza A to which no one or very few will have immunity and which will therefore create sudden widespread outbreaks throughout the world – a pandemic. Knott (2001) outlines the phases of a pandemic in detail and discusses the pandemics that have occurred during the 20th century. Probably the most famous of these was the pandemic of 1918 where between 20% and 40% of the world's population were infected and more than 20 million people died as a result of Spanish flu.

The vaccine

An inactivated vaccine grown on hen's eggs which is therefore contraindicated for those with known anaphylactic hypersensitivity to egg.

It should be given as an intramuscular or deep subcutaneous injection into the deltoid for older children and adults and into the anterolateral thigh for babies and infants. The vaccine will provide 70–80% protection against the circulating strains. Ideally it should be administered between October and November to ensure optimal protection before the flu virus is circulating.

Dosages and schedule (DoH 1996)

- Adults and children aged 13 and over should receive a single dose of 0.5 ml on an annual basis.
- Children aged 4–12 years will need two doses of 0.5 ml separated by 4–6 weeks the first time they receive the vaccine.
- Children aged 6 months to 3 years should receive two doses of 0.25 ml the first time they receive the vaccine.

The high-risk groups that the DoH strongly recommends should be offered annual flu vaccination are people who:

- are living in close proximity, e.g. nursing homes
- are over the age of 65 years
- have chronic heart or respiratory disease including asthma
- have chronic renal failure
- have diabetes
- are immunosuppressed due to disease or treatment, e.g. steroid therapy
- are asplenic.

HEPATITIS

Hepatitis is inflammation of the liver which can have a variety of causes but in relation to vaccination, the most significant is viral. Viral hepatitis can be caused by a number of subtypes and to date these have been categorized as A, B, C, D, E and G. There is no effective treatment for hepatitis and the only hepatitis vaccines presently licensed are for A and B serotypes. However, as hepatitis D can only exist in the presence of the hepatitis B virus, vaccination against hepatitis B will also protect against hepatitis D.

Hepatitis A

This will present as fever, headache, fatigue and generalized weakness which can proceed to nausea, vomiting and right abdominal pain caused by liver inflammation, with jaundice, dark urine, and pale stools. Hepatitis A can be severe, mild or in the case of very young children sometimes subclinical. There is no carrier state to this type of hepatitis, but severity will increase with age and owing to the presence of the virus in the stools during the long incubation period (2–6 weeks), it is always highly infectious.

The exact incidence of hepatitis A is difficult to estimate because of differing patterns of the disease. It is spread mainly by the faecal–oral route and is still endemic in developing countries where hygiene practices are less stringent and it is common practice for raw sewage to be dumped in seas. It can also be transmitted by blood and has been associated with the use of factor VIII and IX concentrates where viral inactivation procedures may not destroy hepatitis A.

Hepatitis A vaccine A single dose of hepatitis A vaccine given intramuscularly into the deltoid will provide protection for up to a year. A booster dose at a year will give protection for a further 10 years from the date of the booster.

Adverse reactions are usually mild and may include transient soreness at the injection site. As with any vaccine, flu-like symptoms such as fever, fatigue and headache may occasionally be reported.

High-risk groups that should receive hepatitis A vaccination (DoH 1996)

- Travellers to developing countries
- Existing liver disease

- Haemophiliacs
- Occupational – laboratory workers exposed to the virus, sewage workers, military personnel
- Persons who practise oral anal sex – may include homosexuals and prostitutes
- Drug abusers

Hepatitis B

Transmitted parenterally and sexually, this illness has an insidious onset and presents with anorexia, vague abdominal discomfort, jaundice, nausea and vomiting; fever may be absent or mild. The incubation period is 40–160 days and about 2–10% of those infected are likely to become carriers with an increased risk of hepatocellular carcinoma.

Globally hepatitis B is considered to be the ninth most common cause of death (Kassianos 2001) and the WHO has recommended that countries introduce hepatitis B as part of the routine childhood schedule. The UK has not yet introduced this; instead the DoH recommends vaccination only for specific groups of people at high risk.

Hepatitis B vaccine The standard schedule consists of three doses of vaccine at day 0, 1 month and 6 months after the first dose.

An accelerated schedule is possible where rapid immunization is required, for example in travellers or post exposure. In this case the third dose can be given 2 months after the first dose and then a further booster at 12 months.

In addition, at the time of writing, the GlaxoSmithKline vaccine Engerix B is the only one licensed to be given as a super-accelerated course of 0, 7 and 21 days with a booster at 12 months.

A blood test should be taken 2–4 months after the last injection to check antibody response; in high-risk individuals such as healthcare workers it is probably worthwhile rechecking these every 5 years. An antibody response of:

- below 10 miu/ml is considered a non-response and the person should be given a repeat course of vaccination and if there is no improvement, specific immunoglobulin should be used in a high-risk situation such as needlestick injury
- between 10 and 100 miu/ml is a poor response and a further dose of the vaccine should be given
- 100 miu/ml and over is a good response.

Adverse reactions are usually mild and may include transient soreness at the injection site. As with any vaccine, flu-like symptoms such as fever, fatigue and headache may occasionally be reported.

High-risk groups that should receive hepatitis B vaccination (DoH 1996)

- At birth to babies born to hepatitis B-positive mothers
- Drug abusers
- Individuals with multiple sexual partners
- Close family contacts of a case or carrier
- Families adopting children from countries with a high prevalence of hepatitis B
- Haemophiliacs
- Chronic renal failure
- Residents in accommodation such as that for those with learning disabilities or prisoners
- Occupational – healthcare workers, embalmers and morticians, ambulance, police, staff working in residential accommodation

KEY PRACTICAL AND PROFESSIONAL ISSUES

BEFORE VACCINATION

Patient group directions

Unless the nurse is able to prescribe vaccines, a patient group direction for each vaccine is required as the authorization for nurses to administer vaccines, which are prescription-only medicines. The DoH has issued guidance on the development of patient group directions (DoH 2000) and this subject is covered in detail in Chapter 22.

Vaccine storage

Only potent vaccines can lead to the development of immunity. Vaccines therefore need to be stored in conditions that maintain potency. Maintaining these ideal conditions as vaccines are moved from one environment to the next is known as the *cold chain*. Any break in the cold chain reduces the length of time that vaccines remain potent.

Storage guidelines (DoH 1996)

- Most vaccines can be stored in the range 2–8°C.
- A specific vaccine fridge is ideal.
- A named person should have responsibility for vaccine storage, with a deputy to cover for absence.
- The contact number for the local community pharmacist should be identified in case of need.

- A maximum/minimum thermometer should be placed in the middle of the fridge.
- Maximum/minimum readings should be recorded every working day and the thermometer reset. If the reading is above or below the recommended level, advice can be sought from the local community pharmacist with responsibility for vaccine storage.
- If a vaccine is allowed to freeze it must be discarded as it will not be potent.
- If the fridge does not automatically defrost, this should be done weekly to prevent build-up of ice which will affect temperature control. Vaccines should be stored in another fridge or insulated container during defrosting.
- The fridge should not be packed too tightly – air should be able to circulate.
- Put oldest vaccines at the front of the shelf so that they are used first and always check the expiry date before use.
- Vaccine vials need to be stored in the manufacturer's box as this protects from light and contains product information.
- Remove only one vial from the fridge at a time – this will prevent repeated warming and cooling of vaccines. However, for clinic sessions it may be more appropriate to keep a small number of vaccines in a cool box to prevent constant opening and shutting of the fridge.
- Opened multidose vials should be discarded 4 hours after opening, but whenever possible use single-dose containers.
- No food, drink or specimens should be stored in the vaccine fridge as this encourages opening and shutting of the fridge and can affect temperature control.
- Vaccines ordered directly from the manufacturers, which arrive by post, should not be accepted if more than 48 hours have elapsed since posting.
- Order realistically to ensure that vaccines can be used before the expiry date. Oral polio vaccine, for example, has a short shelf life.

AT VACCINATION

Assessment of patient suitability for vaccination

Before administration of a vaccine, the nurse must ensure that the patient needs and agrees to vaccination and that there are no contraindications. Issues relating to consent are covered in Chapter 22 on professional accountability.

Contraindications to all vaccination

- Acute illness is a contraindication but minor infections, in the absence of fever or systemic upset, are not contraindications.
- Severe local reaction to a previous dose, such as swelling and inflammation which involves most of the circumference of the arm or anterolateral thigh.
- Severe general reaction to a previous dose, which includes:
  - pyrexia of more than 39.5°C within 48 hours of vaccination
  - high-pitched screaming in babies for more than 4 hours
  - convulsions occurring within 72 hours
  - anaphylaxis
  - bronchospasm or laryngeal oedema.

Contraindications to live vaccines

- Pregnant women – unless the need for vaccination outweighs the possible risk to the fetus, for example in yellow fever.
- High-dose corticosteroids within the previous 3 months.
- Chemotherapy within past 6 months.
- Malignancy such as leukaemia.
- Impaired immunological mechanisms such as hypogammaglobulinaemia.
- Another live vaccine within past 3 weeks. However, except for oral typhoid, live vaccines can be given on the same day.
- Yellow fever and BCG vaccines are not advised for HIV-positive people.
- Gammaglobulin within past 3 months. Normal gammaglobulin from the UK is unlikely to contain yellow fever antibodies and so if there is a significant risk of polio, vaccine can be given on the understanding that the immune response will not be as efficient (DoH 1996).

AFTER VACCINATION

The nurse must be able to give routine advice on side-effects and be able to recognize and manage fainting, convulsions and anaphylaxis.

Fainting

This is common after the vaccination of adults and adolescents but uncommon in young children. Patients may complain of feeling faint, giddy or sick. They become pale with a weak, thready pulse and 'pass out'. If the faint is prolonged they may twitch slightly.

Action Patients should lie down with feet slightly raised. If unconscious they should be placed in the recovery position. Tight clothing should be loosened. Patients should normally recover within 2 minutes, but should remain lying down for at least 15 minutes.

Convulsions

These may occur with no warning, but the patient may have a premonition or aura. Tense rhythmic muscle contractions can be observed and the patient may be incontinent. Afterwards they may feel very sleepy.

Action Call for help. Move furniture to prevent injury. Time the convulsion – if longer than 5 minutes it is an emergency situation and may require intravenous or rectal diazepam. Do not insert anything into the mouth. If possible, put patient into the recovery position.

Anaphylaxis

Anaphylaxis is an allergic reaction following exposure to a substance to which the individual has become hypersensitive. The sooner it occurs after vaccination, the more severe it is likely to be. Patients are therefore often advised to wait in the surgery for 20 minutes after vaccination. If vaccination occurs in the patient's home, an adult who could call for assistance should be available to stay with the patient for 20 minutes after vaccination.

The symptoms of anaphylaxis include:

- the site of injection becoming red, swollen and itchy
- patient complaining of rising anxiety, weakness, giddiness, dyspnoea and feeling hot and itchy
- airway obstruction occurring due to angio-oedema involving the epiglottis and larynx. The patient may show signs of stridor or hoarseness and complain of chest tightness. This can lead to respiratory arrest
- hypotension resulting in decreased consciousness and tachycardia
- severe shock resulting in cardiac arrest.

Nurses involved in vaccination must be able to manage an anaphylactic situation should it occur. A shock pack should be available containing at least three ampoules of adrenaline 1:1000; syringes and needles; airways; and a protocol for administration of adrenaline with reduced child doses listed.

Action Explain to the patient that they are having a reaction to the vaccine and this can be treated. Call for help and get the helper to telephone for an ambulance. Give adrenaline 1:1000 (reduced dose for children) by intramuscular injection (DoH 1996). Raise the patient's legs slightly. If there is no improvement, repeat adrenaline up to three times at 10-minute intervals. If the person is unconscious, insert an airway. Begin resuscitation if necessary.

All cases of anaphylaxis should be observed for at least 6 hours, in case of any delayed reactions, and hospital admission is required (DoH 1996).

Record the incident in the patient's practice notes with the name of the drug that was administered. Complete a yellow card (in the British National Formulary) and send to the Committee on Safety of Medicines.

Between 1992 and 1995, 87 anaphylactic reactions were reported but no deaths occurred. During this period approximately 55 million vaccines were supplied to GP practices and hospitals (DoH 1996).

Although anaphylactic reactions to vaccination are rare, they cannot be predicted and have the potential to be fatal without treatment. **Remember, no one should give vaccinations without access to adrenaline or assistance.**

Disposal and spillage

Vaccines should be disposed of by incineration (DoH 1996).

If a vaccine is accidentally spilt onto the skin, it should be washed off thoroughly with soap and hot water. If any vaccine is splashed into the eyes, they should be irrigated with sodium chloride solution and medical advice sought.

Gloves should be worn and swabs used to mop up spillage on surfaces. Swabs should be disposed of in a bin for incineration and the surface cleaned with a hypochlorite solution.

CONCLUSION

Nurses have a key role in the national vaccination programme and this is recognized and supported by the Department of Health (DoH 1996). The work of nurses in the area of vaccination has been one of the greatest of all health promotion successes. Diseases which were once common, such as diphtheria and polio, are now virtually unknown in this country. Therefore it is understandable that nowadays people seem more concerned about the possible risks associated with vaccines than the morbidity and mortality associated with the diseases. However, as outlined in detail by Kassianos (2001), the bottom line is that in comparison to the diseases, the potential of harm from the vaccinations available as part of our national programme is minimal.

References

American Academy of Pediatrics 2000 The Red Book – the report of the Committee on Infectious Diseases, 25th edn. American Academy of Pediatrics, Elk Grove Village, Illinois

Aszkensay OM, George RC, Begg NT 1995 Pneumococcal bacteraemia and meningitis in England and Wales 1982–92. Communicable Disease Report 5:45–50

Barakk LJ, Manclark C, Cherry J et al 1989 Analyses of adverse reactions to diphtheria and tetanus toxoids and pertussis vaccine by vaccine lot, endotoxin content, pertussis vaccine potency and percentage of mouse gain. Paediatric Infectious Diseases Journal 8:502–507

Conaty S 2000 Meningitec: conjugate meningococcal C vaccine. Prescriber July:51–54

Conrad D, Jenson H 1999 Using acellular pertussis vaccines for childhood immunisation. Postgraduate Medicine 105(7):165–178

DoH 1996 Immunisation against infectious diseases. HMSO, London

DoH 2000 Safety of the meningitis C vaccine programme. Press release by Deputy Chief Medical Officer

DoH 2001a Health information for overseas travel. HMSO, London

DoH 2001b Whooping cough booster vaccine to be given to pre-school children. Press release 2001/0478

DoH 2002 Department of Health immunisation 2001–2 stats bulletin. Department of Health, London

Erikson L 1998 Complications and sequelae of meningococcal disease in Quebec, Canada, 1990–1994. Clinical Infectious Diseases 26:1159–1164

Finn A, Bell F 2000 Time to switch from whole cell to acellular pertussis vaccine? British Medical Journal 320:975

Health Education Authority 1997 A guide to childhood immunisation. HMSO, London

Howard AJ, Dunkin KT, Millar GW 1998 Nasopharyngeal carriage and antibiotic resistance of Haemophilus influenzae in healthy children. Epidemiology and Infection 100:193–203

Kassianos GC 2001 Immunisation: childhood and travel health, 4th edn. Blackwell Science, Oxford

Knott C 2001 Influenza: epidemiology and prevention. Primary Health Care Journal 11(7):27–32

Long S, Welkon C, Clark J 1990 Widespread silent transmission of pertussis in families: antibody correlates of infection and symptomatology. Journal of Infectious Disease 161:480–486

Lopez A, Blumberg D 1997 An overview of the status of acellular pertussis vaccines in practice. Drugs 54(2):189–195

Maple P, Efstratiou A, George R et al 1995 Diphtheria immunity in UK: blood donors. Lancet 345:963–965

Miller E, Waight P 2001 Immunogenicity and reactogenicity of acellular diphtheria/tetanus/pertussis vaccines given as a pre-school booster: effect of simultaneous administration with MMR. Vaccine 19:3904–3911

Montgomery S, Morris D, Pounder R et al 1999 Paramyxovirus infections in childhood and subsequent inflammatory bowel disease. Gastroenterology 116:798–803

PHLS 1999 Meningoccocal factsheet. Public Health Laboratory Service

Reid D, Grist NR 1988 The history of immunisation. Practice Nurse Journal 1(3):130–134

Ryan C 2000 Measles epidemic in Ireland threatens mainland Britain. Nursing Times 96(33):10

Southgate L, Lockie C, Heard S, Wood M 1997 Infection. Oxford Medical Press, Oxford

Taylor B, Miller E, Farrington C et al 1999 Autism and measles, mumps and rubella vaccine: no epidemiological evidence for a causal association. Lancet 353:2026–2029

Vedros NA 1987 The development of meningococcal serogroups. In: Vedro NA (ed) Evolution of meningococcal disease, vol II. CRC Press, Florida, pp33–37

Wakefield A, Murch S, Anthony A et al 1998 Ileal-lymphoid-modular hyperplasia, non specific colitis and persuasive developmental disorder in children. Lancet 351:637–641

WHO 1999a Pertussis vaccines: WHO position paper. Weekly Epidemiological Record 74(18):137–144

WHO 1999b Making a difference. World Health Organization, Geneva

WHO 2000 International travel and health. World Health Organization, Geneva

Resources

World Health Organization (WHO):
www.who.int/
www.who.int/ith/english/risks.htm

Department of Health (DoH):
www.open.gov.uk/doh/
www.open.gov.uk/doh/hat/index.htm

MMR website: www.mmrthefacts.nhs.uk/

Public Health Laboratory Service (PHLS):
www.phls.co.uk
www.phls.co.uk/advice/
www.phls.co.uk/facts/influenza/activity9900/fluact02.htm

Foreign Office: www.fco.gov.uk/

Lonely Planet: www.lonelyplanet.com

Email discussion lists

ISTM (for members only): Bcbistm@aol.com

Practice nurse group: Practicenurse@egroups.com

Travel databases

TRAVAX: www.axl.co.uk/scieh

MASTA: Information from: 01705 553 933

Chapter 6

Travel health

Jeannett Martin

CHAPTER CONTENTS

INTRODUCTION

This chapter outlines the health risks associated with travel abroad and provides practical information relating to the provision of a travel health service within general practice. General issues relating to vaccines are addressed in Chapter 5.

There are over 50.8 million visits abroad by UK residents every year and around 6 million of these are to developing countries (ONS 2002). Less than 5% of illness associated with travel abroad is vaccine preventable and the main risks to health will be those related to behaviour (Steffan & Dupont 1994). A review of the literature (Martin 1996) identified important areas to include when giving travel health advice.

Table 6.1 Levels of risk

Level of risk	Risk factors	Recommendations
Minor	>40 years Obese Previous leg swelling Recent minor injury Varicose veins	Non-alcoholic fluids Walking around plane Ankle-stretching exercises Support stockings
Moderate	Pregnant Hormone therapy Recent major leg injury Family history of thrombophilia	As for minor risk Also consider aspirin before flight
Higher	Previous DVT Known clotting tendency Recent major surgery	As for minor risk Instead of aspirin consider single injection of low-dose molecular heparin before and after flight

FITNESS TO FLY

During ascent atmospheric pressure falls which creates a fall in each constituent gas in the air, the most significant to the traveller being the decrease in the partial pressure of oxygen. Aeroplane cabin pressure is maintained at around 6000 feet in order that the partial pressure of oxygen is at an acceptable level for most travellers.

However, those with an existing oxygen deficiency may develop hypoxia (Harding 1994). Symptoms of hypoxia include euphoria, impaired judgement, incoordination (mental and muscular), cyanosis and in extreme cases death. Smokers will have decreased oxygen-carrying capacity due to the carbon monoxide levels in their blood and consumption of alcohol during a flight can enhance symptoms of hypoxia (Harding 1994).

During ascent the fall in pressure also causes expansion of gases within the body which could rupture recent thoracic or abdominal wounds. On descent total pressure increases and gas inside the middle ear and sinuses contracts. If the eustachian tubes are clear this self-corrects but if they are blocked a pressure differential can develop and there will be severe pain due to barotrauma as the eardrum is drawn inwards (Harding 1994).

Travellers should be advised to contact the airline if they will need additional oxygen during the flight, as this must be booked in advance. The British Lung Foundation (020 7831 5831) will provide advice. In addition, the airline will advise on an individual basis if travellers have special needs or if there are concerns regarding fitness to fly. However, most airlines will consider the following as absolute contraindications for scheduled air travel.

- Pregnancy >35 weeks gestation
- Abdominal surgery <10 days prior to travel
- Chest surgery <2 weeks prior to travel
- Recent cerebral or myocardial infarction
- Uncontrolled cardiac failure
- Severe anaemia
- Severe sinusitis, otitis media or recent ear surgery
- Peptic ulceration <3 weeks prior to travel
- Unstable epilepsy
- Plaster casts unless they can be split prior to flight
- Fractures of mandible with fixed wiring of the jaw
- Communicable disease
- Mental illness without escort and sedation
- Introduction of air into body cavities for diagnostic purposes <7 days prior to travel
- Terminally ill people unlikely to survive the journey

It is thought that the risk of deep vein thrombosis and pulmonary embolism may be increased due to the prolonged immobilization during long-haul flights (over 5 hours), dehydration, the cramped position and pressure of the seat on the popliteal vein (Giangrande 2000). The House of Lords Select Committee on Air Travel (2000) suggested that this syndrome should be described as traveller's thrombosis rather than economy-class syndrome because it is not confined to those travelling economy class. The report categorized travellers' risk as minor, moderate and high and made some recommendations for reducing risk during travel which have been reflected in DoH guidelines (DoH 2001).

JET LAG

Rapid travel across time zones causes a desynchronization of circadian rhythms governed by environmental cues such as the clock hour, light and temperature. Symptoms include insomnia, poor-quality sleep, daytime fatigue, poor concentration, gastrointestinal disturbances. This will persist until the body systems readjust. For business travellers this may have a significant impact on performance.

Adaptation to travel eastward generally takes longer than westward (DoH 2001). Prevention measures include planning arrival to coincide with bedtime, allowing time to readjust before important meetings, taking daytime exercise, avoiding alcohol and caffeine before bedtime.

Melatonin is produced naturally by the pineal gland in hours of darkness. It affects the sleep/wake cycle and its synthesis and secretion are inhibited by bright light. There has been some interest in the use of melatonin to prevent jet lag, but there is little data yet on its safety profile or on when and how much to take. It is available for purchase over the counter (OTC) in America but it is not a licensed drug in the UK or available for purchase here OTC.

ACCIDENTS

Accidents abroad include road traffic accidents relating to poorly maintained vehicles and roads, sports, swimming and diving accidents. They are frequently alcohol related and the highest risk group will be males in their early 20s in whom accidents are the main cause of death abroad (Paixio et al 1991).

Treatment for accidents can involve risks associated with the medical services in developing countries. For example, blood transfusions, needles and syringes can carry the risk of hepatitis B and C, malaria and HIV.

In countries such as Thailand, India or China, rabies is endemic and animal bites must be considered high risk. Bites and scratches should be washed for at least 5 minutes under a running tap to remove all dirt and saliva, then rinsed well before applying povidone iodine or 40% alcohol (gin or whisky is a suitable alternative). The traveller should access medical assistance within 24 hours and if there is any risk at all of rabies then postexposure treatment should be given, consisting of immunoglobulin (20 iu/kg of bodyweight) and a five-dose vaccination course on days 0, 3, 7, 14, 30 if no preexposure vaccination course had been given before travel. If preexposure vaccination had already been administered then two doses of rabies vaccine on days 0 and 3–7 without immunoglobulin can be given (Kassianos 2001).

If travellers wait until return to the UK to seek advice regarding possible rabies risk associated with an animal bite they had abroad then the practice should contact the Public Health Laboratory or its equivalent in Wales, Scotland and Northern Ireland (contact numbers will be in the Green Book (DoH 1996)), for advice and supplies of vaccine for post-exposure treatment.

TRAVELLER'S DIARRHOEA

In developing countries water is often poorly treated and usually unsafe to drink. McIntosh et al (1997) estimated that 40% of travellers from the UK to developing countries will be affected by traveller's diarrhoea and many travellers will be seriously ill with the possibility of long-term complications (Farthing 1995). The majority of traveller's diarrhoea will be bacterial in origin (Farthing 1995), but viruses and protozoa can also be involved.

The pathogenic mechanisms will involve either absorptive dysfunction of the small bowel where enterotoxins bind to intestinal cells and act on biochemical mechanisms of small bowel villi which causes increased loss of sodium chloride and bicarbonate and will present as severe watery diarrhoea. Or there will be invasion and inflammation of mucosa and ulceration of the bowel wall with inflammation and systemic toxicity. Symptoms of this will be fever, severe cramps and blood and mucus in the stool.

Whatever the causative organism, the main risk to health is dehydration. Treatment should focus on rehydration therapy either with commercially available preparations such as Dioralyte or Rehidrat or with an 8:1 sugar-to-salt solution made up using a litre of safe (boiled) water. Loperamide for symptom control can be used for up to 48 hours but not for young children under 12 years or if there is bloody

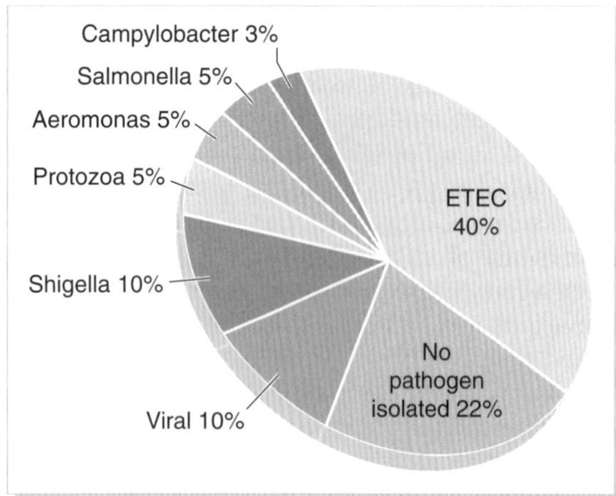

Figure 6.1 Pathogens involved in traveller's diarrhoea (Farthing 1995).

diarrhoea. Medical advice should be sought immediately if bloody diarrhoea (dysentery) is observed or if the person becomes unable to drink. Carbohydrate foods, e.g. bananas, rice and potatoes, can aid recovery and babies should continue to be breastfed.

Absorption of oral contraception can be affected by severe diarrhoea and also by antibiotics required for its treatment. Additional contraceptive precautions, such as condoms, should be used for 7 days after the diarrhoea stops to reduce risk of unplanned pregnancy. In addition, if the woman is taking antibiotics that will extend into the pill-free week she should not have a break between the present and next packet (Kassianos 2001).

Prevention is by ensuring that only safe water is used for drinking, ice and teeth cleaning. This should ideally be boiled but if bottled water is used then carbonated is a safer option than still, as these bottles may have been filled with local tap water.

Also important is to avoid high-risk foods such as:

- shellfish – filter feeders harvested from seas where sewage is dumped
- salads – may be grown in soil fertilized with human manure
- buffet food – kept warm which enables fast multiplication of pathogens
- milk products – often not pasteurized.

Travellers who have preexisting conditions that would be compromised by an episode of severe diarrhoea, e.g. diabetes or immunosuppression, may be recommended to take a supply of Ciproxin abroad with them (Farthing 1995). Ericsson et al (1997) recommended one 500 mg dose of Ciproxin to shorten the severity and duration of an episode of traveller's diarrhoea. In cases of severe diarrhoea they recommended 500 mg bd for 3 days and 500 mg bd for 5 days in dysentery.

SEA AND FRESHWATER BATHING

In developing countries, raw sewage is often dumped in seas and rivers. Swimming in these waters can lead to eye, ear or stomach infections and women water-skiers can develop vaginal infection due to high-speed vaginal douches with sewage-polluted water.

Freshwater lakes in Africa and the Far East, such as Lake Malawi, are frequently contaminated with flatworm schistosomes. The eggs of the worms, excreted by an infected human, hatch in fresh water where they colonize snails. Once mature, they enter the fresh water and penetrate the skin of a human swimming in the water; the worms migrate to the bladder or intestine where they lay their eggs. Bilharzia can be asymptomatic for many years but can cause haematuria, anaemia or even bladder cancer (Bell 1995).

It is advisable for children to wear protective plastic sandals while playing in the sea to reduce the risk of stings and bites from marine animals.

Fish stings can be treated by immersing the affected limb in hot water (45°). Jellyfish stings can be extremely painful and should be inactivated with vinegar. Any adherent tentacles need to be removed very carefully – not with bare hands. The most dangerous jellyfish is the box jellyfish found in the Indian Ocean and this may require treatment with antivenom.

Sea urchin spines can become embedded in feet but it is essential to remove them completely as if left they become badly infected; they may need to be surgically removed.

SUN PROTECTION

Drinking plenty of fluids and remaining indoors during the hottest part of the day will be effective in preventing both heat exhaustion and also heatstroke, which can be an emergency situation.

Exposure to ultraviolet radiation can cause short-term and long-term skin damage. Short-term damage can present initially as sunburn involving redness and soreness or swelling and blistering; tanning then develops in order to protect the skin from further exposure and the skin can also become dry and thickened. Long-term changes include premature ageing and discoloration because of permanent thickening and also an increased risk of malignant melanoma and non-melanotic skin cancer. In the UK there has been a year-on-year increase in malignant melanoma (DoH 2001). Exposure to the sun is a risk factor that could be modified to reduce the incidence of this cancer but would require a shift in attitude towards tanning.

Health education advice relating to sun protection includes the following.

- Wear a hat and T-shirt.
- Avoid sunbathing during the hottest part of the day (11am–2pm).
- Use a sun protection factor (SPF) sunscreen. SPF15 is adequate but needs to be used liberally (about a handful will be enough to cover the body) and frequently (every hour).

SEXUAL HEALTH

Travellers may consume more alcohol than usual while on holiday, which may lower inhibitions and reduce caution towards risks associated with sexual encounters, including sexually transmitted infections (STIs). These include hepatitis B, which globally is the ninth most common cause of death, and HIV whose primary means of spread worldwide is by heterosexual contact.

Condoms provide some protection and women should be encouraged to use these in addition to the oral contraceptive pill to help prevent STIs and to prevent pregnancy if they have traveller's diarrhoea or need antibiotics while abroad. However, travellers should be aware that they ought to buy condoms in the UK before travel as those available abroad may be unreliable or the size too small to be comfortable.

If returned travellers present for advice about possible HIV risk due to unprotected sexual contact abroad, consider referral to the local GUM clinic which can offer pretest counselling, contact tracing and screening for other treatable STIs.

Emergency contraception is not always available abroad and some travellers may choose to take this with them. There are two types available: PC4 (ethinyloestradiol and levonorgestrel) and progestogen only (Levonelle).

Two tablets of PC4 or one tablet of Levonelle should be taken as soon as possible after unprotected intercourse, but within 72 hours. A second dose of two PC4 tablets or one of Levonelle will be required. It is important to then use condoms until the next menstrual period.

ALTITUDE

Appropriate clothing is essential as extreme cold can cause frostbite and hypothermia. In addition, sunscreens and eye goggles will be required to protect against the effects of reflected ultraviolet radiation. Females intending to climb above 4500 metres should discuss contraception 3–6 months before travel as the combined oral contraceptive pill is contraindicated (Kassianos 2001), due to the increased risk of thrombosis at altitude, and a new method may need to be established.

ACUTE MOUNTAIN SICKNESS (AMS)

Symptoms of benign AMS include headache, dizziness, loss of appetite, nausea, vomiting and sleeplessness. Treatment involves rest and acclimatization for 1–2 days. If symptoms persist, descent is essential.

HIGH-ALTITUDE PULMONARY OEDEMA (HAPE)

AMS usually precedes this. HAPE presents with severe breathlessness and a cough. This starts as a dry cough but then becomes bubbly and bloodstained. This is a medical emergency and immediate descent is essential even during the hours of darkness.

HIGH-ALTITUDE CEREBRAL OEDEMA (HACE)

Can be a complication of AMS. Develops over 1–3 days but can kill within 12 hours of onset. Symptoms include confusion, unsteady gait, abnormal behaviour and coma. This is a medical emergency and immediate descent is essential even during the hours of darkness.

Prevention of altitude-related illness is by gradual ascent. Once above 3000 metres, no more than 300 metres should be climbed every day and a rest day scheduled for every 3 days or 1000 metres. Alcohol and sedatives should be avoided.

Prophylactic acetazolamide 250 mg bd starting 1–2 days before ascent (Kassianos 2001) has been used for preventing altitude illness, particularly in those who have to ascend quickly, e.g. mountain rescue teams, but it does not protect against cerebral or pulmonary oedema. Impaired renal function is a contraindication (DoH 2001) and it can cause pins and needles in fingers and toes for the first few days.

Table 6.2 Approximate altitude of some destinations

Destination	Metres	Feet
Addis Ababa	2400	8000
Annapurna (Nepal)	8078	26 504
Ararat (Turkey)	5185	17 011
Cotopaxi (Andes)	5897	19 347
Darjeeling	2200	7000
Etna (Sicily)	3390	11 122
Everest	8850	29 000
Everest base camp	5500	18 000
Hood (Oregon)	3426	11 239
Jungfrau (Switzerland)	4158	13 642
Lassen Peak (California)	3187	10 457
Matterhorn (Alps)	4478	14 692
Mexico City	2300	7500
Mount Kenya	5000	17 000
Olympus (Greece)	2917	9570
Whitney (California)	4417	14 491
Skiing resorts:		
Aspen	2500–3500	8000–11 000
Val d'Isere	1800–3500	6600–11 000
Zermatt	1600–3800	5300–12 500

MALARIA

Malaria is a common tropical disease caused by the parasite plasmodium, which is usually transmitted to humans by the bite of an infected female anopheles mosquito. There are four types of plasmodium: falciparum, vivax, malariae and ovalae. Falciparum is often referred to as malignant malaria due to the associated high risk of mortality; the others are often referred to as benign malaria.

The population of malarial zones who survive their childhood will have immunity but this requires constant reexposure to the parasite and will be lost if they move to a non-malarial area. Malaria is a notifiable disease in the UK and any case diagnosed must be reported to the consultant in communicable disease. In 2000 there were 2069 cases of malaria imported into the UK and 16 deaths (Bradley & Bannister 2001); the majority of these occurred in ethnic travellers who had been to visit friends and relatives in their country of origin and had not taken chemoprophylaxis.

There is no vaccine against malaria, but the *Guidelines for malaria prevention in travellers from the United Kingdom* advise that travellers can reduce their risk of the disease if provided with health education advice on awareness of risk, bite prevention, chemoprophylaxis and recognition of symptoms (Bradley & Bannister 2003). These guidelines are developed by the Advisory Committee on Malaria Prevention; they are available electronically from the Health Protection Agency (HPA) website on

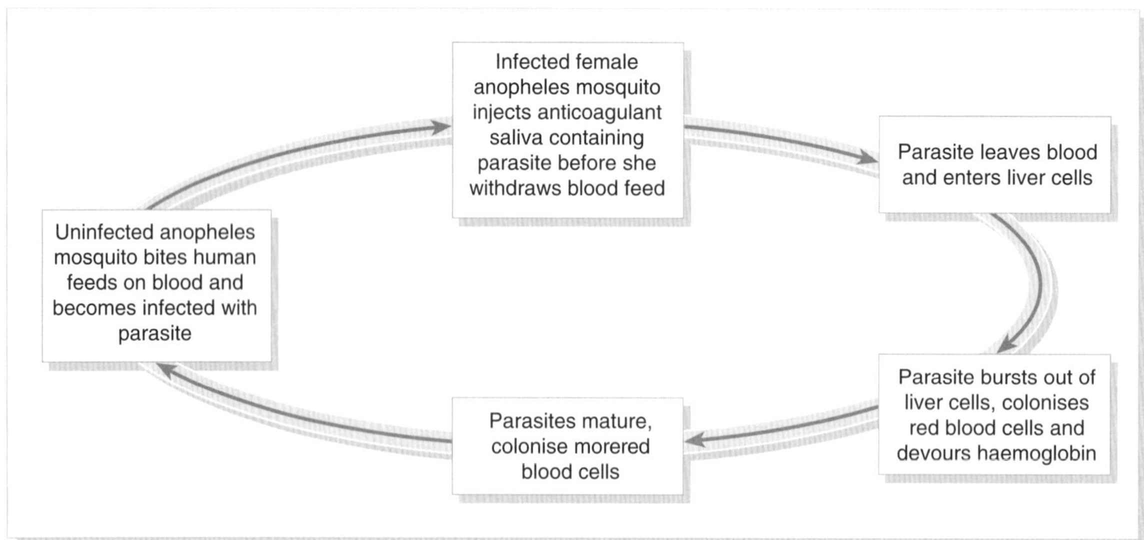

Figure 6.2 Lifecycle of plasmodium.

www.hpa.org.uk/infections/topics_az/malaria/menu/htm.

BITE PREVENTION

There is no evidence that electronic buzzers or vitamin B12 have any protective effect but measures recommended as being effective include the following.

- Insect repellents containing DEET – use according to manufacturer's instructions.
- Covering arms and legs after dusk.
- Avoiding stagnant water where mosquitoes breed.
- Avoiding perfume and dark colours which attract mosquitoes.
- Sleeping under undamaged, permethrin-impregnated bednets.
- Using knockdown sprays.

CHEMOPROPHYLAXIS

Recommendations are based on the destination, season, duration of stay, accommodation, activities, e.g. safari, style of travel, e.g. backpacking, and the drug resistance of the parasites in that area (DoH 2001).

However, all chemoprophylaxis will have contraindications and possible side-effects so it is important to look at the traveller's individual suitability for the recommended chemoprophylaxis. Suitability will depend on age, likelihood of pregnancy, previous experience with antimalarials, family history of epilepsy, concomitant medical conditions and medications.

In areas of no chloroquine resistance the 2003 guidelines advise either chloroquine or proguanil could be recommended. In areas of some resistance a combination of chloroquine and proguanil is recommended, but where there is widespread resistance then the alternatives are mefloquine, doxycycline or

Table 6.3 Malaria chemoprophylaxis

Drug	Contraindications	Side-effects
Chloroquine	Epilepsy Exacerbation of psoriasis	Headaches, convulsions Pruritus, rash, hair loss Blurred vision, dizziness Gastrointestinal problems
Proguanil	Severe renal problems (creatinine >150 μmol/l)	As for chloroquine Aphthous-like mouth ulcers
Mefloquine	Epilepsy, depression Psychiatric illness Cardiac and liver problems Pregnancy 1st trimester & 3 m before pregnancy Breastfeeding, infants <5 kg	Nausea, vomiting, loose stools Headaches, dizziness, abdominal pain Drowsiness, insomnia Nightmares, fatigue, vertigo RARE: depression, suicidal, restlessness, hallucination, psychosis
Doxycycline	Pregnancy and lactation Children <12 years	Diarrhoea, thrush Photosensitivity (3–10%) Teeth discoloration in neonate and young children Oesophagitis May affect absorption of oral contraceptive pill
Malarone	Severe renal failure (creatinine clr <30 ml/min) Pregnancy/lactation (no data) Under 40 kg (no data) Not concurrently with rifampicin/rifambutin/metoclopramide/tetracycline (↓ plasma atovaquone) More than 28 days' stay	Abdominal pain, nausea, anorexia Diarrhoea and vomiting Gastric intolerance, mouth ulcers Headaches, insomnia Anaemia, neutropenia Cough Elevated liver enzymes

Table 6.4 Adult doses and schedules (always check with data sheet) (TRAVAX 2000)

Drug name	Usual dose	Start	Stop
Chloroquine	300 mg weekly	1 week before travel	4 weeks after return
Proguanil	200 mg daily	1 week before travel	4 weeks after return
Mefloquine	250 mg weekly	1 week before travel; if not used previously, 3 weeks before	4 weeks after return
Doxycycline	100 mg daily	3 days before travel	Up to a maximum of 3 months at destination and then 4 weeks after return
Malarone	250 mg atovaquone and 100 mg proguanil per day	1–2 days before travel	Up to a maximum of 28 days at destination and then 7 days after return

malarone and chloroquine and proguanil would only be recommended if none of these can be used.

Advice on chemoprophylaxis for special groups of travellers

Children Can quickly die from malaria. Deterioration is related to rapid increases in parasite density, possibly because of the lower red blood cell mass (Brabin & Ganley 1997). The WHO (2000) strongly advises against young children being taken to malarial zones. If travel is unavoidable strict adherence to preventive measures is essential.

Long-term travellers May be spending several years in a malarial zone. The WHO (2000) recommends that they follow routine advice relating to chemoprophylaxis for the first 1–3 months, but then seek further advice from local healthcare providers familiar with malaria management in non-immune travellers.

Frequent travellers Such as aircrew who make short stops but over a long period of time may decide to use chemoprophylaxis only when visiting high-risk areas. In these cases standby treatment may need to be considered.

Ethnic travellers returning to their country of origin

In areas of very high transmission children who survive are likely to develop immunity to falciparum. This immunity depends on frequent reexposure and will gradually disappear if they leave their home to live in a non-malarial zone. Any children that are born in their new country of residence will not have any immunity passed on to them.

Therefore ethnic minority travellers, and their children, who return home to visit friends and relatives in their country of origin are as likely as any other non-immune tourist to develop malaria if bitten and so do need to take chemoprophylaxis in the same way.

RECOGNITION OF SYMPTOMS

Chemoprophylaxis is not 100% effective and dormant parasites may emerge from the liver after chemoprophylaxis has been discontinued. Malaria most commonly presents as flu-like symptoms which recur every 2–3 days. Fever often has three distinct stages.

- Cold: shivers, rigors, rapid temperature rises
- Hot: flushed, pulse rapid, pyrexial
- Sweating: drenched, temperature drops suddenly

Other possible symptoms include vomiting and diarrhoea (not bloody), delirium, confusion, coma, convulsion, renal failure and jaundice.

In falciparum malaria death can occur very quickly, so the importance of seeking medical advice if symptoms present should not be underestimated. When they contact their doctor, patients should inform the GP that they have been in a malarial area.

DENGUE

This is an arboviral infection, increasing in incidence and transmitted by *Aedes aegypti* which is a daytime biter. The risk to travellers is about 1:1000 (Kassianos 2001) and depends on their level of exposure; there is a lower risk during short visits and in air-conditioned accommodation.

There are four serotypes of the virus (1,2,3,4). The disease can be mild but severity increases with age. Infection will result in lifelong immunity to the serotype contracted but not to any of the others. A second infection after that first exposure, but with another serotype, is much more likely to result in dengue haemorrhagic fever (DHF) which can be life threatening.

Therefore any vaccine developed must be a multivalent that provides protection against all four serotypes, not monovalent as this may leave patients at a higher risk of contracting DHF if they are infected with another serotype after vaccination. So far it has not been possible to combine all four serotypes of dengue in order to produce a vaccine.

Prevention is by strict bite prevention in the same manner as for malarial vectors but as dengue is transmitted by *Aedes aegypti*, these measures need to be followed during the daytime.

VACCINATIONS FOR TRAVELLERS

Details of contraindications, special precautions and schedules for individual vaccines can be obtained from the Green Book (DoH 1996). An excellent additional resource is the textbook on vaccination *Immunisation, childhood and travel health* by George Kassianos (2001).

Travel to northern Europe, North America and New Zealand does not present a very different risk of vaccine-preventable disease from that in the UK, but travellers should be advised regarding updating vaccinations recommended for the UK (DoH 1996). Other destinations may carry additional risk and vaccination should be offered in line with published recommendations (see Table 6.5).

HEPATITIS A

Common in developing countries, highly infectious virus transmitted by the faecal–oral route. Mortality and morbidity relating to hepatitis A increase with age. Although it can be subclinical in children, some children will become ill and, of course, they will all shed the virus during the incubation period of 15–40 days and this may cause outbreaks within the community on their return from abroad. The vaccine (course of two doses) gives protection for 10 years. Specific immunoglobulin for hepatitis A is not now recommended for travellers as some level of protection will be obtained from the vaccine even if travelling soon after vaccination.

CHOLERA

Cholera is spread via contaminated water or food. Seafood has frequently been a source of cholera, particularly raw or undercooked shellfish.

The inactivated oral vaccine now available in the UK is Dukoral from Powderject Pharmaceuticals. Dukoral will provide a protective efficacy against cholera of 80–85% for the first 6 months, reducing to about 63% over a 3-year period. It will also provide some protection against ETEC diarrhoea.

Two doses of vaccine are recommended for adults and children over the age of 6 years. Children from 2 to 6 years should receive three doses. Doses are administered at intervals of at least a week but no more than 6 weeks.

HEPATITIS B

Countries such as Africa, parts of Asia and South America have a high carrier rate. Transmission is by contact with blood and body fluids and the incubation period is between 40 and 160 days.

Unprotected sex with a local contact, blood transfusions or medical treatment with poorly sterilized equipment after an accident, body piercing or tattooing may carry a high risk. Vaccination is available either as a course of three over 6 months or an accelerated course of three over 2 months with a booster at 12 months. A combined hepatitis A and B vaccine is also available.

TYPHOID

Risk is not as high as for hepatitis A, but does increase if sanitation is poor. Transmission is by the faecal–oral route and incubation is between 1 and 3 weeks. About 2–5% of cases will become chronic carriers.

Inactivated injectable vaccines are available which give protection for 3 years. There is also a combined hepatitis A/typhoid vaccine available. The booster for the hepatitis A component is given at the usual time using an ordinary hepatitis A vaccine.

DIPHTHERIA

Still prevalent in developing countries with known outbreaks in Russia. Transmitted by droplet infection. Immunity levels to diphtheria are known to be low in the UK adult population so vaccination should be considered if close contact is expected with the local population, e.g. using public transport. The high-dose vaccine used for young children can cause severe reactions in adults; low-dose combined diphtheria/tetanus vaccine should be used for travellers over 10 years.

MENINGITIS A AND C

Transmitted by droplet infection. The highest risk area is the meningitis belt of Africa during the dry season January to May. The vaccine gives protection for 3 years against A and C strains but no protection against the B strain most commonly found in the UK. Pilgrims to Mecca for the Hajj will be required to produce a certificate of vaccination for meningitis ACWY dated at least 10 days before departure in order to enter the country.

Travellers who have been previously vaccinated with the meningitis C conjugate vaccine as part of the UK schedule may have the A and C vaccine after an interval of 2 weeks. Where meningitis C conjugate vaccine needs to be given after the meningitis A and C then, unless the situation is high risk, there should be an interval of 6 months (DoH 2001).

YELLOW FEVER

Caused by an arbovirus occurring in Africa and South America and spread from monkeys to man (jungle yellow fever) or man to man (urban yellow fever) by daytime-biting mosquitoes. Incubation is 3–6 days.

Some countries require an international certificate of vaccination dated 10 days prior to entry (if travelling from another country where yellow fever is present). The live vaccine can only be given at DoH-approved yellow fever centres and one dose protects for 10 years.

RABIES

A viral infection transmitted by the bite or scratch of an infected mammal. Rabies is present in many countries but endemic in India and Thailand. Once symptoms develop rabies is always fatal. A course of three injections may be advised before travel and is especially important if travellers are unlikely to be able to access medical assistance within 24 hours if bitten.

Full preexposure vaccination does not eliminate the need for treatment if the traveller is bitten. It does, however, reduce the number of postexposure rabies vaccinations required from five to two injections and there will be no need for additional rabies-specific immunoglobulin (Kassianos 2001).

TICKBORNE ENCEPHALITIS

High-risk areas are forested areas of Scandinavia, central and eastern Europe during spring to summer. The virus is transmitted by the bite of an infected tick. Incubation is between 2 and 14 days. Two doses of vaccine are given 1–3 months apart and protect for 1 year; a third dose 9–12 months later will extend protection for 3 years (Kassianos 2001). It is unlicensed in the UK and available on a named patient basis.

JAPANESE B ENCEPHALITIS

Viral infection transmitted by mosquitoes that breed near rice paddies. It occurs in the Far East and south-east Asia mainly around the monsoon season. Although rare, incidence increases in longer stay travellers or those living near breeding sites of the vector. There is a high mortality rate amongst those who become symptomatic and about 30% of survivors have permanent neurological sequelae.

Three doses of the inactivated vaccine are required for longer term exposure but two doses will give short-term protection (DoH 1996). It is an unlicensed vaccine in the UK and available on a named patient basis. Because of the increased risk of an allergic reaction the vaccination course should be completed 10 days before travel and the patient be kept under observation for 30 minutes after vaccination (DoH 1996).

BCG

Tuberculosis is prevalent in Asia, Africa, Central and South America. Testing and then vaccination should be considered for previously unvaccinated travellers, but the vaccine is often in short supply.

Table 6.5 Travel vaccination schedules (Kassianos 2001) (guidance only – individual vaccines may vary slightly so it is important to follow manufacturer's instructions on schedules as outlined in the product information leaflet)

Vaccine	Primary course	Booster	Comments
Diphtheria/tetanus combined	3 doses at monthly intervals	10 yearly for those at risk	Low-dose diphtheria required for travellers over 10 years of age High-dose diphtheria required for children under 10 years of age. This is usually given as part of the childhood schedule at 2, 3, 4 months, preschool and then boosted before school leaving
Hepatitis A	2 doses 6–12 months apart	10 years	Junior hepatitis A vaccine available for children <16 years (<18 years Vaqta). Use vaccine for actual age they are at time of any subsequent doses
Hepatitis B	3 doses at 0, 1, 6 months Accelerated course 0, 1, 2, 12 months. Engerix B only has very accelerated course licensed of 0, 7, 21 days plus 12 months	5 years	Check antibodies 5 yearly for those at high risk; boost if <100 iu
Hepatitis A and B combined	0, 1, 6 months	Hep A (monovalent) at 10 years. Hep B single booster at 5 years	
Japanese B encephalitis	3 doses at 0, 7–14, 30 days	2 years if remaining at risk	Unlicensed vaccine needs to be given on a named patient basis Anaphylactic reaction possible up to 2 weeks postvaccination. Travellers should complete course at least 10 days before departure and remain at surgery for 30 minutes after vaccination A two-dose schedule may give short-term immunity in 80% vaccinees Children under 3 years should receive 0.5 ml by deep subcutaneous injection
Meningitis A and C	Single injection	If at continued risk 3 years for AC Vax and 5 years for Meningivac	
Meningitis ACYW-135	Single injection	3 years if at continued risk	Certificate of vaccination at least 10 days prior to travel required for pilgrims to the Hajj
Rabies	3 doses at 0, 7, 28 days	2–3 years if at continued risk (Rabipur 2–5 years)	Postexposure vaccination If preexposure has been given – 2 doses at 0, 3–7 days If no preexposure has been given – 5 doses at 0, 3, 7, 14, 30 days plus specific rabies immunoglobulin, half infiltrated around bite, the rest IM into the deltoid
Tickborne encephalitis	3 doses at 0, 1–3 and 9–12 months	3 yearly if remaining at risk	Unlicensed vaccine needs to be given on a named patient basis
Typhoid (injectible)	Single injection	3 years if still at risk	
Typhoid (oral)	3 doses – 1 capsule on alternate days	Annual repeat of 3 doses if remaining at risk	Only for travellers >6 years old Must be refrigerated and protected from light
Typhoid and hepatitis A combined	Single dose of combined vaccine followed by a second dose of hepatitis A at 6–12 months	Typhoid at 3 years if remaining at risk Hepatitis A at 10 years	
Cholera/ETEC (oral)	2 doses at an interval of 1–6 weeks for >6 years 3 doses for children 2–6 years	Booster at 2 years Booster at 6 months	Protection against cholera & ETEC 1 week after primary course
Yellow fever	Single injection	10 years if at continued risk	Certificate of vaccination dated at least 10 days prior to departure required for entry to some countries

TRAVELLERS WITH PREEXISTING CONDITIONS

GENERAL ADVICE FOR TRAVELLERS WITH ANY PREEXISTING CONDITION

- Adequate supplies of medication and equipment should be packed in the hand luggage and an extra supply should be taken in case a bag is lost or stolen while abroad.
- Pendants and bracelets can be purchased from the Medic Alert Foundation (see Resources, p.114).
- A summary of their condition and medication should be carried in case of a medical emergency while abroad.
- Appropriate and adequate health insurance is essential.
- Identify location of medical facilities at destination.

DIABETES

Diabetes is not a contraindication to vaccination or malaria prophylaxis. Diabetics are no more or less likely to contract illness while abroad. However, the implications if they do can be more serious than for non-diabetics.

Adequate supplies of medication and equipment such as batteries for the blood testing device should be packed in the hand luggage and an extra supply should be taken in case a bag is lost or stolen while abroad. Glucagon and snacks should be packed for the management of hypoglycaemia if it occurs and a supply of normal blood-testing strips in case the blood glucose monitor fails.

Insulin can be transported and stored in a wide-necked vacuum flask that has been rinsed out with iced water every morning. It will remain stable for up to a month if kept below room temperature (Kassianos 2001) but should be discarded if it becomes discoloured or cloudy, grainy or clumpy.

A letter from the practice may be needed to account to airport authorities for needles and syringes within the luggage, but in any event it is advisable for diabetic travellers to carry some form of summary of their condition and a dose of insulin in case of a medical emergency while abroad. Diabetes UK can provide documentation for this purpose (see Resources, p.114).

Travellers using oral hypoglycaemic agents could consider staying on home time for medication and meals until they can readjust at their destination. Travellers injecting insulin during a journey should not do so until their meal is in front of them as sudden turbulence can delay the distribution of food once it has begun and if the insulin has already been given in anticipation, this could result in hypoglycaemia.

For journeys of up to 8 hours diabetic travellers may decide to keep to home time with their meals and injections and readjust at destination. If travelling for over 8 hours the dose of insulin and timing of injections will need to be adjusted. Kassianos (2001) describes two methods.

1. Omit medium- or long-acting injections and rely on short-acting injections before meals, using 20% of the total daily insulin dose given as short-acting insulin with each of the three meals. Blood glucose should be monitored and minor adjustments made to the insulin depending on results. Once arrived at the destination, the normal regime can be reestablished.
2. For westbound travel increase the time between injections by 2–3 hours twice. The total daily insulin dose may need to be increased by 2–4% for each hour of timeshift. For eastbound travel shorten the time between injections which will result in a lowering of blood sugar so the daily dose of insulin will need to be reduced by 2–4% for each hour of timeshift.

EPILEPSY

Chloroquine and mefloquine are contraindicated as malaria chemoprophylaxis for travellers with epilepsy.

Travellers with epilepsy should be well controlled before travel and should wear an identification disc such as those supplied by the Medic Alert Foundation (see Resources, p.114). All medication should be carried in hand luggage; emergency medication such as rectal diazepam could be taken if necessary but the travelling companion should have instructions as to how and when to administer it.

Crossing time zones will require a readjustment of medication. Kassianos (2001) advises that ideally epileptic travellers should stay on home time until destination and then readjust by shortening the interval between doses rather than extending it.

RESPIRATORY DISEASE

Asthma is the fifth most common inflight illness (Kassianos 2001). Ideally travellers with asthma should carry a spacer device, a supply of oral steroids and a peak flow meter. They should have written instructions on self-management depending on symptoms and peak flow and should ensure that they have adequate supplies of all medication for their time abroad.

Hypoxia can worsen COPD and so travellers with COPD may require oxygen during the flight; if so, this will need to be prebooked via the airline and will usually involve considerable cost as an additional seat needs to be purchased for the cylinder to travel on. The airline will require completion of a MEDIF form by a doctor, which includes information on diagnosis, prognosis, treatment, clinical state and oxygen requirements.

The British Lung Foundation (www.lunguk.org) is a useful source of advice.

HEART DISEASE

To be fit for air travel patients with heart disease should be able to walk 110 metres on the flat at a normal pace without severe breathlessness. Patients with unstable angina, severe heart failure or within 10 days of a myocardial infarction or heart surgery cannot travel by air.

If loop diuretics such as frusemide are omitted by travellers because of concerns about access to the toilet then they may drift into heart failure. As the action of loop diuretics is most evident within the first 4–6 hours, Kassianos (2001) advises that patients can delay taking it until they reach the airport or have boarded the plane.

Traveller's diarrhoea can lead to dehydration and result in hypotension, particularly if patients are taking angiotensin-converting enzyme (ACE) inhibitors and diuretics. Failure to fully excrete the ACE inhibitor may eventually lead to renal failure. Kassianos (2001) advises that these patients should be given instructions that if they lose 3 kg in weight due to vomiting and diarrhoea they should omit the ACE inhibitor and diuretic and seek immediate medical advice.

Changes to diet at the holiday destination can alter gut flora and affect anticoagulant control. Patients on warfarin staying abroad for more than 2–3 weeks should consider having a blood test at destination to check their international normalized ratio (INR). Proguanil can also have an effect on anticoagulant therapy and should not be used in travellers with severe renal disease.

Cardiac patients taking thiazides and amiodarone should be careful about sun protection measures such as wearing a hat and using sunscreens while abroad as photosensitivity may be a problem.

PREGNANCY

Vaccination should generally be avoided during pregnancy and particularly during the first trimester. However, the advice to avoid vaccination during pregnancy is mainly based on lack of data relating to safety, due to an inability to enter pregnant women into vaccine safety trials. Therefore if the woman is unable to postpone her travel and the risk of disease to both the mother and fetus is considered to be high then vaccination may be needed. Advice should be sought from the consultant in communicable diseases before proceeding to recommend vaccination.

Pregnant women are at particular risk of severe malaria (DoH 2001) and should be strongly advised not to travel to malarial zones. However, if they do travel to a malarial zone then they must be extremely careful about prevention of bites and chemoprophylaxis. Proguanil is an antifolate so should be taken with a folate supplement by pregnant women.

INSURANCE

The form E111, which is incorporated within the DoH T6 leaflet *Health advice for travellers* available free from post offices or by phoning 0800 555 777, needs to be completed and authorized at a Post Office and will enable travellers to obtain emergency care in EU countries. *Health advice for travellers* also provides details of those non-EU countries which have reciprocal agreements with the UK.

Healthcare abroad can be extremely expensive and if emergency repatriation after an accident is required it can cost many thousands of pounds. Travellers should ensure that they have adequate health insurance before travel and should read the policy carefully to identify any exclusions. For example, pregnant travellers should ensure that both they and the baby are covered by the policy in the event of delivery abroad.

Travellers with special needs may find that specialist organizations such as Age Concern, British Heart Foundation or Diabetes UK can advise them on the best available insurance.

CONCLUSION

The advice required by travellers will vary depending on their destination and stopovers, duration of stay, activities while away and their past medical and vaccination history. The risk assessment undertaken will be key to the effectiveness of health education advice provided to the individual.

References

Bell D 1995 Tropical medicine, 4th edn. Blackwell Science, Oxford

Brabin B, Ganley Y 1997 Imported malaria in children in the UK. Archives of Disease in Childhood 77:76–81

Bradley D, Bannister B 2003 Guidelines for the prevention of malaria in travellers from the United Kingdom. Communicable Disease and Public Health 6(3):180–199

DoH 1996 Immunisation against infectious disease. HMSO, London

DoH 2001 Health information for overseas travel. HMSO, London

Ericsson C, Dupont H, Mathewson J 1997 Single dose oflaxacin plus lomerimide compared to single dose or three days of oflaxacin in treatment of traveller's diarrhoea. Journal of Travel Medicine 4(1):3–7

Farthing M 1995 Traveller's diarrhoea. Gut 35:1–4

Giangrande P 2000 Thrombosis and air travel. Journal of Travel Medicine 7(3):149–154

Harding R 1994 Aeromedical aspects of commercial airflight. Journal of Travel Medicine 1(4):211–216

House of Lords Science and Technology Committee 2000 Air travel and health. Stationery Office, London

Kassianos GC 2001 Immunisation, childhood and travel health, 4th edn. Blackwell Science, Oxford

Martin J 1996 A descriptive study to explore what advice on health risks associated with travel practice nurses give people who consult them prior to travel to developing countries. Unpublished MA dissertation, University of Reading

McIntosh I, Reed J, Power K 1997 Travellers' diarrhoea and the effect of pre-travel advice in general practice. British Journal of General Practice 47(415):71–75

ONS 2002 Travel trends report. HMSO, London

Paixio M, Dewar R, Cossar J, Covell R, Reid D 1991 What do Scots die of abroad? Scottish Medical Journal 3:114–116

Steffan R, Dupont H 1994 Travel medicine: what's that? Journal of Travel Medicine 1(1):1–3

TRAVAX 2000 www.axl.co.uk/scieh

WHO 2000 International travel and health. World Health Organization, Geneva

Resources

Educational courses available in travel health

MSc in Travel Medicine – Glasgow (0141 330 5617)
Postgraduate Diploma – Royal Free Hospital (020 7830 2999)
RCN/Magister travel health distance learning (01322 427216)
ENB travel health – Staffordshire (01785 229 684)
Travel medicine course – Lancaster (01524 384 604)
Travel medicine short course – LSHTM (020 7299 4648)
Tropical medicine for nurses – LSHTM (020 7299 4648)
Yellow fever training – NaTHNaC (020 7387 9300 ext 5943)

Telephone advice lines for the public

Malaria Reference Laboratory – 0891 600350
Hospital for Tropical Diseases – 09061 337733
Liverpool School of Tropical Medicine – 0891 172111
MASTA – 0891 224100

Useful telephone numbers

Diabetes UK – 020 7323 1531
British Heart Foundation – 020 7935 0185
British Lung Foundation – 020 7831 5831
Age Concern – 020 8679 8000
British Epilepsy Society – 0800 800 5050
British Red Cross (loan of equipment) – 020 7235 5454
Royal Association for Disability and Rehabilitation (RADAR) – 020 7250 3222
Medic Alert Foundation – 020 7833 3034
Foreign & Commonwealth Office – 020 7270 4129
British Travel Health Association – 0141 300 1174

Telephone advice lines *only* for health professionals

Malaria Reference Laboratory – 020 7636 3924
NaTHNaC – 020 7380 9234
TRAVAX – 0141 300 1130
Aventis Pasteur MSD Vaccine Information Service – 07000 766 73 847

Databases

TRAVAX: www.axl.co.uk/scieh
MASTA: www.masta.org/index.html

Useful websites

Centre for Disease Control: www.cdc.gov/travel/index.htm
Department of Health: www.open.gov/travel/index.htm
World Health Organization: www.who.int/
Foreign Office: www.fco.gov.uk
Fit for Travel: www.fitfortravel.scot.nhs.uk
Health Protection Agency: www.hpa.org.uk
National Travel Health Network and Centre: www.nathnac.org

APPENDIX 1 EXAMPLE RISK ASSESSMENT FORM

Name			
Age			
Past and current medical conditions			
Any current medications			
Any present febrile illness			
Women: Possibility of pregnancy Oral contraception			
Any reactions to previous vaccinations			
Any allergies			
Countries to be visited (including stopovers)			
Date of departure			
Length of stay			
Type of visit, e.g. package holiday, safari			
Reason for travel			
Type of accommodation			
Activities planned while abroad, e.g. scuba diving			
Previous vaccinations • Tetanus • Polio • Typhoid • Meningitis C • Meningitis A & C • Hepatitis A • Hepatitis B • Yellow fever • Cholera/ETEC	**Date last given**	**Any reaction**	**Recommended for this trip**
Malaria advice required YES/NO		Malaria leaflet given YES/NO	
State which health education leaflets given to pt			
Name of nurse		Date form completed	

APPENDIX 2 EXAMPLE OF PREVISIT PATIENT INFORMATION LEAFLET

This leaflet provides you with information about your appointment with the nurse for advice and vaccination before you travel abroad

1. **Before vaccination the nurse will ask you:**
   - what vaccinations you have had in the past
   - if you have had yellow fever vaccination within the past 3 weeks
   - if you feel unwell or feverish
   - if you suffer from any existing medical condition
   - if you are allergic to anything such as antibiotics or eggs
   - if you are pregnant or planning a pregnancy
2. **How the vaccines may affect you afterwards**
   - Many people suffer no ill effects at all after vaccination
   - Some may feel faint after vaccination
   - Very rare is the possibility of a severe reaction to the vaccine – this can be treated by adrenaline so we advise all patients to wait in the practice for 15 minutes after vaccination
   - A few people may feel unwell a few hours after vaccination. These symptoms may resemble flu and come on suddenly a few hours after vaccination; they are usually mild and will disappear within a day or so
   - Your arm may feel sore and swollen after vaccination. This should wear off within a couple of days but after tetanus vaccination your arm may remain sore and stiff for up to a week
   - It is advisable not to drink alcohol for 24 hours after vaccination
   - No vaccines give 100% protection
3. **Other health risks associated with travel – most are not vaccine preventable**
   - *Malaria* – is the most important disease hazard facing travellers to tropical areas
   - *Sun* – can permanently damage your skin
   - *HIV* infection – is a worldwide problem
   - *Accidents* – are the main cause of death in overseas travellers and most can be prevented

All these and other health risks will be discussed and are covered in the T6 leaflet which the nurse will give you

Enjoy your trip and stay fit and healthy

Acknowledgement: based on a patient information leaflet designed by Ursula Shine

APPENDIX 3 GUIDELINES ON CHARGING NHS PATIENTS (KASSIANOS 2001)

No charge can be made for travel health advice given to NHS patients as this would put the practice in breach of the GP's terms of service which require that patients are given health advice. In addition, practices cannot make a charge to travellers for vaccination where payment for this service is included in the GMS global sum, e.g. typhoid and hepatitis A. The practice cannot choose to opt out of this service and then charge their NHS patients privately for a service they would have been entitled to under the NHS.

A private script can be issued and a direct charge made to travellers:

- if travelling abroad for over 3 months (one month's supply should be given on FP10)
- for malaria chemoprophylaxis
- for drugs to be used abroad in anticipation of an illness (if providing drugs: no charge for script)
- for administration of vaccination course not available on NHS, e.g. Japanese B encephalitis
- for travel cancellation certificate
- for passport countersignature
- for fitness to travel certificate
- for freedom from infection certificate.

APPENDIX 4 FIRST AID KIT FOR TRAVEL ABROAD

Sterile medical kits are available from pharmacies. These include syringes, needles, injection swabs and an intravenous giving set.

Other useful items include:

- disinfectant/cleaning solution
- dressings
- plasters
- scissors
- tweezers
- disposable gloves
- insect repellent
- sunscreen
- calamine
- antimalarials
- standby antibiotics
- antibiotic cream
- analgesia
- antihistamines
- antacids
- antidiarrhoeals
- laxatives
- rehydration powders
- ear/eye drops
- Canesten pessaries for vaginal thrush
- emergency contraception
- condoms
- sanitary supplies

SECTION 2

Disease management

SECTION CONTENTS

Chapter 7

Asthma

Trisha Weller

CHAPTER CONTENTS

DEFINITION

Asthma is an inflammatory disease of the airways which causes variable air flow obstruction. It affects both the large and the small airways (bronchioles). As a result of inflammatory changes the airways become hyperresponsive (i.e. twitchy and sensitive) and are affected by a variety of stimuli or trigger factors. In asthma airways obstruction is reversible either spontaneously or in response to treatment. In some patients with chronic or poorly controlled asthma, the airway response is reduced and the airway obstruction becomes irreversible and fixed.

PREVALENCE

Asthma is very common and is increasing in the developed world. In the UK asthma affects about 5–7% of the general population and 10–15% of children and is the most common chronic disease of childhood (National Asthma Campaign 2001). Asthma is more common in boys than in girls (approximately a ratio of 2:1) but during adolescence and into adulthood the sex differential evens out. Many children 'grow out' of their asthma during childhood. A long-term study in Melbourne, Australia, which followed children with asthma from age 7 years through to age 42 years, reported that asthma can recur (Phelan et al 2002). Those with persistent and severe asthma during childhood were more likely to have asthma throughout their adult life.

The National Asthma Campaign now estimates there are approximately 5 million asthma sufferers in the United Kingdom (National Asthma Campaign 2001). A general practice with a patient list size of 10 000 patients is likely to have approximately 600 patients with current asthma. Many of these can be cared for within primary care, but if the asthma is difficult to control or the diagnosis is uncertain, more specialist expertise and treatment will be required. Many general practices have nurses trained in asthma management and the British Guideline on the Management of Asthma (BTS/SIGN 2003) acknowledges the importance of this.

Asthma causes considerable morbidity and is still a cause of death in just over 1500 people a year (BTS 2002). The death rate has declined from 2000 deaths a year a decade ago, but many deaths are still preventable. Greater awareness of the disease, more prompt diagnosis and improved medication, as well as asthma management guidelines for health professionals, have probably contributed to this fall, but there are still improvements that can be made. Analysis of mortality data suggests that frequently both patients and doctors fail to recognize the severity of symptoms or their significance, patients delay seeking help and there is inadequate preventive therapy as well (Mohan et al 1996).

ATOPIC AND NON-ATOPIC ASTHMA

The terms 'extrinsic' and 'intrinsic' asthma were previously used to differentiate between the two main types of asthma. Atopic (allergic) or non-atopic (non-allergic) asthma respectively are now the preferred terms but not all patients fit neatly into one category; 15–20% of the population are atopic (i.e. they have an exaggerated response to an allergic trigger factor), 90% of childhood asthma is due to an allergic response, often to more than one trigger but in the adult population only 30% of asthma has an allergic basis.

A detailed medical history and some simple investigations will often identify which category is appropriate. Table 7.1 illustrates the main differences between the two.

It is important to have a basic understanding of what happens at a cellular level when there is

Table 7.1 Differences between atopic and non-atopic asthma

Atopic asthma (extrinsic)	Non-atopic asthma (intrinsic)
• Predominantly affects children	• Affects adults
• Episodic	• Persistent symptoms
• Often history of atopy	• Rarely allergic
• Family history of atopic illness	• Few identifiable trigger factors
• Identifiable triggers	• Little or no atopic family history
• Good prognosis	• Tendency towards aspirin allergy and nasal polyps

exposure to an allergic trigger factor in order to appreciate the need for appropriate treatment. This allergic process will be explored in greater detail on p.124.

PATHOPHYSIOLOGY

Before considering what happens to the airways in asthma, it is worth revisiting the respiratory system as a whole.

- The respiratory system begins at the nose, *not* in the lungs.
- Air is breathed in through the nose and is warmed, filtered and moistened before passing into the lungs. The nose is lined with ciliated columnar epithelial tissue (ciliated mucous membrane).
- Air passes down through the pharynx, larynx and trachea.
- The trachea is supported by cartilage and bands of smooth muscle. It is also lined with ciliated columnar epithelium which contains mucus-secreting goblet cells.
- At the carina the trachea divides and two main bronchi are formed.
- One bronchus passes into each of the two lungs.
- Each lung is divided into lobes – two in the left and three in the right.
- The bronchi are lined with ciliated columnar epithelial tissue as in the rest of the respiratory tract. The left and right bronchi are again supported by cartilage and smooth muscle.
- Each bronchus further subdivides into bronchioles: terminal bronchioles and respiratory bronchioles. There is no supporting cartilage in the bronchioles but smooth muscle is present and they are lined with ciliated columnar epithelium.
- The respiratory bronchioles lead into the alveoli ducts and finally the alveoli, which consist of a single layer of flattened epithelial cells.
- A capillary network of blood vessels surrounds the alveoli.
- Gas exchange occurs during respiration across the alveolar and capillary membranes.

THE ALLERGIC PROCESS

In asthma a reaction to a trigger factor or irritant causes changes within the airway mucosa. These changes result in:

- contraction of the bronchial smooth muscle, resulting in airway narrowing
- inflammation and oedema of the epithelial and submucosal layers
- excess mucus production.

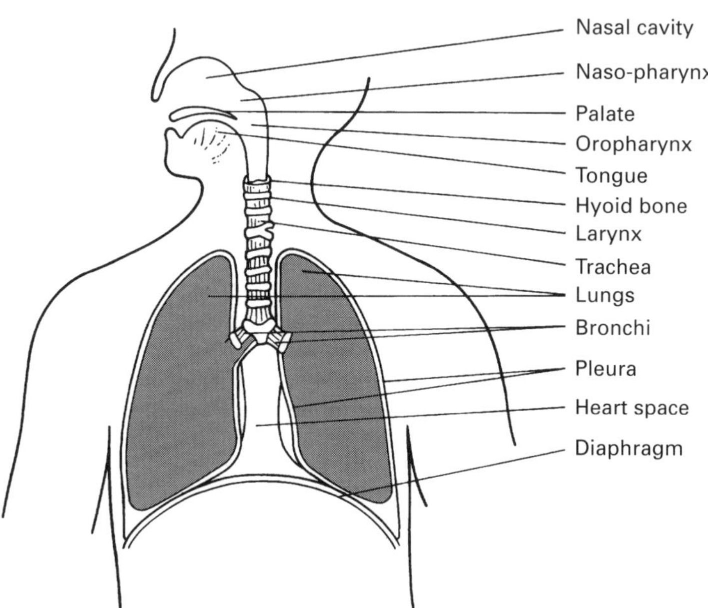

Figure 7.1 The respiratory tract. (From Watson R 2000 *Anatomy and physiology for nurses*, with permission of Elsevier Ltd.)

This response can cause the airways to become very sensitive or irritable and this is known as bronchial hyperreactivity. Some of the triggers of these airway changes are due to an exaggerated allergic response to trigger factors such as pollens, house dust mites or cats.

In atopic individuals, exposure to specific allergens will result in the immune system producing immunoglobulin E (IgE) in excessive amounts, which then attaches to mast cells in the submucosa. This process is known as sensitization.

On reexposure, the allergen binds to the attached IgE molecules, causing the mast cells to degranulate. Mast cells are found in the skin and mucosal surfaces and are part of the body's defence mechanism against foreign matter such as bacteria and parasitic infection. Degranulation of the mast cells releases chemical messengers or mediators such as histamine, prostaglandins and platelet-activating factor. Release of histamine causes nerve irritation and increased permeability of cell walls, leading to swelling and vasodilatation, and results in symptoms such as those of asthma. Initial exposure to an allergen followed by reexposure causes a priming of this allergic response.

Non-atopic asthma is not a result of an allergic response and there are often no clearly identified trigger factors except for a viral infection. Other chemical mediators are involved in this inflammatory response but the mechanism is not clearly understood. In some it is possible that late-onset asthma is a reoccurrence of childhood asthma that may have been long forgotten or perhaps not previously diagnosed or treated (Phelan et al 2002).

TRIGGER FACTORS

Viral infections are the most common trigger of asthma symptoms, especially in children. Other common allergic trigger factors include:

- house dust mite
- pollens and fungal spores
- animals, e.g. cats, dogs, horses, rabbits
- feathers.

Food substances play only a small part in triggering asthma symptoms, but it is important to remember that anaphylactic reactions to food substances such as peanuts can and do occur.

In addition to allergic trigger factors, there are many other triggers of asthma. Respiratory symptoms can be provoked by changes in air temperature, laughter, stress and exercise. Inhaled irritants such as environmental tobacco smoke (ETS) and the pollutant effects of fuel emission also cause respiratory symptoms. ETS is a confirmed airway irritant and a known cause of lung cancer. ETS causes respiratory symptoms, especially in young children, and smoking cessation advice to parents and carers is essential.

Other causes of respiratory symptoms include the use of beta-blockers and non-steroidal anti-inflammatory drugs (NSAIDs). These drugs cause cellular changes by either inhibiting or blocking normal responses. Only some individuals are susceptible to these effects.

Exposure to trigger factors in the work environment can cause occupational asthma. If occupational exposure is identified as the *cause* of asthma, early removal from the causative agent can result in a resolution of the asthma symptoms. Exposure for longer than 6 months is likely to result in chronic asthma symptoms.

Occupational triggers include:

- isocyanates (in adhesives, paint, foam, rubber, printing)
- colophony fumes (from soldering)
- platinum salts (in platinum refining)
- epoxy resins (in adhesives, paint and plastic)
- proteolytic enzymes (in detergents)
- grain or flour dust
- wood dust.

ASTHMA SYMPTOMS

WHEEZE

Often described as noisy breathing or a whistling sound. This sound is heard because air is trying to force its way out of narrowed airways. Wheezing is usually expiratory but in acute severe asthma wheezing may be both inspiratory and expiratory. Wheezing is not always the predominant asthma symptom. In some languages or local dialects, the word 'wheeze' may not be recognised or even understood (Cane et al 2000).

COUGH

Particularly night time and early morning, after exercise and following upper respiratory tract infections (URTIs). The cough is spasmodic, dry or productive. In children cough may be the predominant symptom, although all children will cough at some time even if they do not have asthma (Munyard & Bush 1996). Cough alone is not diagnostic of asthma.

CHEST TIGHTNESS

This is due to bronchoconstriction, causing a feeling of tightness around the whole of the chest. Chest tightness may cause pain which is often felt in the sternal area. Response to a short-acting bronchodilator may help confirm that the chest tightness is asthma rather than cardiac based.

SHORTNESS OF BREATH

Exertional symptoms are common, especially in children, but are frequently underreported. Shortness of breath may occur because of lack of fitness and obesity (Chinn & Rona 2001, Von Mutius et al 2001). In the elderly shortness of breath may be a symptom of diseases other than asthma. Alternative diagnoses should be excluded and chest X-ray, electrocardiograph and some routine blood tests may be required. An alternative diagnosis should be sought if there is a failure to respond to treatment.

It is important to recognize that the patient with asthma may present with only some of the possible symptoms. However, a careful history may reveal others. In young children with mild asthma, symptoms may be present only during an asthma exacerbation. Coughing, usually at night and often causing night-time disturbance and reduced exertional tolerance, is a common symptom.

DIAGNOSIS AND OBJECTIVE TESTING

The correct diagnosis of asthma depends on taking a detailed medical history from the patient and/or carer. In addition, some appropriate diagnostic tests will enable the diagnosis of asthma to be confirmed. In children under 6 or 7 years of age a history and a trial of asthma therapy can confirm or refute the diagnosis of asthma.

PEAK EXPIRATORY FLOW RATE

Peak flow meters are widely used in general practice to confirm the diagnosis of asthma. They are available as low or standard range meters and are prescribable on an FP10 prescription. The peak expiratory flow (PEF) measures the maximum amount of air an individual can expel in a forced blow in 10 milliseconds, starting from full inhalation. The measurement obtained relates only to airflow in the large airways and is therefore a less sensitive diagnostic tool than spirometry. An abnormally low PEF reading may indicate that a patient has asthma, but a normal reading does not exclude asthma! Asthma is a dynamic disease in that it is variable and may be intermittent in severity.

When recording peak flow readings, the patient should ideally be asked to stand up, in order to inhale and exhale as deeply as possible. Three separate peak flow readings should be performed and the best (i.e. the highest) of the three is recorded as the actual PEF reading. If this is the first time that PEF readings have been performed the actual reading obtained is compared to predicted PEF readings for those of a similar age and height. Thereafter previous best values should be used. Charts are available with predicted values and are calculated on age, sex and height. In children these predicted values are based on height alone until puberty, when gender is important because of the differences in growth rate. Predicted values are based on Nunn and Gregg nomograms.

There are several different makes of peak flow meters. Ideally the same peak flow meter should always be used because readings obtained will all vary slightly, not only between different makes but between meters of the same make. If a patient has a PEF meter at home, it is important to advise them to read the instruction sheet for information as to the care and maintenance of the device. Many of the pharmaceutical companies provide blank peak flow charts with space for symptom charting, free of charge.

SERIAL PEF MONITORING

Because asthma is a variable disease it is helpful to obtain recordings at different times of the day. Recording PEF levels in the morning and evening will reflect the normal diurnal pattern where the PEF is highest in the evening and lowest in the morning. The main diagnostic feature in asthma is a marked increase in this diurnal peak flow variation; that is, the peak flow rate recorded in the mornings is significantly lower than in the evenings. A diurnal variation of at least 20% between the highest and the lowest PEF readings on three or more days in a week and over a 2-week period will confirm the diagnosis of asthma (BTS/SIGN 2003). A variation of approximately 5% is normal even in non-asthmatics.

Recording a PEF more often than twice a day can become an onerous chore but it is useful to have more frequent readings where occupational causes are suspected. A 2-week recording of PEF is probably as much as most patients will tolerate! The differences between work and rest day PEF readings may be a more reliable assessment tool where occupational asthma is suspected (Anees et al 2002).

REVERSIBILITY TESTS

Asthma is a reversible airways disease, so if a PEF is lower than previous best or predicted readings, administering a bronchodilator drug can improve the readings obtained.

To carry out a reversibility test, a baseline PEF is performed (i.e. the highest of three sequential blows). An inhaled bronchodilator drug such as a beta-2 agonist (i.e. salbutamol or terbutaline) is administered. The dose normally used is either salbutamol 200–400 micrograms or terbutaline sulphate 250–500 micrograms, according to age and size of the patient. A large volume spacer with a metered dose inhaler or dry powder inhaler devices are suitable for administering the bronchodilator. Alternatively 2.5 mg salbutamol via a nebulizer can be used. The PEF readings should be repeated 15–20 minutes later. A 20% improvement from the baseline readings will demonstrate reversibility and confirm the diagnosis of asthma (BTS/SIGN 2003).

Some individuals, especially the elderly, require larger doses of medication via a nebulizer to demonstrate reversibility.

It is important to view this test as only part of the investigative procedure: it may confirm the diagnosis, but a negative result does not exclude asthma. Not only is asthma dynamic but the test may have been carried out at a time of day when there was no bronchoconstriction. It is important to remember that a bronchodilator will have no effect on airway narrowing due to inflammation and oedema.

STEROID TRIAL

An oral steroid trial is useful where there is minimal response to a bronchodilator reversibility test and where the diagnosis is still unclear. In adults a trial of 30 mg prednisolone for 14 days is sufficient (BTS/SIGN 2003). Baseline PEF readings before and after the steroid course are necessary and if possible every morning and evening for the duration of the course. An improvement of 20% in PEF readings will confirm the diagnosis of asthma. If no improvement in PEF occurs, it is possible the patient may have irreversible airways disease, e.g. chronic obstructive pulmonary disease (COPD), or other more sinister pathology such as lung cancer.

In children a steroid trial is rarely if ever performed. Instead oral steroids are used as a trial of treatment to gain rapid control of respiratory symptoms. A course of prednisolone for a few days may be sufficient to improve symptoms and lower doses are more usual than in adults.

EXERCISE TOLERANCE TEST

If a patient records normal PEF values but reports intermittent symptoms made worse by exertional activity, it may be helpful to perform an exercise tolerance test to confirm the diagnosis of asthma. Exercise in most asthmatics will produce bronchoconstriction. An exercise tolerance test is not conducted on an individual unused to exercise or who has an abnormally low PEF prior to starting the test. In the elderly an exercise test is rarely if ever performed to confirm a diagnosis of asthma.

An exercise tolerance test consists of the following.

1. Initial PEF recording (best of three).
2. Exercises (i.e. run) for 6 minutes. This can be conducted either indoors, e.g. using stairs or treadmill, or outdoors.
3. The PEF is measured after exercise and at 10-minute intervals, for 30 minutes post exercise (BTS/SIGN 2003). If the PEF falls by 20% during this period, this is indicative of asthma. The bronchoconstriction usually reverses spontaneously, but sometimes the patient may need a bronchodilator such as salbutamol or terbutaline to reverse this exertional effect.

An exercise test can be carried out at home by someone who is well motivated and who understands the test procedure. A home exercise test is especially useful when symptoms occur after more than 6 minutes of exercise.

SPIROMETRY

The ideal diagnostic test to confirm asthma is spirometry, together with a full medical history.

Spirometry measures airflow within the small airways, which in asthma are affected by bronchoconstriction. Spirometers are becoming more widely used in general practice but there are still important issues around both correct spirometry technique and interpretation of the results. A single spirometry reading is of no value. Three readings should be measured sequentially and there should be no more than a 5% variation between the three readings to be a valid result. Asthma causes a decrease in both PEF and forced expiratory volume in 1 second (FEV_1). Spirometry results should be compared to the European Coal and Steel normal values (BTS/SIGN 2003).

Spirometry measurements can be used as an alternative to PEF readings when undertaking diagnostic tests. They can also be used at the beginning and end of an oral steroid trial. A positive test result is indicated by a 15% change from baseline FEV_1 and at least a 200 ml change.

Children under the age of 6 or 7 are usually unable to perform either PEF or spirometry tests reliably and repeat test manoeuvres are often inaccurate. Symptom monitoring is usually preferable in this age group and is as effective as PEF and spirometry testing for monitoring asthma (Gibson 2000, McGrath et al 2001, Yoos et al 2002).

OTHER TESTS

It is not necessary to perform routine chest X-rays (CXR) if asthma is suspected but they should be performed if the clinical picture is unclear and to exclude other more serious pathology. X-rays may show hyperinflation and bronchial wall thickening, both of which are suggestive of asthma, but a CXR is not a diagnostic test for either asthma or COPD.

Skin prick tests (SPT) are useful to confirm the presence of atopy but should be performed only by those trained in their use. They cannot predict who will develop respiratory symptoms of asthma or indeed rhinitis. SPT can help identify specific asthma triggers which may be beneficial when trying to offer practical allergy avoidance advice.

NON-DRUG MANAGEMENT OF ASTHMA

The treatment for asthma will depend on the severity of the disease at any given time and on the trigger factors. Non-drug treatment options, such as smoking cessation, are essential when caring for someone with asthma.

NON-ALLERGIC TRIGGER FACTORS

Upper respiratory tract infections

A URTI is the most common trigger factor for all those with asthma and is virtually impossible to avoid. Infections are often relatively mild as with viral infections causing the 'common cold'. It is appropriate to advise what action if any to take at the onset of URTI. This advice will include monitoring of respiratory symptoms and peak flow measurements and for some, a temporary increase in asthma treatment. While there is no good clinical evidence that temporarily increasing treatment is effective (BTS/SIGN 2003, Garrett et al 1998), there may be benefit to some asthma patients (Charlton et al 1994). However, if adherence to therapy is variable increasing inhaled steroid medication may be of some clinical benefit to individual patients. Increased airway hyperreactivity makes it more likely that other trigger factors contribute to worsening symptoms as well.

Smoking

There is evidence that smoking during pregnancy is associated with an increased incidence of respiratory symptoms in the preschool child (Lewis et al 1995). Mothers who smoke during pregnancy are at increased risk of having smaller birthweight babies who will consequently have airways of a smaller calibre (Gilliland et al 2000). In addition, mothers who smoke and are atopic are at increased risk of having a child with asthma (Dezateau et al 1999). Smoking cessation advice needs to be given at every opportunity.

Exercise

Exercise is a common trigger of asthma and causes bronchoconstriction. It is often underreported or trivialized. All exercise should be encouraged because activity is part of a normal healthy lifestyle.

Increased activity increases the respiratory rate with the result that the airways cool and dry, especially with mouth breathing. Exercise in a warm and moist environment such as in an indoor heated swimming pool is less likely to cause asthma symptoms than exercising outdoors in cold, dry air such as in cross country running and cycling. This is because the inhaled air is already moist, warm and at a constant temperature and this lessens the likelihood of exercise-induced bronchospasm.

Preexercise bronchodilator therapy will prevent exercise symptoms occurring. Planned activities are easier to pretreat, but unplanned activities, as in childhood play, are less so. Obesity and subsequent reduced activity is known to increase the likelihood of respiratory symptoms, especially in childhood (Chinn & Rona 2001, Von Mutius et al 2001).

DRUG TRIGGERS OF ASTHMA

About 10–11% of asthmatics are allergic to aspirin and other NSAIDs. According to an Australian study, the prevalence in non-asthmatics was only 2.5% (Vally et al 2002). Adults who are NSAID intolerant often have rhinitis, nasal polyps and non-allergic asthma (McGeehan & Bush 2002, Vally et al 2002). It is more common in those with severe disease (Mygind et al 1996), but NSAID intolerance is rarely seen in children.

People with asthma should be generally advised to avoid aspirin or NSAID-based analgesics, but not all asthma sufferers are affected. The general advice needs to be viewed in the context of the individual patient as some patients have used NSAIDs for years without problems. Paracetamol is a safer alternative although there have been reports that it may contribute to morbidity (O'Shaheen et al 2000).

Beta-blocker eye drops are normally the drug of choice for glaucoma sufferers. Some of the drug is absorbed systemically and can cause bronchoconstriction in susceptible individuals or even an asthma attack, because it blocks beta-2 receptor sites. When taking a history from an older patient, remember to ask about any eye drops they are instilling. A change to alternative treatment may need to be considered. Eye drops are not necessarily viewed as a medication by the patient.

It is important to check and document what medications the patient is taking, both prescribed and over the counter (OTC). Don't forget that cough is a well-documented side-effect of ACE inhibitor antihypertensive therapy but this does not cause bronchoconstriction.

ALLERGIC TRIGGER FACTORS

Allergic trigger factors can sometimes be avoided, but this is often difficult. It may be more appropriate to use regular 'preventer' asthma therapy to control the airway hyperreactivity. Alternatively preexposure bronchodilator therapy may be indicated if there are infrequent symptoms and the allergic trigger factor is known.

House dust mite

About 80% of children with asthma are allergic to the house dust mite (HDM) and it is the commonest allergic trigger in the UK. It is virtually impossible to eradicate HDM and they thrive in carpets, soft furnishings and especially bedding.

Advice as to the reduction of HDM must be practical and acceptable to the patient and family. The most benefit will be gained by concentrating efforts to limit exposure in the bedroom. The following recommendations may be of some benefit.

- Vacuum regularly, preferably with a machine that returns very low amounts of dust to the room, i.e. a vacuum cleaner with a HEPA filter.
- Use pillows and duvets which can be washed.
- Carry out regular damp dusting of bedroom furniture.
- Change the bedlinen weekly.
- Use flooring that is easy to keep clean and dust free, e.g. vinyl, lino or wood flooring.
- Use simple roller blinds as an alternative to curtains which trap the dust.
- Limit the number of soft toys, especially around the bed.
- Wash soft toys regularly and occasionally put in the freezer overnight to kill the mite.
- Avoid making the bed in the presence of the asthma sufferer.

While individuals may make attempts to live in a 'dust mite-free' environment, it is not possible to avoid all contact with HDM. Allergen-impermeable covers for mattresses, pillows and bed quilts have not shown improved asthma control in adults (Custovic et al 2002).

Animals

Cat and dog allergens are frequent triggers of asthma and eye and nose symptoms (rhinoconjunctivitis). Cat allergens are produced mainly in the salivary glands, as well as in the skin. They are deposited on the cat fur when cats lick their fur. Dog allergens are found in saliva, shed skin (dander) and in urine. Allergens are found in the urine in animals such as mice, rats, guinea pigs and hamsters.

It is very difficult to know if the family pet is the culprit and it may be necessary to arrange a trial separation period in order to confirm the trigger. Interestingly it may be that an individual is allergic to one particular animal only. Asthma sufferers often state that their own pet causes them no problems but other similar animals do.

Getting rid of the pet used to be the standard advice when asthma was diagnosed. The stress resulting from the removal of a beloved family pet may well provoke an asthma exacerbation. If pet allergy is suspected, it is more usual now to recommend keeping the pet out of the bedroom, as well as minimal handling. Severe asthma may warrant a different approach and replacement of the pet should be considered very carefully.

Regular bathing and combing of animals such as dogs and cats may reduce the allergen load, but there is little clinical evidence that respiratory symptoms improve.

Pollen

Pollens originate from several sources: trees, grass and weeds. Their seasons are spring, summer and autumn respectively. Timothy and rye grasses are the major culprits for grass pollen allergy in the United Kingdom. Commonly known as hayfever, symptoms are at their highest in June and July. Birch, hazel, oak, elm and plane trees produce pollen grains that can also trigger hayfever symptoms. A good clinical history may identify the offending pollen source.

Hayfever symptoms vary and may affect the nose, eye and respiratory tract. If wheezing occurs the more accurate diagnostic name is pollen-induced asthma which requires antiasthma treatment. If respiratory symptoms do not occur at any other time, starting antiasthma treatment a few weeks before the offending pollen season and continuing for the duration can be effective in controlling this type of asthma.

It is difficult to avoid grass pollen, but it may be sensible to avoid grass cutting and visits to the countryside at peak pollen times. The pollen count is reported daily in the newspapers during the summer months and is worth noting as part of monitoring and managing respiratory symptoms.

Food

Food allergy is not a common trigger factor for asthma, although some parents of younger asthmatics believe that it is. A detailed clinical history may help identify the offending foods but sometimes further investigations and tests are required. Some individuals are especially sensitive to certain foodstuffs and these should be avoided. Foods which contain eggs, milk, wheat, nuts and shellfish can cause allergic reactions. Tartrazine (yellow food colouring) and sulphites used as a preservative in alcoholic drinks can also trigger asthma in some individuals.

If food is suspected to be the cause of asthma, then it is important that the individual is referred for specialist advice. It is unwise to introduce an elimination diet without full nutritional advice; however, allergy services are few and far between in the UK. It is worth noting that food allergy more commonly gives rise to skin rashes than respiratory symptoms.

OCCUPATIONAL ASTHMA

Occupational asthma is now the most common industrial lung disease in the developed world with more than 400 reported causes (BTS/SIGN 2003). Occupational asthma may account for about 10% of adult-onset asthma. Occupational asthma is caused by factors associated with the individual's workplace and symptoms are frequently worse during the working week, although with persistent exposure this is not always the case.

Avoidance is not easy and may be impossible without a change of employment. Certain substances are now legally recognized as triggers of industrial asthma and industrial compensation is available. However, it is not always easy to prove cause and effect and compensation claims are not always met. Ideally all patients with a suspected occupational cause should be referred to an occupational chest physician for a diagnosis and confirmation of the offending trigger.

It is possible that there is a critical period of sensitization to an allergic trigger factor. It may be that the early identification and removal from an industrial trigger will increase the chances of avoiding long-term or chronic asthma problems. There should therefore be no delay in investigating these problems when they arise.

DRUG TREATMENT OF ASTHMA

The stepped approach to asthma drug treatment is outlined in the BTS/SIGN guidelines (BTS/SIGN 2003). Treatment guidelines should be followed and adjusted according to age and asthma severity.

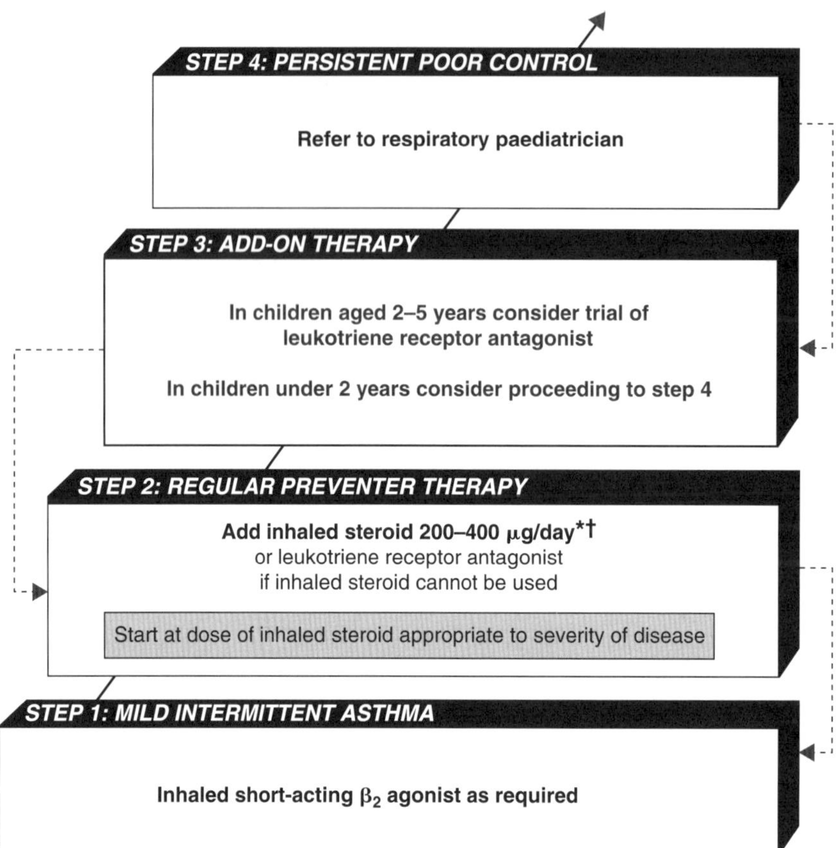

Figure 7.2 Summary of stepwise management in children less than 5 years (BTS/SIGN 2003). (Reproduced with permission from the BMJ Publishing Group.)

Drug therapies can be divided loosely into three categories:

- relievers
- preventers
- acute savers.

RELIEVERS

Relievers are drugs that relax bronchial smooth muscle. These drugs provide symptomatic relief but do not treat the underlying pathology. They should not be used as the mainstay treatment for asthma. They are classified into the following groups:

- beta-2 agonists
- anticholinergics
- methylxanthines.

Beta-2 agonists

These drugs stimulate the beta-2 receptor sites which results in relaxation of bronchial smooth muscle. Side-effects include tremor, peripheral dilatation, palpitations and headaches. However, in recommended doses, these side-effects are minimal. There are two types of beta-2 agonists: short and long acting.

Short acting These are used for the immediate relief of symptoms. When inhaled they have an almost instant effect with optimum effect occurring within 10–15 minutes and lasting for up to 4 hours. These drugs may be inhaled, injected or taken orally. They can also be administered by a nebulizer.

Examples of short-acting bronchodilators are:

- salbutamol (Airomir, Asmasal, Pulvinal salbutamol, Salamol, Salbulin, Ventolin)
- terbutaline (Bricanyl).

Long acting These have a similar effect on the beta-2 receptor sites but for a much longer period – up to 12 hours. In asthma they should be used in conjunction with preventive therapy (BTS/SIGN 2003). There are both inhaled and oral beta-2 agonist

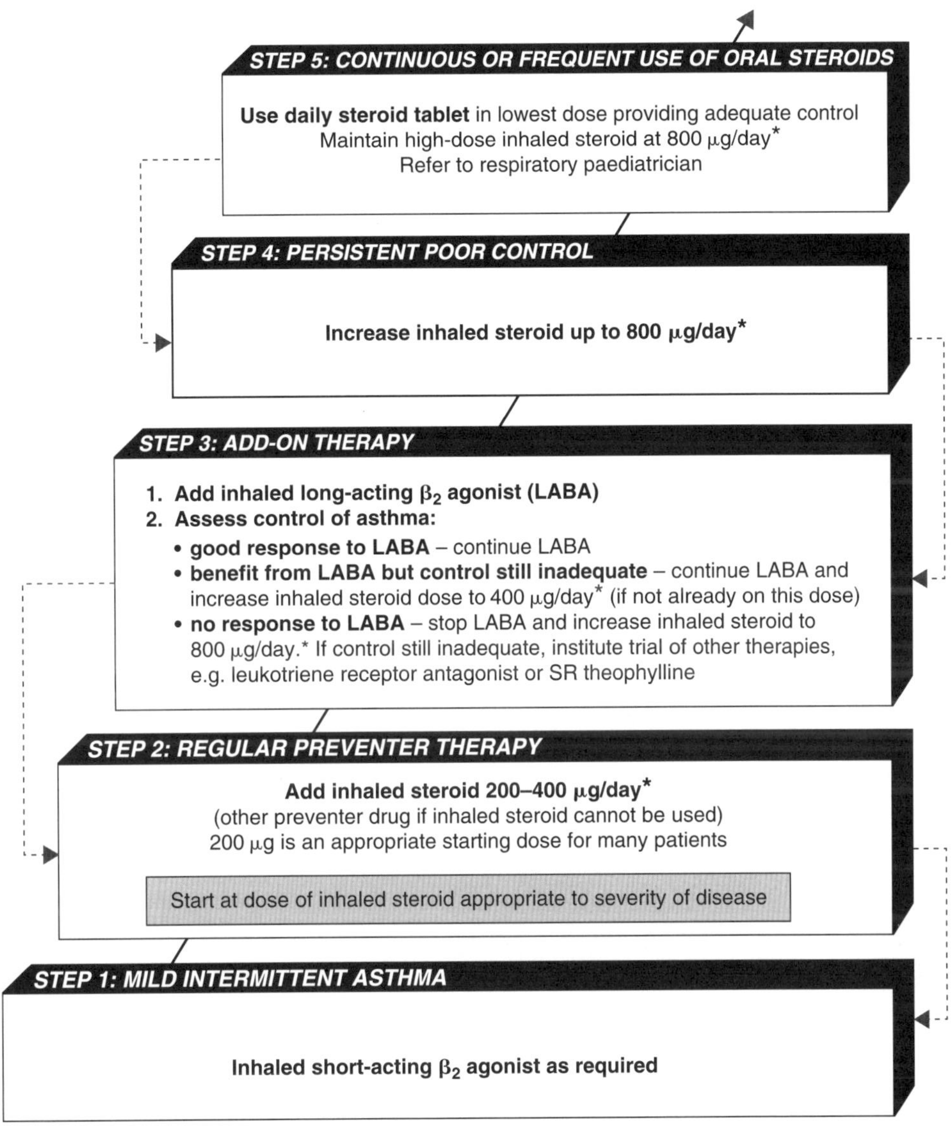

Figure 7.3 Summary of stepwise management in 5–12 year olds (BTS/SIGN 2003). (Reproduced with permission from the BMJ Publishing Group.)

preparations but oral therapies are used less frequently.

Examples of inhaled long-acting beta-2 agonists are:

- salmeterol (Serevent). This has a product licence from 4 years of age
- formoterol (e.g. Oxis). This has a product licence from 6 years of age.

In addition, these products are available in combination with the inhaled steroids of fluticasone (as Seretide) and budesonide (as Symbicort) respectively.

An example of an oral long-acting beta-2 agonist is bambuterol (Bambec) which is not recommended for children.

Anticholinergics

Anticholinergic drugs inhibit the bronchoconstricting effect of the parasympathetic nervous system as well as reducing mucous secretions.

In the very young anticholinergic drugs were thought to be more effective than beta-2 agonists but a review of the evidence does not support this

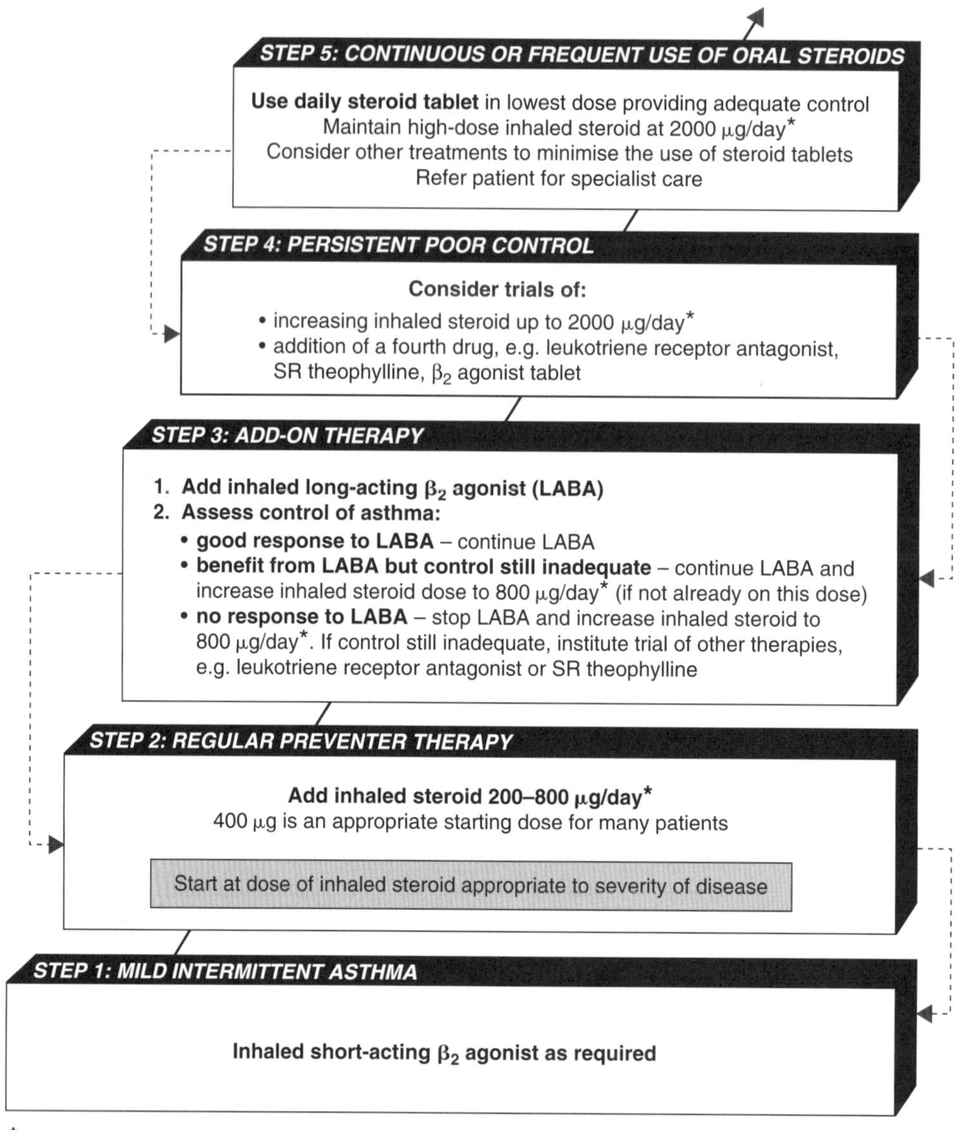

Figure 7.4 Summary of stepwise management in adults (BTS/SIGN 2003). (Reproduced with permission from the BMJ Publishing Group.)

(Everard & Kurian 1999). The Asthma Guideline advocates their use in the treatment of acute severe asthma but only in addition to a short-acting beta-2 agonist (BTS/SIGN 2003).

In the elderly, in whom there is often a pattern of mixed airways disease, anticholinergic medications are often more effective than beta-2 agonists alone. Subsequently they are used in combination with salbutamol (a short-acting beta-2 agonist) (Combivent) in proven COPD.

Onset of action of anticholinergic drugs is slower than in beta-2 agonists, taking about 30–40 minutes to be effective. Side-effects include dry mouth, urinary retention and constipation. These drugs are available only in inhaled or nebulized form.

Examples of anticholinergic drugs are:

- ipratropium bromide (Atrovent)
- tiotropium (Spiriva), only for COPD.

Methylxanthines

The way in which these drugs work is unclear, but they do relax smooth muscle and inhibit the release of mediators from mast cells.

Side-effects such as nausea, vomiting and headaches are common, but these drugs have the potential for serious side-effects. Side-effects are more likely if blood levels are above 20 mg/l and overdosage is potentially fatal. The aim is to keep the therapeutic blood levels between 10 and 20 mg/l so serum levels should be carefully monitored.

Individual absorption rates are unpredictable and subsequently methylxanthines are not viewed as a first-line therapeutic option in this country. However, they are useful for those with more difficult asthma and they do have the benefit that they are inexpensive but need to be considered in line with BTS/SIGN Asthma Guideline recommendations (BTS/SIGN 2003).

In an acute attack of asthma the administration of aminophylline is unlikely to offer any advantage over inhaled bronchodilators or systemic steroids (Parameswaran et al 2001, Yung & South 1998).

Examples of methylxanthines are:

- theophylline (Nuelin, Slo-phyllin, Theo-dur, Uniphyllin continus)
- aminophylline (Phyllocontin continus).

PREVENTERS

Preventers are prophylactic therapies which are taken on a regular basis to control the inflammatory process of asthma.

Inhaled steroids

Inhaled steroids are the preventer drug treatment of choice for asthma (BTS/SIGN 2003). Unlike short-acting bronchodilators, inhaled steroids have no immediate effect on symptoms. This needs careful explanation to the patient as they may not start to have any noticeable effect for several days. Inhaled steroids reduce inflammation and mucus hypersecretion and subsequent bronchiole hyperreactivity of asthma.

Inhaled steroids are usually taken twice a day, the dose depending on the age of the patient and the severity of the asthma. A more recent inhaled corticosteroid is a once-a-day treatment taken at night, but it can be started as a twice-daily regime if necessary.

High doses of inhaled steroids are known to have systemic side-effects and adrenergic effects have been reported (Todd et al 2002). A report from the Medicines Control Agency (now the Medicines and Healthcare Products Regulatory Agency (MHRA)) does not single out any specific inhaled steroid but instead concludes it is a class effect of corticosteroids (Medicines Control Agency 2002).

The aim of asthma management is to effect maximum control with the minimum of medication. If control is not achieved in adults at 800 micrograms inhaled steroid per day, additional medication should be considered (BTS/SIGN 2003). If asthma control is not achieved at 400 micrograms beclometasone per day (or equivalent) in children less than 5 years of age, they should be referred to a respiratory paediatrician for further advice and confirmation of the asthma diagnosis. In children aged 5–15 years inhaled steroid therapy can be increased up to 800 micrograms per day of beclometasone (or equivalent) for persistent poor asthma control. Referral to a respiratory paediatrician for advice may be necessary if this fails to control asthma symptoms or the diagnosis is in doubt.

In children there are ongoing concerns that inhaled steroids may cause growth delay. The concerns of carers need to be listened to and addressed sensitively. However, poorly controlled asthma is more likely to delay growth during puberty than affect the ultimate height achieved. Agertoft's study reports minimal growth effects as a result of long-term inhaled steroids (Agertoft & Pedersen 2001). Monitoring the child's growth velocity is important and should be continued until growth is complete. Measurement should take place at regular intervals and be recorded on centile measurement charts (Fig. 7.5). Ideally height measurement should be done using the same measuring device each time and by the same individual for an accurate record of growth rate (Voss & Bailey 1994).

Inhaled steroids, especially in high doses, can cause hoarseness, sore throats and oral candidiasis. The use of a volume spacer device will reduce the oropharyngeal deposit as well as washing out the mouth after using the inhaler, preferably rinsing and spitting.

Examples of inhaled steroids are:

- beclometasone (Beclazone, Becloforte, Becotide, Pulvinal beclometasone, Qvar)
- budesonide (Pulmicort)
- fluticasone (Flixotide)
- mometasone (Asmanex).

Leukotriene receptor antagonists

These drugs are different from other asthma therapies in that they are oral preparations.

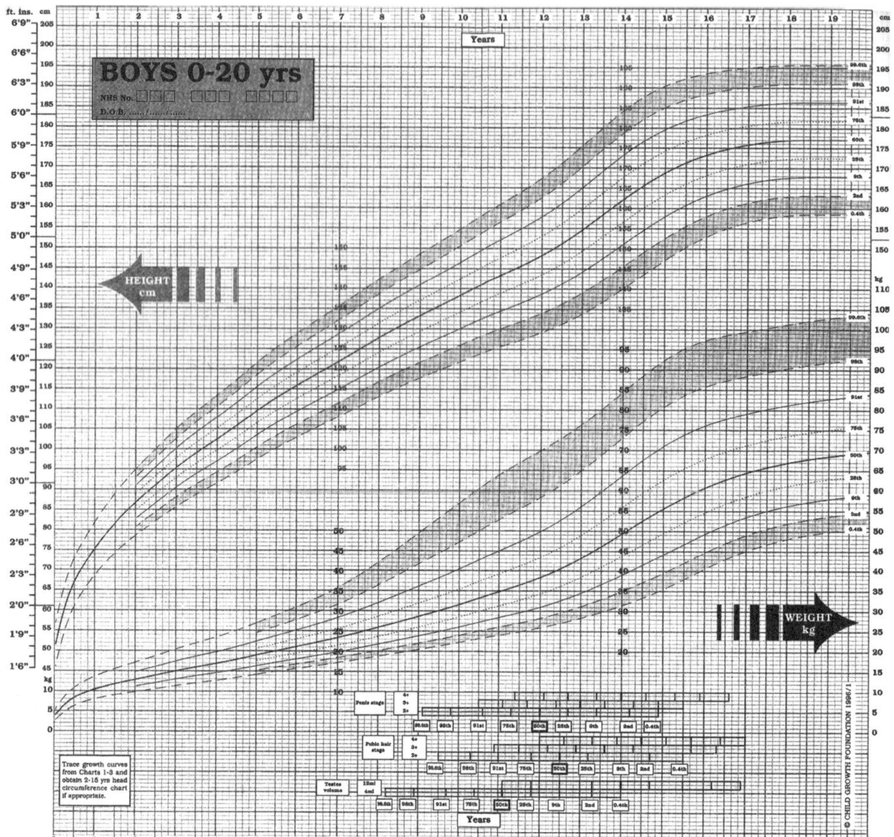

Figure 7.5 Example of a boy's centile growth chart. (Copyright Child Growth Foundation. This chart may not be reproduced in any form whatsoever and is for illustrative purposes only.)

Anti-leukotriene medications block the leukotriene receptor sites, inhibiting cytokine responses that cause both early and late symptoms in asthma.

Examples of leukotriene receptor antagonists (LTRAs) are:

- montelukast (Singulair) – once daily
- zafirlukast (Accolate) – twice daily.

Montelukast has a licence from 6 months of age, while the zafirlukast licence is from 12 years. LTRAs are not effective in everybody and often a trial of treatment will be necessary to determine whether the patient responds to this treatment or not. In children less than 5 years, LTRAs have been shown to be effective (Knorr et al 2001).

Rather than increasing the dose of inhaled steroids above 400 micrograms per day in children or 800 micrograms per day in adults, additional therapies such as long-acting beta-2 agonists, LTRAs or slow-release theophyllines should be considered. (BTS/SIGN 2003).

Non-steroidal antiinflammatory drugs

These drugs stabilize mast cells and therefore prevent the release of chemical mediators which cause bronchial constriction. They are less effective than inhaled corticosteroids and a systematic review reported no benefit from cromoglicate in children (Tasche et al 2000). Cromoglicate is no longer recommended as an alternative preventer therapy to inhaled corticosteroids at Step 2 of the guideline (BTS/SIGN 2003), but it is still effective in preventing exercise-induced asthma in children over 5 years old (BTS/SIGN 2003). Exercise-induced symptoms are usually an expression of poorly controlled asthma.

Examples of NSAIDs are:

- nedocromil sodium (Tilade) – from 6 years
- cromoglicate (Intal, Cromogen).

Regular oral steroids

Poorly controlled asthma may require daily oral steroids if other therapies, e.g. inhaled steroids, long-acting beta-2 agonists, LTRAs and theophyllines, fail to control symptoms. Any medication failing to be of benefit after a trial of about 6 weeks should be stopped (BTS/SIGN 2003). The dose of oral steroids should be titrated to the lowest dose required to control symptoms.

In paediatric practice regular oral steroids are given on alternate days because of the reported reduction in side-effects (Balfour-Lynn 1987); however, there are no randomized controlled studies to support what is accepted clinical practice. Long-term oral steroid use should only be initiated by a paediatric respiratory physician and should be avoided if possible because of the potential for serious side-effects, which include:

- Cushing's syndrome
- diabetes
- hypertension
- osteoporosis
- adrenal crisis.

ACUTE SAVERS

These drugs are used during and following an acute exacerbation of asthma:

- systemic steroids
- high-dose bronchodilators
- oxygen.

Systemic steroids

In acute asthma, systemic steroids are effective in reducing mucosal oedema, mucus hypersecretion and bronchial hyperreactivity. Short courses of oral steroids are required to gain rapid control of poorly controlled asthma and following an acute attack. As a general rule, if an asthma patient requires high doses of a bronchodilator either by large volume spacer or nebulizer, a short course of oral steroids should be given. A PEF recording of 50% of predicted or best requires a course of oral steroids. Used short term, the potential for side-effects is minimal and any risks are outweighed by the benefits to the patient. Underuse of systemic steroids is a major reason for deaths from asthma.

Systemic steroids are usually given orally but are occasionally administered by the parenteral route. Onset of action from administration of the drug is the same, provided the medication can be swallowed and retained. Benefits become apparent within 3–4 hours (BTS/SIGN 2003).

High-dose bronchodilators

Beta-2 agonists via a large volume spacer device are as effective as those administered by nebulization (BTS/SIGN 2003, Dewar et al 1999). High doses (up to 20 doses in adults and 10 doses in children) are required and repeated as often as necessary. Monitoring the patient continually is essential and failure to improve requires urgent referral to the emergency services with possible hospital admission. In severe asthma attacks, the addition of nebulized ipratropium bromide to a short-acting bronchodilator is helpful (BTS/SIGN 2003).

Oxygen

Patients with acute severe asthma are hypoxaemic. Oxygen saturation levels should be monitored using a pulse oximeter. A pulse oximeter is a simple, easy-to-use, non-invasive oxygen measuring device. Oxygen saturations of at least 92% must be achieved and high concentrations of inspired oxygen should be administered to all patients with acute asthma (BTS/SIGN 2003). This raises important issues for primary care where this equipment may not be available.

INHALER DELIVERY SYSTEMS

Asthma medications are usually administered via the inhaled route. There are several benefits:

- drug delivery to the site of action
- rapid onset of action of drug
- smaller doses required than with oral therapy
- minimal side-effects
- can be effective in acute asthma.

There are many inhaler devices available. Nurses involved in asthma care must ensure they are familiar with the various devices in order to be able to advise and instruct patients on how to use the device effectively. Difficult-to-control asthma may be simply due to poor inhaler technique and/or an inappropriate choice of delivery system. Regular checking of inhaler technique at each visit ensures it is part of routine asthma care.

The National Institute for Clinical Excellence (NICE) advocates the use of a spacer and metered dose inhaler as the preferred inhaler device for children under 5 years of age (NICE 2000). Inhaled steroids for children 5–15 years should be administered via a spacer and metered dose inhaler as the

1. Shake the inhaler.
2. Hold the inhaler upright. Open the cap.
3. Breathe out gently. Keep the inhaler upright, put the mouthpiece in the mouth and close lips and teeth around it (the airholes on the top must not be blocked by the hand).
4. Breathe in steadily through the mouthpiece. DON'T stop breathing when the inhaler "puffs" and continue taking a really deep breath.
5. Hold the breath for about 10 seconds.
6. After use, hold the inhaler upright and immediately close the cap.
7. For a second dose, wait a few seconds before repeating steps 1–6.

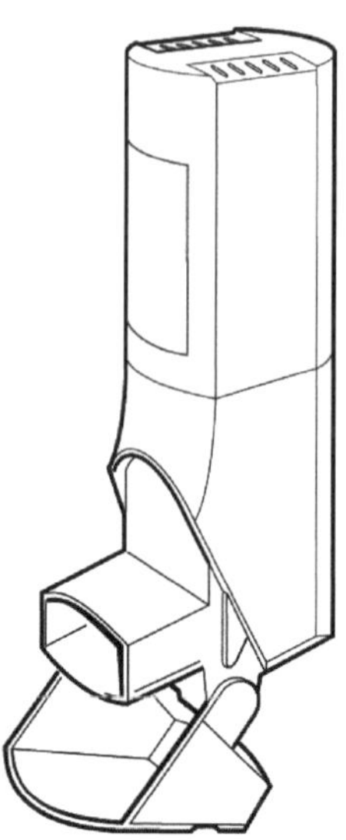

Figure 7.6 Easi-Breathe (an example of a breath-activated device). (Copyright National Respiratory Training Centre.)

preferred option (NICE 2002). Any appropriate device is recommended for bronchodilator use in this age group.

INHALER DEVICES

- Metered dose inhalers
- Breath-actuated devices, e.g. Autohaler, Easibreathe
- Dry powder inhalers, e.g. Accuhaler, Clickhaler, Diskhaler, Pulvinal, Twisthaler, Turbohaler

Spacer devices include:

- Able spacer
- Aerochamber
- Nebuchamber
- Nebuhaler
- Pocket Chamber
- Volumatic.

These spacer devices are available on prescription, with the option of prescribing a facemask as well. Facemasks attached to the spacer device are required to administer inhaled asthma medications to children under approximately 3 years of age.

1. Remove the mouthpiece cover from the inhaler.
2. Attach the facemask to the spacer mouthpiece. The Laerdal mask attaches to the Volumatic and the Nalato mask to the Nebuhaler.
3. Shake the inhaler and insert into the spacer device.
4. Tip the spacer to an angle of about 45° to enable the valve to remain open.
5. Apply the mask to the child's face covering nose and mouth with as tight a seal as possible.
6. Press the inhaler canister once to release a dose of the medication. Keep the mask on the child's face for 5 or 6 breaths or for as long as they will tolerate it.
7. Wait for 30 seconds before repeating steps 3–6.
8. When using this method to administer inhaled steroids, remember to wash the child's face after each treatment.

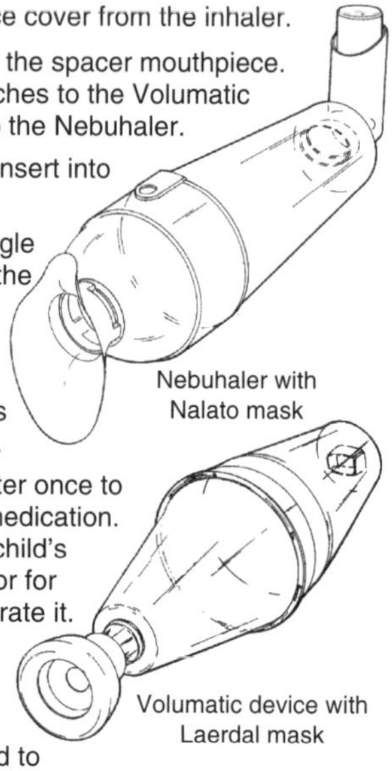

Nebuhaler with Nalato mask

Volumatic device with Laerdal mask

Figure 7.7 Spacer with mask – Volumatic and Nebuhaler (large volume spacer with facemask for young children). (Copyright National Respiratory Training Centre.)

1. Unscrew and lift off white cover.
2. Hold main body of Turbohaler upright. Twist the red base as far as it will go in both directions. A clicking sound will be heard.
3. Breathe out away from the Turbohaler mouthpiece.
4. Put the mouthpiece between the lips and teeth and breathe in as deeply as possible.
5. Remove the Turbohaler from the mouth and breathe out.
6. For further doses repeat steps 2–5.
7. Replace white cover.
8. The dose counter changes from a white background to a red one once it has the number 20 in the window. When the 0 on the red background reaches the middle of the window the device is empty.

NB: Before a new device is used for the first time, prepare the inhaler as in steps 1 and 2, and repeat step 2. This is the initial priming. Thereafter follow instructions 1–8.

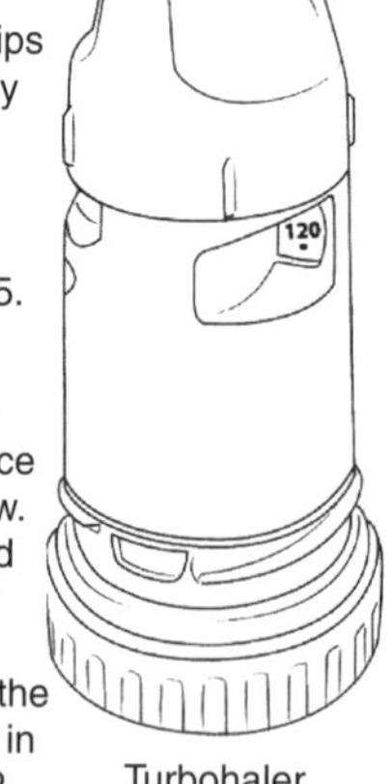

Figure 7.8 Turbohaler for combination therapy (example of dry powder device with numerical counter). (Copyright National Respiratory Training Centre.)

A tight seal between the facemask and face is essential to maximize drug administration (Everard 1992) and if the child cries whilst receiving inhaled medication the amount of medication inhaled will

1. Put 2 parts of the spacer device together.

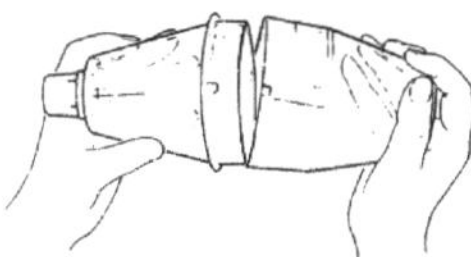

2. Remove the mouthpiece cap from the metered dose inhaler.

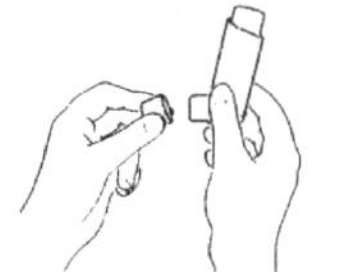

3. Shake inhaler and insert into flat end of spacer

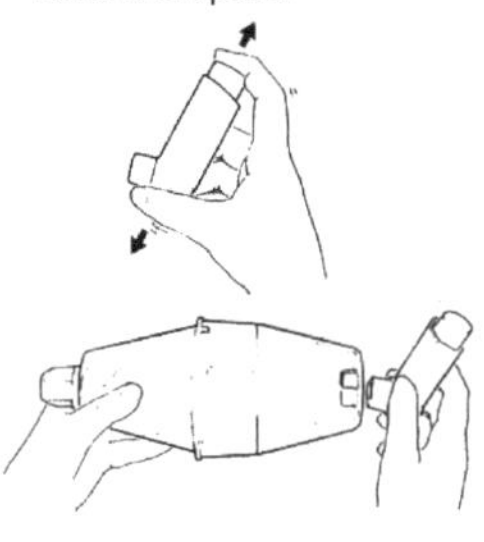

4. Place spacer mouthpiece in patient's mouth and press inhaler canister once to release a dose of the short acting bronchodilator medication. (If unable to use the mouthpiece, attach facemask to the mouthpiece end and place over nose and mouth ensuring a good seal).

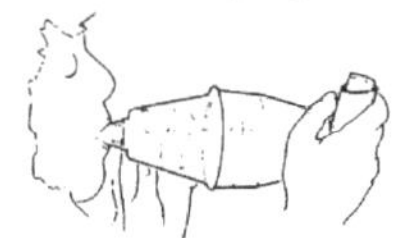

5. Only one dose of medication should be actuated at a time
6. Ask the patient to breathe in and out through the spacer device for 4 or 5 breaths.
7. Remove mouthpiece from patient's mouth.
8. For effective relief of symptoms in acute asthma repeat steps 4–7. Up to 20 puffs (actuations) of a short acting bronchodilator may be required for adult patients (up to 10 puffs for children).
9. Shake the inhaler canister gently between actuations. This can be done with the canister still inserted in the spacer device.

If there is no immediate improvement or the patient's condition continues to deteriorate, seek urgent medical help. Whilst waiting for emergency assistance repeat above steps.

Figure 7.9 Spacer used in an emergency (acute asthma). (Copyright National Respiratory Training Centre.)

Multiple breath technique

1. Remove the cap.
2. Shake the inhaler and insert into the device.
3. Place the mouthpiece in the mouth.
4. Start breathing in and out slowly and gently. (This will make a 'clicking' sound as the valve opens and closes).
5. Once the breathing pattern is well established, depress the canister leaving the device in the same position and continue to breathe (tindal breathing) several more times.
6. Remove the device from the mouth.
7. Wait about 30 seconds before repeating steps 2–6.

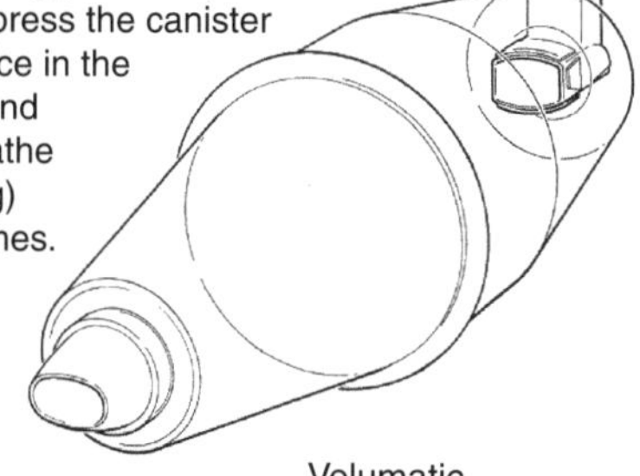

Figure 7.10 Volumatic multiple-breath technique (example of large volume spacer). (Copyright National Respiratory Training Centre.)

1. Remove the cap.
2. Shake the inhaler.
3. Breathe out gently.
4. Put the mouthpiece in the mouth and at the start of inspiration, which should be slow and deep, press the canister down and continue to inhale deeply.

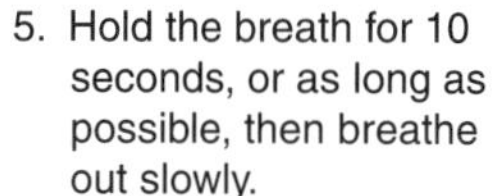

5. Hold the breath for 10 seconds, or as long as possible, then breathe out slowly.
6. Wait for a few seconds before repeating steps 2–5.

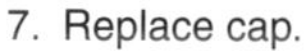

7. Replace cap.

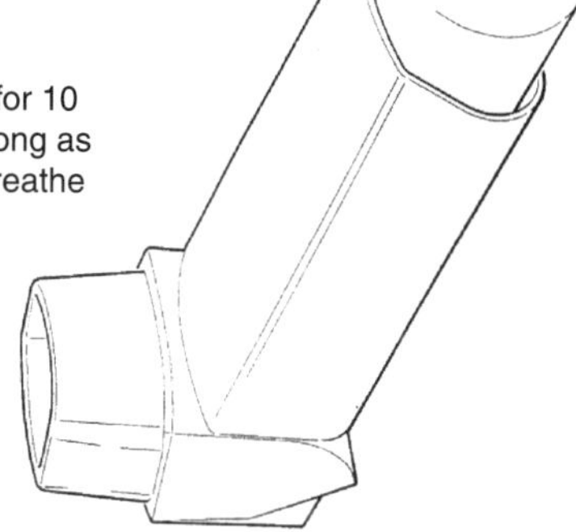

Figure 7.11 Metered dose inhaler. (Copyright National Respiratory Training Centre.)

be reduced (Iles & Edmunds 2002). The Babyhaler device is available but is not prescribable.

RECOGNIZING POOR CONTROL

It is important that asthma sufferers and their carers appreciate when asthma is worsening and out of control. In most cases, asthma control deteriorates for a period of time before a severe attack occurs.

The following is a list of signs and symptoms that indicate worsening and poorly controlled asthma:

- increase in respiratory symptoms
- sleep disturbance
- decrease in exercise tolerance
- increased use of bronchodilators
- decline in efficiency of bronchodilators
- fall in peak flow to 70% or below of previous best
- increased diurnal variation in peak flow.

These symptoms require an urgent review of treatment and clinical management to prevent further deterioration. In the current asthma guidelines there are various algorithms for the management of acute asthma across the different age ranges (Figs 7.12, 7.13).

Many deaths from asthma are preventable, but delay can be fatal. Factors leading to poor outcome include:

- Doctors failing to assess severity by objective measurement
- Patients or relatives failing to appreciate severity
- Under use of corticosteroids

Regard each emergency asthma consultation as for acute severe asthma until it is shown to be otherwise.

Assess and record:

- Peak expiratory flow (PEF)
- Symptoms and response to self-treatment
- Heart and respiratory rates
- Oxygen saturation (by pulse oximetry, if available)

Caution: *Patients with severe or life-threatening attacks may not be distressed and may not have all the abnormalities listed below. The presence of any should alert the doctor.*

Moderate asthma	**Acute severe asthma**	**Life-threatening asthma**
INITIAL ASSESSMENT		
PEF > 50% best or predicted	**PEF 33–50% best or predicted**	**PEF < 33% best or predicted**
FURTHER ASSESSMENT		
• Speech normal • Respiration < 25 breaths/min • Pulse < 110 beats/min	• Can't complete sentences • Respiration ≥ 25 breaths/min • Pulse ≥ 110 beats/min	• SpO_2 < 92% • Silent chest, cyanosis, or feeble respiratory effort • Bradycardia, dysrhythmia or hypotension • Exhaustion, confusion or coma
MANAGEMENT		
Treat at home or in surgery and ASSESS RESPONSE TO TREATMENT	**Consider admission**	**Arrange immediate ADMISSION**
TREATMENT		
• High dose β_2 bronchodilator. – Ideally via oxygen-driven nebulizer (salbutamol 5 mg or terbutaline 10 mg) – Or via spacer or air-driven nebulizer (1 puff 10–20 times) If PEF > 50–75% predicted/best: • Give prednisolone 40–50 mg • Continue or step up usual treatment If good response to first nebulized treatment (symptoms improved, respiration and pulse settling, and PEF >50%) continue or step up usual treatment and continue prednisolone	• Oxygen 40–60% if available • High dose β_2 bronchodilator: – Ideally via oxygen-driven nebulizer (salbutamol 5 mg or terbutaline 10 mg) – Or via spacer (1 puff β_2 agonist via a large volume spacer and repeat 10–20 times) or air-driven nebulizer • Prednisolone 40–50 mg or IV hydrocortisone 100 mg • **If no response in acute severe asthma: ADMIT**	• Oxygen 40–60% • Prednisolone 40–50 mg or IV hydrocortisone 100 mg immediately • High dose β_2 bronchodilator and ipratropium: – Ideally via oxygen-driven nebulizer (salbutamol 5 mg or terbutaline 10 mg and ipratropium 0.5 mg) • Or via spacer (1 puff β_2 agonist via a large volume spacer, repeated 10–20 times) or air driven nebulizer
Admit to hospital if any: • Life threatening features • Features of acute severe asthma present after initial treatment • Previous near fatal asthma Lower threshold for admission if: **afternoon or evening attack, recent nocturnal symptoms or hospital admission, previous severe attacks, patient unable to assess own condition, or concern over social circumstances.**	**If admitting the patient to hospital:** • Stay with patient until ambulance arrives • Send written assessment and referral details to hospital • Give high dose β_2 bronchodilator via oxygen-driven nebulizer in ambulance	**Follow up after treatment or discharge from hospital:** • **GP review within 48 hours** • Monitor symptoms and PEF • Check inhaler technique • Written asthma action plan • Modify treatment according to guidelines for chronic persistent asthma • Address potentially preventable contributors to admission

Figure 7.12 Management of acute severe asthma in adults in general practice (BTS/SIGN 2003). (Reproduced with permission from the BMJ Publishing Group.)

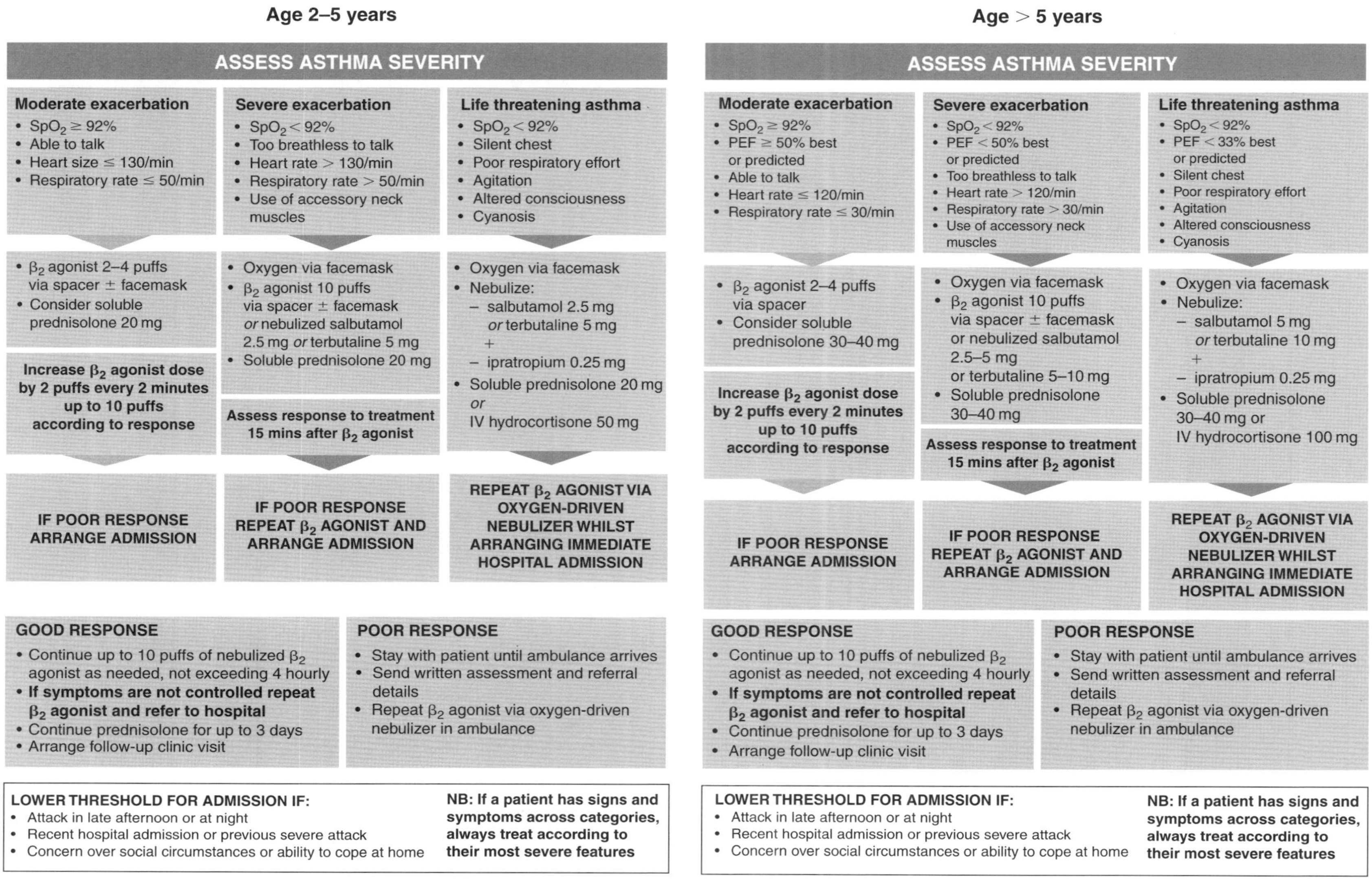

Age 2–5 years

ASSESS ASTHMA SEVERITY

Moderate exacerbation	Severe exacerbation	Life threatening asthma
• $SpO_2 \geq 92\%$ • Able to talk • Heart size ≤ 130/min • Respiratory rate ≤ 50/min	• $SpO_2 < 92\%$ • Too breathless to talk • Heart rate > 130/min • Respiratory rate > 50/min • Use of accessory neck muscles	• $SpO_2 < 92\%$ • Silent chest • Poor respiratory effort • Agitation • Altered consciousness • Cyanosis
• β_2 agonist 2–4 puffs via spacer ± facemask • Consider soluble prednisolone 20 mg	• Oxygen via facemask • β_2 agonist 10 puffs via spacer ± facemask *or* nebulized salbutamol 2.5 mg *or* terbutaline 5 mg • Soluble prednisolone 20 mg	• Oxygen via facemask • Nebulize: – salbutamol 2.5 mg *or* terbutaline 5 mg + – ipratropium 0.25 mg • Soluble prednisolone 20 mg *or* IV hydrocortisone 50 mg
Increase β_2 agonist dose by 2 puffs every 2 minutes up to 10 puffs according to response	**Assess response to treatment 15 mins after β_2 agonist**	
IF POOR RESPONSE ARRANGE ADMISSION	**IF POOR RESPONSE REPEAT β_2 AGONIST AND ARRANGE ADMISSION**	**REPEAT β_2 AGONIST VIA OXYGEN-DRIVEN NEBULIZER WHILST ARRANGING IMMEDIATE HOSPITAL ADMISSION**

GOOD RESPONSE

- Continue up to 10 puffs of nebulized β_2 agonist as needed, not exceeding 4 hourly
- **If symptoms are not controlled repeat β_2 agonist and refer to hospital**
- Continue prednisolone for up to 3 days
- Arrange follow-up clinic visit

POOR RESPONSE

- Stay with patient until ambulance arrives
- Send written assessment and referral details
- Repeat β_2 agonist via oxygen-driven nebulizer in ambulance

LOWER THRESHOLD FOR ADMISSION IF:

- Attack in late afternoon or at night
- Recent hospital admission or previous severe attack
- Concern over social circumstances or ability to cope at home

NB: If a patient has signs and symptoms across categories, always treat according to their most severe features

Age > 5 years

ASSESS ASTHMA SEVERITY

Moderate exacerbation	Severe exacerbation	Life threatening asthma
• $SpO_2 \geq 92\%$ • PEF ≥ 50% best or predicted • Able to talk • Heart rate ≤ 120/min • Respiratory rate ≤ 30/min	• $SpO_2 < 92\%$ • PEF < 50% best or predicted • Too breathless to talk • Heart rate > 120/min • Respiratory rate > 30/min • Use of accessory neck muscles	• $SpO_2 < 92\%$ • PEF < 33% best or predicted • Silent chest • Poor respiratory effort • Agitation • Altered consciousness • Cyanosis
• β_2 agonist 2–4 puffs via spacer • Consider soluble prednisolone 30–40 mg	• Oxygen via facemask • β_2 agonist 10 puffs via spacer ± facemask or nebulized salbutamol 2.5–5 mg or terbutaline 5–10 mg • Soluble prednisolone 30–40 mg	• Oxygen via facemask • Nebulize: – salbutamol 5 mg *or* terbutaline 10 mg + – ipratropium 0.25 mg • Soluble prednisolone 30–40 mg or IV hydrocortisone 100 mg
Increase β_2 agonist dose by 2 puffs every 2 minutes up to 10 puffs according to response	**Assess response to treatment 15 mins after β_2 agonist**	
IF POOR RESPONSE ARRANGE ADMISSION	**IF POOR RESPONSE REPEAT β_2 AGONIST AND ARRANGE ADMISSION**	**REPEAT β_2 AGONIST VIA OXYGEN-DRIVEN NEBULIZER WHILST ARRANGING IMMEDIATE HOSPITAL ADMISSION**

GOOD RESPONSE

- Continue up to 10 puffs of nebulized β_2 agonist as needed, not exceeding 4 hourly
- **If symptoms are not controlled repeat β_2 agonist and refer to hospital**
- Continue prednisolone for up to 3 days
- Arrange follow-up clinic visit

POOR RESPONSE

- Stay with patient until ambulance arrives
- Send written assessment and referral details
- Repeat β_2 agonist via oxygen-driven nebulizer in ambulance

LOWER THRESHOLD FOR ADMISSION IF:

- Attack in late afternoon or at night
- Recent hospital admission or previous severe attack
- Concern over social circumstances or ability to cope at home

NB: If a patient has signs and symptoms across categories, always treat according to their most severe features

Figure 7.13 Management of acute asthma in children in general practice (BTS/SIGN 2003). (Reproduced with permission from the BMJ Publishing Group.)

Date of assessment:
Date of birth: Age: Sex:
Occupation: Current: Past: Retired:
Height: Weight: BMI Centile measurement (under 16 years):
Smoking status: Current: Ex: Non-smoker:
Family members smoking:
Year/age onset of symptoms:
Age/year of diagnosis:
Previous hospital admissions (dates):
Family history of atopic disease:
History of atopic disease:
Trigger factors/provocation:
URTI:
Allergies (list):
Exercise:
Seasonal:
Emotion:
Other:
Past treatments for asthma:
Current treatments (including dose frequency, delivery device):
Current symptoms:
Wheeze:
Cough day:
Cough night:
Dyspnoea:
Sputum:
Nasal symptoms
Current URTI:
Tests: Peak flow: Best ever peak flow: Predicted:
Reversibility test: Pre: Post:
Exercise tolerance test:
PEF Pre: PEF Post: 10 min: 20 min: 30 min:
Other:
Date last chest X-ray: Result:
Home peak flow meter: Diary card:
Personal Action Plan:

Figure 7.14 Example of information contained within an asthma assessment form.

ASTHMA MANAGEMENT IN GENERAL PRACTICE

The aim of structured asthma care is to improve asthma control by reducing symptoms, preventing acute attacks and improving quality of life issues. Asthma care should be proactive and not reactive to asthma crises. An asthma review is also an opportunity to collect data to support Quality Indicator information for the new General Medical Services (GMS) contract. A structured approach to asthma care requires a practice protocol to be developed as well as identifying training needs for health professionals within the practice.

A PRACTICE PROTOCOL

- Identify asthma patients and establish a practice asthma register. The GMS contract requires an asthma register to be established once the diagnosis of asthma has been confirmed by objective tests. Asthma diagnostic criteria are determined according to the BTS/SIGN Asthma Guideline (2003).

- Establish a call and recall appointment system.
- Initial assessment procedure.
  Determine which diagnostic tests are appropriate:
  - *Reversibility testing*. These tests may require the administration of different bronchodilators. Patient Group Directions (PGD) may be required to administer these drugs (NHSE 2000).
  - *Exercise test*. A short-acting bronchodilator should be made available during this test procedure in case of any exacerbation of asthma symptoms. A Patient Group Direction may be required.
  - *Steroid trial*. A protocol should clearly identify which patients should have a steroid trial, the dose required and the length of the trial.
  - *Peak flow meters*. Not all patients need peak flow meters. Patients with more severe disease, frequent course of oral steroids or hospital admission for asthma should be prescribed their own peak flow meter and supplied with diary cards for logging any recordings made. Long-term monitoring is notoriously unreliable.
  - *Symptom monitoring* is helpful in young children.
- Educational input on asthma.
  Patients need to have a basic understanding of what asthma is. This information needs to be modified to suit age, language, comprehension and cultural differences.
- Treatment should be prescribed according to the British Guideline on the Management of Asthma (BTS/SIGN 2003), taking local prescribing policies into account. Any treatment decisions made outside these guidelines should be justified.
- Inhaler device selection. The most appropriate devices for individual patients should be chosen. Recommendations as to choice should follow NICE guidelines in the under-15 age groups (NICE 2000).
- All patients should have an Asthma Action Plan. There is good evidence that personalized action plans improve asthma outcomes (BTS/SIGN 2003).
- Review/follow-up visits. Follow-up time intervals should be planned with the patients. Children on inhaled steroids should be seen on a regular basis (3–6 monthly) in order to reassess medication needs and to reduce to the lowest possible medication to control asthma symptoms. Height should be monitored regularly until growth is complete.
- Telephone support. Contact by telephone to question the patient about their asthma symptoms may enable some clinic visits to be foregone. Pinnock et al (2003) reported that more patients were reviewed and had shorter consultation times with telephone consultations. Additionally they found that there was no clinical disadvantage to the patient or loss of patient satisfaction. However, telephone consultations are no substitute for direct patient contact in times of worsening or acute asthma.
- Email. This form of communication may be suitable for contacting patients whose asthma is well controlled and could be complementary to face-to-face consultation. It may appeal to teenagers and those who find it difficult to attend for regular asthma review because of work commitments.

EMERGENCIES AND EMERGENCY PROTOCOL

The practice should have an emergency asthma protocol which should be updated on a regular basis. This should include:

1. Initial assessment of the acute attack
   - PEF, pulse, respiratory rate, oxygen saturation levels, colour and use of accessory muscles.
2. Treatment policy should be clearly stated and include:
   - What can be given? What route of administration ? How much? How often? By whom?
   - Supplemental oxygen: flow rates should be specified as a guide.

The protocol should be dated, signed, individual names specified as appropriate and the protocol should be updated regularly. When assessing the patient, any information obtained should be clearly documented and signed with a clearly identifiable signature.

EQUIPMENT

Minimal equipment is required to run an asthma clinic.

- Peak flow meters (standard and low reading)
- Disposable one-way mouthpieces

- Height chart (centile charts)
- Predicted peak flow values (children and adults)
- Peak flow monitoring charts
- In-check dial and one-way mouthpieces
- Placebo inhaler devices
- Bronchodilator medication for reversibility tests
- Asthma Action Plans. These can be obtained from the National Asthma Campaign (NAC) or from pharmaceutical companies free of charge
- Educational material. The NAC have excellent informative literature on asthma (see Resources below).

EDUCATION AND TRAINING

The extent of a nurse's involvement in asthma care will vary according to professional expertise and GP support. The nurse must not take on roles for which she/he is not competent and has not been trained (NMC 2002). Nurse-run asthma care has reported reduced school and work absence, reduced exacerbation rates and improved symptom control (Hoskins et al 1999). Observation suggests that practice nurses with an asthma diploma level course may achieve better asthma outcomes for their patients (Dickinson et al 1997). The BTS/SIGN Guideline advocates that in primary care, people with asthma should be reviewed regularly by a nurse with training in asthma management.

NURSE'S ROLE

One way of looking at the nurse's role is to divide it into minimum, medium and maximum involvement. At each level it is critical that a referral process is established between the nurse and the doctor.

Minimum role

1. Compile and update asthma register in the practice.
2. Record peak flow measurements.
3. Teach and correct inhaler device technique.
4. Basic patient education.

Nurse and doctor both see the patient on each occasion.

Medium role

1. Explain and teach peak flow monitoring.
2. Carry out objective tests such as reversibility and exercise testing.
3. Provide more detailed patient education and counselling.
4. Identify poor asthma control.

Nurse-run asthma management programme with doctor seeing selected patients (e.g. those whose asthma is not controlled).

Maximum role

1. Carry out assessments and regular follow-up of patients.
2. Take a formal medical history.
3. Formulate a written Asthma Action Plan with the patient.
4. Alter medication dosage according to protocols.
5. Give advice to patients by telephone and email.
6. See patients in an acute asthma emergency according to emergency asthma protocol

Nurse-run asthma management programme, with doctor available for advice.

PATIENT EDUCATION

It has been assumed that if patients are better educated about their asthma, then their adherence to medication regimens will improve. However, this is only one aspect of adherence, which is a complex issue.

Asthma education is important to enable asthma patients to monitor their asthma safely and effectively. However, not all want the same amount of information or detail about asthma and it is important to tailor information specifically to each patient.

All those with asthma should have some information about the following.

- A basic understanding of what having asthma means.
- Recognize what triggers their asthma symptoms.
- Understand why medications may be needed and what they do.
- Recognize symptoms of deteriorating asthma and know what action to take.
- Recognize what an asthma attack is and what to do.
- The importance of seeking help.

Small amounts of information can be given over a period of time and it is important that the health professional does not go into information overdrive! Knowledge can be confirmed and reinforced

ACTION PLAN Be in control			
Symptoms are:	**Peak Flow is:**		**Action is:**
No symptoms		→	Normal – continue your treatment or talk to your doctor/nurse about taking less treatment
Getting a cold, symptoms during daytime and/ or nightime		→	Take .... of ....(times a day) and blue inhaler for relief of symptoms
Out of breath Blue inhaler does not help		→	Continue as above and start steroid tablets .... mg x .... and contact ....
Too breathless to speak		→	This needs emergency action straight away. See back page

Figure 7.15 Personal Action Plan (NAC) (BTS/SIGN 2003). (Reproduced with permission from the BMJ Publishing Group.)

by asking the patient about specific aspects of the disease and correcting their knowledge if necessary. Allowing the patient to ask questions and addressing their concerns is an important part of any asthma consultation.

There are numerous leaflets, videos and other educational aids available about asthma, but they should be used in conjunction with face-to-face dialogue. The National Asthma Campaign provides some excellent literature which can be obtained from their website free of charge (www.asthma.org.uk). The NAC's Point of Diagnosis Pack for primary care provides excellent basic information for newly diagnosed asthma patients and there is a pack for parents of newly diagnosed children as well. These booklets are available free of charge.

ASTHMA ACTION PLANS

Asthma is a chronic disease and therefore it is essential that asthma sufferers are not passive recipients of care.

Written instructions are essential for each patient, but the extent of 'self-management' will vary (BTS/SIGN 2003). An Asthma Action Plan may contain simple instructions such as what medication to take and when and advice to contact the doctor in an emergency. Others will want more detailed action plans and greater involvement in their asthma care, some monitoring their peak flow readings and initiating a course of oral steroids in an emergency.

Asthma Action Plans, produced by the NAC (Fig. 7.15), are available from all major respiratory pharmaceutical companies. These materials are available to support the Asthma Guideline.

FREQUENCY OF CLINIC CONSULTATIONS

How frequently people with asthma should be reviewed will depend on individual patient needs and the severity of the disease, as well as the organisational and administrative issues in the surgery. The following is a guide only.

- Newly diagnosed asthma – every few weeks until control established.
- Children on inhaled steroids – every 3–6 months and to monitor their growth velocity.
- Adults on preventive treatment – every 3–6 months, depending on severity and control of symptoms.
- If there is a specific annual trigger only, i.e. hayfever – see on annual basis before the specific trigger season starts.

AUDIT

Asthma is a dynamic condition and therefore improved outcomes of disease management may not always be seen over a short period of time. The following are examples of what may be monitored within the practice. It is not an inclusive list.

- Number of patients on the asthma register
- The number of children diagnosed with asthma
- The number with a specific objective measure to confirm the diagnosis of asthma
- The number prescribed inhaled steroids
- Those on high doses of inhaled steroids
- The number on long-acting bronchodilators, leukotrienes, etc.
- Numbers of short-acting bronchodilators prescribed to individual patients each month
- Those with persistent asthma symptoms
- Identifying the numbers of patients at each step of the Asthma Guideline
- Emergency treatment with either high-dose bronchodilators via a spacer device or nebulizer
- Home nebulizer use and maintenance arrangements
- Emergency visits to A&E or out-of-hours services
- Emergency hospital admissions
- Courses of oral steroids

CONCLUSION

Good asthma care can benefit both the patient and their family by reducing asthma symptoms and contributing to an improved quality of life. Asthma care is dependent on a partnership agreement with the patient and/or carer and the willingness to take the treatment agreed. The practice nurse who is trained in asthma management is ideally placed to contribute to improving asthma within primary care.

References

Agertoft L, Pedersen S 2001 Effect of long-term treatment with inhaled budesonide on adult height in children with asthma. New England Journal of Medicine 343(15):1064–1069

Anees W, Blainey D, Huggins V, Robertson K, Burge PS 2002 Differences in indices of peak expiratory flow variability between workers with occupational asthma and irritant (grain dust) exposed health individuals. Thorax 57(iii):56

Balfour-Lynn L 1987 Effect of asthma on growth and puberty. Pediatrician 14:237–241

British Thoracic Society 2002 The burden of lung disease. Munro & Forster Communications, London

British Thoracic Society (BTS)/Scottish Intercollegiate Guideline Network (SIGN) 2003 British guideline on the management of asthma. Thorax 58 (suppl 1)

Cane RS, Ranganathan SC, McKenzie SA 2000 What do parents of wheezy children understand by wheeze? Archives of Disease in Childhood 82:327–332

Charlton I, Antoniou AG, Atkinson J et al 1994 Asthma at the interface: bridging the gap between general practice and a district hospital. Archives of Disease in Childhood 70(4):313–318

Chinn S, Rona RJ 2001 Can the increase in body mass index explain the rising trend in asthma in children? Thorax 56(11):845–850

Custovic A, Forster L, Matthews E et al 2002 The effect of mite allergen control by the use of allergen-impermeable covers in adult asthma: the SMAC Trial. Thorax 57 (suppl 111):45–46

Dewar AL, Stewart A, Cogswell JJ, Connett GJ 1999 A randomised controlled trial to assess the relative benefits of large volume spacers and nebulisers to treat acute asthma in hospital. Archives of Disease in Childhood 80:421–423

Dezateau C, Stocks J, Dundas I, Fletcher ME 1999 Impaired airway function and wheezing in infancy: the influence of maternal smoking and a genetic disposition to asthma. American Journal of Respiratory & Critical Care Medicine 159:403–410

Dickinson J, Hutton S, Atkin A, Jones K 1997 Reducing asthma morbidity in the community: the effect of a targeted nurse-run asthma clinic in an English general practice. Respiratory Medicine 91:634–640

Everard M 1992 Drug delivery from holding chambers with attached face mask. Archives of Disease in Childhood 67:580–585

Everard ML, Kurian M 1999 Anti-cholinergic drugs for wheeze in children under the age of two years (Cochrane Review). The Cochrane Library, Issue 4. Update Software, Oxford

Garrett J, Williams S, Wong C, Holdaway D 1998 Treatment of acute asthmatic exacerbations with an increased dose of inhaled steroid. Archives of Disease in Childhood 79:12–17

Gibson PG 2000 Monitoring the patient with asthma: an evidence-based approach. Journal of Allergy & Clinical Immunology 106(1 Pt 1):17–26

Gilliland FD, Berhane K, McConnell R, Gauderman WJ, Vora H, Rappaport EB 2000 Maternal smoking during pregnancy, environmental tobacco smoke exposure and childhood lung function. Thorax 55:271–276

Hoskins G, Neville RG, Smith B, Clark RA 1999 The link between nurse training and asthma outcomes. British Journal of Community Nursing 4:222–228

Iles R, Edmunds AT 2002 Crying significantly reduces absorption of aerolised drug in infants. Archives of Disease in Childhood 31:163–165

Knorr B, Franchi LM, Bisgaard H et al 2001 Montelukast, a leukotriene receptor antagonist for the treatment of persistent asthma in children aged 2 to 5 years. Pediatrics 108(3):1–10

Lewis S, Richards D, Bynner J, Butler N, Britton J 1995 Prospective study of risk factors for early and persistent wheezing in childhood. European Respiratory Journal 8:349–356

McGeehan M, Bush RK 2002 The mechanisms of aspirin-intolerant asthma and its management. Current Allergy & Asthma Reports 2(2):117–125

McGrath AM, Gardner DM, McCormack J 2001 Is home peak expiratory flow monitoring effective for controlling asthma symptoms? Journal of Clinical Pharmacy & Therapeutics 26(5):311–317

Medicines Control Agency 2002 Inhaled corticosteroids and adrenal suppression in children. Current Problems in Pharmacovigilance 28:7

Mohan G, Harrison BDW, Badminton RM, Mildenhall S, Wareham NJ 1996 A confidential enquiry into deaths caused by asthma in an English health region: implications for general practice. British Journal of General Practice 46:529–532

Munyard P, Bush A 1996 How much coughing is normal? Archives of Disease in Childhood 74:531–534

Mygind N, Dahl R, Pedersen S, Thestrup-Pedersen K 1996 Essential allergy, 2nd edn. Blackwell Science, Oxford

National Asthma Campaign 2001 Out in the open. Asthma Journal 6(3):supplement

NHSE 2000 Patient Group Directions (England only). Department of Health, London

NICE 2000 Guidance on the use of inhaler systems (devices) in children under the age of 5 years with chronic asthma. National Institute for Clinical Excellence, London

NICE 2002 Inhaler devices for routine treatment of chronic asthma in older children (aged 5–15 years). National Institute for Clinical Excellence, London

NMC 2002 Code of professional conduct. Nursing & Midwifery Council, London

O'Shaheen S, Sterne JAC, Songhurst CE, Burney PGJ 2000 Frequent paracetamol use and asthma in adults. Thorax 55(4):266–270

Parameswaran K, Belda J, Rowe BH 2001 Addition of intravenous aminophylline to beta-2-agonists in adults with acute asthma (Cochrane Review). The Cochrane Library, Issue 3. Update Software, Oxford

Phelan PD, Robertson CF, Olinsky A 2002 The Melbourne Asthma Study: 1964–1999. Journal of Allergy & Clinical Immunology 109(2):189–194

Pinnock H, Bawden R, Proctor S et al 2003 Accessibility, acceptability, and effectiveness in primary care of routine telephone review of asthma: a pragmatic, randomised controlled trial. British Medical Journal 326(7387):477–479

Tasche MJ, Uijen JH, Bernsen RM, De Jongste JC, Van Der Wouden JC 2000 Inhaled disodium cromoglycate (DSCG) as maintenance therapy in children with asthma: a systematic review. Thorax 55(11):913–920

Todd GRG, Acerini CL, Ross-Russell R, Zahra S, Warner JT, McCance D 2002 Survey of adrenal crisis associated with inhaled corticosteroids in the United Kingdom. Archives of Disease in Childhood 87:457–461

Vally H, Taylor ML, Thompson PJ 2002 The prevalence of aspirin intolerant asthma (AIA) in Australian asthmatic patients. Thorax 57(7):569–574

Von Mutius E, Schwartz J, Neas LM, Dockery D, Weiss ST 2001 Relation of body mass index to asthma and atopy in children: the National Health and Nutrition Examination Study III. Thorax 56(11):835–838

Voss ID, Bailey BJR 1994 Equipping the community to measure children's height: the reliability of portable instruments. Archives of Disease in Childhood 70:469–471

Yoos HL, Kitzman H, McMullen A, Henderson C, Sidora K 2002 Symptom monitoring in childhood asthma: a randomized clinical trial comparing peak expiratory flow rate with symptom monitoring. Annals of Allergy, Asthma & Immunology 88(3):283–291

Yung M, South M 1998 Randomised controlled trial of aminophylline for severe acute asthma. Archives of Disease in Childhood 79:405–410

Resources

Useful addresses

National Asthma Campaign (NAC)
Providence House
Providence Place
London N1 0NT
Tel: 020 7226 2260
www.asthma.org.uk

Education and training

National Respiratory Training Centre
The Athenaeum
10 Church Street
Warwick CV34 4AB
Tel: 01926 493313
Fax: 01926 493224
www.nrtc.org.uk

Child growth foundation growth charts supplied by:

Harlow Printing Limited
Maxwell Street
South Shields
Tyne and Wear NE33 4PU

Further reading

NRTC 2003 Simply asthma. A pocket book. National Respiratory Training Centre, Warwick

Chapter 8

Chronic obstructive pulmonary disease

Rachel Booker

CHAPTER CONTENTS

INTRODUCTION

Chronic obstructive pulmonary disease (COPD) is a common condition encountered in general practice. There are currently around 600 000 people in the UK with diagnosed COPD, but because it tends to present in the late, severe stages of the disease process this is probably an underestimate of its true prevalence. It causes around 30 000 deaths per year in the UK and is projected to become the fifth most common cause of death worldwide by 2020 (Murray & Lopez 1996).

The slowly progressive nature of COPD results in considerable morbidity and disability. Many sufferers are forced to give up work early, disrupting long-held retirement plans, causing loss of productive life and financial hardship. Currently COPD costs around £331 million per year in state benefits and results in the loss of 21.9 million working days (BTS 2001).

As the disease progresses sufferers often become housebound, socially isolated and dependent. Depression and loss of self-esteem are common. Despite knowledge of the devastating effects COPD has on patients and their families it has, until recently, been the 'Cinderella' of respiratory medicine and has received little attention. However, the publication of national and international guidelines on the management of COPD has increased interest and research in this neglected area. This may lead to improvements for patients.

DEFINITIONS

COPD is defined as:

> *A chronic, slowly progressive disorder characterized by airflow obstruction (reduced FEV_1 and FEV_1/FVC*

ratio) that does not change markedly over several months. Most of the lung function impairment is fixed, although some reversibility can be produced by bronchodilator (or other) therapy. (BTS 1997a)

COPD is an umbrella term encompassing several disease processes.

- Chronic bronchitis
- Small airway disease (also known as chronic bronchiolitis)
- Emphysema
- Chronic asthma that has become irreversible

Chronic bronchitis is defined as: 'The production of sputum on most days for at least 3 months in at least 2 consecutive years – in the absence of other causes for excess sputum production' (MRC 1965). This definition describes a set of symptoms that is common amongst smokers. Many smokers develop a 'smoker's cough', but it is known that only 15–20% develop the airflow obstruction that is the primary feature of COPD.

Small airway disease refers to the pathological changes that result in permanent narrowing and distortion of the small, 2–5 mm airways. These include:

- inflammatory changes in the airway wall
- inflammatory exudates
- fibrosis and smooth muscle hypertrophy
- goblet cell hyperplasia
- occlusion of the airway with mucus and exudates. This can be particularly prominent during exacerbations and further increases airflow obstruction.

Emphysema is defined as: 'A condition of the lung characterized by abnormal, permanent enlargement of the air spaces distal to the terminal bronchiole, accompanied by destruction of their walls' (Snider et al 1985). This definition describes a pathological process that is largely associated with cigarette smoking. Cigarette smoke is an irritant and, in some people, results in an imbalance between destructive and protective enzymes in the lungs, causing a loss of alveolar tissue. This loss of alveolar tissue has several important consequences.

- **Loss of lung elasticity.** The natural elastic properties of the lung provides some of the driving force behind exhalation and helps to expel air from the alveoli at the end of a breath. Elastic recoil of the lungs helps to support the small airways and prevent them from collapsing during exhalation.

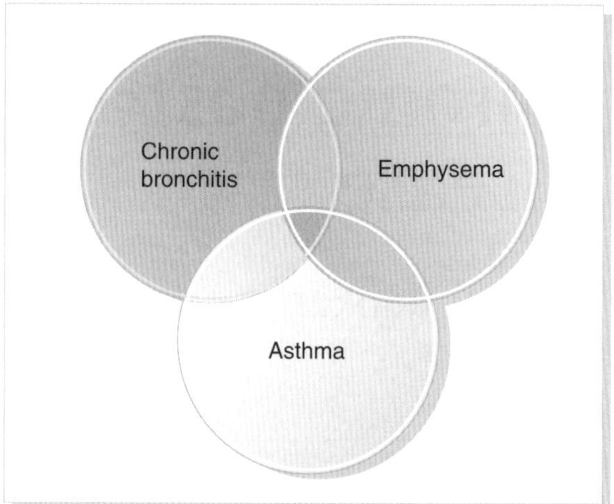

Figure 8.1 The overlapping spectrum of COPD.

- **Loss of alveolar capillary interface.** Reduction in the surface area of the lungs reduces the ability to exchange oxygen and carbon dioxide efficiently.

Thus emphysema can result in both disrupted gas exchange and airflow obstruction.

Asthma is defined as: 'A chronic inflammatory condition of the airways, leading to widespread, variable airways obstruction that is reversible spontaneously or with treatment' (BTS 1997b). Long-standing asthma can result in permanent remodelling of the airways and loss of reversibility.

The duration and severity of the asthma are important risk factors and there is increasing evidence that the underuse of effective antiinflammatory treatments increases the risk of developing fixed airflow obstruction.

In summary, there are a number of different pathological processes that go to make up the spectrum of COPD. In practice, all these processes may be occurring at the same time in the same patient and patients may demonstrate features of all of them (Fig. 8.1).

LONG-TERM CONSEQUENCES

Chronic disruption of airflow results in abnormal gas exchange and reduced oxygen levels – hypoxaemia. The normal response to hypoxaemia is to increase the respiratory rate to correct the blood gases. However, some people have a more responsive respiratory drive than others. Those with a responsive respiratory drive will continue to breathe harder and harder as the disease progresses and, whilst they will manage to keep their oxygen levels within reasonably normal limits, they will be acutely breathless.

Patients who are severely breathless are often underweight. The increased work of breathing results in increased energy expenditure. Breathlessness also impedes patients' ability to cook, shop and eat and they may be unable to meet their energy requirements. Weight loss results and this is associated with increased mortality.

Those with a less responsive respiratory drive tolerate a degree of hypoxaemia and will be less breathless. However, the long-term consequences of chronic hypoxaemia shorten life expectancy considerably. These patients develop complications involving the heart – cor pulmonale.

Cor pulmonale is complex and incompletely understood. It is a syndrome characterized by:

- chronic hypoxaemia
- renal hypoxia with consequent disruption of fluid balance mechanisms
- oedema
- pulmonary hypertension
- right ventricular strain, hypertrophy and eventual failure.

Why there are individual differences in the responsiveness of the respiratory drive is not understood, but it is thought that there are genetic or familial factors involved.

CAUSES OF CHRONIC OBSTRUCTIVE PULMONARY DISEASE

CIGARETTE SMOKING

Overwhelmingly, the most important cause of COPD is cigarette smoking with 90% of cases being due to smoking. However, not all smokers are at risk of developing COPD.

Fifteen to 20% of smokers suffer an accelerated decline in lung function as a result of their smoking habit (Fletcher & Peto 1977). Forced expired volume in 1 second (FEV_1) reaches maximum value by the age of 25 years and normally declines at the rate of 25–30 ml a year after the age of 35–45 years. In 'at-risk' smokers the rate of decline can be double or more the normal rate (Fig. 8.2).

Unfortunately this loss of lung function occurs in the so-called 'silent area' of the lungs – airways 2–5 mm in diameter – and is asymptomatic until at

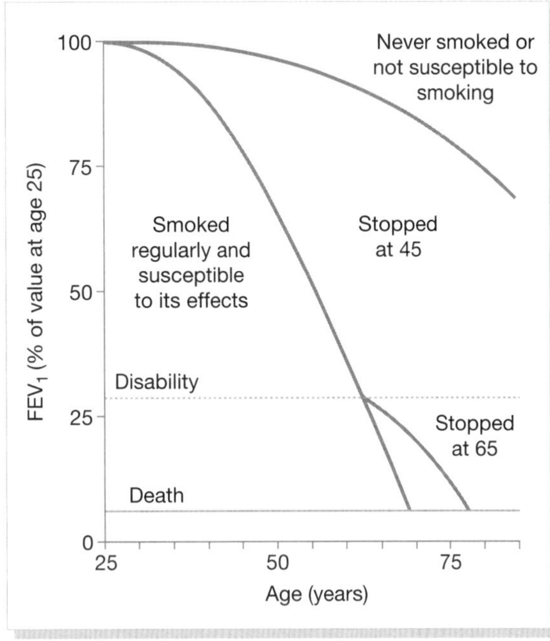

Figure 8.2 Influence of smoking on airflow obstruction.

least half the FEV_1 at 25 years of age is irretrievably lost. Patients therefore have lost considerable lung function by the time they present with symptoms. If they can be persuaded to stop smoking the rate of decline will revert to that of a non-smoker or non-susceptible smoker. Even when symptoms of COPD have developed, worthwhile salvage of lung function and life expectancy can still be achieved.

IT IS *NEVER* TOO LATE TO STOP SMOKING!

AGE AND SEX

Because COPD is slowly progressive, increasing age is a risk factor. Currently there are more males than females with COPD but whilst the rate of COPD in men is stable and may be declining, the rate in women is increasing, reflecting changes in women's smoking habits.

LOWER SOCIO-ECONOMIC STATUS

COPD is more prevalent in lower socio-economic groups. Whilst these groups have higher smoking rates this would not seem to be the only causative factor.

Antioxidant vitamins, such as vitamin C, are thought to be protective of lung function and a diet low in these vitamins may be associated with decreased lung function and increased risk of COPD. Crowded, damp housing may increase the risk of repeated respiratory infection.

Thus, not only high levels of smoking but also poor housing, poor diet and 'risky' occupations (see below) are all thought to contribute to the high levels of COPD in these groups.

BRONCHIAL HYPERRESPONSIVENESS (BHR)

BHR is a feature of asthma but is also present in smokers. Increased 'twitchiness' of airway muscle is thought to result in muscle hypertrophy and airway obstruction.

LOW BIRTHWEIGHT AND INFECTION IN INFANCY

Pregnancy and the first 3 years of life are periods of rapid lung growth and development. If the fetus is malnourished in utero lung function will be reduced at birth. Children who have severe lower respiratory tract infection in infancy and early childhood also suffer an 'insult' during a period of rapid lung growth and development.

Unfortunately lung development does not 'catch up' after such insults and when the child reaches adulthood the lung function is likely to be reduced. They will then have less to lose during the ageing process.

Low birthweight and childhood respiratory infections are thought to be independent risk factors for reduced lung function in adult life and are more common in children whose mothers smoke.

OCCUPATION

Some occupations carry an increased risk of COPD.

- Coal mining – coal miners who develop COPD are now eligible for compensation, although the rate of compensation awarded is adjusted to take account of smoking habit
- Welders – welding fumes contain many noxious gases
- Cotton processing
- Farming
- Steel foundry workers

Any occupation involving dusty, dirty working conditions may be a risk factor for the development of COPD, but only coal miners are currently eligible for compensation. Information about compensation can be obtained from the Employment Medical Advisory Service, part of the Health and Safety Executive.

AIR POLLUTION

Air pollution in the UK is largely due to vehicle emissions and since the 1950s and the advent of Clean Air legislation, the level of heavy particulate pollution has fallen dramatically. Whilst vehicle emission pollution is a respiratory irritant and will worsen existing COPD, it is not currently thought to be a causative factor. Heavy particulate pollution in industrial cities in the Third World, however, is thought to cause COPD in non-smokers.

ALPHA 1 ANTITRYPSIN DEFICIENCY

Alpha 1 antitrypsin is a protective enzyme that neutralizes a destructive elastase. Deficiency is a rare, inherited cause of emphysema. Although it accounts for less than 1% of cases of COPD it should be suspected if patients present under the age of 40 years, if they have a light smoking history and if they have a strong family history of severe COPD at a young age. It can be detected with a blood test.

PRESENTATION AND HISTORY

The most important presenting symptoms of COPD are slowly progressive breathlessness on exertion, cough (with or without sputum production), wheeze and repeated winter chest infections.

Asthma and COPD share many common features and asthma can occur at any age, regardless of smoking history. Differentiating between the two can be difficult but there are some discriminating features. Those that are particularly useful are highlighted in bold type in Table 8.1.

Breathlessness on exertion is slowly progressive but some patients will state that their symptoms started with a chest infection and that they have not recovered since then. Close questioning will often reveal that they have unconsciously adapted their lives to their breathlessness prior to this and the infective episode was 'the straw that broke the camel's back'. Questions such as: 'Before you had this infection were you able to walk briskly, keeping up with your friends?' and 'Were you able to walk and carry on a conversation at the same time?' may

Table 8.1 Differences between the presentation and history of asthma and COPD

Asthma	COPD
H/O asthma or childhood wheeze or chestiness	No history of asthma or childhood wheeze
Positive family history of asthma or atopy (eczema, rhinitis, etc.)	No family history of asthma or atopy
Previous H/O atopic disease	No H/O atopic disease
Allergic triggers (cat, house dust, etc.) or symptoms that are worse in summer	No clear exacerbating factors apart from upper respiratory tract viral infections
Variable symptoms that come and go. Cough and wheeze often prominent	**Slow, insidious onset of shortness of breath on exertion with no 'good days and bad days'**
Waking at night with cough/wheeze	No nocturnal disturbance with respiratory symptoms
Morning symptoms persist for several hours	Morning cough clears rapidly after producing sputum
Sputum 'thick and tacky' and difficult to clear – green/yellow with exacerbations	Sputum grey and mucoid. Easy to clear. Mucopurulent and increased volume during exacerbations
Non-smoker or genuinely light smoking history	**Significant smoking history – usually >20 pack-years**
Symptoms started <40 years	**Symptoms develop >45 years**
Good response to bronchodilators	Modest response to bronchodilators

H/O = history of

reveal the slowly progressive symptoms that are suggestive of COPD.

It is important to elicit an accurate smoking history. Pack-years are probably the best way of estimating an individual's tobacco exposure, calculated by the equation:

$$\frac{\text{Number smoked per day}}{20} \times \text{Number of years smoked}$$

A significant smoking history for COPD is greater than 20 pack-years, although a light smoking history does not preclude it. COPD does occur, rarely, in light or non-smokers.

Box 8.1 Differential diagnoses to consider in COPD

- Asthma
- Cardiac disease:
  - left ventricular failure
  - angina
  - valve disease
- Lung cancer
- Anaemia
- Bronchiectasis
- Fibrotic/interstitial lung disease

Smokers are also at risk of other smoking-related diseases such as ischaemic heart disease and lung cancer. It is most important that, before a patient is labelled as suffering from COPD, alternative causes for the symptoms are excluded.

People with mild, early COPD are unlikely to be known to their GP. Mild COPD may present as repeated winter 'chest infections'. A high index of suspicion in smokers and ex-smokers who present with infections every winter may improve the rate of diagnosis.

ASSESSMENT

SPIROMETRY

COPD may be suggested by the history but spirometry is essential for the early and accurate diagnosis of COPD.

Peak expiratory flow rate (PEFR), whilst extremely helpful for monitoring the variable, diffuse airflow obstruction that is typical of asthma, is less useful for detecting the small airway obstruction of COPD. It can significantly underestimate the degree of obstruction in COPD and may be normal in mild and moderate disease.

FEV_1 is the measurement of choice.
In COPD:

- the FEV_1 is less than 80% of the predicted value
- the FEV_1 does not improve to over 80% of the predicted value after administration of bronchodilators or steroids
- the FEV_1/FVC ratio is less than 70%.

Spirometers are becoming more widely available in general practice. There are a wide variety of spirometers available, in various price ranges and relying on different technologies to obtain the result. However, there are national guidelines on the features a spirometer should incorporate.

- It should be possible to accurately check the calibration at regular intervals.
- A hard copy of the results should be available.
- There should be a printout of the volume time graph of sufficient size to enable manual checking of the results and the technical acceptability of the blow (slow start to the blow, early stoppage, etc.).
- A visual display of the blow, in order to check the accuracy of the patient's technique, is helpful.
- A flow volume trace is optional.

If spirometry is used in general practice:

- the personnel using spirometers must have appropriate, recognized training in what constitutes an acceptable technique and how to obtain it
- there must be someone competent in the basic interpretation of results.

If these conditions are not available in the practice then referral for lung function testing is needed. Some areas have open access to lung function laboratories but others require the patient to be referred to the chest physician. In other areas the primary care trust runs a spirometry and COPD assessment service.

The technique for spirometry is difficult for patients to master and poorly performed spirometry is worse than useless. It may lead to inaccurate diagnosis and inappropriate treatment, missed diagnosis, inappropriate referral or failure to refer those patients who require secondary care.

REVERSIBILITY TESTING

Reversibility testing used to be recommended as a routine diagnostic procedure (BTS 1997a). However, there are several difficulties with this approach.

Box 8.2 Classification of disease severity

Disease severity	FEV_1 (% predicted FEV_1)
Mild airflow obstruction	50–80% predicted
Moderate airflow obstruction	30–50% predicted
Severe airflow obstruction	Less than 30% predicted

- The degree of reversibility previously cited as significant was not evidence based.
- COPD patients can show significant, spontaneous variability in response to a single dose of bronchodilator. This variability could result in a 'positive' response on one day and a 'negative' one the next.
- A reversibility test does not predict long-term symptomatic response to treatment. Bronchodilator reversibility testing is therefore unhelpful in determining which therapy to give the patient for long-term use.
- Trials of corticosteroids do not accurately predict which patients will benefit from long-term inhaled corticosteroids.

Evidence-based guidelines from The National Institute for Clinical Excellence (NICE) no longer recommend routine reversibility testing. **The diagnosis of COPD can generally be made on the basis of a thorough clinical history, and spirometric evidence of airflow obstruction.** The response to a therapeutic trial of bronchodilators of several weeks' duration can then be assessed objectively with spirometry and subjectively in terms of symptomatic response. COPD is unlikely if:

- the FEV_1 and FEV_1/FVC ratio return to normal with therapy
- the patient reports a dramatic improvement in their symptoms with therapy.

The role of reversibility testing is to help differentiate between asthma and COPD where the history is not clear. Reversibility tests should be performed when the patient is clinically stable. Reversibility can be tested with bronchodilators and/or steroids.

- Measure FEV_1 before and 15 minutes after 2.5–5 mg salbutamol or 5–10 mg terbutaline via nebulizer, or four puffs salbutamol or terbutaline via large volume spacer.

Or

- Measure FEV_1 before and 30 minutes after 250–500 μg ipratropium bromide via nebulizer, or four puffs ipratropium bromide via large volume spacer.

Or

- Measure FEV_1 before and 30 minutes after both drugs in combination.

And/or

- Measure FEV_1 before and after a trial of 30 mg prednisolone a day for 2 weeks.

An improvement in the FEV_1 of 400 ml or more is highly suggestive of asthma.

To calculate percentage change in FEV_1 in reversibility testing:

$$\frac{\text{Posttest FEV}_1 - \text{Pretest FEV}_1}{\text{Pretest FEV}_1} \times 100$$

EXCLUDING ALTERNATIVE DIAGNOSES

Chest X-ray

Middle-aged and elderly smokers who present with respiratory symptoms should have a chest X-ray in order to help exclude:

- lung cancer (most but not all lung cancers will be visible on chest X-ray by the time patients present with symptoms)
- ventricular failure and pulmonary oedema
- pulmonary fibrosis.

Chest X-ray cannot confirm a diagnosis of COPD. A hyperinflated picture may support a diagnosis of COPD but it should be remembered that this is also seen in uncontrolled asthma.

ECG or echocardiography

Should be considered if there is:

- a history of ischaemic heart disease or hypertension – particularly in the diabetic patient
- a previous history of valve disease
- doubt about the diagnosis.

Full blood count

- To exclude anaemia as a cause of breathlessness.
- To detect secondary polycythaemia (this can occur in COPD as a result of chronic hypoxaemia).

ASSESSING DISABILITY AND HANDICAP

COPD, by definition, causes irreversible airflow obstruction and large improvements in lung function with therapy should not be expected. Improvements in the level of disability and handicap that patients experience are, however, achievable. It is important to take some baseline measure of how the disease impacts on a patient's life in order to assess any response to interventions.

Assessment of disability

'Disability' refers to the impact that a disease has on a patient's ability to work and carry out normal activities of daily life.

Six-minute walk The distance a patient can walk, indoors on the flat, over a 6-minute period is measured. A practice walk is allowed and a standardized method of encouragement is used. Measurements are taken after the second walk.

This is often not practical in a general practice setting.

Shuttle test This test is most often used for assessment before and after a rehabilitation programme and is well validated, sensitive and reproducible. The patient walks between two cones, 10 metres apart, each circuit of the cones being a 'shuttle'. The speed of the walk is dictated by 'beeps' from a tape recording and gets progressively faster. The number of shuttles completed before the patient is forced to stop is counted.

Medical Research Council Dyspnoea Scale Patients grade their breathlessness on a scale of 0–5 depending on the activity that induces it (Table 8.2).

This is a quick and easy test but is relatively insensitive to change. Its main use is as a baseline measure of disability and to assess disease progression on an annual basis.

Oxygen cost diagram This visual analogue scale (Fig. 8.3) allows the patient to place a mark on a 10 cm line against an activity, beyond which they would become breathless.

This too is quick and easy to use and has the advantage of being sensitive to change. It can be used to assess response to treatment.

Borg Scale Patients grade their breathlessness performing a particular activity according to the intensity of the sensation. This too is a sensitive tool and can be used to assess response to treatment.

0 Nothing at all
0.5 Very, very slight (just noticeable)

Table 8.2 MRC Dyspnoea Scale

Grade	Degree of breathlessness related to activities
0	Not troubled by breathlessness except on strenuous exercise
1	Short of breath when hurrying or walking up a slight hill
2	Walks slower than contemporaries on the level because of breathlessness or has to stop for breath when walking at own pace
3	Stops for breath after walking about 100 m or after a few minutes on the level
4	Too breathless to leave the house or breathless when dressing or undressing
5	Breathless at rest

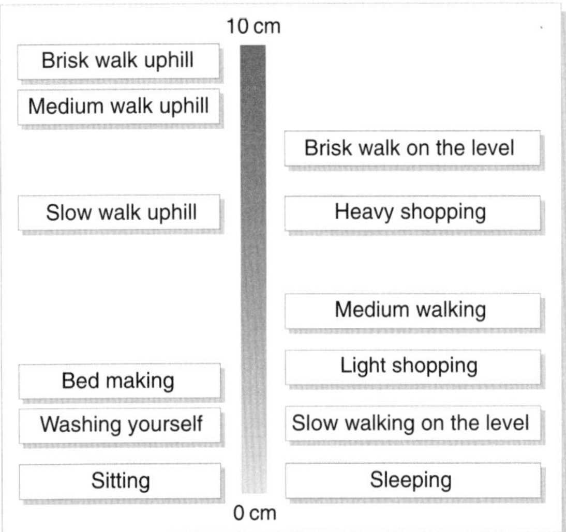

Figure 8.3 Oxygen cost diagram.

1	Very slight
2	Slight (light)
3	Moderate
4	Somewhat severe
5	Severe (heavy)
6	
7	Very severe
8	
9	Very, very severe (almost maximal)
10	Maximal

Assessing health status

'Health status' (handicap) is the term used to describe the 'global' impact of COPD on a patient. It encompasses areas such as the degree of control and mastery over their condition that patients feel and the emotions that it engenders. Health status is individual and is poorly related to lung function. Some patients with very severe COPD are little handicapped by it and vice versa.

Health status can be improved by both drug and management interventions.

Health status can be measured using a variety of questionnaires, such as the Chronic Respiratory Disease Index Questionnaire (CRDIQ), the St George's Respiratory Questionnaire (SGRQ) and the Breathing Problems Questionnaire (BPQ). However, these were developed as tools for research and some are time consuming to administer and complicated to score. Few are practical for everyday use.

Some questions that may help in assessing how patients cope with their disease and serve to generate discussion include:

- How confident do you feel about dealing with your illness?
- Do you feel upset or frightened by your attacks of breathlessness?
- Do you feel in control of your breathlessness?
- How tired does your illness make you feel?
- Does your illness make you feel 'down' or depressed?

It is most important that nurses who care for COPD patients work closely with their GP colleagues. These older smokers often suffer from multiple pathologies and present diagnostic and management problems. A team approach will give these patients the best possible care.

MANAGEMENT

Management of COPD can best be divided into five main areas.

- Prevention of disease progression
- Relief of symptoms, reduction of disability and improvement of health status:
  - with drug therapy
  - with other approaches
- Prevention and treatment of exacerbations
- Improvement of life expectancy
- Terminal care

PREVENTION OF DISEASE PROGRESSION

Smoking cessation

This is the only intervention that slows progression of COPD. It must be actively encouraged and patients should be offered support to attempt to stop. The use of nicotine replacement therapy or bupropion has been shown to considerably increase the chances of success and should be encouraged.

Steroids

Recent large, randomized placebo-controlled trials have shown that inhaled steroids do not slow the decline of lung function in COPD at any stage of the disease (Burge et al 2000, LHSRG 2000, Pauwels et al 1999, Vestbo et al 1999).

Oral steroids also have no effect on lung function decline. The side-effects of maintenance oral steroids in this group of patients are very significant and long-term oral steroid use is not indicated.

Future developments

New drugs that may affect disease progression are currently being developed, but the mainstay of prevention is, and is likely to remain, smoking cessation.

RELIEF OF SYMPTOMS, REDUCTION OF DISABILITY AND IMPROVEMENTS IN HEALTH STATUS

Drug therapy

Bronchodilators The cornerstone of COPD treatment is bronchodilator therapy. The same bronchodilators as are used in asthma are effective but they are needed in higher doses and more regularly for the treatment of COPD.

Response to bronchodilators varies between individuals. The most effective drug or combination of drugs needs to be determined on an individual basis following therapeutic trials of several weeks. The best way to assess the outcome of a therapeutic trial is to use a measure of disability, such as the oxygen cost or Borg Scale. Assessment of outcome in terms of lung function lacks logic since it is unlikely to alter significantly. If a patient is able to:

- walk further
- do more or do the same but more quickly
- get less breathless
- feel better

the trial can be considered positive.

Both short-acting beta 2 stimulants and anticholinergic bronchodilators have been shown to be effective. Anticholinergic bronchodilators may be particularly useful since increased cholinergic tone is thought to be an important factor in the airflow obstruction of COPD.

Combinations of short-acting beta 2 stimulants and anticholinergics may provide the best symptom relief for some patients. Patients with moderate and severe disease often need to take bronchodilators both regularly and on a prn basis. They are often prescribed for use at doses outside their licence. They are generally safe and well tolerated and patients should be reassured about this.

The long-acting beta 2 stimulant salmeterol has been shown to be effective in reducing symptoms and is licensed for use in COPD. Tiotropium, a long-acting anticholinergic with a duration of action of 24 hours is licensed for use in COPD. Long-acting beta 2 stimulants and tiotropium provide improvements in lung function, prolonged symptom relief and reduce the frequency of exacerbations. They appear to be more effective than short-acting agents and the NICE guideline (NCCCC 2004) recommends that they be considered in patients who experience symptoms despite the use of short-acting agents.

Inhaler devices The same consideration should be given to selection of inhaler devices for COPD patients as is given to asthma patients. Factors such as portability and patient acceptability should be considered. Large-volume spacers can be particularly useful, especially in severe disease, but they are not portable and if patients are to be encouraged to maintain social contacts and activity a smaller, portable, discreet device may be more acceptable.

In severe disease nebulizers may be the most effective way of delivering high-dose bronchodilators. However, the patient should be assessed by a specialist before long-term nebulized therapy is recommended. Nebulized therapy is expensive and

Box 8.3 Nebulizer trial

Weeks 1–2	400 µg salbutamol + 80 µg ipratropium bromide qds via spacer
Weeks 3–4	2.5–5 mg salbutamol qds via nebulizer
Weeks 5–6	250–500 µg ipratropium bromide qds via nebulizer
Weeks 7–8	Combination of 2.5–5 mg salbutamol + 250–500 µg ipratropium bromide qds via nebulizer

Assess response to each arm of the trial. A positive response is an improvement in disability or well-being or a 15% improvement in the mean PEFR.

compressors and nebulizers are not available on prescription. The provision of centrally organized nebulizer services that assess and supervise patients, provide and maintain equipment is not yet universal.

For many patients multiple doses of bronchodilator administered from a standard inhaler device can provide the same symptomatic relief as a nebulizer and may be cheaper and more convenient.

Other approaches

Pulmonary rehabilitation Breathlessness induces panic and anxiety, which then results in activity avoidance. This in turn reduces general fitness and increases breathlessness. The COPD patient is in a downward spiral of breathlessness, activity avoidance, worsening general fitness and increasing breathlessness. Dependence and social isolation increase. The sufferer frequently loses self-esteem and becomes withdrawn, depressed and hopeless.

Breathlessness is not intrinsically harmful and patients can become 'desensitized' to their breathlessness if they are encouraged to exercise. They become fitter, able to do more and experience reduced symptoms, improved health status and disability. This is the cornerstone of pulmonary rehabilitation.

Pulmonary rehabilitation consists of an individually prescribed exercise programme, combined with education to improve understanding and self-management skills. It is highly effective at reducing disability and improving health status in COPD and has also been shown to reduce emergency admissions. Carers are usually actively encouraged to participate and rehabilitation sessions also become social and supportive events.

Most rehabilitation programmes are hospital based, although more primary care-based programmes are being set up. Programmes usually last for between 6 and 9 weeks with patients attending 2–3 sessions a week. Each session contains an element of exercise and an education session. Patients are also expected to complete a programme of exercise at home.

At the end of the programme patients are either discharged back to primary care or are graduated to a self-help group, such as a local British Lung Foundation Breathe Easy group.

It is a sad fact that the provision of pulmonary rehabilitation is still patchy and there are many areas of the country without access to a secondary or primary care-based programme. The role of the practice nurse is to channel appropriate patients to existing programmes and to support and encourage 'graduates' to continue with the exercise and lifestyle changes they have undertaken during pulmonary rehabilitation.

Where there is no access to pulmonary rehabilitation practice nurses should encourage and support patients to remain as active as possible. Simply reassuring COPD patients that it is safe for them to get breathless and encouraging them to take some form of regular exercise, a daily walk at their own pace or stair climbing every day for example, can be helpful.

A Borg Scale can be used to help and encourage patients. They should be encouraged to exercise between 3 and 5 on the Borg Scale.

NICE recognise the benefits of rehabilitation and state that programmes should be available for all suitable patients and for all patients who consider themselves functionally disabled by their disease; generally MRC dyspnoea scale 3 and above. It is hoped that this recommendation will provide the impetus to improve the provision of this highly effective service.

Short-term oxygen Oxygen is often given to patients with severe COPD to relieve severe breathlessness or to 'preoxygenate' before a bout of exercise. There is no good research to support this practice and there is likely to be a considerable placebo response.

The following are suggestions for assessing suitability for short-term oxygen (RCP 1999).

- Oxygen saturation decreases to 86% or less on exercise.
- A 10% improvement in walking distance on oxygen.
- A 10% reduction in a visual analogue breathlessness score on oxygen.

Many patients who fit these criteria are likely to fit the criteria for long-term oxygen as well (see below).

PREVENTION AND TREATMENT OF EXACERBATIONS

Vaccination against influenza and pneumococcal pneumonia

Influenza vaccination has been shown to reduce mortality from COPD and should be actively encouraged. Specific data for the effectiveness of pneumococcal vaccination in COPD are limited. However, the Department of Health and NICE recommend that it is offered to patients suffering from chronic lung disease and the vaccine is safe. It should only be given once. Booster doses are not needed.

Recent research into inhaled steroids

There is evidence (Burge et al 2000) that high doses of inhaled fluticasone – 1000 μg per day – reduce the number of exacerbations, and the consequent accelerated decline in health status, in patients with severe COPD.

NICE recommend the use of long-term inhaled steroids for patients who have:

- an FEV_1 less than 50% predicted
- experienced two or more exacerbations requiring treatment with oral steroids and/or antibiotics in the previous 12 months.

Inhaled steroids will generally be added to long-acting bronchodilators. Combinations of inhaled steroid and long-acting beta 2 agonists are licensed for use in COPD.

The most effective dose of inhaled steroids has yet to be determined. Metaanalysis suggests that moderate to high doses are needed and that low doses are not effective (Alsaeedi et al 2002). Further dose-ranging studies are needed to definitively determine the optimum dose.

There are few data on the long-term side effects of high dose inhaled steroids on this population of elderly, immobile smokers. NICE recommend that consideration be given to the use of osteoporosis prophylaxis; particularly when there are other risk factors for osteoporosis present.

Self-management advice

There is very limited evidence that self-management plans, such as have been used for asthma, are effective in reducing exacerbations in COPD. However, informing patients and their carers of the signs and symptoms that should lead them to seek medical advice is advocated by NICE.

- Increase in sputum volume
- Increase in sputum purulence
- Increasing breathlessness or wheeze
- Development or worsening of ankle oedema

Some physicians give patients a supply of antibiotics and/or steroids to keep at home so that they can initiate treatment promptly without having to wait to see a doctor.

Education to empower patients and improve feelings of control is likely to be helpful and is generally well received by patients and their carers.

Bronchodilators in exacerbations

Bronchodilators should be increased during an exacerbation. Patients should be encouraged to use higher doses, more regularly and the addition of other bronchodilators, e.g. anticholinergics, may be needed. Large-volume spacers can be helpful but nebulizers are not usually necessary.

Antibiotics in exacerbations

Antibiotics are recommended if the patient has increased sputum purulence during an exacerbation. They are not indicated if this is not the case, except if there are clinical signs of pneumonia or a chest X-ray shows consolidation.

Antibiotics should be prescribed in line with local protocols and in short courses.

Oral steroids in exacerbations

Oral steroids are indicated in the following circumstances.

- If the exacerbation is associated with a significant increase in breathlessness which interferes with daily activities.
- For all patients requiring hospital admission.

Prednisolone should be given in short courses of 30 mg per day for 1–2 weeks. If exacerbations are frequent and the patient has an FEV_1 below 50% predicted, consideration should be given to commencing long-term inhaled steroids to reduce the frequency of exacerbations.

Patients who require frequent short courses of oral steroids, should be monitored for osteoporosis and considered for osteoporosis prophylaxis.

IMPROVEMENT OF LIFE EXPECTANCY

Smoking cessation

Reduces the rate of decline of lung function and improves life expectancy.

Long-term oxygen therapy (LTOT)

Used to treat chronic hypoxaemia. It can reduce pulmonary hypertension and improve life expectancy. Ankle oedema, exercise tolerance, appetite, general mental ability and quality of life may also improve considerably. Patients who have experienced cor pulmonale have only a 30% 3-year survival without LTOT. Improvements in life expectancy can be very substantial if LTOT is given to patients at an appropriate stage in their disease. To facilitate this NICE recommend that pulse oximetry be recorded in all patients with moderate to severe COPD (FEV_1 50% predicted or less) as a routine.

Patients who have presented with ankle oedema and/or cyanosis and who:

- are taking optimum bronchodilator therapy
- have oxygen saturation <92%
- are currently stable (more than 4 weeks after their last exacerbation)

should be considered for referral for arterial blood gases.

The criteria for LTOT are:

- FEV_1 less than 1.5 litres
- PaO_2 <7.3 kPa

or

- PaO_2 7.3–8 kPa + evidence of pulmonary hypertension or nocturnal hypoxaemia

Patients who continue to smoke are not usually considered for LTOT. The lung function will continue to decline at an accelerated rate in such patients and since their haemoglobin will be taken up with carbon monoxide, they are unlikely to benefit from treatment. They are also a fire hazard.

Arterial blood gases need to be taken twice, breathing air, over a 3-week period.

LTOT needs to be given for a minimum of 15 hours a day if it is to improve life expectancy. The flow rate needs to be determined by the chest physician and must not be exceeded. These patients may suffer a depressed respiratory drive and carbon dioxide retention if too much oxygen is given.

The most cost-effective and convenient method of delivering LTOT is with an oxygen concentrator. In Scotland the oxygen concentrator is prescribed by the chest physician. In England, Wales and Northern Ireland the GP prescribes LTOT following recommendation by the chest physician. The company with the contract for delivering services to patients in each region is listed in the British National Formulary. They are responsible for supplying and maintaining the concentrator. The cost of the electricity used for running the concentrator is reimbursed directly to the patient.

TERMINAL CARE

The inexorably progressive nature of COPD means that patients will eventually reach the end-stage of their disease. Most will no longer be able to attend the GP surgery and practice nurse involvement in their care may be confined to an advisory and supportive role as the 'respiratory expert' in the nursing team. The district nursing service is likely to be most closely involved at this stage.

It is important for both patients and their carers that all avenues of extra support, both financial and practical, for day-to-day care have been explored. Other agencies, such as Macmillan nursing services or palliative care nursing teams, could also be usefully involved at this stage. NICE recommend that the full range of palliative care services, including hospice care, should be made available to COPD patients, but unfortunately care and support for terminally ill COPD patients is still woefully inadequate in most areas of the country.

CONCLUSION

The early detection of mild COPD with active support to stop smoking may prevent the development of severe, symptomatic disease. However, there has been a great deal of nihilism surrounding the treatment of symptomatic COPD and health professionals have often felt that there was nothing that could be done. There is no longer any justification for such attitudes. Like other chronic, debilitating illnesses, COPD patients often benefit from the holistic care that properly trained nurses can give. Whilst it is not possible to reverse lung damage and return patients to complete health, there is a great deal that can be done to improve disability, reduce symptoms, improve health status and enable patients and their families to have the best attainable quality of life.

References

Alsaeedi A, Sin DD, McAlister FA 2002 The effects of inhaled corticosteroids in chronic obstructive pulmonary disease: A systematic review of randomized placebo-controlled trials. American Journal of Medicine 113:59–65.

BTS 1997a BTS guidelines on the management of chronic obstructive pulmonary disease. Thorax 52 (suppl 5):S1–S28

BTS 1997b British guidelines for asthma management. Thorax 52 (suppl 2):S1–S24

BTS 2001 The burden of lung disease. www.brit-thoracic.org.uk/publi/publications.html

Burge PS, Calverley PMA, Jones PW, Spencer S, Anderson JA, Maslen TK 2000 Randomised, double blind, placebo controlled study of fluticasone propionate in patients with moderate to severe chronic obstructive pulmonary disease: the ISOLDE trial. British Medical Journal 320:1297–1302

Fletcher C, Peto R 1977 The natural history of chronic air-flow obstruction. British Medical Journal I:1645–1648

LHSRG (Lung Health Study Research Group) 2000 Effect of inhaled triamcinolone on the decline in pulmonary function in chronic obstructive pulmonary disease. New England Journal of Medicine 343(26):1902–1909

Medical Research Council 1965 Definition and classification of chronic bronchitis for clinical and epidemiological purposes. Lancet i:775–779

Murray C, Lopez A 1996 Evidence-based health policy – lessons from the Global Burden of Disease Study. Science 274:740–743

National Collaborating Centre for Chronic Conditions (NCCCC) 2004 Chronic obstructive pulmonary disease: National Clinical Guideline for management of chronic obstructive pulmonary disease in adults in primary and secondary care. Thorax 59 (suppl 1)

Pauwels R, Lofdahl C, Laitinen L et al 1999 Long-term treatment with inhaled budesonide in persons with mild chronic obstructive pulmonary disease who continue smoking. New England Journal of Medicine 340:1948–1953

RCP 1999 Domiciliary oxygen therapy services. Royal College of Physicians, London

Snider G, Kleinerman J, Thurlbeck W, Bengazi S 1985 The definition of emphysema: report of the National Heart and Blood Institute, Division of Lung Diseases workshop. American Review of Respiratory Diseases 132:82–185

Vestbo J, Sorensen T, Lange P et al 1999 Long-term effect of inhaled budesonide in mild and moderate chronic obstructive pulmonary disease: a randomized controlled trial. Lancet 353:343–345

Resources

British Lung Foundation. Tel: 020 7831 5831. The BLF runs Breathe Easy groups for patients

British Thoracic Society. www.brit-thoracic.org.uk

Global Initiative for Chronic Obstructive Lung Disease (GOLD Initiative). www.gold.copd.com

National Institute for Clinical Excellence. www.nice.org.uk

Training

National Respiratory Training Centre (NRTC), The Athenaeum, 10 Church Street, Warwick CV34 4AB. Tel: 01926 493313. email: enquiries@nrtc.org.uk. Prospectus: www.nrtc.org.uk

The NRTC offers 'Essential Skills' training days in COPD and spirometry and assessed COPD courses at diploma (L2) and degree (L3) as stand-alone modules or as part of a DipHE or BSc(Hons) programme accredited by the Open University.

Respiratory Education and Training Centre, University Hospital Aintree, Training and Development Centre, Lower Lane, Liverpool L9 7AL. Tel: 0151 529 2598. email: info@respiratoryetc.com. Website: www.respiratoryetc.com

Chapter 9

Diabetes

Marilyn Gallichan

CHAPTER CONTENTS

Diabetes is a chronic disorder of metabolism in which the blood glucose is persistently raised. This is caused by a deficiency of insulin secretion by the pancreas and/or by insulin resistance, a reduction in tissue sensitivity to insulin. It has been estimated that the number of adults with diabetes worldwide will rise from 135 million in 1995 to 300 million in the year 2025 (King et al 1998). It affects at least 3% of the UK population, with an average age at diagnosis of 51–52 (Diabetes UK 2000). The estimated UK incidence is 1.7 new diagnoses per 1000 population per year (Gatling et al 2001) or three a year for each GP with an average list size.

In the past, most care for people with diabetes was provided by hospital specialist teams. However, changes to GP contracts, and health promotion payments from 1990, recognized and encouraged the already increasing role of primary care. Since then, there has been an even greater shift of responsibility to primary care. Children, and most people with type 1 diabetes, are still usually referred to hospital for all their diabetes care, but most routine care for adults with type 2 diabetes is provided in general practice. Practice nurses play a key role in care provision and coordination, liaising with other professionals as required, including the GP, the diabetes specialist nurse, dietitian, chiropodist, district nursing team, social workers, counsellor and diabetologist.

CLASSIFICATION OF DIABETES

Type 1 diabetes, formerly known as insulin-dependent diabetes, accounts for about 10% of cases in Europe and North America and can arise at any age. In most cases an autoimmune mechanism destroys the insulin-producing beta cells in the pancreatic islets of Langerhans. People with type 1 diabetes are dependent on injections of insulin to survive.

Type 2 diabetes, formerly known as non-insulin dependent diabetes, usually arises in middle or old age but is increasingly seen in younger people. It is much more common than type 1, accounting for about 90% of the diabetic population of Europe and North America, and is thought to be due to a combination of impaired insulin secretion and resistance to the action of insulin at its target cells. In most cases, it is a progressive disease in which insulin production declines over time and/or insulin resistance increases. About 10–20% of people with type 2 diabetes are able to achieve adequate blood glucose control through diet and exercise alone (UKPDS 1998), but the majority soon progress to monotherapy with an oral hypoglycaemic agent, then to a combination of two and sometimes three oral agents, before eventually requiring insulin treatment. Because of its slow onset, milder symptoms and the ability of patients to survive without insulin injections, type 2 was once considered to be a mild form of diabetes. However, it is now recognized that this is a serious condition in which quality of life and life expectancy are reduced because of a greatly increased risk of cardiovascular disease, as well as the same long-term complications as type 1 diabetes.

RISK FACTORS FOR DIABETES

People in the following categories are at increased risk of developing type 2 diabetes:

- people over 40 years of age
- people of Asian and Afro-Caribbean origin
- individuals who are overweight
- those with a family history of diabetes
- women with a history of gestational diabetes or any woman who has had a large baby (over 4 kg in weight).

Up to 50% of people with newly diagnosed diabetes already have evidence of diabetic tissue damage (UKPDS 1998), so it is hoped that the incidence of complications will be reduced by earlier diagnosis of diabetes. National guidelines for targeted population screening for type 2 diabetes are currently under development by the National Screening Committee but, in the meantime, opportunistic screening of people in the above categories is recommended.

Table 9.1 Differences between type 1 and type 2 diabetes

Type 1	Type 2
Onset at any age	Usually middle-aged or elderly at onset
Sudden onset of symptoms	Slow and insidious onset
Tend to be lean, with recent unexplained weight loss	Tend to be overweight (60% are obese at diagnosis)
Severe symptoms at diagnosis	Mild symptoms or may be diagnosed before symptoms develop
Ketonuria	Ketonuria unlikely
No long-term diabetic complications at diagnosis	Long-term complications often present at diagnosis
Insulin treatment essential	Insulin treatment optional
C-peptide absent or low	C-peptide present
Islet cell antibodies present	No islet cell antibodies

OTHER TYPES OF DIABETES

Diabetes is sometimes caused by other endocrine disorders (e.g. Cushing's syndrome, acromegaly) or by pancreatic disease (pancreatitis or haemochromatosis). It can be induced by drugs, especially steroids, and to a lesser extent by diuretics and beta-blockers and is also associated with a number of genetic syndromes (e.g. cystic fibrosis).

GESTATIONAL DIABETES

Another less common type of diabetes is gestational diabetes, which arises during pregnancy. Although it usually disappears on delivery of the baby, these women are at increased risk of developing diabetes later in life.

MATURITY-ONSET DIABETES OF THE YOUNG (MODY)

This is a rare genetic type of diabetes characterized by autosomal dominant inheritance, non-insulin dependence and a young age of onset, often before the age of 25.

SYMPTOMS

The classic symptoms of diabetes, weight loss, excessive thirst and urination, are usually severe in type 1 diabetes and can progress quickly to ketoacidosis and diabetic coma. Symptoms may be mild or absent in type 2 and clinicians should be alert to the possibility of diabetes in patients presenting with any of the symptoms shown in Box 9.1.

Box 9.1 Symptoms of diabetes

Recent weight loss (very rapid in type 1)
Polyuria, nocturia
Glycosuria
Tiredness
Blurred vision
Poor wound healing
Urine infections
Genital irritation or thrush
Boils, carbuncles or abscesses
Depression or irritable mood

DIAGNOSIS

A diagnosis should never be made on the basis of glycosuria or capillary blood glucose alone, although these may be useful screening methods. A laboratory plasma glucose estimation is essential. In the presence of classic diabetic symptoms, a single fasting plasma glucose over 7 mmol/l, or random plasma glucose over 11.1 mmol/l, is sufficient for a diagnosis of diabetes. In the absence of symptoms, the test should be repeated on another day, as at least two results in the diabetic range are required for a diagnosis.

A fasting plasma glucose of 6–7 mmol/l is termed impaired fasting glycaemia (IFG) and requires an oral glucose tolerance test (OGTT) to exclude or confirm a diagnosis of diabetes. An OGTT is also indicated when random plasma glucose results are 7.8–11.1 mmol/l. To perform an OGTT the patient continues his or her usual unmodified diet before

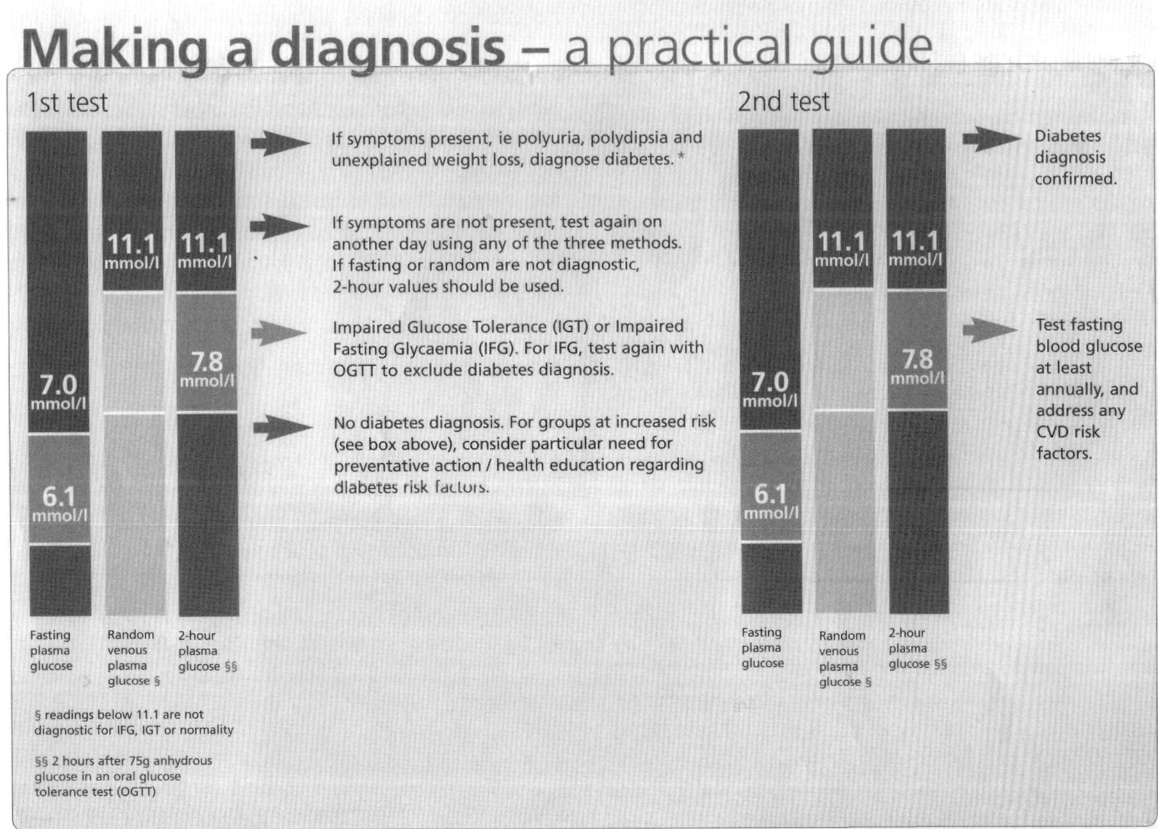

Figure 9.1 Making a diagnosis – a practical guide. © Diabetes UK. Reproduced from *Diabetes Update* (Summer 2000) with the kind permission of Diabetes UK.

fasting overnight for 10–12 hours, taking only water to drink.

- At time zero, take a venous blood sample for laboratory glucose estimation.
- Then give 75 g glucose (anhydrous) dissolved in 300 ml of water or an equivalent which provides 75 g glucose, e.g. 140 ml Maxijul made up to 300 ml with water.
- Patients must not eat, smoke or exercise throughout the duration of the test.
- A further venous blood sample is taken 120 minutes after the glucose drink.

If the 2-hour postglucose value is above 11.1 mmol/l, diabetes is diagnosed. A 2-hour value of 7.8–11.1 mmol/l signifies impaired glucose tolerance (IGT). People with IFG or IGT need assessment and appropriate treatment of cardiovascular risk factors, as well as a test for fasting plasma glucose at least annually.

It is usually evident from the presenting signs and symptoms whether the patient has type 1 or type 2 diabetes. The rapid onset of symptoms in a lean patient and the presence of ketonuria would be diagnostic of type 1 diabetes. Type 2 diabetes is characterized by the slow onset of milder symptoms and, even though they may have lost some weight prior to diagnosis, these people are usually still overweight.

MANAGEMENT

INITIAL MANAGEMENT

People diagnosed with type 1 diabetes need urgent (same day) referral to the specialist diabetes team. Hospital admission will be required for those sick enough to require intravenous rehydration and correction of acidosis but, increasingly, newly diagnosed type 1 patients, including children in some parts of the UK, are managed as outpatients, with the support of diabetes specialist nurses.

The pressing need of most people with newly diagnosed type 2 diabetes is for information, rather than medication. They can usually be managed in primary care from the start and it is often helpful for partners/carers to be involved as much as possible, with the patient's agreement. In many cases it is the role of the practice nurse to explain to the patient (and partner or carer) the implications of the diagnosis of diabetes, giving as much information as requested initially and arranging a follow-up appointment, usually within the next week, for further information giving, when the patient has recovered from the initial shock of the diagnosis. Oral hypoglycaemic medication is not usually introduced unless a trial of lifestyle and dietary changes for at least 2 months has failed to achieve satisfactory glucose levels.

AIMS OF MANAGEMENT

The aims are to relieve symptoms associated with diabetes and to prevent or delay the progression of long-term complications. Management consists of a combination of education, healthy eating, appropriate medication and structured monitoring and surveillance for the early identification and treatment of cardiovascular risk factors and other complications.

Education

Guidance from the National Institute for Clinical Excellence (NICE 2003) recommends that structured patient education is made available to all people with diabetes at the time of diagnosis and then as required, based on a formal, regular assessment of need. It favours education by a multidisciplinary team to groups of people with diabetes, family members and carers, but recognizes that this approach is not suitable for all. Diabetes education needs to incorporate both information giving and self-care skills and should include personalized goal setting (Naqib 2002). Leaflets, videos and computer-based multimedia packages can all assist with this process.

Essential education topics include the following:

- understanding diabetes/implications of diagnosis
- effective use of prescribed medication
- dietary advice
- footcare advice
- smoking and support to quit
- self-monitoring of glucose
- cardiovascular risk factor awareness and management
- what care to expect/importance of regular review (BP, retinal screening, etc.)
- exercise
- hypoglycaemia
- action to take when unwell.

Other topics to be addressed as appropriate:

- family planning and pregnancy advice
- driving

- employment
- state benefits
- insurance
- travel and holidays.

Healthy eating

Diabetes UK recommends that every newly diagnosed patient should have the opportunity to see a state-registered dietitian, but it is important that practice nurses are able to reinforce this advice at follow-up appointments. The high-fibre, low-fat, low-sugar diet recommended for people with diabetes is based on the same healthy eating advice that applies to the population as a whole. While it is wise to restrict fatty and very sweet products, no foods are completely banned. Choosing foods which reduce fluctuations in blood glucose levels will reduce the risk of microvascular complications and restricting fat intake is thought to reduce the risk of macrovascular complications. Regular meals and snacks will reduce the risk of hypoglycaemia for those on diabetes medication. Recent guidance from Diabetes UK (Diabetes UK 2003a) emphasizes that nutritional advice should be provided in the context of wider lifestyle changes, particularly physical activity (see p.178) and makes the following recommendations.

- Lose weight if overweight. A reasonable target is 10 kg weight loss or, if weight loss is not achieved within the first 3–6 months, the goal should be to avoid further weight gain. A reduced fat intake, combined with daily physical exercise, should be tried first and if this fails, an energy prescription to reduce daily energy intake by 500 kcal. It is recommended that the use of very low calorie diets should be restricted to special cases (e.g. BMI >35) in experienced centres.
- Regular meals containing complex carbohydrate (high in cereal fibre, e.g. wholegrain bread, and/or soluble fibre, e.g. porridge, beans, peas and lentils).
- Increase energy from complex carbohydrate to 50–55%.
- Reduce energy from fats:
  - less than 10% daily energy intake from saturated fat (e.g. fat on meat, butter)
  - not more than 10% from polyunsaturated fatty acids (e.g. vegetable fat spreads)
  - 10–20% from monounsaturated fatty acids (e.g. olive oil).
- At least one portion of fish per week (preferably oily), but fish oil supplements are not recommended.
- Plant sources of n-3 fatty acids, e.g. rapeseed oils, nuts, green leafy vegetables.
- Protein not more than 1 g per kg bodyweight. Protein reduction may slow the rate of progression to renal failure.
- Reduce salt to 6 g daily, especially in hypertensive patients.
- Sugar should not exceed 10% of daily energy intake.
- Special 'diabetic' foods are not recommended. They are expensive, offer no advantage over 'ordinary' products and may have a laxative effect.
- Alcohol should be restricted in people with peripheral neuropathy but otherwise is acceptable in moderation. Patients need to be aware of its potential to contribute to hypoglycaemia and should be advised to follow alcohol with food containing carbohydrate. Alcohol can also contribute significantly to overall calorie intake.

Foods with a low glycaemic index can help to prevent both hypoglycaemia and high glucose levels. The glycaemic index (GI) is a ranking of foods based on their overall effect on blood glucose levels (Brand-Miller et al 1998) (Box 9.2). Slowly absorbed foods have a low GI rating, whilst foods that are more quickly absorbed will have a higher rating. For instance, 30 g of carbohydrate in bread does not have the same effect on blood glucose as 30 g of carbohydrate in fruit or in pasta.

Box 9.2 The GI rating of common foods. Source: Diabetes UK. www.diabetes.org.uk/faq/GI.htm

Low GI	*Medium GI*	*High GI*
Apples, oranges, pears, peaches	Honey	Glucose
Beans and lentils	Jam	White and wholemeal bread
Pasta (all types made from durum wheat)	Shredded Wheat	Brown rice
Sweet potato, peeled and boiled	Weetabix	White rice, cooked
Sweetcorn	Ice cream	Cornflakes
Porridge	New potatoes, peeled and boiled	Baked potato
Custard	White basmati rice, cooked	Mashed potato
Noodles	Pitta bread	
All Bran, Special K, Sultana Bran	Couscous	

It is acknowledged that standard nutritional advice has little or no supporting evidence and there is increasing professional interest in alternative approaches. For example, the DAFNE study (DAFNE 2002) has revived carbohydrate counting in type 1 diabetes, which was in vogue until the 1990s. Adjusting their own insulin dose before each meal, according to planned physical activity and the carbohydrate content of the food in front of them, allows these patients complete dietary freedom. The Atkins low carbohydrate diet (Atkins 1999) is also gaining credence, especially in type 2 diabetes. Short-term results have been encouraging, in terms of weight loss, glucose control and lipid levels, but there is currently little evidence to support its long-term efficacy and safety (Eisenstein et al 2002).

DRUGS USED IN DIABETES

Most people with diabetes eventually require a cocktail of prescribed drugs, including glucose-lowering medication, antihypertensives, lipid-lowering agents, aspirin and possibly weight-reducing drugs and/or hormone replacement therapy. This chapter will deal only with drugs to reduce blood glucose.

ORAL HYPOGLYCAEMIC AGENTS

Oral hypoglycaemic agents are indicated when satisfactory blood glucose levels cannot be achieved through attention to diet and physical activity. Most people with type 2 diabetes require medication soon after diagnosis, but a few can maintain adequate glucose control without drugs for many years. Oral agents achieve their glucose-lowering effect through different modes of action. Some stimulate the pancreas to increase insulin secretion: these are known as insulin secretagogues. Some reduce insulin resistance by enhancing the action of insulin and others slow down the absorption of glucose from the gut. Initial treatment is usually with a single agent (monotherapy) but, because of their different ways of working, combination therapy, with drugs from different groups, can be very effective when monotherapy is no longer sufficient.

- The most common initial treatment is metformin. If this is contraindicated or not tolerated, a glitazone may be prescribed for overweight people, or a sulphonylurea for people who are not overweight.
- When monotherapy is no longer sufficient, treatment is with a combination of any two of these, according to tolerance, weight and any contraindications (i.e. metformin + glitazone, metformin + sulphonylurea or glitazone + sulphonylurea).
- Triple therapy with all three agents is currently unlicensed in the UK.

INSULIN SECRETAGOGUES

Drugs in this group stimulate the pancreatic beta cells to secrete insulin. Side-effects are rare, but they carry the risk of hypoglycaemia. Since they promote weight gain, they are not the agents of choice for first-line treatment of obese patients but are widely used by the non-obese and overweight people who are intolerant of metformin.

Sulphonylureas

Sulphonylureas are derived from sulphonamides and were developed in the 1950s following the accidental discovery of the hypoglycaemic effect of these antibacterial agents. They can be expected to reduce the fasting glucose by 2–3 mmol/l. Although tolbutamide is safe and effective, most of the other older agents in this class have been superseded. Chlorpropamide and glibenclamide, in particular, are noted for their long half-life and renal excretion, and have been implicated in cases of profound hypoglycaemic coma especially in the elderly. Gliclazide and glipizide are examples of sulphonylureas in common use. Traditionally sulphonylureas have been taken in divided doses, but some of the newer agents, glimepiride (Amaryl) and gliclazide (Diamicron MR), are formulated to be taken once daily. However, apart from convenience, they offer no advantage over other sulphonylureas, in terms of glucose control and potential for weight gain.

Prandial glucose regulators

These tablets are taken a few minutes before meals, stimulating insulin secretion to reduce postprandial hyperglycaemia. Owing to their short duration of action, they have a lower risk of hypoglycaemia than sulphonylureas and there may be less weight gain. Repaglinide (NovoNorm) can be used as monotherapy or in combination with metformin, but is not recommended for people aged over 75.

Table 9.2 Oral hypoglycaemic agents

Class	Insulin secretagogues		Insulin enhancers		Agents to delay glucose absorption	
	Sulphonylureas	**Prandial glucose regulators**	**Biguanides**	**Thiazolidinediones (glitazones)**	**Alpha-glucosidase inhibitors**	**Guar gum (bulking agent)**
Preparations	Gliclazide (Diamicron) Glimepiride (Amaryl) Gliquidone (Glurenorm) Glipizide (Glibenese, Minodiab) Tolbutamide	Repaglinide (NovoNorm) Nateglinide (Starlix)	Metformin (Glucophage)	Pioglitazone (Actos) Rosiglitazone (Avandia)	Acarbose (Glucobay)	Guarem
Characteristics	Risk of hypoglycaemia Long duration of action Cause weight gain Side-effects rare	Reduced risk of hypoglycaemia Rapid onset and short duration Side-effects rare	No risk of hypoglycaemia No weight gain GI side-effects common Rare but fatal side-effect: lactic acidosis	No risk of hypoglycaemia Side-effects rare, but heart and liver function must be monitored	No risk of hypoglycaemia GI side-effects, especially flatulence	No risk of hypoglycaemia
Options for combination therapy	Licensed for monotherapy Can be used with metformin or glitazone Also triple combination with metformin and acarbose Can be combined with insulin	Use repaglinide as monotherapy or combine with metformin Nateglinide not licensed for monotherapy – use only with metformin	Monotherapy or combined with sulphonylurea or glitazone Also in combination with insulin	Monotherapy or combined with metformin or sulphonylurea. Not licensed in combination with insulin	Monotherapy or combined with other oral hypoglycaemic agents	Use as adjunct to any hypoglycaemic medication

Nateglinide (Starlix) is licensed to be used only in combination with metformin.

AGENTS TO ENHANCE INSULIN SENSITIVITY

Metformin

Metformin is the only biguanide licensed for use in the UK. Like the sulphonylureas, it can reduce fasting glucose levels by 2–3 mmol/l, and has the added advantages that it does not normally cause hypoglycaemia or weight gain. It acts by enhancing peripheral glucose uptake and reducing glucose production by the liver. Unfortunately gastrointestinal side-effects are common and, for a significant minority, intolerable, but these can be minimized by starting with just one tablet daily taken with or after food, and slowly increasing the dose as tolerance develops. The dose is often limited to the amount the patient is able to tolerate. As metformin is not metabolized and is excreted by the kidneys, it should be avoided in patients with renal impairment. The NICE (2002b) recommends restricting this treatment to patients whose creatinine level is not greater than 130 μmol/l. Because of lactic acidosis, the rare but potentially fatal side-effect of metformin treatment, it should be avoided in patients with cirrhosis, alcoholism or heart failure.

Thiazolidinediones (glitazones)

Introduced in the late 1990s, the thiazolidinediones are the newest class of oral hypoglycaemic agent. They reduce insulin resistance by enhancing sensitivity to insulin in the liver, adipose (fat) tissue and skeletal muscle. They increase the uptake and storage of glucose and reduce breakdown of triglycerides. Rosiglitazone (Avandia) and pioglitazone (Actos) are licensed for monotherapy and can be used with metformin or a sulphonylurea, but cannot be used with insulin. The first thiazolidinedione to be introduced was quickly withdrawn because of its association with severe liver damage, so patients treated with these agents should be monitored to check that they do not develop liver problems. (LFTs every 2 months for first year, and periodically thereafter.)

AGENTS TO DELAY GLUCOSE ABSORPTION

Acarbose (Glucobay), taken with the first mouthful of food at meal time, delays carbohydrate digestion and glucose absorption by inhibiting the digestive enzyme alpha-glucosidase. The associated malodorous flatulence, abdominal bloating and diarrhoea can be minimized by gradually building up the dose to a therapeutic level over a period of several weeks. Those able to tolerate this product can expect a 0.5% HbA1c reduction (Holman et al 1999). Though not licensed for use with insulin, it can be used as monotherapy or in triple combination with metformin and a sulphonylurea. Hypoglycaemia is not a risk in monotherapy with acarbose but may arise in combination treatment with a sulphonylurea and needs to be treated with glucose, since the absorption of sucrose (ordinary sugar) would be hindered by acarbose.

Guar gum (Guarem) is not commonly used, but can be a useful adjunct to other treatments if tolerated. A soluble fibre preparation, supplied in granular form, it is to be taken with 200 ml of liquid before meals. It delays gastric emptying and hence glucose absorption and has a similar side-effect profile to acarbose.

COMBINATION THERAPY

Sulphonylureas can be combined with other oral agents or with insulin, but would not be used with a prandial glucose regulator because of their similar modes of action. However, although metformin and the glitazones both belong to the group of drugs that enhance insulin sensitivity, these can be used in combination because they have different modes of action. A product combining a glitazone and metformin in a single tablet (Avandamet) is also available. The glitazones can be used with either metformin or a sulphonylurea, but NICE (NICE 2002a) guidance recommends that a glitazone combination is not tried unless glucose control remains unsatisfactory with a sulphonylurea/metformin combination. In this case, since triple combination of metformin, a glitazone and a sulphonylurea is not currently licensed, either the sulphonylurea or metformin should be discontinued. The glitazones require a period of at least 4 weeks to achieve maximum effectiveness so, for most people, substituting a glitazone for metformin or a sulphonylurea means that glucose control deteriorates initially.

INSULIN TREATMENT

Everyone with type 1 diabetes, and a significant proportion of those with type 2, requires daily injections of insulin, but how does one choose from the 38 preparations currently available in the UK? Although there is clear evidence of the benefits of good glucose control (DCCT 1993, UKPDS 1998), little evidence exists to suggest that any particular insulin regimen is more likely than another to achieve it. It is more a question of finding the most appropriate, acceptable and effective individualized regimen from the many available options. MIMS, the monthly index of medical specialities, always carries a very useful chart which tabulates the species, onset, peak activity and total duration of each insulin available. The range includes porcine, bovine and synthetic ('human') preparations, which may be short, medium or long acting, or a stable mixture of short and medium acting.

Box 9.3 Factors that influence choice of insulin regimen

Type 1 or type 2 diabetes
Individual glycaemic targets (depending upon age, duration of diabetes, general health status and social factors)
Eating patterns
Patterns of physical activity
Individual glucose profile
Patient preference (e.g. species of insulin, number of injections, injection device)
Mental ability
Manual dexterity

Basal/bolus regimen

Most people with type 1 diabetes, and some people with type 2, are encouraged to follow a basal/bolus multiple injection regimen, to mimic endogenous insulin secretion as closely as possible and to offer the most flexibility of routine. A once (or twice) daily injection of medium or long-acting insulin (e.g. Insulatard, Humulin I) is given, to imitate the 24-hour daily basal insulin secreted by the pancreatic islet cells in the non-diabetic individual. This is supplemented with a bolus of short-acting insulin (e.g. Human Actrapid, Humulin S) before each main meal, just as the non-diabetic pancreas would secrete sufficient insulin to deal with the glucose produced every time food is consumed. This regimen allows for variations in the timing of meals and adjustment of the dose injected, according to the carbohydrate content.

The recently developed insulin analogues are particularly appropriate for use in this way. Lantus (insulin glargine) is the first insulin preparation to resemble physiological basal insulin, in that it has no peak of activity. This reduces the risk of hypoglycaemia, especially at night. The very rapid-acting insulin analogues, Humalog (insulin lispro) and NovoRapid (insulin aspart), are ideal for bolus injections before meals. Because of their very rapid onset of action, they can be injected immediately before meals, which is more convenient than waiting for the recommended 30 minutes between injecting traditional rapid-acting insulin and eating a meal.

Twice-daily mixed (biphasic) insulin

Some people with type 1 diabetes, and many with type 2, can achieve good glycaemic control with a twice-daily injection of a mixture of short and medium-acting insulin (e.g. the Humulin M and Mixtard ranges). These are available with different ratios of short and medium-acting insulin, to cater for different glycaemic patterns, and are suitable for people whose daily routine and food consumption are fairly constant.

Once-daily medium or long-acting insulin

It is not usually possible to achieve a blood glucose profile close to the normal range with only one injection daily, but this may be of secondary importance for some patients. For example, the aim of treatment for a frail elderly person living alone might simply be to avoid the symptoms of hyperglycaemia and the risks associated with hypoglycaemia.

Combination treatment with insulin and oral hypoglycaemic agents

A few years ago, the common practice was for all oral hypoglycaemic agents to be discontinued when people with type 2 diabetes reached the point when insulin was required, but it is now recognized that there are benefits from using a combination of oral agents and insulin. Metformin is usually continued with insulin, to reduce the risk of weight gain associated with insulin treatment. If metformin is not tolerated or contraindicated, a sulphonylurea can be continued in combination with insulin. The simplicity of a once-daily injection can help to persuade some patients to accept insulin treatment but, in the long term, this is rarely sufficient for good glycaemic control for the whole 24-hour period, including the periods between meals.

Presentation of insulin preparations

It is crucial that the patient's prescription states not only the correct name of the insulin preparation but also the appropriate presentation for the chosen injection method. Insulin is supplied in three different presentations:

- 10 ml vials for use with insulin syringes and needle-free injectors
- preloaded (disposable) injection devices, each containing 3 ml insulin
- 3 ml cartridges for reusable injection pens.

Some preparations are available in all three forms, a few are presented only in vials and others only in cartridges or preloaded injection devices. The 3 ml cartridges from different manufacturers are not uniform in shape and must be matched with a compatible injection pen.

Injection devices

The development of injection devices over the last two decades has made injections very simple and much more acceptable. Although a few people with long-standing diabetes continue to use an insulin syringe, most prefer an injection pen device. Injection devices are available on prescription but the choice of device is sometimes restricted by the choice of insulin preparation. Needle-free delivery devices, which blast insulin through the skin in very fine jets, are cumbersome and noisy in operation but invaluable for people of all ages with absolute needle phobia. The Novo Penmate (Novo Nordisk), for use with the NovoPen, and Autoinject 2 (Owen Mumford), for use with a plastic syringe, are useful injection aids for those with lesser degrees of needle phobia, but are not available on prescription. At approximately £2200 plus £1000 per year for consumables, insulin pumps for continuous infusion of insulin are expensive and not in common use, but their popularity is growing.

Injection technique For maximum efficacy, insulin should be injected into the subcutaneous adipose (fat) tissue. If the injection is too shallow, it can cause local irritation and delay in absorption. If it is too deep and penetrates muscle tissue, the injection may be more painful and the insulin may be absorbed too quickly. Modern, short insulin needles allow an injection administered at an angle of 90° to

Box 9.4 Prescribable injection devices

Glass syringe (0.5 ml or 1 ml with separate 12 mm needles)
Preset glass syringe (1 ml with separate 12 mm needles)
0.3 ml disposable plastic syringe (with fixed 8 mm or 12 mm needle)
0.5 ml disposable plastic syringe (with fixed 8 mm or 12 mm needle)
1 ml disposable plastic syringe (with fixed 12 mm needle)
Reusable injection pens (e.g. NovoPen, Autopen) for 3 ml cartridges
Reusable Innovo device for 3 ml cartridges
Disposable injection devices (e.g. Flexpen, Optipen, Innolet device)
Medical House Insulin jet needle-free injection system (mhi-500)

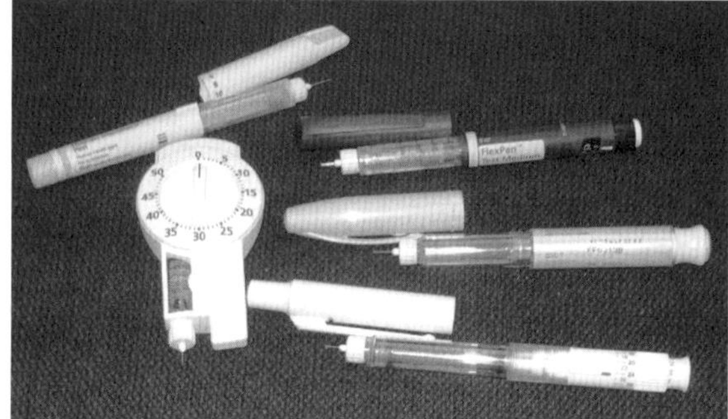

Figure 9.2 Preloaded (disposable) insulin injection devices.

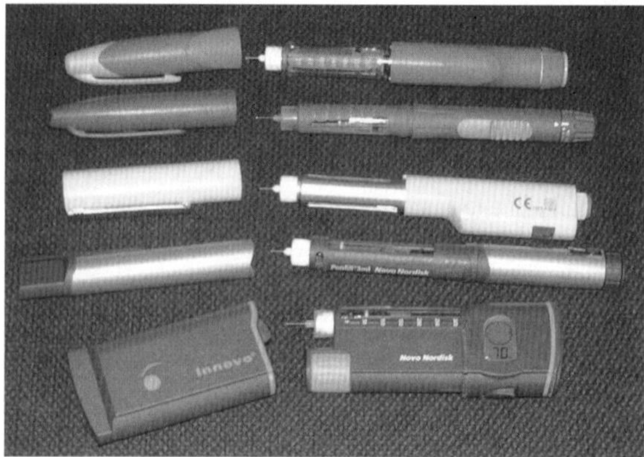

Figure 9.3 Reusable insulin injection devices.

deliver the insulin correctly. If injecting an area well covered in fat, a pinch-up is unnecessary but when injecting into a lean area, the skin and fat should be pinched up, to pull it away from the muscle. The injection can then be administered into the centre of the pinched-up skinfold. To ensure that the whole injection is delivered, the needle should not be withdrawn for 6–10 seconds after completing the injection and the skinfold should be held until after withdrawal of the needle. This helps to prevent leakage of insulin from the injection site and dripping from the needle when the injection is complete.

The rate of insulin absorption varies between different injection sites, being absorbed most rapidly from the abdomen. It is therefore recommended that injections given at the same time each day should be into the same general area (e.g. abdomen or thigh), but not at exactly the same spot.

Repeated insulin injections into the same small areas causes lipohypertrophy, an overgrowth of hardened fatty tissue (Fig. 9.4). Not only can this be unsightly, but it also leads to erratic and unpredictable insulin absorption. It is therefore important for patients to vary their injection sites as much as possible, avoiding any areas that have become hard, to allow the tissue to recover and regain its original shape.

Disposal of sharps Patients need information about the local policy for the collection and disposal of sharps from their homes. Sharps bins (for disposal of used syringes, needles and lancets from finger-pricking devices) and needle clipping devices (for the safe removal and storage of needles from insulin syringes) are available on prescription in England and Wales. Needle clipping devices are available in Scotland and Northern Ireland. In some areas filled sharps bins are returned to GP surgeries, clinics or hospitals for incineration. In other parts of the UK they are collected from patients' homes by the county council. For up-to-date advice, see also Diabetes UK's position statement (Diabetes UK 2003a).

Animal versus 'human' insulin

From 1923 until 1981, the only source of insulin for injection was the pancreas of slaughtered cattle or pigs. When synthetic 'human' insulin, produced by genetic engineering, became available in 1981, it received an enthusiastic welcome. There had been concerns that animal disease might unexpectedly reduce the pancreas supply, but here was an infinite source of insulin for injection, which it was assumed would be less allergenic than preparations derived from animal sources. There was widespread conversion of existing patients from animal to 'human' insulin and since that date, it has been usual practice for new patients to be routinely treated with a 'human' preparation.

However, ever since its launch, small numbers of people have reported problems which they attribute to 'human' insulin. The most specific complaint is a change in hypoglycaemic awareness, but other non-specific problems have also been reported, including weight gain, mood swings and joint pains. Understandably, the greatest anxiety amongst insulin-treated patients arises following newspaper stories with emotive headlines. Every time 'human' insulin receives adverse media publicity, a significant number of worried patients are keen to switch from 'human' to animal preparations.

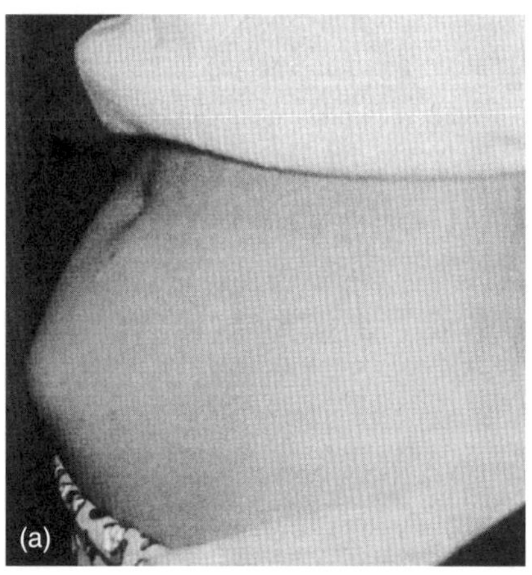

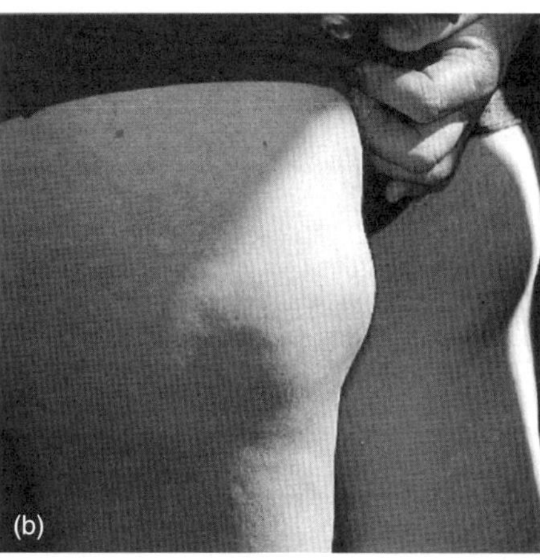

Figure 9.4 (a,b) Examples of lipohypertrophy ('lipos'). Reproduced by permission of Becton Dickinson.

It is acknowledged that 'human' insulin was introduced for routine treatment without adequate comparison of its efficacy, compared with animal preparations. However, patients should be reassured that none of the large reviews of studies comparing animal and human insulin has found any evidence of clinical difference between them (Airey et al 2000, Nellemann Jorgensen et al 1994, Richter & Neises 2002).

Nurses have a professional duty to support patients in their treatment choice, even if it is not the decision they would have made themselves. Some people are keen to try all the latest treatments and technologies, while others prefer to stick with those that have been tried and tested for many years. Some people do not wish to use genetically engineered products, while others avoid using products derived from animal sources. When patients have the opportunity to discuss the advantages and disadvantages of transferring to animal insulin, most choose to continue with their current 'human' insulin regimen, because the advantage of using their preferred injection device or current insulin mixture outweighs any potential disadvantage.

Compared with 'human' insulin, there is a limited range of animal insulin preparations and compatible injection devices. Nevertheless, for the small minority of individuals who choose treatment with animal insulin, there is a choice of 10 different porcine or bovine preparations, many of which are available in cartridges to fit the Autopen injection device, available on prescription.

ACUTE DIABETIC COMPLICATIONS (HYPOGLYCAEMIA AND HYPERGLYCAEMIA)

The short-term diabetic complications arise when hypoglycaemic medication is either in excess of the body's requirements (hypoglycaemia) or inadequate (hyperglycaemia).

HYPOGLYCAEMIA

Hypoglycaemia (plasma glucose below 3.5 mmol/l) is a very common side-effect of treatment with insulin or with oral hypoglycaemic agents that stimulate insulin secretion, especially the sulphonylureas. It can be asymptomatic, mild, moderate or severe. Intermittent mild hypoglycaemia, especially before lunch and before the evening meal, is an inevitable consequence of adequate insulin treatment, but about 25–30% of insulin-treated patients suffer one or more severe hypoglycaemic episodes (requiring the assistance of others) per year. It also carries the additional risks of hypothermia, injuries sustained from falls and, especially in the elderly, hypoglycaemia-induced heart attacks and strokes. Hypoglycaemia creates as much anxiety in insulin-treated patients as the fear of blindness and other long-term complications (Williams & Pickup 2002).

Box 9.5 Symptoms of hypoglycaemia

Autonomic	*Neuroglycopaenic*	*Other*
Pallor	Headache	Weakness
Sweating	Loss of concentration	Tingling lips
Trembling	Loss of coordination	Nightmares
Tachycardia	Slurred speech	
Palpitations	Double/blurred vision	
Anxiety	Aggressive behaviour	
Irritability	Confusion	
Hunger	Drowsiness	
	Seizures	
	Coma	

Autonomic symptoms are the body's first response to low blood glucose levels but if the glucose level continues to fall, the brain is deprived of glucose, leading to neuroglycopaenic symptoms. Non-specific symptoms may include tingling lips, weakness or nightmares. Some people with diabetes, especially those with poor glycaemic control, experience symptoms of hypoglycaemia even when the blood glucose is within the normal range. This is because of adaptation of the brain to chronic hyperglycaemia. Similarly, and especially in patients who strive the hardest to maintain normal glucose levels, the brain may adapt to subnormal glucose levels, so that the autonomic warning symptoms of hypoglycaemia do not arise until after brain function has been affected by neuroglycopaenia, when it is too late for the patient to take corrective action. Awareness of hypoglycaemia diminishes with duration of diabetes but can often be restored by relaxing glycaemic control to avoid low blood glucose for a few weeks.

Hypoglycaemia arises when there is an excess of insulin or a shortage of carbohydrate and is often precipitated by physical exercise. The consumption of large amounts of alcohol, especially if not followed by food, can cause hypoglycaemia by suppressing gluconeogenesis (the formation of new glucose from stored fat and protein). Some medications for co-existing conditions can exert a hypoglycaemic effect, for example aspirin and fluoxetine (Prozac). Likewise, other medications cause raised blood glucose (e.g. steroids), so that a dosage reduction could contribute to hypoglycaemia. Impaired renal or liver function can delay excretion of insulin and other hypoglycaemic agents, while increased blood flow, because of hot conditions or exercise of the injected limb, can increase the absorption rate of insulin.

Box 9.6 Factors contributing to hypoglycaemia

Accidental or deliberate overdose of insulin or oral agent
Forgotten or delayed meal
Insufficient carbohydrate
Unanticipated exercise, including spring cleaning, gardening, sexual intercourse
Drug interactions
Large amounts of alcohol
Renal or liver impairment
Hot weather/sauna/hot bath
Different injection site/depth
Lipohypertrophy at injection site
Exercise of injected limb

Mild hypoglycaemia is treated with two or three glucose tablets, a small glass of fresh fruit juice or a sugary drink containing about 10 g of carbohydrate (e.g. two tablespoons of Lucozade or a drink containing two teaspoons of sugar). This should be repeated if symptoms persist after 10 minutes. If a meal is not yet due, a substantial snack should be taken, to avoid a recurrence of hypoglycaemia. If the patient is uncooperative but conscious, it may be possible to squeeze Hypostop into their mouth. This is a dextrose gel available on prescription and supplied in squeezable sachets with a nozzle. The unconscious patient should be placed in the recovery position and, after confirming hypoglycaemia with a capillary glucose test, an injection of glucagon may be administered by anyone trained to do so or intravenous glucose may be administered by a physician. When the patient is sufficiently recovered, a carbohydrate snack will be required to prevent a relapse.

Prevention of hypoglycaemia

When a patient has recovered from an episode of hypoglycaemia, they should try to establish the cause, in order to use forward planning to reduce the risk of a similar event in the future. The insulin dose or the timing of meals and snacks may need to be adjusted.

HYPERGLYCAEMIA

The symptoms of hyperglycaemia are of course the same symptoms that lead to a diagnosis of diabetes and they can return, gradually or suddenly, especially in patients whose glycaemic control is not monitored and treated accordingly.

Box 9.7 Causes of hyperglycaemia

Infection or illness
Medication, especially steroids; also diuretics
Chronic or acute inadequacy of insulin or oral hypoglycaemic medication
Large volumes of sweet drinks to quench thirst
Emotional stress

Symptoms can develop very quickly in type 1 diabetes, because of the absolute insulin lack. Thirst, polyuria and lethargy are quickly followed by nausea and vomiting, induced by the build-up of ketones from fat breakdown. If sufficient insulin is not administered at this stage, dehydration and ketosis can lead to coma and death from diabetic ketoacidosis. Type 2 diabetes is usually less dramatic but nevertheless, uncontrolled hyperglycaemia can lead to hyperosmolar non-ketotic coma (HONK) and death.

Prevention of hyperglycaemic coma

The single most effective way to reduce the incidence of diabetic coma is by improved education for patients, relatives and health professionals. It needs to be understood that illness usually raises the blood glucose and that insulin and oral hypoglycaemic agents should therefore *not* be omitted, even when no food is being taken. Very serious consequences follow the omission of insulin injections by people who believe they are suffering from food poisoning, when in fact they are developing ketoacidosis. Self-monitoring of blood glucose is more important

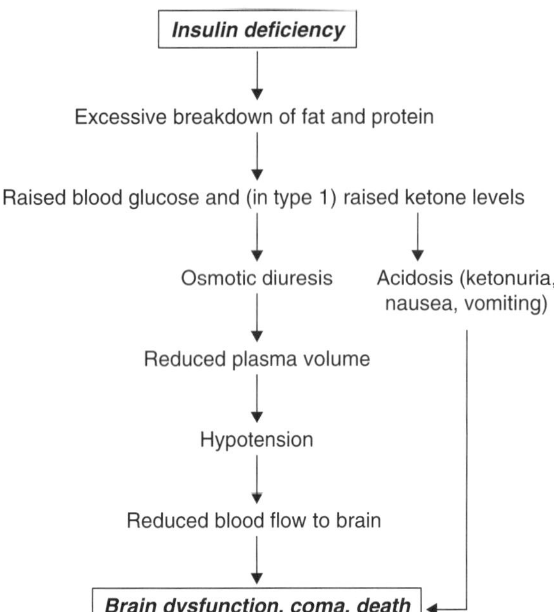

Figure 9.5 The succession of events in uncontrolled hyperglycaemia.

during illness than at any other time. In the case of vomiting, accompanied by low blood glucose levels, it would be correct to reduce the insulin dose, to avoid hypoglycaemia. However, if the blood glucose is raised, a higher dose than usual may be required, even if the patient has little or no appetite. A persistently raised blood glucose level, especially in the presence of heavy ketonuria, is a clear indication for increased insulin therapy. Urgent hospital admission is required for patients with hyperglycaemia, heavy ketonuria and vomiting.

LONG-TERM DIABETIC COMPLICATIONS AND RISK REDUCTION

Even though they may have no symptoms of hyperglycaemia, people whose blood glucose is above the normal range for many years are susceptible to a number of serious long-term diabetic complications. Genetic susceptibility, hypertension and hyperlipidaemia also play a major part, as does smoking, which greatly increases the risk of all diabetic complications. Many diseases are seen more frequently in people with diabetes, including joint disorders and skin conditions, but the three major categories of diabetic complications are large vessel disease (macrovascular), small vessel disease (microvascular) and neuropathy.

It was always assumed that good glycaemic control would reduce the risk of diabetic complications and two landmark studies have provided conclusive evidence that this is in fact the case. The Diabetes Control and Complications Trial (DCCT 1993), a 10-year American multicentre study, followed 1400 subjects with type 1 diabetes for a mean of 6.5 years each, comparing a conventionally treated group (achieving only moderate glycaemic control) with a more intensively treated group (achieving improved glycaemic control). Clinically important retinopathy, nephropathy (indicated by urine albumin excretion) and neuropathy were all reduced by at least one third in the group with tighter glucose control. Similarly, the United Kingdom Prospective Diabetes Study (UKPDS 1998) clearly demonstrated the benefits of tighter glucose control in type 2 diabetes. This 20-year study followed 5000 newly diagnosed patients from 23 centres, who were randomly allocated to different treatment groups. A difference in HbA1c of just 1% between conventionally treated patients (HbA1c 7.9%) and the more intensively treated group (7.0%) was associated with a 24% reduction in microvascular complications (see Monitoring in diabetes, p.177, for a definition of HbA1c). Another major finding of this study, perhaps of even greater importance, was that tight blood pressure control in type 2 diabetes led to a marked reduction in both microvascular and macrovascular complications, including a 44% reduction in the risk of strokes.

Box 9.8 Primary and secondary macrovascular risk reduction

Smoking advice and support to quit
Aspirin
BP control
Lipids – control with diet + lipid-lowering medication if necessary
Blood glucose control
Foot screening and preventive care
Weight – achievement and maintenance of ideal bodyweight
Coronary artery bypass
Carotid endarterectomy
Angioplasty of femoral arteries

MACROVASCULAR COMPLICATIONS

Coronary artery disease, stroke and peripheral vascular disease are all 2–4 times more common in people with diabetes than in the non-diabetic population and are the most frequent cause of morbidity and mortality in diabetes. As well as causing enormous personal suffering, macrovascular disease accounts for 80% of the cost of diabetic care.

Footcare

Foot ulceration is the most common reason for hospital admission in diabetes and the amputation rate is more than 15 times higher in people with diabetes than in the general population (Diabetes UK 2001). Predisposing factors are a more aggressive atherosclerosis (leading to ischaemia) and neuropathy (leading to loss of pain perception and muscle/tendon imbalance). The uninjured foot will not necessarily develop problems, but any physical trauma is a potential cause of trouble and can rapidly lead to infection and ulceration. Precipitating factors are:

- puncture wounds from an ingrowing toenail, a foreign body in the shoe or careless footcare
- localized pressure from tight shoes
- friction caused by loose footwear that allows the foot to slip
- heat, for example from bath water, a hot water bottle or walking barefoot across hot sand
- cold weather causing chilblains.

However, much of this suffering is preventable if patients take care to protect their feet and report problems early. People who have peripheral vascular disease and/or neuropathy need education to increase their awareness of their vulnerability to foot problems. Because of the absence of pain, they may fail to notice foot lesions or fail to appreciate their seriousness. For example, they may continue to walk on an injured foot, causing further harm. People with diabetes are often told they must 'look after their feet', but many do not understand exactly what this means in practice. The importance of simple routine care and daily foot inspection cannot be overestimated.

The practice nurse should take every opportunity to reinforce these simple instructions and to ask patients about their feet and examine them. The nurse will take care of minor foot lesions, requesting early treatment with antibiotics if signs of infection are present and referral to a wound care specialist nurse or chiropodist/podiatrist if appropriate. It is important to try to establish the cause of the injury, so that a future occurrence can be prevented. Foot assessment should always include palpation of foot pulses and a 10 g monofilament test for neuropathy. Active lesions, deformities, callus, colour and foot temperature should also be noted. All patients with a high risk of ulceration, as well as some patients with a moderate risk, will need referral to a state-registered chiropodist/podiatrist.

Box 9.9 Routine foot self-care for people with diabetes

Daily inspection of feet for breaks in skin, inflammation or swelling
Check shoes for foreign bodies
Avoid walking barefoot, including bathroom visits during the night
Well-fitting leather shoes with stout soles to protect feet (not slip-ons)
Wool or cotton socks changed daily
Wash feet daily (but don't soak) and dry carefully, especially between the toes
Trim toenails to the shape of the toe
Seek treatment for corns and calluses from state-registered podiatrist
Test water temperature and take care with hot water bottles (not too hot and not placed next to skin)

MICROVASCULAR COMPLICATIONS

Retinopathy

Diabetic retinopathy is the commonest cause of visual loss and blindness in people of working age in the Western world. It is related to duration of diabetes, poor glycaemic control, hypertension and smoking and can accelerate following a rapid dramatic improvement in glycaemic control, for example during pregnancy. As retinopathy is usually asymptomatic until the disease process is advanced, screening is essential (by fundoscopy through dilated pupils), so that appropriate early laser treatment can be given if required.

Background → Pre-proliferative
↓
Advanced diabetic retinopathy ← Proliferative

Retinopathy is primarily a disease of the retinal capillaries, which later extends to larger vessels. It is classified according to the features seen on ophthalmoscopy, indicating the stage of its development. Background retinopathy is the first stage of retinopathy: microaneurysms (dots), exudates and retinal vein dilatation are visible, but there is no visual loss unless the macula is involved. These changes may resolve and disappear, but can progress to pre-proliferative retinopathy, characterized by signs that new vessels are about to form, such as large blot haemorrhages and venous dilatation or looping. Early referral to a specialist ophthalmologist is required at this stage, before the disease progresses to sight-threatening proliferative retinopathy. Bleeding into the vitreous from the newly formed prolific and fragile retinal blood vessels found in the proliferative stage can cause sudden and dramatic visual loss in type 1 diabetes. These haemorrhages usually clear with time, but can persist. In advanced diabetic retinopathy there is persistent vitreous haemorrhage, which can lead to retinal detachment. Visual loss in type 2 diabetes is usually associated with macular oedema: it develops more gradually, but is less responsive to laser treatment.

Prevention and treatment

- Strict blood glucose control but once retinopathy is established, it may advance, even if glucose control is good.
- Strict control of hypertension.
- Low-dose aspirin or clopidogrel or dipyridamole to reduce platelet stickiness.
- Stop smoking.
- Advise patients to report 'floaters' (may be haemorrhage) or progressive blurring of vision (may be macular oedema), but this is not to be confused with the intermittent blurring associated with fluctuations in blood glucose levels.
- Laser treatment: this is most effective when applied before any visual loss.
- Vitrectomy (surgery to replace contents of the vitreous chamber of the eye).

Nephropathy

Diabetic nephropathy, which affects about 30% of people with diabetes (both type 1 and type 2), is defined by persistent proteinuria, declining glomerular filtration rate (GFR) and rising blood pressure. Proteinuria may be intermittent for many years but once persistent proteinuria has developed, renal function usually declines gradually but progressively towards end-stage renal failure. Nephropathy is usually preceded by a long period of hyperglycaemia but, as with retinopathy, other contributory factors are also thought to be important, especially hypertension and genetic predisposition. The early stages of the disease are asymptomatic but oedema, headache, nausea and vomiting, tiredness, hiccoughs, foamy urine and pruritus arise in advanced nephropathy, signalling the impending need for dialysis. Diabetic nephropathy is a marker for cardiovascular disease, a common cause of death in these patients.

Nephropathy is already at an advanced stage by the time protein can be detected by a dip-stick in urine. However, during the long stage of incipient nephropathy, while there is insufficient protein in the urine to register on a dip-stick, microalbuminuria (traces of protein in the urine) can be measured by sensitive immunoassay. This is of great significance, as it has been shown that medical intervention at

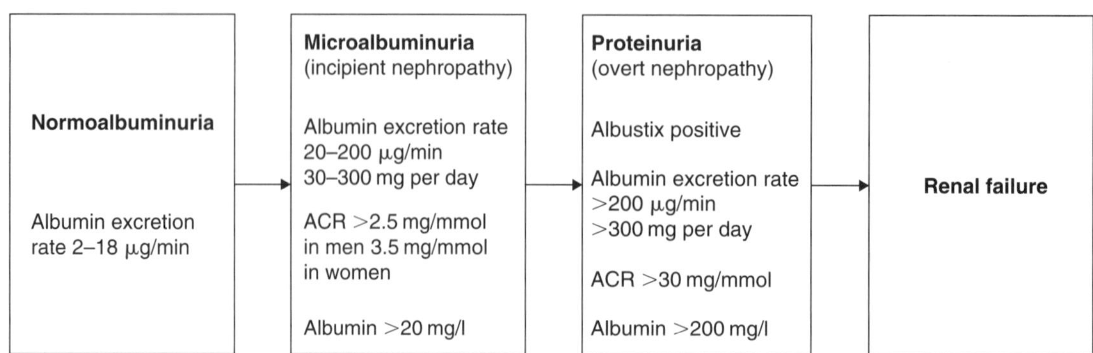

Figure 9.6 Stages of diabetic nephropathy.

this stage can slow the progression to proteinuria (Lewis et al 1993). The urinary albumin excretion rate (UAE) can be assessed with timed urine collections but because of the practical difficulties with this method, the urinary albumin/creatinine ratio (ACR), expressed as mg albumin/mmol creatinine, in an early morning sample of urine is widely accepted as an alternative screening method.

Prevention and treatment

- Strict blood glucose control.
- ACE inhibitor, even in patients with normal blood pressure, because these agents reduce intraglomerular pressure as well as systemic blood pressure (Williams & Pickup 2002).
- Early effective control of hypertension – NICE target <135/75 mmHg.
- Stop smoking.
- Address other cardiovascular risk factors, especially hyperlipidaemia.
- Moderate protein restriction.
- Renal replacement (haemodialysis, continuous ambulatory peritoneal dialysis (CAPD) or renal transplant).

NEUROPATHY

Sensory neuropathy

The commonest type of diabetic neuropathy is distal (peripheral) symmetrical neuropathy, usually affecting the feet in a stocking distribution and, more rarely, also the hands and arms. This arises insidiously over many years and can lead to numbness, hypersensitivity (e.g. to bedclothes or the normal pressures of walking), burning or tingling sensations that are usually worse at night and sometimes excruciating pain. Episodes may last for months or years. Treatments which may alleviate these symptoms include transparent dressings (e.g. Opsite film or spray), Axsain cream, tricyclic antidepressants (e.g. amitriptyline) and gabapentin (Neurontin).

Motor neuropathy

One or both thighs may be affected by diabetic amyotrophy, which causes continuous pain, with wasting and weakening of the quadriceps, but slow recovery over many months is usual. When motor neuropathy has weakened the muscles in the foot, minor trauma can lead to Charcot arthropathy (chronic destruction, deformity and inflammation of the joints and bone).

Autonomic neuropathy

Common manifestations of autonomic nerve damage are postural hypotension, gustatory sweating (induced by eating), other abnormal sweating, diarrhoea (often nocturnal) and erectile dysfunction. Gastroparesis (delayed gastric emptying and vomiting) and bladder dysfunction are rarer.

MONITORING IN DIABETES

For optimum health with this chronic lifelong condition, structured monitoring and screening for complications are essential, so that treatment to reduce risk factors can be introduced or adjusted at the earliest opportunity.

Well-being

A sense of well-being is essential for effective self-care but, with so many physiological assessments to monitor, it is all too easy for clinicians to fail to assess the patient's psychological needs. Practice nurses are ideally placed to provide psychological support, but should recognize that there will be a few people with more challenging psychological problems, who will require referral to a counsellor or psychotherapist.

Cardiovascular risk factors

These should be assessed at least annually, including blood glucose control, blood pressure, a full lipid profile (HDL and LDL cholesterol, and triglycerides), family history of cardiovascular disease and abdominal adiposity, albumin excretion rate and smoking status. A risk assessment chart, e.g. the Joint Societies' charts in the British National Formulary, is useful in type 2 diabetes but these are not appropriate for type 1 diabetes.

Blood glucose control

This is assessed by HbA1c (glycated haemoglobin) every 2–6 months (normal for most laboratories <6.0%) and also by fasting plasma glucose (normal <6 mmol/l) or random plasma glucose (normal <7.8 mmol/l), self-monitoring of capillary glucose and/or self-monitoring of urine (normal = no glycosuria). The usual aim would be to achieve results as near to the normal range as possible, but for some individuals (e.g. terminally ill or frail elderly patients), it is more appropriate to aim for freedom from hypoglycaemia and from the osmotic symptoms of hyperglycaemia.

Blood pressure

BP should be monitored on an annual basis if it is below 140/80 mmHg. For persistently raised BP, at or above 140/80 mmHg, more frequent measurements are required and antihypertensive drugs should be introduced, according to NICE guidance (NICE 2002b). Achieving blood pressure results as near to target as possible often requires a combination of several antihypertensive agents.

Lipids

Total cholesterol, low-density lipoprotein (LDL), high-density lipoprotein (HDL) and triglycerides are measured, using a fasting blood sample if feasible, when diabetes is diagnosed, and annually if the total cholesterol is less than 5.0 mmol/l and triglycerides are less than 2.3 mmol/l. Recommendations for management of people with an adverse lipid profile are outlined in the NICE (2002b) guideline H. A low-fat diet, and weight loss if overweight, would be the first line of treatment, with the addition of lipid-lowering agents if necessary. No pharmacological treatment is currently recommended when the total cholesterol is less than 5.0 mmol/l and triglycerides are less than 2.3 mmol/l, but recent results from a large randomized controlled trial suggest that this threshold should be lowered (HPSCG 2003).

Weight, body mass index (BMI) and waist measurement

Overweight and obesity are usually measured by the BMI, with normal or healthy weight classified as BMI 18.5–24.9 kg/m^2, overweight as 25–29.9 and obese as levels over 30. Waist circumference is also a very important predictor of cardiovascular disease. A waist measurement greater than 88 cm in women and 102 cm in men is a simple indicator of increased risk (Lean et al 1998).

Renal function tests

An annual blood test for serum creatinine is required for all patients with diabetes and if a dipstick test for urinary protein is negative, an early morning urine sample should be screened for microalbuminuria. After a positive microalbuminuria result, a midstream specimen of urine should be analysed to exclude infection as a cause. If microalbuminuria or proteinuria is present, the test should be repeated twice more, within a month where possible (NICE 2002c). Because albumin excretion can vary from day to day, the albumin excretion rate must be outside the normal range in at least two of the three samples for a diagnosis of microalbuminuria to be made.

Smoking status

This should be reviewed and smoking cessation advice offered as appropriate.

Retinal screening

Local retinal screening programmes should offer annual examination of both fundi through dilated pupils, using a retinal camera or slit-lamp indirect ophthalmoscopy (NICE 2002d).

Visual acuity

Annual test corrected with pinhole if worse than 6/9.

Assessment of the feet

This includes inspection for callus, active lesions, colour and temperature, and assessment of foot sensation and pulses. All patients with a high-risk foot, as well as some patients with a moderate-risk foot, will need referral to a state registered podiatrist.

Injection sites

Injection sites of insulin-treated patients should be inspected regularly. Lipodystrophy commonly goes unnoticed.

Review of diet

See p.165.

Exercise

The benefits of regular exercise are even more relevant to people with diabetes than to the general population. As well as assisting with weight loss, lipid and blood pressure control, exercise increases insulin sensitivity, reducing the requirement for insulin and/or oral hypoglycaemic medication. Patients should be given information about local facilities, such as swimming, keep fit groups and walking clubs. Recommendations need to be realistic, taking into account individual limitations and preferences. The British Heart Foundation recommends building up to 30 minutes of moderate intensity activity on five or more days of the week and defines moderate intensity as sufficient exercise to cause people to breathe harder and feel warmer (BHF 2002). A simple goal could be to try to increase activity by two minutes each day.

SELF-MONITORING OF GLUCOSE BY PEOPLE WITH DIABETES

Since home blood testing equipment became widely available in the early 1980s, it has been widely assumed that glucose self-monitoring, preferably of blood glucose, is desirable or even essential for everyone with diabetes. But present evidence suggests that this may not be the case (Coster et al 2000). Some patients give up self-monitoring if they cannot see its purpose, while others feel guilty, helpless and frustrated in the face of unsatisfactory results which they feel powerless to improve. Self-monitoring tests are often inaccurate and unreliable, and inappropriate and unhelpful testing is widespread. If home monitoring of glucose is to serve a useful purpose, the patient must know why, when and how to test and how to interpret the results. Avoiding inappropriate and unnecessary tests will result in enormous cost savings to the NHS, as well as increasing the psychological well-being of people with diabetes.

Purpose of home monitoring

Home glucose monitoring should be performed only if it serves an identified purpose which is clear to both the patient and the nurse or doctor. This may be:

- to provide patients with information about their day-to-day glycaemic control, enabling them to make appropriate adjustments to their diet or diabetic medication, especially in relation to strenuous exercise or activities involving potential danger, e.g. driving
- to provide the nurse or doctor with information about patients' day-to-day glycaemic control, enabling them to give appropriate treatment advice, e.g. following a raised HbA1c measurement
- to detect hypoglycaemia. Home monitoring of blood glucose can confirm or rule out hypoglycaemia.

Glucose monitoring methods

The monitoring method should depend upon the purpose of monitoring and the patient's manual dexterity, visual and cognitive ability, and personal preference.

Urine testing This remains a useful method of monitoring glycaemic control, especially among older patients with type 2 diabetes, when the aim of treatment is not strict normoglycaemia. Urine tests should ideally remain negative for glucose, indicating, in patients with a normal renal threshold, that the blood glucose level has not risen above 10 mmol/l.

Blood testing Self-monitoring of blood glucose is the method of choice for younger patients, and for most patients treated with insulin. It is particularly helpful during pregnancy and for women planning pregnancy, and is the only method which can detect hypoglycaemia. As treatment decisions are made on the basis of these results, it is essential that their accuracy is assessed, either by direct observation of the performance of a test or by asking the patient to complete a blood spot series for laboratory analysis. Ideally, most blood test results should be within the normal range (4–8 mmol/l). However, the risks of hypoglycaemia must be balanced against the risks of hyperglycaemia, especially in the elderly, and an appropriate individual target range should be decided.

No self-monitoring Some patients may prefer not to measure their glucose levels at all, choosing rather to rely on regular laboratory estimations of HbA1c to monitor glycaemic control.

Timing and frequency of tests

The patient and doctor or nurse should agree on the most appropriate timing and frequency of home monitoring tests, including additional tests during illness or a change of treatment. Many people with type 1 diabetes need to test several times a day every day, adjusting the dose of soluble insulin at each mealtime, to achieve optimum glycaemic control. However, this is not necessary for the majority of people with type 2 diabetes, even those treated with insulin, as they are not susceptible to such wide fluctuations in blood glucose.

Individual plan

An individual home monitoring plan should be agreed with the patient. This should include the timing and frequency of tests, and a review date. Regular reviews of the plan will prevent the performance of unnecessary tests after the need for them has passed. The patient should be able to perform the test accurately, according to the manufacturer's instructions, and must know what results to expect and what action to take if the results are outside the expected range.

Box 9.10 Suggested plans for self-monitoring of glucose

Non-insulin treated diabetes

- Test before breakfast and 2 hours after the main meal on one day per week or fortnight
- Test after meals on one day per week during dose adjustment of prandial glucose regulators

Insulin-treated diabetes

- Test once a day, varying the time of the test from day to day, e.g. before breakfast on Monday, mid-morning on Tuesday, before lunch on Wednesday, and so on (taking occasional days off testing)
- Test before breakfast, lunch and evening meal and at bed-time on one day per week, and after meals on another day
- Occasional tests at 2 or 3 am may also be useful

Basal/bolus insulin regimen

- Tests before and 1–2 hours after the same meal are used to estimate the optimum dose of soluble insulin
- Basal insulin is adjusted according to tests before breakfast
- Occasional tests at 2 or 3 am may also be useful

Blood glucose meters

There is a bewildering assortment of portable blood glucose meters for home blood testing, each compatible only with its own specific test strips, available on prescription. Meters are not supplied on the NHS but can be purchased for as little as £10 and are often supplied by the manufacturers, free of charge, for practice nurses and diabetes specialist nurses to supply to patients at their discretion. Each meter has its own advantages and disadvantages, and the most appropriate device depends upon the individual requirements of the patient. An active young person may choose a very small pocket-size device, while an older person with poor vision and manual dexterity would prefer a device with a larger, clearer display of the result and test strips that are easier to handle (e.g. Accu-chek Advantage by Roche). Others may choose a device capable of storing results that can be uploaded into a computer program for analysis. People who have difficulty obtaining a finger-prick sample will achieve more accurate results with a device whose test strips require a smaller size drop of blood and the option of alternative site testing, such as the forearm (e.g. One Touch Ultra by Lifescan or Freestyle by Therasense). New devices are continually coming onto the market, but regularly updated information on the available range can be found on Diabetes UK's website.

FUTURE POSSIBILITIES

People with diabetes look forward to the day when they will know their prevailing blood glucose level without the need to prick their finger (or alternative site). The currently available continuous glucose monitoring devices can sometimes identify unrecognized hypoglycaemia, but are expensive and of limited practical use. A successful non-invasive blood glucose monitoring method has yet to be developed. Likewise, the search continues for new ways to deliver insulin painlessly and in a more physiological manner. Trials involving transplants of islet cells (extracted from the pancreas of cadavers), injected into the portal vein of people with type 1 diabetes, are a very exciting development. In several successful operations the transplanted cells have continued to secrete insulin, in response to prevailing blood glucose levels. However, several pancreases are needed to treat one person with diabetes, potent immunosuppressive drugs are required for life and insulin secretion from the transplanted islet cells may become deficient or cease altogether.

DNA technology, therefore, may eventually prove to be a more realistic option and animal experiments are very encouraging. For instance, in the future, it may be possible to take cells from the liver of a person with type 1 diabetes, modify the cells using DNA technology and inject them back into the patient's liver, where they will function as islet cells, secreting insulin in response to blood glucose levels.

THE NATIONAL SERVICE FRAMEWORK (NSF) FOR DIABETES

The National Service Framework for diabetes is the sixth NSF introduced by the government

(DoH 2001, 2003). By setting 12 national standards for England, the Framework aims to improve the care of people with diabetes and make it consistent across the country. It gives most of the responsibility to primary care trusts (PCTs) and emphasizes the need for practice-based diabetes registers, systematic call and recall for regular review of patients, and close cooperation between primary care and specialist services, with clear referral criteria and pathways of care. The Royal College of Nursing has published a practical guide to the diabetes NSF, which summarizes the 12 standards and offers practical tips for achieving them (RCN 2003).

Wales will use the same standards as England, with its own delivery strategy (NHS Wales 2003). Scotland has published its own Diabetes Framework with slightly different priorities (NHS Scotland 2002), but the overall content is very similar to England's. Northern Ireland's follows the Scottish approach (Diabetes UK 2003b).

THE STANDARDS

Standard 1: Preventing type 2 diabetes

This standard aims to reduce the number of people who develop diabetes. It is primarily concerned with increasing public awareness and providing targeted support and information to people who are at high risk of developing the disease (see Risk factors for diabetes on p.162).

Standard 2: Identifying people with diabetes

Standard 2 aims to identify people who don't know they have diabetes, so that early intervention and education can reduce the risk of diabetic complications.

Standard 3: Empowering people with diabetes

This standard encourages people with diabetes (and their carers) to be involved in decision making. Patient education and the provision of patient-held records, which should include an agreed care plan, are key to this aim.

Standard 4: Clinical care of adults with diabetes

A team approach is required to achieve this standard, which aims to optimize the quality of life for people with diabetes and to reduce their risk of long-term complications. It relies upon establishing and implementing clear guidelines and protocols and on the continuing education of all healthcare professionals involved in the diagnosis and care of people with diabetes.

Standards 5 and 6: Clinical care of children and young people

These standards aim to meet the special needs of children and young people, ultimately enabling them to manage their diabetes effectively. Children, young people and their families should receive high-quality care and support and there should be a smooth transition from paediatric to adult diabetes services. Although the majority of care for these groups is provided by the secondary care multidisciplinary paediatric team, practice nurses, GPs, school nurses and health visitors also have an important role.

Standard 7: Diabetic emergencies

Education of patients and the general public will form a key part of the work to achieve this standard, which aims to ensure that acute diabetes-related complications are recognized promptly and treated by appropriately trained healthcare professionals.

Standard 8: Caring for people in hospital

To ensure consistently good-quality care for people with diabetes admitted to hospital for any reason, hospital staff need continuing education and support from the specialist diabetes team.

Standard 9: Diabetes and pregnancy

The aim of this standard is for women with preexisting diabetes or who develop diabetes in pregnancy to have a positive experience of pregnancy and childbirth and have healthy babies. This requires identification of patients who are at risk of developing diabetes during their pregnancy and provision of high-quality preconception and antenatal care, especially meticulous blood glucose control. Guidance for screening pregnant women is awaited from the National Screening Committee, but in the meantime local protocols should be followed.

Standards 10, 11 and 12: Detecting and managing complications

These standards aim to minimize the impact of diabetic complications through early detection and effective management. This requires integrated service provision and clear referral criteria, and may involve the development of highly specialized secondary care services.

Acknowledgements

The author is grateful to several professional colleagues for their valuable comments on the manuscript, especially Christopher Soper, diabetes specialist nurse; Maggie Shepherd, diabetes research fellow; Becky Nute, diabetes specialist nurse; Sarah O'Brien, diabetes nurse consultant; Samantha Bell, podiatrist; Simon Fleming, consultant biochemist; and Anna Bell, dietitian.

References

Airey CM, Williams DRR, Martin PG et al 2000 Hypoglycaemia induced by exogenous insulin – 'human' and animal insulin compared. Diabetic Medicine 17:416–432

Atkins RC 1999 Dr Atkins new diet revolution. Vermillion, London

BHF (British Heart Foundation) 2002 Physical activity and diabetes. Patient advice leaflet. Orderline for health professionals 01604 640016

Brand-Miller J, Foster-Powell K, Colagiuri S, Leeds A 1998 The GI factor: the glucose revolution, 2nd edn. Hodder, London

Coster S, Gulliford MC, Seed PT, Powrie JK, Swaminathan R 2000 Monitoring blood glucose control in diabetes mellitus: a systematic review. Health Technology Assessment 4(12):iv

DAFNE Study Group 2002 Training in flexible, intensive insulin management to enable dietary freedom in people with type 1 diabetes: Dose Adjustment for Normal Eating (DAFNE) randomised controlled trial. British Medical Journal 325:746

DCCT (Diabetes Control and Complications Trial) Research Group 1993 The effect of intensive treatment of diabetes on the development and progression of long-term complications in IDDM. New England Journal of Medicine 329:977–986

Diabetes UK 2000 Fact sheet no 2. Diabetes: the figures. Available online at: www.diabetes.org.uk/infocentre/fact/fact2.htm

Diabetes UK 2001 Fact sheet no 3. Diabetes: cost and complications. Available online at: www.diabetes.org.uk/infocentre/fact/fact3.htm

Diabetes UK 2003a Nutritional subcommittee of the Diabetes Care Advisory Committee of Diabetes UK. The implementation of nutritional advice for people with diabetes. Diabetic Medicine 20:786–807

Diabetes UK 2003b Safe disposal of needles and lancets (sharps). Position statement. Available online at: www.diabetes.org.uk/infocentre/state/sharps

Diabetes UK 2003c Report of the Northern Ireland Task Force on Diabetes. Available online at: www.diabetes.org.uk/n.ireland/execsummary.doc

DNSG (Diabetes and Nutrition Study Group) of the European Association for the Study of Diabetes 2000 Recommendations for the nutritional management of patients with diabetes mellitus. European Journal of Clinical Nutrition 54:353–355

DoH 2001 National Service Framework for diabetes: standards. Department of Health, London

DoH 2003 National Service Framework for diabetes: delivery strategy. Department of Health, London

Eisenstein J, Roberts SB, Dallal G et al 2002 High-protein weight-loss diets: are they safe and do they work? A review of the experimental and epidemiological data. Nutrition Reviews 60:189–200

Gatling W, Guzder RN, Turnbull JC et al 2001 The Poole diabetes study: how many cases of Type 2 diabetes are diagnosed each year during normal health care in a defined community? Diabetes Research and Clinical Practice 53:107–112

Holman RR, Cull CA, Turner RC 1999 A randomized double-blind trial of acarbose in type 2 diabetes shows improved glycemic control over 3 years (UK Prospective Diabetes Study 44). Diabetes Care 22(6):960–964

HPSCG (Heart Protection Study Collaborative Group) 2003 MRC/BHF Heart Protection Study of cholesterol-lowering with simvastatin in 5963 people with diabetes: a randomised placebo-controlled trial. Lancet 361:2005–2016

King H, Aubert RE, Herman WH 1998 Global burden of diabetes, 1995–2025: prevalence, numerical estimates and projections. Diabetes Care 9:1414–1431

Lean ME, Han TS, Seidell JC 1998 Impairment of health and quality of life in people with large waist circumference. Lancet 351:853–856

Lewis EJ, Hunsicker LG, Bain RP, Rhode RD 1993 The effect of angiotensin converting enzyme inhibition on diabetic nephropathy. New England Journal of Medicine 329:1456–1462

Naqib J 2002 Patient education for effective diabetes self-management: report, recommendations and examples of good practice. Diabetes UK, London

Nellemann Jorgensen L, Dejgaard A, Pramming SK 1994 Human insulin and hypoglycaemia: a literature survey. Diabetic Medicine 11:925–934

NHS Scotland 2002 Scottish Diabetes Framework. Available online: www.scotland.gov.uk/library5/health.sdf-00.asp

NHS Wales 2003 The Diabetes National Service Framework Standards for Wales. Available online: www.wales.nhs.uk/sites/documents/334/diabetes-standards-wales.pdf

NICE 2002a Inherited clinical guideline G. Management of Type 2 diabetes: management of blood glucose. National Institute for Clinical Excellence, London

NICE 2002b Inherited clinical guideline H. Management of Type 2 diabetes. Management of blood pressure and blood lipids. National Institute for Clinical Excellence, London

NICE 2002c Inherited clinical guideline F. Management of Type 2 diabetes. Renal disease – prevention and early management. National Institute for Clinical Excellence, London

NICE 2002d Inherited clinical guideline E. Management of Type 2 diabetes: Retinopathy – screening and early management. National Institute for Clinical Excellence, London

NICE April 2003 Guidance on the use of patient education models for diabetes. Technology appraisal 60. National Institute for Clinical Excellence, London

RCN 2003 An RCN guide to the National Service Framework for diabetes. Available from RCN Direct (0845 772 6100) or online: www.rcn.org.uk/direct. Publication code 002 011

Richter B, Neises G 2002 'Human' insulin versus animal insulin in people with diabetes mellitus. Cochrane Library, Issue 3, Oxford. Available online: www.update-software.com/cochrane/abstract.htm

UKPDS (UK Prospective Diabetes Study Group) 1998 Intensive blood glucose control with sulphonylureas or insulin compared with conventional treatment and risk of complications in patients with Type 2 diabetes (UKPDS 33). Lancet 352:837–853

Williams G, Pickup JC (eds) 2002 Handbook of diabetes, 2nd edn. Blackwell Publishing, London

Resources

Diabetes education and training for practice nurses

Training courses in diabetes range from local half-day workshops to a Master's degree in diabetes. Ask your PCT, local health board, local diabetes clinical lead or diabetes specialist nurse what training is available in your area. The prospectus of your local university will advertise diabetes modules which count towards a diploma or degree and there is also a variety of distance learning opportunities. A comprehensive list of courses, with contact details, can be found online at www.diabetes.org.uk/infocentre/inform/courses.doc

If you subscribe to Diabetes UK as a professional member, you will receive several mailings each year, keeping you up to date with new developments in diabetes care and advertising courses and conferences. Members of the RCN can join the diabetes nursing forum, at no additional cost (RCN Direct: 0845 772 6100 or www.rcn.org.uk/direct).

Recommended reading

Diabetes and Primary Care, published quarterly by SB Communications Group (tel: 020 7627 1510)

Useful websites

Diabetes UK: www.diabetes.org.uk
American Diabetes Association: www.diabetes.org
National Institute for Clinical Excellence: www.nice.org.uk
Scottish Intercollegiate Guidelines Network: www.sign.ac.uk
Diabetes in Scotland: www.diabetesinscotland.org
Diabetes journals: www.diabetesjournals.org
Royal College of Nursing: www.rcn.org.uk/diabetes

Chapter 10

Epilepsy

Marion M Welsh

CHAPTER CONTENTS

There are few chronic conditions which impact as vividly and dramatically as epilepsy and have such far-reaching consequences from the biopsychosocial perspective (Brown et al 1998). This chapter discusses the key concepts related to the practice nurse's role in responding to the needs of patients with epilepsy, focusing upon interventions and implications for practice. The interventions discussed have two main aims: to improve the quality of life of people with epilepsy and to raise the profile of the condition by challenging and tackling the inequality it evokes (Allen 1996). This incorporates three discrete but interrelated levels of care: biomedical, health promotion and challenging social inequalities using a holistic model (Doise 1982) which is conceptually underpinned by working in partnership with clients, families, carers and other multidisciplinary members and agencies (Crawford & Nicholson 1999).

Historically, epilepsy can be summarized as 4000 years of ignorance, superstition and stigma followed by 100 years of knowledge, superstition and stigma (Kale 1997). Not surprisingly, then, modern literature on epilepsy consistently mentions the need to improve not only the negative social impact of the condition, but also health service provision at all levels of care (Allen 1996, Brown et al 1998, Joint Epilepsy Council 1999). Clear deficiencies exist within primary healthcare and consistently identified is the need for structured care, particularly for those patients who do not attend acute neurological services (Davis 2002, Joint Epilepsy Council 1999). The potential for significant improvement within a patient-led primary healthcare service clearly exists, as those affected have unique, distinctive and unmet healthcare needs.

EPILEPSY: THE BIOMEDICAL CONDITION

Normal brain physiology is governed by the activity of millions of well-orchestrated neurones. A sudden and temporary disruption along the neural pathway causes a rapid and excessive discharge of electrical activity within the grey matter. This consequently affects neurological function and clinically manifests as a seizure (Lanfear 2002, Patten 1993).

Epilepsy is a condition characterized by paroxysmal, recurrent and unprovoked seizures which may be partial or generalized, depending on which part of the brain is affected, resulting in variable disturbances of consciousness, behaviour, emotion, motor function, perception or sensation (Appleton & Gibbs 1998). For many patients, seizure activity entails rare, brief episodes of bodily dysfunction, in which they experience intermittent loss of control. For others it means frequent seizures, which significantly affect the quality of their lives.

The term 'epilepsy' does not denote a definitive disease process but succinctly conveys a condition which encompasses a wide variety of seizure disorders and syndromes. An international classification exists (Box 10.1; CCTILE 1981) for seizure typology and delineation which is crucially important in determining the appropriate pharmacological treatment, management and prognosis outcomes.

Box 10.1 Seizure classification

1. Partial seizures

Simple (consciousness not impaired)

- With motor symptoms
- With sensory symptoms
- With autonomic symptoms
- With psychic symptoms

Complex (with impaired consciousness)

- Beginning as simple
- Progressing to complex partial
- Impairment of consciousness only with automatisms

2. Generalized seizures

Absence seizures

- Typical
- Atypical

Myoclonic

Tonic clonic

Tonic

Clonic

3. Unclassified epileptic seizures (inadequate/ incomplete data)

AETIOLOGY AND EPIDEMIOLOGY

Approximately 40% of epilepsy cases are symptomatic, with definable causes related to tumour, infection, brain injury, degenerative disorders, metabolic disturbance, recreational drug and alcohol misuse (Lanfear 2002). The remaining 60% of cases are either idiopathic, where no causal factor is identified, or cryptogenic, where the cause is suspected but remains unconfirmed (Russell & Hanscomb 1997).

Epilepsy is not a benign condition, a fact often unrecognized by professionals. Mortality is 2–4 times higher than that of an age-matched population without epilepsy. There are 1000 epilepsy-related deaths each year and associated causes include status epilepticus, suicide and accidents. Another cause relates to the phenomenon of sudden unexplained death in epilepsy (SUDEP), associated with acute respiratory arrest, the peak incidence of which is in early adulthood (Hanna 2002). Associated morbidity has been the subject of a Government-funded audit, which aimed to establish whether inadequacies in standards of care contributed to morbidity outcomes. The conclusions drawn placed a damning indictment on the levels of service provision (Reynolds 2001). The inferences become more acute when comprehension of epidemiological perspective is included.

Epilepsy is acknowledged as a serious, common, neurological condition which affects up to 50 million people worldwide and does not discriminate between age, gender, race, intellect or social class (Reynolds 2001). In the UK, figures suggest that approximately 1 in 140–200 people has active epilepsy (Crawford & Nicholson 1999) and that 420 000 people have the condition; 35 000 people are diagnosed each year and 100 people will have their first seizure today. GPs will, on average, have 10–12 patients with epilepsy on their list. These figures emphasize the numerical significance of epilepsy within the general practice setting.

Epilepsy can occur at any age, yet has been traditionally understood as a condition more commonly presenting in childhood (Kurtz et al 1998, Neville 1997). However, population trends now suggest a shift towards the elderly, with a decline in the childhood figures (Cockerell et al 1995, Everitt & Sander 1998). This evidence is based on increased rates of stroke, which can precipitate epilepsy, and consequently represents a valid argument based on the concept of an ageing population.

Epilepsy is also known to be higher within specific patient population groups, for example patients with learning disabilities, where the incidence is approximately 1 in 5 and increases proportionally with the severity of disability (Brown et al 1998, Loughran & O'Brien 2001). Thus a continuum exists within the primary care setting, from those who have epilepsy to those who have epilepsy with severe learning disabilities. Precise epidemiological data on epilepsy are difficult to establish as diagnosis has particular nuances and is generally a retrospective event which makes obtaining an accurate diagnosis a common problem (Davis 2002).

ESTABLISHING DIAGNOSIS

Initially, specialist neurological referral is indicated in order to establish a diagnosis and advise on the appropriate treatment. Potentially anyone can have a seizure given the right circumstances so it is important to comprehend that a single seizure episode is not diagnostic of epilepsy (Davis 2002). Evidence suggests that up to 35% of patients who have a history of epilepsy have been misdiagnosed, as various conditions, in particular syncope, pseudo-seizures and panic disorders, can mimic epilepsy (Brown et al 1998, Dornan 2000, Zaidi et al 1998). Overdiagnosis of epilepsy is not uncommon and consequentially can impose a dual penalty on the patient, with failure to treat or manage an undiagnosed disease/disorder and the unnecessary treatment of the patient without epilepsy, together with the raft of subsequent implications which accompany this diagnosis (Brown et al 1998). Cautionary notes therefore exist stressing the importance of establishing an accurate diagnosis based upon a reliable history or witness accounts and always considering the possibility of differential diagnosis (Brodie & French 2002).

Even when seizure activity is clearly visible to aid diagnosis, for example in a generalized seizure, in other cases consciousness levels may remain unaffected. This is particularly true within the context of partial attacks where seizure activity can be subtle, diffuse and difficult to recognize and may require diagnostic support. Numerous investigative procedures are available and their function is to support, not establish, diagnosis. Their utility is individually assessed with a view to revealing any underlying pathology and assisting in seizure classification (Brodie & French 2000).

- Blood tests: to exclude the presence of metabolic disorders
- Electroencephalogram (EEG): to detect abnormal electrical brain activity
- Neuroimaging: involving CT and MRI scanning to determine structural/vascular pathology, particularly relevant with management of elderly patients where vascular insufficiency is suspected
- Videotelemetry: conducted within specialized units, this involves continuous EEG monitoring and the use of video, in order to simultaneously capture and record seizure activity.

TREATMENT OF EPILEPSY

Individuals who experience a single seizure clearly merit further investigations but treatment is not generally considered at this juncture. The indications to commence treatment are evidence of two seizures close together within one year, an episode of status epilepticus (prolonged seizure activity of 30 minutes, managed as a clinical emergency) or diagnosis of an underlying brain disorder or syndrome (Taylor 1996).

Anti-epilepsy drugs (AEDs) remain the mainstay of treatment and the pharmacological choices are generally governed by seizure classification. The pharmacological issues for both patients and professionals represent a vast and complex field (Kwan & Brodie 2001, Prevett & Duncan 1995, Smithson & Kaufman 1997). The primary aim of drug treatment is to provide optimal seizure control without unacceptable drug-induced side-effects. A variety of pharmacological treatments exist (Box 10.2, 10.3), either as mono or combined therapy, which can provide up to 80% of patients with good seizure control without unacceptable side-effects (Crawford 1999, Feely 1999, Mead 1995). For the remaining 20% of patients

Box 10.2 Established AEDs

Drug	Year
Bromide	1870
Phenobarbitone	1912
Phenytoin	1938
Primadone	1952
Ethosuximide	1955
Carbamazepine	1963
Sodium valproate	1973
Clonazepam	1974
Clobazam	1979

Box 10.3 Newer AEDs

Vigabatrin	1989
Lamotrigine	1991
Gabapentin	1993
Toprimate	1995
Tiagabine	1999
Oxcarbazepine	2000
Levitoracetam	2000

the law of diminishing returns prevails and their epilepsy will remain refractory despite pharmacological interventions (Brodie & French 2000).

Contemporary prescribing tends to avoid phenobarbitol and its analogue, primadone, due to their overtly sedative effects which are less well tolerated. However, evidence confirms that most of the older established AEDs, despite their well-established track records, may also demonstrate adverse cognitive consequences, with complaints of sedation, tremors and depression to varying degrees (Kwan & Brodie 2001, Smithson & Kaufman 1997). Prescribing can present a double-edged sword in terms of limiting seizure activity but inducing negative effects on the quality of life. Some patients with epilepsy also demonstrate a greater propensity for cognitive and behavioural dysfunction, prior to initiating treatment, which may compound underlying problems (Kwan & Brodie 2001).

In contrast, newer drugs introduced within the last decade have more favourable outcomes, in terms of comparable efficacy and significantly fewer drug-induced behavioural and cognitive problems. Despite limited empirical evidence at this stage, authoritative sources suggest that clinicians should adopt a more holistic and individualized approach to prescribing which acknowledges potential negative sequelae (Allen 1996, Crawford 1999, Crawford & Nicholson 1999, Prevett & Duncan 1995).

Key issues for practice nursing include a knowledge of pharmacology which is required to underpin care, centring on the needs of the individual patient (Welsh 2001). Pertinent issues are numerous and predominantly relate to drug interactions which may reduce the efficacy of both the AEDs and other prescribed preparations; for example, in patients attending for travel healthcare, concomitant use of mefloquine (Lariam) for antimalarial prophylaxis would affect serum concentrations by lowering plasma levels of AEDs and increasing seizure activity. This drug should be avoided and alternative therapy sought (Walker et al 1993), with clear explanation regarding the inherent implications of an increased malarial risk due to the necessity to opt for less efficacious treatment.

Concordance issues abound within this context with strategies required to work in partnership with patients on agreed healthcare outcomes (Blenkinsopp et al 2002). Evidence suggests that many patients do not comply with medication for a variety of reasons (Mead 1995) and consequently issues surrounding medication become an important focus for the practice nurse to develop a partnership approach in patient care. Good communication skills are powerful therapeutic tools in translating the complexities of epilepsy and its treatment for patients with differing capacities for understanding and from varied societal backgrounds. Undoubtedly this presents a significant challenge, especially with issues of pharmacology, highlighting the required knowledge base and skills to articulate potential problem areas.

The opportunity to interact with patients can present itself within the confines of ritualistic therapeutic drug monitoring. As a routine activity, this is rarely indicated for the majority of well-controlled patients and appears as an unnecessary catalyst for inappropriate changes in drug dosage (Crawford 1999, Crawford & Nicholson 1999, Prevett & Duncan 1995). If the patient's seizure activity is well controlled and they remain side-effect free, even when this exceeds the upper therapeutic limit, then a limited approach is required. The adage is to treat the patient and not a therapeutic blood level. This is pertinent within the context of the significantly less sedative action of the newer AEDs. The major indications to undertake monitoring of blood levels are (Mead 1995, Prevett & Duncan 1995):

- to check compliance in the event of continuing seizures; this may be particularly relevant in patients with learning disabilities who have recurrent seizures and have communication difficulties
- to confirm dose-related side-effects, i.e. oversedation
- to monitor patients who are unwell, pregnant or contemplating pregnancy.

Other haematological investigations, in particular liver function tests and folic acid levels, may be undertaken prior to commencing treatment and annually thereafter, with use of the established AEDs (Crawford 1999). The specifics of recommended serological studies should be evaluated in light of guidance from pharmaceutical data sheets and audit review. Nevertheless, the value of attempting to preempt blood dyscrasias or acute hepatic problems as a routine activity appears unconvincing (Crawford 1999).

Cost-effective prescribing has now become common practice throughout the UK and in most areas of pharmacological treatments the shift from branded to the generic equivalent goes unnoticed. However, some authors suggest that seizure control may be compromised by switching brands of medication (Crawford et al 1996), inducing changes in drug bio-availability and precipitating seizure activity. Consistent proprietary prescribing is advocated unless under clinical assessment, as retitration may be required.

PHARMACOLOGY AND WOMEN'S ISSUES

Particular care is required in the management of women with epilepsy, as they require information on a raft of related subjects along a continuum which ranges from the menarche to the menopause (Box 10.4). A survey of women members of the British Epilepsy Association (BEA) supports this premise as it highlighted that women receive inadequate information regarding contraceptive and preconceptional advice (Madden 1999). Guidelines were subsequently published specifically aimed at improving the care of women with epilepsy (British Epilepsy Association 1999).

Box 10.4 Women with epilepsy

- Sexual development
- Sexuality
- Menstruation
- Contraception
- Fertility
- Pregnancy
- Motherhood
- Menopause

Women of child-bearing age merit special consideration as they have particular issues and health needs which need to be addressed and significantly relate to pharmacology issues. For instance, if women are taking enzyme-inducing therapy, such as carbamazepine, then oral contraceptives need to be prescribed at the higher dose of 50 μg in order to maintain efficacy. This has inherent implications for nurses who are eligible to prescribe from the Nurse Prescriber's Extended Formulary (BMA/RPS 2002–3). Nurse prescribing, within this context of health promotion (Blenkinsopp et al 2002), would normally also include folic acid supplements preconceptionally and during pregnancy to prevent neural tube defects but the Nurse Prescriber's Formulary (p.440) clearly states that women on AEDs 'need individual counselling by their doctor before starting folic acid', the rationale being that it needs to be prescribed at a higher dose and for a longer period. This endorses an approach which advocates that specialist preconceptional counselling be a mandatory service provision (Brown et al 1998). The importance of this service also becomes pertinent when considering that many of the older AEDs have a potential teratogenic effect with reported abnormalities including spina bifida, cardiac anomalies and cleft lip and palate (BMA/RPS 2002–3, Rosser & Wilson 1999). In contrast, the new-generation drugs, in particular lamotrigine, are being viewed optimistically as non-teratogenic and female friendly (Brodie & French 2000).

Given the significant contribution practice nursing makes to women's healthcare, the implications are plainly evident regarding the pharmacological knowledge base which underpins care and how this may require subsequent referral to the most appropriate healthcare professional. Specific information for women needs to be introduced at an early age so that women can make an informed choice about contraceptive methods and promptly access preconceptual care.

WITHDRAWAL OF MEDICATION

The natural history of epilepsy suggests that remission can occur in some individuals (Jacoby 1997). However, attempted withdrawal of medication has significant implications for the individual's lifestyle and life circumstances. A trial withdrawal of medication, which can be contemplated after two or more seizure-free years, necessitates stopping driving from the commencement of the withdrawal period and thereafter for up to 6 months after stopping treatment. Any subsequent seizure would cause a driver to forfeit their licence until they had been seizure free again for 1 year (Walsh 1999). Such considerations place patients in a dilemma, as this may impact on issues other than independence regarding transport difficulties, e.g. potential loss of employment and income, self-esteem and quality of life.

A prudent approach is recommended regarding attempted withdrawal of medication with neurologist referral to discuss and supervise outcomes (Prevett & Duncan 1995).

ALTERNATIVES TO DRUG TREATMENT

Surgical interventions (Box 10.5) have become more widely available in recent years and are considered when up to five drugs have been tried over a period of 3–5 years and patients continue to experience very frequent disruptive seizures (Harkness 1996, Neville 1997). To be effective the epileptogenic focus must, if possible, be identified, removed or disconnected from other non-epileptogenic tissue.

Box 10.5 Epilepsy surgery

- Temporal lobectomy
- Corpus callosotomy
- Hemispherectomy
- Stereotactic treatment
- Gamma knife

Positive surgical outcomes have demonstrated significantly reduced or complete cessation of seizure, permitting individuals to interact more positively with society and achieve personal development (Harkness 1996). However, the psychosocial impact of a lifetime with refractory epilepsy may never be overcome.

Another approach which may be considered is vagal nerve stimulation. This is a neurophysiologic treatment which requires the insertion of a pacemaker-sized implant in the left upper chest. Although the mechanism is not clearly understood, pulsed nerve stimulation of the vagus nerve occurs every 3–5 minutes, affecting parts of the brain which are believed to generate excessive electrical activity. This device can also be magnetically triggered by patients who experience an aura, to abort an impending seizure (Brodie & French 2000).

Other alternative treatments whose evidence base still requires validation include a ketogenic diet (high fat), behaviour therapy, herbalism, homeopathy and aromatherapy. Few cautions exist within nursing and medical texts regarding the use of aromatherapy but it is not innocuous and essential oils for massage, aromatic baths, vaporization, inhalation, compresses and mouthwashes should only be used under the assessment and direction of a qualified aromatherapist. Specifically, rosemary, sage, fennel and hyssop are inappropriate for use in patients with epilepsy because of their stimulating effect on the central nervous system, potentially precipitating seizure activity (Wildwood 1996).

GENERAL PRACTICE MANAGEMENT AND PRACTICE NURSE INTERVENTION

Following initial diagnosis and treatment by a neurologist, general practice has been deemed the most appropriate setting for ongoing care for the vast majority of patients with epilepsy. Despite this, in comparison with services for other chronic conditions, service provision for patients has been evaluated as fragmented and occupying a low profile (Joint Epilepsy Council 1999). Whilst GPs accept a role in epilepsy management (Smithson & Kaufman 1997), many demonstrate a low or moderate interest in it. The perception is that some GPs lack confidence in managing epilepsy (Jacoby 1997) and feel that care should be the domain of acute neurology services. Yet the reality is that neurologists with an interest in epilepsy are sparse and demands on this service often outstrip supply (Roberts 2000).

Evidence confirms that the healthcare needs of patients with epilepsy are inadequately met (Dornan 2000, Madden 1999, Marshall 1998, Ridsdale et al 1997, SIGN 1997). Their principal requirements for continuing information and support are similar to other groups of patients who suffer with chronic conditions (Crawford & Nicholson 1999). Supporting this are the recorded higher rates of A&E admission for epilepsy, in comparison with other chronic diseases, highlighting an unenviable and unique position.

Practice nurses have demonstrated the provision of high-quality care in other chronic disease management fields (Jacoby 1997) and clearly have transferable skills which can be applied to epilepsy care. Underpinning this approach is the need for professional education, relevant not just for the practice nurse but for all members of the primary healthcare team (SIGN 1997). Quality care requires planning, structuring and adopting across the interface of all service provision and increasingly practices have demonstrated their intention to review epilepsy care and develop competency in management and ongoing support.

The crux of primary healthcare management should focus upon what patients with epilepsy have a right to expect. Succinctly this can be viewed as:

- no seizures
- no dose-related side-effects
- freedom from interference in everyday life by the medical process
- involvement in treatment decisions.

AUDIT, GUIDELINES AND PROTOCOLS

Undertaking an initial practice-based audit will demonstrate the present standard of care, which can provide a platform to generate discussion and involvement on adopting a structured approach to feasible improvements (Appendix 1). Audit criteria have been suggested by the Scottish Intercollegiate Guidelines Network (SIGN 1997) which produces comprehensive evidence-based guidelines for general practice. These guidelines were reviewed and updated in 2003. The inaugural launch of NICE guidelines for epilepsy is not anticipated until June 2004.

Reviewing the current evidence regarding standards and quality in care is an important initial step as is the ability to critically appraise the literature. In order to help patients help themselves to a better quality of life, general practices must continue to assess care via clinical audit and evaluation of current research (Smail 1997, Thomas 1997). Audit record templates can be constructed to aid continuing audit and easy access to patient details for all the primary care team.

The development of chronic disease management services often occurs at the behest of the GP concerned and this highlights the importance of undertaking health needs assessment in partnership with this particular population. A number of key documents and guidelines have been published in recent years supporting this approach and highlighting the importance of improving epilepsy services (Brown et al 1998, Epilepsy Advisory Board 2000, Joint Epilepsy Council 1999, Madden 1999, SIGN 1997).

Primary care groups/local healthcare cooperatives produce evidence-based guidelines from which practices may operate or they may choose to develop their own, based on current good practice. A collaborative approach with acute neurology services and with specialist nurses in epilepsy should also be considered in the development of protocols for the effective management of epilepsy (Hart 1995, Russell 1997). This also recognizes that responsibilities and levels of care will vary depending on the interest and competencies of those involved.

For specific patients, particularly children and those with refractory epilepsy, the most appropriate referral and management should be undertaken within an acute specialist unit (Brodie & French 2000). A significant number of patients with epilepsy will remain within general practice care (Ambury 1997).

The cornerstone of epilepsy management is clearly drug treatment but it is all too easy to allow drug-maintained patients to drift into the background of general practice. These patients are distinctly different from other populations whose condition demands long-term drug treatments, e.g. hypertensive patients, and must be considered a special group. The ability and potential to function normally, to have a driver's licence, to face employment issues, the risk of having a child with an abnormality all depend on their medication and their overall well-being. Therefore epilepsy is a condition with an enormous emotive element which strengthens the argument for a structured approach which acknowledges and incorporates the wider implications.

Establishing a co-ordinated care programme is the key to improving care (Laville 1998) and practice nurses with appropriate knowledge and skill can provide education and support for patients on understanding epilepsy and its management. Practices may have a large enough population to hold specific disease clinics which can be efficient by allowing for protected time and ease of administration.

An appropriate starting point would be to invite patients to attend for an annual review and a management record card can be instrumental in explaining investigations, how prescribed drugs work, efficacy, reporting dose-related side-effects, how to manage missed doses and drug interactions (Appendix 2). Consolidating patient information promotes communication between the service user and provider and in so doing, acknowledges the concept of a partnership approach (Appendix 3). Undertaking an annual review will provide the opportunity not only to consider the principles of drug treatment but also to focus on other areas of concern within psychosocial care. This reinforces the concept that epilepsy management extends far beyond the scope of seizure treatment (Porter & Chadwick 1997). Evidently, role intervention includes assessing individual need and providing advice on the many associated topics and incorporating these as part of a management strategy (Box 10.6). This

Box 10.6 Management issues

- Understanding epilepsy
- Investigations
- Understanding medication
- Co-prescribing and drug interactions
- Safety issues
- Employment, access to specialist advice
- Pathways to specialists
- Driving, legal implications
- Preconception, contraception and pregnancy
- Parenting
- Exemption from prescription charges
- Support groups
- Good record keeping

can be augmented by a range of excellent materials available from various support organizations, which can also be accessed by patients (see Resources).

The nurse can become an accessible resource for individuals and families by facilitating their understanding of the condition, teaching first aid approaches to seizures (Appendix 4), highlighting treatment and lifestyle implications and assisting with issues of advocacy and empowerment (Laville 1998). This service could also be accessed by patients, families and carers who do attend the acute sector and who may at times require access to an informed professional. The practice nurse is also ideally placed to interface with other community disciplines, acute and social services within a co-ordinated epilepsy service, aiming to improve quality of life and reduce associated morbidity (Carnwell 1998, Joint Epilepsy Council 1999). Knowledge of the condition's psychological impact is significantly important and highlights the complexities of community nursing (National Society for Epilepsy 2002) as it embraces the biopsychosocial concept by using a flexible, eclectic approach.

Correlating this to individual epilepsy care suggests the need to provide accessible and relaxed environments and develop a rapport with patients by using effective channels of communication (Roberts 2000). Use of counselling skills which facilitate discussion of fears, anxieties, misunderstandings or misconceptions associated with epilepsy (Laville 1998) can assist the individual to focus upon what they *can* do, rather than what they cannot.

Of importance is the ability to gauge the patient's level of understanding and build on their interpretation of epilepsy. This is especially important for patients with learning disabilities who may not attend specialist services and lack the ability to confidently articulate within general practice (Loughran & O'Brien 2001) and therefore may necessitate liaison with colleagues within the learning disabilities team.

Fundamentally the nursing interventions discussed contribute to promoting the health of patients with epilepsy, considered a definitive aspect of nursing practice (Piper & Brown 1998). Interestingly this premise also presents the unique opportunity to subliminally contribute to prevention at a primary level (Brown et al 1998). Initiatives aimed at reducing rates of stroke, preventing accidents and alcohol and drug misuse are areas in which the practice nurse already plays a key role. Practice nurses also need to demonstrate skills in communication, listening, counselling, leadership and teaching (UKCC 1998), which are commensurate with specialist-level practice in order to promote health within the management of epilepsy.

ADOLESCENTS AND PARENTS

Interacting with individuals within specific, age-related groups dictates a need to be perceptive, especially when dealing with adolescents who, in growing older, may become less dependent on hospital clinics and more able to access primary care services. At this stage of personal development it is common for adolescents to face many problems. Epilepsy not only magnifies these but also introduces new ones (Smith 1998). Issues of self-awareness and deviations from peer group norms assume great importance: epilepsy can be disastrous for an adolescent's self-esteem and sense of identity. Mood swings and rebellious behaviour may also surface (Marshall 1998). Studies suggest that adolescents are more at risk of lowered self-esteem and isolation, which then becomes socially disabling (Appleton et al 1997, O'Donohoe 1994). Psychological problems can destabilize emotional well-being and potentially reduce seizure control, hence referral to psychology services may be necessary (Appleton & Gibbs 1998). Adolescents with chronic conditions need the opportunity to discuss difficulties associated with their condition and the adolescent process (Gay 1997), empowering them to confidently adopt a positive stance in dealing with epilepsy, to find out more about it and take control.

Major trigger factors can uniquely affect this group and awareness of these issues is significantly important as these relate to sleep deprivation, missing meals, stresses associated with exams, alcohol and recreational drug use (Brodie & French 2000). The latter two issues can cause significant anxiety, particularly for parents. Regarding use of alcohol, it is accepted that minimal amounts (up to two units) should not cause problems (Lanfear 2002) providing medication is not stopped and a responsible approach is adopted. However, recreational drug use should be avoided.

Adolescence is about gaining independence but parents will have played a major role in helping to manage their child's epilepsy and this may continue to foster an attitude of dependency within the adolescent. Practice and school nursing services can act as valuable sources of information and support for both the adolescent and the parents. The optimum relationship established should be one of healthy interdependence (Williams 1999). The needs of the family that has a child with epilepsy change over time and this requires recognition.

For many parents, the initial response to their child's diagnosis of epilepsy is one of grief and anxiety, of which the latter is a constant emotion. Parents can have a tendency to overprotect and this may inhibit the realization of the full potential of their child; a balanced approach is not always easy to achieve. The opportunity to access a skilled and sensitive professional who can help support them through this process (O'Donohoe 1994) can be invaluable. Their knowledge of support groups, national and local associations, as well as networking with other members of the multidisciplinary health and social work teams to provide support structures, is crucially important to the well-being of the whole family (Appleton et al 1997).

THE SOCIAL ACTION PERSPECTIVE

Social action perspectives for practice nursing include countering inequality and social injustice linked with epilepsy but firstly it must be considered why social action is relevant and appropriate. There are few chronic health conditions which terrify and frighten more than epilepsy (O'Donohoe 1994, Smithson & Kaufman 1997), based on a lack of knowledge and understanding of how to deal with it. Some authors speculate (Laybourn & Hill 1991) that societal discomfort originates with negative public perceptions, arising from the minority of people with epilepsy and severe learning disabilities whose condition is more observable and less well controlled. Society then develops a stereotypical view based on visualizing the worst end of the epilepsy continuum, which is then indiscriminately applied to everyone with epilepsy.

Public misunderstanding of epilepsy induces fear, often the precursor of social stigma which leads to prejudice and discrimination in school, work and community environments. This stimulates the individual's fear, precipitating social isolation which in turn can trigger further seizures and so perpetuate problems which have no direct correlation with the disease process (Allen 1996).

According to the British Epilepsy Association (Fearn 1996), members confirmed prejudices throughout the social strata: difficulties with teachers, finding places at colleges, victimization at work and, regrettably, lack of support from healthcare professionals. Subsequently many suffer depression, resulting in a downward spiral of life circumstances (Allen 1996, Russell & Hanscomb 1997). Often expounded is the concept that people with epilepsy suffer more from societal attitudes than from the condition (Kale 1997). This negativity also permeates to UK charitable donations. In 1996 over £200 m was raised for cancer and £9 m for leprosy, of which Britain had no new cases, but only £2 m for epilepsy, despite there being 420 000 people in the UK with the condition. This undoubtedly reflects the perception that epilepsy is connected with mental health problems and evidently less emotive.

If community nursing practice is functioning effectively, the potential for marginalization and discriminatory attitudes towards this patient group should be recognized and challenged. Practice nurses can make significant contributions by raising the profile of epilepsy (Welsh 2001) and one need only examine the management of asthma in practice nurse-led clinics to appreciate the improvement both clinically and socially (Cohen 1995). Interacting with community groups and schools provides opportunities to challenge misconceptions and fears in those who teach and employ, thereby attempting to tackle issues of discriminatory practice (Allen 1996).

EDUCATION AND EMPLOYMENT

Students with epilepsy should expect to be treated with equity and teaching staff must be aware that to do otherwise is morally reprehensible. The variability of the condition means that children will be differently affected and broad discrimination will affect their learning potential.

Educational establishments should facilitate access to knowledgeable and skilled advisors regarding accurate information on employment and careers. This should be an early intervention and, as with any individual, primarily based upon abilities and skills and only then should their epilepsy be considered. The law does, however, govern some employment options, some related to driving, and restricts the individual, for example, from joining the armed forces or police, piloting aircrafts or driving heavy goods vehicles. The spectrum of careers options which is available far exceeds those which are not (Welsh 2001). The current financial budget for epilepsy is £2 billion per annum, of which 65% is paid in unemployment and welfare benefit, underpinning, perhaps, discrimination associated with employment opportunity (Brown et al 1998, Smithson & Kaufman 1997). Important issues relate to an awareness of equal opportunities legislation and facilitating access to disability advisory services. Patients with epilepsy which remains difficult to control and does preclude employment and driving may be able to claim certain benefits and further advice can be sought by contacting their local benefits agency, welfare rights worker or the local citizens' advice bureau.

SERVICE PROVISION

Comprehensive and extensive research aimed at assessing the quality of existing service provision at national and regional level confirms a fragmented service, lacking vital resources (Joint Epilepsy Council 1999). It describes as 'basic' the service provision within some parts of the country, identifying gaps in management and minimal service provision. Variations in care provided, particularly between urban and rural areas, have been debated by clients and healthcare professionals. Patients in rural areas, for example, have access to fewer neurology services, fewer local physicians with an interest in neurology and fewer, if any, epilepsy specialist nurses (Joint Epilepsy Council 1999).

Not only is this patient group socially disadvantaged in terms of public perception and stigma, they are also disadvantaged and socially excluded regarding service provision (Joint Epilepsy Council 1999). Reasons why patients with epilepsy, who arguably require more attention, receive less remain unclear.

Nevertheless, opportunities exist to empower and encourage patients to influence and develop new services and improve existing ones through partnership approaches. Opportunities exist for practice nurses and the wider primary healthcare team to provide services built on their knowledge and skill which empower and encourage patients. They can also be proactive in campaigning for improved epilepsy service at strategic primary care group/local health care council level.

CONCLUSION

Epilepsy is the most common, chronic, neurological condition where patients strive not only to control their symptoms and survive, but also to lead normal lives despite the problems associated with their condition and its treatment.

The medical treatment of seizure control, whilst undeniably crucial, defines only a small proportion of the life experiences of the person with epilepsy. Society's attitudes foster feelings of low self-esteem, dependence, stigmatization and discrimination for people with epilepsy. As a result, those with the condition may demonstrate higher rates of psychosocial problems. If individuals and health professionals openly challenge public misconceptions and fear of epilepsy, a cascade effect may occur which could counteract the stigma and inequality that coexist with this condition.

There are substantial deficiencies and inequalities in epilepsy care evident at national, local and general practice level. For the majority of patients, the chronicity of the condition merits ongoing management, information and support which can be facilitated in general practice within a holistic structured patient-centred service. This permits acute neurology services to appropriately manage refractory cases and specialized groups.

Practice nurses have a pivotal role to play in delivery of healthcare for patients with epilepsy, supported by collaborative working and acknowledging the important contribution of other multi-agency professionals and the patients' families and carers. This requires the practice nurse to be perceptive, innovative and skilled in interpersonal communication, playing a major role in improving the quality of life for patients with epilepsy and raising the profile it currently occupies within the healthcare agenda.

The challenge for practice nursing is to drive forward improvements for patients with epilepsy by responding and contributing to their health and social care needs. Comprehension of the key issues regarding management, the negative psychosocial impact and the need to support patients in developing positive attitudes to life choices are important concepts and interventions for the practice nurse caring for patients with epilepsy.

References

Allen D 1996 Opening Pandora's box. Nursing Standard 11(9):22–23

Ambury T 1997 Out of the shadows. Scottish Medicine 16(6):4–5

Appleton R, Chapel B, Beirne M 1997 Your child's epilepsy: a parent's guide. Class Publishing, London

Appleton RE, Gibbs J 1998 Epilepsy in childhood and adolescence, 2nd edn. Dunitz, London

Blenkinsopp A, Paxton P, Blenkinsopp J 2002 Nurse prescribers: staying safe when prescribing. Primary Health Care 12(7):35–37

British Epilepsy Association 1999 We can campaign: women with epilepsy speak out. BEA, London

British Medical Association, Royal Pharmaceutical Society 2002–3 Nurse Prescribers' Formulary (incorporating British National Formulary) No. 43. BMA, London

Brodie MJ, French J 2000 Management of epilepsy in adolescents and adults. Lancet 356:323–329

Brown S, Betts T, Crawford P 1998 Epilepsy needs revisited: a revised epilepsy needs document for the UK. Seizure 7:435–446

Carnwell R 1998 Conceptual models for practice. In: Blackie C (ed) Community health care nursing. Churchill Livingstone, Edinburgh, pp105–124

CCTILE (Commission of Classification and Terminology of the International League against Epilepsy) 1981 Proposal for revised clinical and electroencephalographic classification of epileptic seizures. Epilepsia 22:289–501

Cockerell O, Eckle I, Goodridge D 1995 Epilepsy in a population of 6000 re-examined: secular trends in first attendance rates, prevalence and prognosis. Journal of Neurology, Neurosurgery and Psychiatry 58:570–576

Cohen P 1995 Epilepsy aim. Practice Nurse 10(4):244

Crawford P 1999 Monitoring requirements with antiepileptic drugs. Prescriber 10(22):122–123

Crawford P, Hau W, Chapel B 1996 Generic prescribing for epilepsy: is it safe? Seizure 5(1):1–5

Crawford P, Nicholson C 1999 Epilepsy management. Professional Nurse 14(8):565–569

Davis J 2002 Improving care for the patient with epilepsy. In: Muncey T, Parker A (eds) Chronic disease management. Palgrave, London, pp231–244

Doise W 1982 L'explication en psychologie sociale. PUF, Paris

Dornan C 2000 Managing epilepsy. Nursing Times 96(19):37–38

Epilepsy Advisory Board 2000 Epilepsy care: making it happen. BEA, Leeds

Everitt AD, Sander JW 1998 Incidence of epilepsy is now higher in elderly people than children. British Medical Journal 316(7133):780

Fearn H 1996 Understanding epilepsy. Healthlines 31(26):26

Feely M 1999 Drug treatment of epilepsy. British Medical Journal 318(7176):106–109

Gay MJ 1997 Talking sense with adolescents. Asthma Journal 2(1):19–20

Hanna N 2002 The National Sentinel Audit of Epilepsy-Related Death: epilepsy death in the shadows. Stationery Office, London

Harkness W 1996 The surgical option. Presentation of paper at Growing up with Epilepsy conference. BEA, Leeds

Hart Y 1995 Epilepsy: clinical management. Practice Nursing 6(19):19–22

Jacoby A 1997 Age related considerations. In: Engle J, Pedley TA (eds) Epilepsy: a comprehensive textbook, vol 2. Lippincott-Raven, Philadelphia, pp1121–1130

Joint Epilepsy Council 1999 Service development kit. Epilepsy Task Force, London

Kale R 1997 Bringing epilepsy out of the shadows. British Medical Journal 315(7099):2–3

Kurtz Z, Tookey P, Ross E 1998 Epilepsy in young people: 23 year follow up of the British national child development study. British Medical Journal 316(7128):339–342

Kwan P, Brodie MJ 2001 Neuropsychological effects of epilepsy and antiepileptic drugs. Lancet 357:216–221

Lanfear J 2002 The individual with epilepsy. Nursing Standard 16(46):43–53

Laville L 1998 Switching the management of epilepsy to primary care. Nursing Times 94(19):52–53

Laybourn A, Hill M 1991 Children with epilepsy and their families: needs and services, a review and discussion. Scottish Office, Edinburgh

Loughran SJ, O'Brien D 2001 Health care, epilepsy and learning disabilities. Nursing Standard 15(22):33–34

Madden V 1999 Women with epilepsy are not getting pregnancy advice. British Medical Journal 318(7195):1374

Marshall F 1998 Your child: epilepsy. Element Books, Shaftesbury

Mead M 1995 Keys to epilepsy care. Practice Nurse 9(5):370–372

National Society for Epilepsy 2002 Epilepsy and leisure. NSE, London

Neville BGR 1997 Fortnightly review: epilepsy in childhood. British Medical Journal 315(7113):924–930

O'Donohoe N 1994 Epilepsies of childhood, 3rd edn. Butterworth-Heinemann, Oxford

Patten JP 1993 Diseases of the nervous system and voluntary muscles. In: Hawkins RL (ed) Treatment and prognosis: medicine, 2nd edn. Butterworth-Heinemann, Oxford, pp97–120

Piper SM, Brown PA 1998 The theory and practice of health education applied to nursing: a bi-polar approach. Journal of Advanced Nursing 27(2):383–389

Porter J, Chadwick D 1997 Overview: general approaches to treatment. In: Engle J, Pedley TA (eds) Epilepsy: a comprehensive textbook, vol 2. Lippincott-Raven, Philadelphia, pp1101–1102

Prevett MC, Duncan JS 1995 Anti-epileptic drugs. Update 51(9):507–511

Reynolds E 2001 ILEA/IBE/WHO global campaign 'Out of the Shadows': global and regional developments. Epilepsia 42(8):1094–1110

Ridsdale L, Robins D, Cryer C 1997 Feasibility and effects of nurse run clinics for patients with epilepsy in general practice: randomised controlled trial. British Medical Journal 314(7074):1120

Roberts P 2000 Establishing a nurse led counselling clinic for people with epilepsy. Primary Health Care 10(1):22–26

Rosser EM, Wilson LC 1999 Drugs for epilepsy have teratogenic risks. British Medical Journal 318(7193):129

Russell A 1997 How nurses can support people with epilepsy. Nursing Times 93(27):50–51

Russell A, Hanscomb A 1997 Epilepsy: the most common serious neurological condition. Nursing Times 93(21):52–55

SIGN (Scottish Intercollegiate Guidelines Network) 1997 Diagnosis and management of epilepsy in adults. Scottish Intercollegiate Guidelines Network, Edinburgh

Smail J 1997 Shifting the boundaries in practice nursing. In: Gastrell P, Edwards J (eds) Community health nursing. Baillière Tindall, London, pp259–271

Smith PEM 1998 The teenager with epilepsy. British Medical Journal 317(7164):960–961

Smithson H, Kaufman G 1997 Improving your epilepsy service. Practice Nurse 14(5):321–323

Taylor MP 1996 Managing epilepsy in primary care. Blackwell Science, Oxford

Thomas E 1997 Evidence based primary health care nursing. In: Gastrell P, Edwards J (eds) Community health nursing. Baillière Tindall, London, pp198–206

UKCC 1998 Standards for specialist education and practice. UKCC, London

Walker E, Williams G, Raeside F 1993 ABC of healthy travel, 4th edn. BMJ Publishing, London

Walsh M 1999 The nervous system. In: Walsh M, Crumbie A, Reveley S (eds) Nurse practitioners: clinical skills and professional issues. Butterworth-Heinemann, Oxford, pp54–72

Welsh M 2001 The practice nurse's role in the management of epilepsy. British Journal of Community Nursing 6(3):112–117

Wildwood C 1996 Aromatherapy. Bloomsbury, London

Williams C 1999 Needs of teenagers with chronic disability. British Medical Journal 318:945

Zaidi A, Clough P, Scheepers B 1998 Treatment resistant epilepsy or convulsive syncope. British Medical Journal 317:869–870

Resources

The National Society for Epilepsy
Chalfont Centre for Epilepsy
Chalfont St Peter
Gerrards Cross
Buckinghamshire SL9 0RJ
Tel: 01494 601 3000
Helpline: 01494 601 4000
Website: www.epilepsynse.org.uk

Epilepsy Action
New Anstey House
Gate Way Drive
Yeadon
Leeds LS19 7XY
Tel: 0113 201 8800
Fax: 0113 391 0300
Email: epilepsy@epilepsy.org.uk

Epilepsy Action Scotland
48 Govan Road
Glasgow G51 1JL
Tel: 0141 427 4911
Fax: 0141 419 1709

Wales Epilepsy Association Cyf
15 Chester Street
St Asaph
Denbighshire LL17 0RE
Tel/fax: 01745 584444
Helpline: 08475 413 774

British Epilepsy Association (N Ireland)
Graham House
Knockbracken Health Care Park
Saintfield Road
Belfast BT8 8BH
Tel: 02871 799355

Brainwave (ROI)
Irish Epilepsy Association
249 Crumlin Road
Dublin
Tel: 003531 455 7500
Fax: 003531 445 7013
Email: brainwave@iol.ie

Continued professional development in epilepsy education

Irene Hamill, Epilepsy Specialist Nurse
Institute of Neurological Sciences
Southern General Hospital
Govan Road
Glasgow G51 4TF
Tel: 0141 201 2556
Fax: 0141 201 2509
Short course for practice nurses

Professional Diploma in Epilepsy Care (Distance Learning)
Centre for Community Neurological Studies
Leeds Metropolitan University
Calverley Street
Leeds LS1 3HE
Tel: 0113 283 5981
Fax: 0113 283 3124

APPENDIX 1 EPILEPSY AUDIT

NAME	Mr A Green	Ms B Gray	Mr C White	Mrs D Brown
Date of birth	04/03/75	28/02/79	02/02/55	01/08/25
Date of review	30/06/98	30/06/98	30/06/98	30/06/98
Age at onset	19	13	birth	68
Life event prior to onset	motorbike accident	✕	neonatal hydrocephalus, severe hypoxia	stroke
Date last seen by secondary care for epilepsy	✕	24/04/97	✕	02/01/94
Seizure description in notes	✔	ABS, GTCS, Myoclonic jerks	✕	✕
Classification in notes	SPS → CPS	JME	✕	✕
Learning difficulty/brain injury or disease	haematoma left temporal	✕	severe LD, hemiparesis	initial speech loss, now recovered
EEG	✔	✔	✕	✔
CT	✔	✕	✕	✔
MRI	✕	✕	✕	✕
Record of seizure frequency in notes	✕	✔	✕	✕
Seizure free (since ...)	?	✔ 1993	✕	✕
Current AEDs	CBZ-R	VPA	PHT, PB CBZ	PB
Dose ..../.../..../....	400/400	500/500	200/200, 60/90 200/200/200/200	30/30
Side-effects	✕	2 stone weight gain	unknown	✕
AEDs tried in past	✕	✕	VPA, PRM	✕
Phenytoin level in last year	N/A	N/A	✕	N/A
Considered for surgery	✕	✕	✕	✕
Child-bearing potential	N/A	✔	N/A	N/A
Advice given and note recorded on contraception & pregnancy	N/A	✕	N/A	N/A
Advice given and note recorded on driving regulations	✔	✔	✕	✕
Action 1	diary given	advice re C & P	diary given	diary given
2		treatment options	rationalize present AEDs	?further specialist review
3		advice re withdrawal of AEDs	PHT level	advice re driving
4			specialist review	treatment options
5			seizure description	seizure description

APPENDIX 2 MANAGEMENT RECORD CARD

Name: d.o.b. ID

Epilepsy/seizure details

Age at onset ______________

Seizure type(s) (e.g. tonic-clonic, absence) ______________

Epilepsy syndrome (if known, e.g. JME) ______________

Cause of epilepsy ______________

Precipitating factors ______________

Any pattern ______________

Witnessed account obtained? (if yes, from whom?) ______________

Has the patient experienced non-epileptic seizures? ______________

Complications of epilepsy (e.g. cognitive decline, status) ______________

Other conditions/long-term medication ______________

____

Investigations	Date	Place	Result
EEG			
CT			
MRI			
Video telemetry			
Other			

If seizures controlled, date of last seizure ______________

Previous antiepileptic medication

Drug name	Date stopped	Max dose	Reason stopped

Has the patient had any of the following:	Yes	No
Assessment for surgery?	☐	☐
Psychological treatment?	☐	☐
Psychiatric treatment?	☐	☐

Consultants involved in care ______________

Acetazolamide/Diamox (AZM), carbamazepine/Tegretol (CBZ), clobazam/Frisium (CLB), clonazepam/Rivotril (CLZ), ethosuxamide/Zarontin (ESM), gabapentin/Neurontin (GBP), lamotrigine/Lamictal (LTG), levitoracetam/Keppra (LEV), oxcarbazepine/Trileptal (OCBZ), phenobarbitone (PB), phenytoin/Epanutin (PHT), primidone/Mysoline (PRM), sodium valproate/Epilim (VPA), tiagabine/Gabatril (TGB) topiramate/Topamax (TPM), vigabatrin/Sabril (VGB)

APPENDIX 3 PATIENT INFORMATION

Name ______________________ d.o.b. ______________ ID ______________

Diagnosis made (date) ______________ by (name) ______________

Basic information	Yes	N/A	Initials	Date
Has the patient/carer been:				
informed of diagnosis?	☐		____	____
told what epilepsy is?	☐		____	____
told what the seizures are like, their name and syndrome?	☐		____	____
given a basic information booklet?	☐		____	____
given first aid information?	☐		____	____
given information on legal restrictions for driving?	☐		____	____
Medication				
Has the patient been told:				
the purpose of medication?	☐	☐	____	____
the importance of compliance?	☐	☐	____	____
about possible side-effects?	☐	☐	____	____
about drug interactions, e.g. with the oral contraceptive pill?	☐	☐	____	____
that medication is free of charge on the NHS?	☐	☐	____	____
Does the patient/carer know what to do if:				
a dose is missed?	☐	☐	____	____
vomiting occurs?	☐	☐	____	____
a trip abroad is planned?	☐	☐	____	____
Lifestyle				
Has guidance been given on:				
leading an active and independent life? (avoiding overprotection)	☐		____	____
moderate alcohol intake?	☐		____	____
regular and sufficient sleep?	☐		____	____
safety in the home (e.g. fires, bathing, stairs, cooking)?	☐		____	____
safety/risk for sport (e.g. swimming, cycling, riding)?	☐		____	____
implications for social and sexual relationships?	☐		____	____
informing schools, employers, insurance companies, etc?	☐		____	____
SUDEP?	☐		____	____
Parenthood				
Has advice been given on:				
fertility, pregnancy and parenthood?	☐	☐	____	____
the importance of pregnancy planning?	☐	☐	____	____
medication during pregnancy?	☐	☐	____	____
Ongoing dialogue				
Has the patient/carer been:				
encouraged to return with questions?	☐		____	____
encouraged to keep a record of seizures?	☐		____	____
encouraged to report changes in seizure pattern to GP?	☐		____	____
given a contact card?	☐		____	____
Further help				
Is the patient/carer aware of where to get additional support/information?	☐		____	____

APPENDIX 4 MANAGEMENT OF SEIZURES

MANAGEMENT OF PARTIAL SEIZURE

The management of minor seizure activity may require differing action depending on the behaviour being exhibited.

- With abrupt falls, ensure the person has not sustained any injury.

If prolonged confusion is apparent:

- protect from obvious danger, for example wandering into traffic
- a light touch should be used to guide the individual
- dissuade other people from crowding around
- speak gently to the person in reassuring tones
- stay with the individual until they are able to resume normal activities
- convulsive episodes may occur at the end of a minor attack so be aware of this possibility.

MANAGEMENT OF CLONIC-TONIC SEIZURE

Do

- Stay calm, check time, note length of seizure
- Make the person comfortable lying down, gently assist to floor if sitting
- Place item of clothing or cushion to protect the head if you can
- Loosen tight clothing
- Remove nearby objects which may cause injury, including glasses if worn
- Minimize the number of people crowding around
- Once movements have stopped, if possible, place person on their side in recovery position
- Check airway is clear
- Allow person to regain consciousness in their own time – this may take some time
- Provide privacy and offer assistance if the person has been incontinent
- Stay with the person until fully recovered or until they can be escorted home
- They may require time to resume normal activities after a period of quiet rest or sleep

Do not

- Put anything into the person's mouth or attempt to force teeth apart
- Attempt to constrain convulsive movements
- Give any food or fluids until fully conscious
- Move the person unless in a dangerous position

Chapter 11

Heart disease in primary care

Susan H Simpson

CHAPTER CONTENTS

INTRODUCTION

This chapter addresses the issues of prevention and treatment of heart disease in primary care. As the population ages, heart disease becomes more prevalent and as treatment becomes more effective, more people are living longer with heart disease. It is therefore essential that people receive advice and interventions for the primary prevention of heart disease and if they have already developed symptoms, secondary prevention strategies should include treatment with drugs proven to reduce mortality and morbidity.

Therapies for heart disease have developed considerably in the last 10 years, yet many patients do not receive the evidence-based treatments which have been shown to maintain and improve quality of life. These include not only drug treatment but also health education and support to modify risk factors and comply with prescribed therapies. Coronary heart disease is the main focus for such strategies but people with chronic conditions such as heart failure, atrial fibrillation and congenital heart disease should also benefit from the expertise of the primary care team.

CORONARY HEART DISEASE

The incidence of coronary heart disease (CHD) in the UK remains high in spite of a fall of 5.2% in deaths from heart disease and stroke in 2000. The latest figures show circulatory disease, including stroke, to be the cause of death in 33% of men and 20% of women under 65 years of age (DoH 2001a). For this reason, the government has identified prevention of CHD as a priority and the *Saving lives* document (DoH 1999a) sets a target of reducing the death rate from heart disease and stroke amongst those under 75 by at least two-fifths by 2010, saving up to 200 000 lives.

The National Service Framework (NSF) for CHD (DoH 2000) presents a comprehensive strategy for the prevention and treatment of CHD. It acknowledges the wide inequalities in health that exist in the UK, as the reduction in death rates from CHD has been mainly amongst the more affluent in society: the less well off have benefited very little. Through the NSF, healthcare professionals in both primary and secondary care are charged with developing robust protocols and efficient service delivery models to address the prevention and treatment of heart disease in the UK.

PATHOPHYSIOLOGY OF CORONARY ARTERY DISEASE

The two main coronary arteries form the first branches off the aorta just above the aortic valve. These arteries provide the blood supply to the myocardium. The coronary arteries are a unique arterial system as, after branching, the arteries join together again forming a crown around the heart; hence the term 'coronary', like a coronet. This acts as a 'back-up' system, for if one artery becomes narrowed or blocked, it is possible for the part of the artery distal to this blockage to fill in a retrograde fashion (backwards) (Marieb 2001).

Atherosclerosis affects coronary as well as other arteries in the body causing them to become narrowed. This process takes place over many years but evidence of this disease process has been noted in people as young as 20 (Bhattacharyya & Libby 1997). Yellow fatty streaks appear in the lining of the arteries, especially in areas where they branch. These fatty streaks comprise white blood cells which have migrated into the vessel wall and ingested low-density lipoproteins (LDL), forming what are known as 'foam cells' which are present in the fatty streaks. These foam cells secrete substances that attract smooth muscle cells to migrate into the lining of the artery, forming the fibrous plaque that, as it grows, slowly narrows the artery.

It is unusual for symptoms to develop unless the diameter of the coronary artery has been narrowed by at least 70%, as at this point the oxygen supply to the myocardial cells is significantly reduced. This occurs particularly during exercise, exertion or during emotional upset, for as the heart rate increases in response to these stressors, the oxygen demand of the heart also increases. When the myocardial cells' demand for oxygen outstrips their supply, they become ischaemic, which is manifest by the onset of central chest pain, radiating down the left arm and into the jaw – the classic sign of angina pectoris.

People who develop symptoms of angina at rest or who are woken with chest pain are suffering from unstable angina and require urgent hospitalization for investigation and treatment, as these symptoms are often a precursor to a myocardial infarction (MI). In this instance, the fibrous plaque may have partially occluded a significant part of a coronary artery, for example the main stem of the left coronary artery, or an atherosclerotic lesion is complicated by vasoconstriction, reducing the oxygen supply further (Sabatine et al 1997).

Within the core of the fibrous plaque are various factors which promote the formation of thrombotic lesions. These factors are normally separated from the blood by a fibrous cap that forms over the lesion. However, these caps can rupture, causing the blood to clot on the site of the fibrous plaque, leading to an acute thrombosis. This completely blocks the artery, leading to MI, which is when an area of myocardium is starved of its blood supply, and can lead to sudden death. Should the patient survive the initial event, without intervention this area of muscle will be replaced by fibrous tissue, which adversely affects the function of the heart and can lead to heart failure. The use of fibrinolytic agents, recombinant tissue plasminogen activator (rTPA) or streptokinase, given within 6 hours of the onset of chest pain aims to break down the thrombosis and restore a blood supply to the damaged myocardium, minimizing long-term damage (DoH 2000). It is important that people with diagnosed CHD should be informed that they need to get to a hospital emergency department should they experience chest pain that is not relieved by rest, three nitroglycerin tablets or sprays within 15 minutes of onset.

> Primary care teams contacted by a patient with the symptoms of a suspected myocardial infarction should call for an ambulance *before* attending to the patient in person.

If thrombolysis is administered as soon as possible after the onset of pain, it is more effective in revascularizing the myocardium. For this reason the NSF

(DoH 2000) sets a standard to be achieved by April 2003, that patients presenting at hospital with an MI should receive thrombolysis within 20 minutes of arrival.

CHD RISK FACTORS

It is well known that fat plays an important part in the process by which coronary artery disease develops. However, it should not be assumed that all fat in the diet is bad, for some actually helps to protect against atherosclerosis. Fat is transported around the body in water-soluble complexes called lipoproteins. LDL is the main means of transporting cholesterol, whereas high-density lipoproteins (HDLs) are involved in the transport of cholesterol *away* from the cells to the liver. There is a direct relationship between the level of cholesterol in the blood (and LDL) and the risk of developing CHD. However, high levels of HDL (present in olive oil) protect against developing CHD (RCP 2000).

Genetics play a big part in the way an individual's metabolism deals with fat. There are huge differences in the prevalence of CHD according to ethnic origin, which cannot be explained by diet and lifestyle alone. People from South Asia, particularly Bangladesh, have a 50% higher risk of heart disease than the overall average for the UK and those from West Africa and the Caribbean have 50% less (Wild & McKeigue 1997).

Although our genes play a part in the risk of developing CHD, adopting a healthy lifestyle can greatly reduce this. Even those with a genetic abnormality known as hypercholesterolaemia, in which blood cholesterol levels are very high, can lower their risk of an early MI by adopting a low-fat diet, increasing the amount of exercise they take and not smoking.

As well as ethnic differences, there are also stark differences in the incidence of CHD between geographical areas in the UK and social classes. People living in the north of England have a much higher incidence than those in the south, with death rates from CHD in Salford for those under 65 being three times those of people living in the London Borough of Kingston and Richmond (DoH 2000). Men under 65 in social class V (unskilled) have almost twice the mortality rate from CHD of the national average and have 2.5 times the risk of dying of a man in social class I (professional) (BHF 1999). The NSF Standard One states: 'The NHS and partner agencies should develop, implement and monitor policies that reduce the prevalence of coronary risk factors in the population, and reduce inequalities in risks of developing heart disease' (DoH 2000).

The known risk factors for CHD have largely been discovered through a longitudinal research study that commenced in 1948, which studied the health of the population of Framingham, Massachusetts. Some of the major milestones in the study are listed below (HLBI 2001).

- **1960** Cigarette smoking found to increase the risk of heart disease
- **1961** Cholesterol level, blood pressure and electrocardiogram abnormalities found to increase the risk of heart disease
- **1967** Physical activity found to reduce the risk of heart disease and obesity to increase the risk of heart disease
- **1970** High blood pressure found to increase the risk of stroke
- **1976** Menopause found to increase the risk of heart disease
- **1978** Psychosocial factors found to affect heart disease
- **1988** High levels of HDL cholesterol found to reduce risk of death

In addition to the factors identified above, the risk of people with diabetes developing CHD is 2–5 times that of non-diabetics (DoH 2000).

Smoking, diet, high serum cholesterol and lack of exercise are of course modifiable CHD risk factors yet the *Saving lives* document (DoH 1999a) identifies poverty, unemployment, bad housing and social isolation as major determinants of health and illness. When giving healthy living advice, it is essential to take into account how these four factors will affect an individual or family's ability to respond and act upon information given.

Stress is commonly believed to be a contributing factor in the development of CHD and hypertension, yet it is notoriously difficult to quantify. However, research known as the Whitehall Study has attempted, through a longitudinal study of civil servants, to look at the link between stress and ill health, particularly cardiovascular disease. Although civil servants are far from the poorest in society, it was discovered that those in the higher grades lived longer than people in lower grades, with known risk factors accounting for only one third of the difference in mortality rates (Van Rossum et al 2000). The Whitehall II Study has demonstrated a link between CHD and stress at work, particularly related to having low control over your work and how it is organized. If this is compounded with poor support networks through friends and family, this increases risk further (UCL 2001). Therefore although it is commonly believed that those in high-powered careers are more likely to succumb to CHD, as can be seen, it is in fact those with lower status jobs, and incomes, who are most at risk.

As psychosocial factors play a large part in an individual's susceptibility to heart disease, the DoH (1999b) has identified the most vulnerable in society as 'those without social networks, the socially excluded, the economically disadvantaged, and some minority ethnic groups' (p.8). These people are least likely to access services and care, so the document charges 'Nurses, midwives and health visitors ... to adapt their practice to reach and target these groups to make services and care more accessible' (p.8).

PRIMARY PREVENTION OF CHD

Nurses can help prevent CHD by targeting individuals at different times in their lifespan, commencing with advice during pregnancy and to young mothers to promote healthy living in future generations. However, for lifestyle advice to be successful it is essential that an individualized approach to health promotion is taken. Four stages to this have been identified (Schofield 1997).

1. Eliciting the patient's views, beliefs and readiness to change.
2. Explaining the nature of and reasons for the advice.
3. Negotiating and agreeing goals.
4. Supporting the patient to achieve and maintain change.

Smoking cessation

Smoking by the population as a whole has declined markedly since it became widely accepted in the mid-1970s that it was a major cause of lung cancer. However, there are variations according to social class. In 1996 only 10% of men and women in social class I smoked, in contrast to 45% of men and 38% of women in social class V. The most worrying trend was that between 1994 and 1996 the number of women who smoked actually increased and again, this was most noticeable among women from lower social classes. Amongst secondary school pupils more girls than boys are regular smokers (BHF 1999).

Since the Framingham study it has been known that smoking doubles the risk of developing CHD and recently it has been discovered that some people are more susceptible to the effect of smoking than others. If a smoker has the apolipoprotein E4 gene, his risk of developing CHD is quadrupled (Humphries et al 2001). But no matter how long someone has smoked, within 4 years of quitting, their risk of developing CHD has returned to almost the same as someone who has never smoked; therefore every effort should be made to encourage patients to access support to enable them to quit. The NSF Standard Two states: 'The NHS and partner agencies should contribute to a reduction in the prevalence of smoking in the local population'.

It has been identified that risk of CHD can be directly related to events that occur even before birth (DoH 2000). The exact mechanism of this is not understood but low birthweight babies tend to have higher rates of CHD later in life than those with an average or above average birthweight. Low birthweight is associated with maternal deprivation and smoking during pregnancy, so nurses and midwives need to ensure that women are aided to give up smoking ideally before embarking on a planned pregnancy, or to quit as soon as possible. Currently 24% of women smoke during pregnancy and the aim is to reduce this number to 18% by 2005 (DoH 1999a). Nicotine replacement therapy for pregnant women is a priority; women can be referred to the smoking cessation service and a special national telephone service to help pregnant women to quit smoking has been set up (DoH 2001b).

A priority for action is to prevent children and young adults taking up smoking (DoH 1999a). The banning of tobacco advertising is intended to lower the profile of cigarette smoking, but peer pressure still plays a large part in a child's decision to smoke. A strategy to maintain a group of 10–15 year olds as non-smokers has proved successful (except in girls aged 14–15), whereby information about smoking was sent under the signature of their general practitioners (Fidler & Lambert 2001). Brief motivational interventions have recently been shown to be effective and can be carried out as part of any consultation. In this, young people are helped to examine their beliefs about their behaviour; they are then given individual feedback reinforcing any self-motivational statements made (Lowe 2000).

Nurses should use opportunistic visits by patients to address the issue of smoking and nicotine replacement therapy should be offered to all smokers unless there is a medical contraindication (DoH 2000).

Dietary advice

Being overweight puts an extra strain on the heart and increases the risk of developing high blood pressure. If people are clinically obese, this adversely affects all aspects of their health, including increasing their risk of CHD. Although the population may appear to be more diet conscious than ever, the number of people whose body mass index is in excess of 30 (the clinically obese) has continued to rise. Between 1987 and 1997 the number of men in this category increased from 6% to 17% and the number of women from 12% to 19% (BHF 1999).

Adopting a healthy diet can aid weight loss and also reduce serum cholesterol levels, which should be below 5 mmol/l. However, over a quarter of men and women in the UK have levels in excess of this (BHF 1999). For every reduction of 1% in the serum cholesterol level, the risk of CHD falls by 2%. Alcohol consumption also needs to be addressed as this can increase triglyceride levels, which potentiates the adverse effects of raised cholesterol levels, although drinking in moderation, be it wine or beer, has been shown to reduce the risk of CHD. People who are teetotal have as high a risk of heart disease as those who drink in excess of the maximum recommended 28 units for men and 21 for women (Rimm 1999).

The main principles of healthy eating are as follows (NHS Direct 2001).

- Eat a variety of foods, including one portion of fish (preferably oily) per week.
- Eat plenty of foods rich in starch and fibre (rice, pasta and potatoes) and at least five portions of fruit and vegetables each day.
- Don't eat too much fat and generally avoid fried food. Choose lean cuts of red meat, or chicken. Avoid animal fats for cooking; if possible, use olive oil (high in HDLs). Choose dairy foods which have a lower fat content, e.g. semi-skimmed milk, Edam cheese, low-fat spreads.
- Don't eat sugary foods too often.

Good nutrition is vital, but problematic for people on low incomes and those who live in areas of social deprivation (DoH 2000). Nurses offering advice should take into account the availability of foods in the local economy and practical advice is needed to enable people to turn health education messages into practice.

The diet of children and young people is a cause for concern, as it tends to contain too much sugar, salt and fat, and this can lead to problems in the future with obesity, diabetes and hypertension as well as CHD. Education of parents regarding a suitable diet for young children should be included in child health clinics and guidelines have been set for nutritional standards of school meals. The National Curriculum also includes the teaching of the principles of nutrition and food preparation to young people (DoH 1999a).

It is suggested that focusing efforts on prevention of weight gain is more efficient and effective than attempting to help an individual lose weight. The main periods of life when weight is more likely to be gained in men are between the ages of 35 and 40 and after marriage and in women, between the ages of 15 and 19, during pregnancy and the menopause. The socially deprived and those from an Afro-Caribbean or South Asian background are also more likely to put on weight (DoH 2000). For those people who would benefit from weight loss, referral to a support group is helpful. It is difficult to lose weight by diet alone and a programme of exercise should also be included (NHS Direct 2001).

Exercise

Levels of exercise amongst adults in Britain is low, with only 37% of men and 25% of women undertaking the recommended activity level of 30 minutes brisk walking, cycling or dancing for 5 or more days per week. It is recommended that children participate in moderate intensity exercise for one hour a day; however, in England only 55% of boys and 39% of girls aged under 15 take such exercise daily. The number of girls undertaking regular exercise declines rapidly after the age of 8 with only one in five girls aged 15 undertaking the recommended level of exercise (BHF 2000).

The benefits of regular exercise include the prevention or delay in the development of high blood pressure, weight reduction or maintenance and improvement in mental health, and it halves the risk of developing CHD (DoH 2001c).

Children especially should be encouraged to undertake regular exercise. Although motivation to exercise tends to be high amongst young people, many see costs as prohibitive and they feel they have no time due to demands of homework

(Mulvilhill et al 2000). The National Curriculum provides for only 1.5 hours of exercise per week, so it is essential that children are encouraged to join in out-of-school sport or dance activities; even walking or cycling to school could provide adequate levels of exercise (DoH 1999a). The government, through its transport policies, is encouraging local authorities to ensure safe routes for walking and cycling, thereby reducing the incidence of children being driven to school (DTLR 1998).

Encouraging adults to undertake regular exercise has been shown to be most effective if the activity can be carried out as part of daily life and when assessing lifestyle, nurses can make practical suggestions as to how this could be achieved (Hillsdon & Thorogood 1996). Liaison between primary healthcare staff and leisure service personnel is to be encouraged and the development of referral systems that ensure assessments and exercise programmes are delivered by appropriately trained individuals is paramount. For this reason the Exercise Referral Systems quality assurance framework has been developed (DoH 2001c).

Hypertension

The effective management of hypertension is essential to reduce cardiovascular disease, including stroke. As few patients have any symptoms of high blood pressure, routine screening should be offered to all patients a minimum of every 5 years (DoH 2000).

Blood pressure should be measured in the sitting position after the patient has rested for 5 minutes, with the arm at heart level and cuff adjusted for arm circumference. A device with validated accuracy that is properly maintained and calibrated should be used. Blood pressure should be taken twice each visit, recorded to the nearest 2 mmHg, with diastolic pressure recorded as the disappearance of the sounds (phase V). Blood pressure is considered to be raised if it is above 140/85 (BHS 2000), the assessment of which is shown in Table 11.1.

All people with hypertension should be examined and undergo some routine investigations to discover if there is a specific cause, e.g. renal disease, or if they have developed complications, e.g. left ventricular hypertrophy (BHS 2000). Investigations include:

- urine strip test for blood and protein
- serum electrolytes and creatinine
- plasma glucose
- serum total: HDL cholesterol ratio
- 12-lead ECG.

Table 11.1 Assessment of hypertension

BP measurement	Remarks
Diastolic BP >110 mmHg	Repeat weekly over 3 weeks. If sustained, treat
Systolic BP >160 mmHg and/or diastolic BP >100 mmHg	Lifestyle advice, assessment of other risk factors, repeat monthly for 3 months, and if sustained, treat
Systolic BP 140–159 mmHg and/or diastolic BP 85–99 mmHg	Lifestyle advice, assessment of other risk factors, repeat 2 monthly for 6 months. Treat depending upon risk score

If any of these investigations is abnormal it is appropriate for the patient to be referred for specialist advice. However, the majority of patients (90%) have essential hypertension, which is not related to any specific underlying disease, the risk factors being similar to those for the development of CHD. Therefore non-drug treatment involves similar lifestyle advice as should be given to any other patient: stop smoking, reduce alcohol consumption, dietary interventions and take regular exercise.

Various trials have shown no important differences in efficacy and patient acceptability between the main drugs used for antihypertensive therapy. These include thiazide diuretics, alpha-blockers, calcium antagonists, ACE inhibitors and beta-blockers. However, differences have been noted related to age and ethnic group. Elderly people and those from Afro-Caribbean and South Asian ethnic groups do not respond well to ACE inhibitors or beta-blockers when used alone and require additional drug(s) to be added (BHS 2000).

Recommendations for commencing antihypertensive therapy are as follows (BHS 2000).

- Start with lowest recommended dose of a drug.
- If *partially effective but well tolerated* increase dose (except thiazide diuretics).
- If *ineffective or partially effective* change drug or add a drug with a complementary action (see Table 11.2). If not well tolerated, change drug to another class.
- Allow an interval of at least 4 weeks to observe the full response, unless it is necessary to lower blood pressure more urgently.
- More than one drug will be required to achieve optimal BP control in most patients.

Table 11.2 Logical drug combinations (BHS 2000)

	Diuretic	Beta-blocker	Calcium channel blocker	ACE inhibitor	Alpha-blocker
Diuretic	–	✓	–	✓	✓
Beta-blocker	✓	–	✓*	–	✓
Calcium channel blocker	–	✓*	–	✓	✓
ACE inhibitor	✓	–	✓	–	✓
Alpha-blocker	✓	✓	✓	✓	–

* Verapamil + beta-blocker = absolute contraindication

As most patients with hypertension have no symptoms, compliance with drug therapy can be a problem. It is therefore essential that patients are informed of the risks of untreated or inadequately treated high blood pressure. Nurse-led hypertension clinics in primary care can provide the time for effective patient education to take place, which leads to an increase in well-controlled hypertension (Bandolier 2001).

QUANTIFYING RISK OF CHD

The NSF states clearly that one of the highest priorities in healthcare should be identifying and treating people who are at the greatest risk of developing CHD. Standard Four states:

> *General practitioners and primary healthcare teams should identify all people at significant risk of cardiovascular disease but who have not yet developed symptoms and offer them appropriate advice and treatment to reduce their risks.*

Significant risk is quantified as the chance of a cardiac event being greater than 30% over 10 years (DoH 2000).

Most patient records held in primary care do not contain adequate information to quantify coronary risk and therefore these data need to be collected systematically (McManus et al 2000). The NSF states that in order to achieve this all patients over the age of 16 should have the following information in their GP records and these should be updated 5 yearly:

- personal history of serious illness
- family history of premature CHD, i.e. father/brother before 55, mother/sister before 65
- family history of diabetes, hyperlipidaemia, hypertension, stroke or cancers
- smoking habit
- blood pressure
- height and weight (with BMI calculated)
- alcohol intake
- level of physical activity.

Recording of basic data will give some idea of coronary risk but to define an individual's specific susceptibility to CHD, a coronary risk assessment tool should be used. The Coronary Risk Assessment is available as a chart and as a computer program (BHS 2000) and other risk assessments approved by the NSF include the third edition of the Sheffield Risk Table (Wallis et al 2000), the European Risk Chart (Second Joint Task Force 1998) and the New Zealand Table (Anderson et al 1991). A recent programme has been developed to calculate risk of death from CHD that compares an individual's results with an average of people of the same age and sex (Pocock et al 2001).

In order to calculate risk, additional information regarding serum cholesterol and diabetes/plasma glucose levels is required. It is not necessary to fast patients prior to routine cholesterol testing. However, should the blood lipid levels be found to be raised, subsequent testing should be fasting (see Table 11.3).

Those with familial hyperlipidaemia should be referred for specialist advice (DoH 2000). It is estimated that the prevalence of this is 1 in 500 of the population and only one-quarter are diagnosed early in life. The remainder tend to be diagnosed in middle age, by which time significant cardiovascular disease has developed, and the risk of a coronary event by the age of 60 is 50% in men and 30% in women (Neil et al 2000).

Table 11.3 Blood lipid assessment

Cholesterol measurement	Remarks
Total cholesterol <5 mmol/l	Reassure and repeat in 5 years
Total cholesterol 5–7.9 mmol/l	If diagnosed with cardiovascular disease, repeat in 1 month, and if raised, treat. Without cardiovascular disease, give dietary advice and repeat in 3 months. Decision to treat based on cardiovascular risk score
Total cholesterol >8 mmol/l	Repeat in 1 month and if still raised, treat

NB: Repeat measurements should be fasting

Table 11.4 Statins

	Dose	Maximum (for use in hypercholesterolaemia)
Atorvastatin	10 mg once daily	80 mg once daily
Cerivastatin	100 μg once daily	100 μg
Fluvastatin	20–40 mg at night	40 mg twice daily
Pravastatin	10 mg at night	40 mg at night
Simvastatin	20 mg at night	80 mg at night

INTERVENTIONS FOR PEOPLE AT RISK OF CHD

Following assessment of the patient, an appropriate level of advice and treatment can be planned. For patients with a risk higher than 30% the following interventions should be standard.

- Advice about how to stop smoking, including advice on the use of nicotine replacement therapy.
- Information about modifiable risk factors and personalized advice about how they can be reduced.
- Advice and treatment to maintain blood pressure below 140/85.
- Prescribe statins to lower serum cholesterol to either 5 mmol/l or by 30% (whichever is greater).
- Meticulous control of blood pressure and blood glucose in people with diabetes.

Dietary advice can reduce serum cholesterol by 5% but most patients with high cholesterol levels will require treatment with statins (see Table 11.4). They work to reduce serum cholesterol by inhibiting the synthesis of cholesterol by the liver. They reduce the total cholesterol by 20% and have been demonstrated to reduce the risk of death due to CHD by 28% (Shepherd et al 1995).

ORGANIZATION OF CHD PRIMARY AND SECONDARY PREVENTION IN PRIMARY CARE

The NSF suggests three main methods of delivering systematic care for the prevention of CHD (DoH 2000).

1. Routine consultation, but this must be structured by the use of a specific protocol.
2. Nurse-led specialized 'practice cardiac prevention clinics' in general practice.
3. Nurse-led 'multipractice or PCT cardiac prevention clinics' where patients at high risk of cardiac events from more than one practice are invited.

Standard Three of the NSF states that 'General practitioners and primary care teams should identify all people with established cardiovascular disease and offer them comprehensive advice and appropriate treatment to reduce their risks'. It is suggested that these patients with preexisting CHD should also be managed in the cardiac prevention clinics where they will be offered, in addition to the interventions listed above, appropriate drug therapy including aspirin, beta-blockers and ACE inhibitors. It has been demonstrated that patients managed in this way are more likely to be prescribed appropriate drug therapy, less likely to be admitted to hospital and have an improved quality of life and functional status. However, the impact on reducing the risk of recurrent cardiac events remains uncertain at present (McAlister et al 2001).

First, patients with established cardiovascular disease need to be identified from practice records. Searching for patients prescribed nitrates can identify up to 70% of patients with angina. There should also be opportunistic identification using routine consultations and letters from hospital outpatient departments, as well as hospital discharge summaries. In addition, a search can be carried out through practice databases for the Read codes shown in Table 11.5.

Once a register of patients with preexisting CHD has been established this will need to be extended to those whose risk of CHD events over the next 10 years is greater than 30%.

Table 11.5 Read codes for cardiovascular disease

Condition	Read 4-byte set	Read 5-byte set
CHD	G4	G3
Angina pectoris	G44	G33
Acute MI	G41	G31
Heart failure	G6A	G58
Atrial fibrillation	G67	G573
Stroke	G75	G66
Peripheral vascular disease	G81	G70

STABLE ANGINA

The development of angina pectoris pain is a common occurrence in the UK with up to 20 000 people each year developing this for the first time (BHF 2000). Standard Eight of the NSF states that 'People with symptoms of angina or suspected angina should receive appropriate investigation and treatment to relieve their pain and reduce their risk of coronary events'.

People with suspected angina should be considered for hospital referral for investigation and treatment. Rapid-access chest pain clinics have been established in many hospitals and provide a 'one-stop shop' for assessment of patients (Jain et al 1997). Patients should be seen within 2 weeks of referral (DoH 2000), and a diagnosis made if necessary by means of an exercise stress test. Should this be positive, the patient will be stratified into high or low risk. High-risk patients will be investigated further and may be offered revascularization. Low-risk patients should be offered treatment to relieve symptoms, including sublingual nitrates and usually beta-blockers and/or calcium antagonists. These patients can then be reviewed regularly in primary care and offered lifestyle advice, treatment to maintain blood pressure below 140/85 mmHg and statins to lower cholesterol. Low-dose aspirin (75 mg daily) is an essential part of management of patients with stable angina and is as effective in preventing vascular events as higher doses (Antithrombotic Triallists' Collaboration 2002).

CARDIAC REHABILITATION

Coronary heart disease causes considerable psychological morbidity in people even when their actual physical limitations are few. Many patients with CHD, even after revascularization, are afraid to take any exercise, including sexual activity, in case it damages their heart. These anxieties are understandable and so it is essential that patients are offered support, supervision and education designed to help them with lifestyle modification and exercise training. This not only improves their psychological well-being but reduces their risk of dying over 3 years by 20–25% (O'Connor et al 1989).

Cardiac rehabilitation is defined by the World Health Organization (WHO 1993) as:

> *... the sum of activities required to influence favourably the underlying cause of the disease, as well as the best possible, physical, mental and social conditions, so that they (people) may, by their own efforts, preserve, or resume when lost, as normal a place as possible in the community. Rehabilitation cannot be regarded as an isolated form or stage of therapy but must be integrated within secondary prevention services of which it forms one facet.*

The following categories of people with CHD have been shown to benefit from cardiac rehabilitation (DoH 2000).

- Following acute MI
- Before and after revascularization (CABG and angioplasty)
- Stable angina
- Heart failure (not NYHA Class 4 – see Box 11.2)

Box 11.1 Stages of cardiac rehabilitation

Phase One:	Prehospital discharge
Phase Two:	Early postdischarge period (up to 6 weeks)
Phase Three:	Four to six weeks after acute cardiac event
Phase Four:	Long-term maintenance of changed behaviour

Primary care teams should encourage such patients to access local programmes, as uptake varies from 15% to 59%, and participation is affected by such practical issues as transport and accessibility (Pell et al 1996).

Phase One of cardiac rehabilitation should begin before discharge from hospital following an acute cardiac event or revascularization procedure. It should involve the patient's family and include education on lifestyle modifications, employment, sexual activity and medication. A written individual plan should be given to each patient documenting how individual needs can be met, including information about local cardiac support groups and rehabilitation programmes (DoH 2000).

It is during the early postdischarge phase that patients require support from their primary care team. Families find this a particularly stressful time, as the impact of their loved one's cardiac event becomes more apparent. Patients and their partners often use 'protective buffering' in which they do not discuss their fears in order to protect each other from worry (Stewart et al 2000) and play down the significance of their heart condition (Thompson et al 1995). Patients and their family often feel vulnerable and afraid and have concerns which they did not consider prior to discharge; they may feel they have not received adequate support from healthcare professionals (Stewart et al 2000). The lifestyle modification advice given in hospital must now be implemented and they often require practical advice to do so. The nurse in primary care is in a position to assist the family to make the necessary emotional and practical adjustments to their lives after the cardiac event. Encouragement should also be given to people to attend formal Phase Three rehabilitation programmes, particular emphasis being given to those least likely to want to participate, including women, the elderly and those from minority ethnic groups (DoH 2000).

During Phase Three, support is offered by the multidisciplinary rehabilitation team which should include people experienced in:

- provision of advice about exercise and exercise supervision, and who can modify exercise appropriately to the individual
- lifestyle modification
- psychological interventions
- advanced life support.

On completion of the exercise programme, primary care teams should be provided with details of the patient's progress, so they are enabled to take over their care in Phase Four and ensure follow-up in the cardiac prevention clinic.

HEART FAILURE

Heart failure is a clinical syndrome caused by a reduction in the heart's ability to pump blood around the body. Most cases of heart failure in the UK are due to CHD and about a third are due to hypertensive heart disease (DoH 2000).

The symptoms of heart failure include:

- oedema in the feet, ankles and legs and if the patient's mobility is restricted, this can also manifest in the sacral area and genitalia. Ascites can cause abdominal swelling
- shortness of breath due to pulmonary oedema which restricts activity and may wake patients at night as they are unable to lie flat. They may also have a persistent (unproductive) cough
- poor appetite and nausea which can result from abdominal distension and venous congestion
- fatigue which is a common complaint and can be due to a lack of sleep, breathlessness, poor appetite and muscle weakness due to poor perfusion.

Heart failure can be of varying severity from Class 1, causing little effect to the individual, to Class 4 in which patients are very disabled by their shortness of breath (Box 11.2).

Box 11.2 NYHA classification of heart failure

1 Ordinary physical activity does not cause undue dyspnoea or fatigue
2 Slight limitation of physical activity, comfortable at rest, but ordinary activity results in fatigue or dyspnoea
3 Marked limitation of physical activity, comfortable at rest but less than ordinary activity results in symptoms
4 Unable to carry out any physical activity without discomfort, symptoms present even at rest

Heart failure causes a significant economic burden on the NHS. It was estimated in 1991 that £337 m was spent on care and treatment (1.2% of total health costs) of which 63% was attributable to hospitalization (Hobbs et al 2000). Although the death rates from ischaemic heart disease are falling in the UK, the incidence of and mortality from heart failure are increasing due to an ageing population and increased survival following MI (Kannal et al 1994). Overall prevalence is 3–20 per 1000 population, although in those over 75 years of age this rises to 100 in 1000 (10%) (Davis et al 2000). Every general practitioner will have at least 20 patients affected by heart failure (Hobbs et al 2000).

Heart failure accounts for 5% of all medical admissions to hospital; readmission rates are the highest for any common condition (estimated at 50% over 3 months) and survival rates are worse than those for breast or prostate cancer (DoH 2000).

There is evidence that optimal diagnosis, treatment and ongoing support of patients with heart failure can reduce morbidity and mortality (DoH 2000). However, many people with heart failure are not adequately treated and there is evidence that some people who have been diagnosed on the basis of clinical signs do not have heart failure (Wheeldon et al 1998). Although signs and symptoms are important in diagnosis, more objective tests based on assessed cardiac function, chest X-ray, ECG and echocardiography should be used (European Society of Cardiology 2001).

A marker which could be used for diagnosis of heart failure in primary care is brain natriuretic peptide (BNP). In response to stretch, the atria release a hormone, atrial natriuretic peptide (ANP), and the ventricles BNP. The level of these hormones increases in the presence of heart failure where there is an increase in volume and pressure inside the heart (Jackson et al 2000). Increased BNP levels have been found to have a prognostic as well as diagnostic value (Koglin et al 2001) with those patients with high levels at greatest risk of serious cardiovascular events.

The NSF states that primary care teams and hospitals should work together to put in place models of care so that they use a systematic approach to:

- identify people at high risk of heart failure (e.g. people who have had an MI or who have high blood pressure)
- assess and investigate people with suspected heart failure
- provide and document the delivery of appropriate advice and treatment
- offer regular review to people with established heart failure.

TREATMENT OF HEART FAILURE

The standard treatment for heart failure is with ACE inhibitors and diuretics and recently the use of beta-blockers has been recommended (when commenced under controlled conditions). However, it is recognized throughout Europe that the underprescribing and underdosing of ACE inhibitors and beta-blockers in heart failure is a continuing problem, contributing to the morbidity and mortality of this patient group (European Society of Cardiology 2001). Therefore concise practical recommendations are needed to ensure patients benefit from these proven therapies (McMurray et al 2001a). It is now considered appropriate for ACE inhibitor therapy for patients with heart failure to be commenced in primary care if they can be closely monitored (Fig. 11.1). However, initiation of beta-blockade and its subsequent up-titration should only be undertaken in a specialist environment and patients with NYHA class 4 should only have beta-blockade commenced following recommendation by a consultant cardiologist.

Drug therapy for heart failure

ACE inhibitors There is powerful evidence from clinical trials supporting their use as first-line therapy in all patients with reduced LV systolic function, i.e. ejection fraction of less than 40–45%. These drugs can increase survival, reduce hospital admissions and improve NYHA class and quality of life. These should be up-titrated to the dosages shown to be effective in large controlled trials. The benefit is greatest in those patients with the worst heart failure.

Diuretics Diuretics are essential for symptomatic treatment when fluid overload is present and should always be administered in combination with ACE inhibitors if possible. Mild heart failure can be treated with a thiazide diuretic but loop diuretics are usually necessary. Potassium-sparing diuretics should only be used if hypokalaemia persists despite ACE inhibitor therapy. In advanced heart failure (NYHA Class 3–4) spironolactone is recommended in low dose (25 mg daily), with regular checks on blood chemistry as this can cause hyperkalaemia.

Beta-blockers Recommended for all patients with stable heart failure on standard treatment of diuretics and ACE inhibitors. Initial doses should be small, up-titration slow and adapted to individual response. Although beta-blockers were once thought to be contraindicated in patients with heart failure, several randomized controlled trials have shown conclusively that they increase survival, reduce hospital admissions and improve NYHA class and quality of life when added to standard therapy of diuretics, digoxin and ACE inhibitors.

Digoxin Does not reduce mortality but can be useful in reducing persistent heart failure symptoms despite standard treatment with diuretics and ACE inhibitors. Digoxin is indicated in atrial fibrillation.

Specialist nurse-led heart failure clinics have been shown to substantially reduce readmission rates in the UK (Blue et al 2001). Up-titration of drug therapy

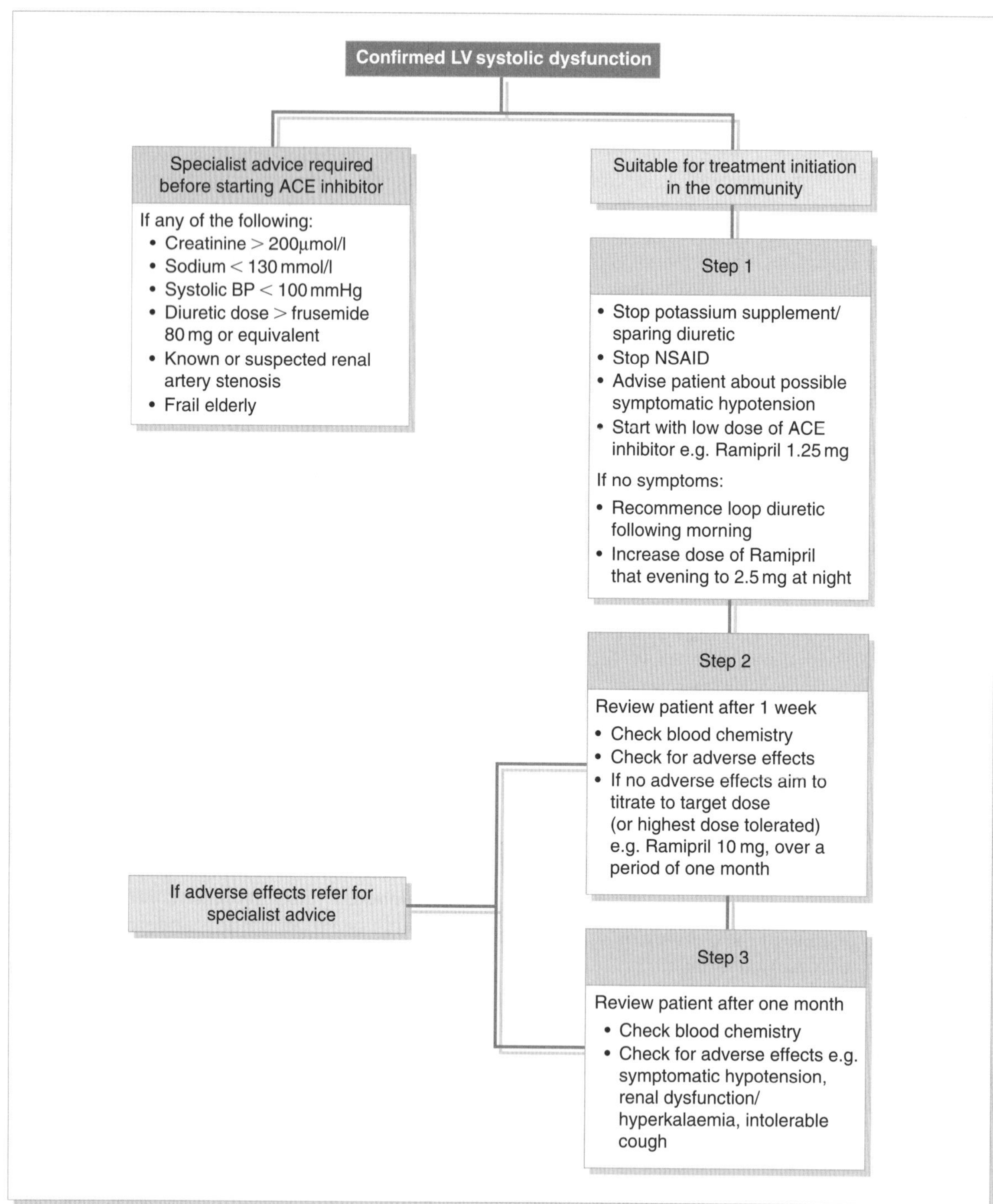

Figure 11.1 Primary care algorithm for the use of an ACE inhibitor in heart failure (adapted from SIGN 1999).

can be undertaken in these clinics but just as important is the emphasis placed upon encouraging patient compliance by education about their medication, as non-compliance is a major cause of readmission as well as increased morbidity and mortality (Evangelista & Dracup 2000). In particular, strategies to encourage maximum patient participation in self-monitoring their condition should be implemented.

PATIENT EDUCATION IN HEART FAILURE

Daily weight

Patients should be encouraged to weigh themselves at the same time every day and record this in a patient diary or 'passport'. Explanations should be given that this is to monitor their fluid status and any increase of 1 kg (2–3 lb) in 24 hours, sustained over 2–3 days, could indicate fluid retention. In such circumstances advice should be sought from their GP or nurse, especially if this is associated with increasing shortness of breath, persistent cough and increased swelling of the ankles. Some patients may be suitable for managing their own diuretic therapy in relationship to their weight or to restrict their fluid intake to 1500 ml/24 hours.

Diet

Advice should be given about healthy eating and strategies to reduce salt intake should be discussed, as salt retention by the kidneys can exacerbate heart failure (Jackson et al 2000). Patients should be encouraged not to add extra salt once their food is cooked and to try to avoid processed foods which often have a high salt content. Patients who are obese should be encouraged to lose weight as this reduces the workload of the heart. This can be difficult in those people who have a low exercise tolerance and specialist advice should be sought from a dietitian. In severe heart failure cachexia is common, due to a feeling of nausea or abdominal fullness caused by ascites. Small, frequent meals should be encouraged together with nutritional supplements to increase calorie intake.

Alcohol

A high intake of alcohol can be a cause of heart failure (alcoholic cardiomyopathy) and in these circumstances patients should be encouraged to stop completely. However, all patients with heart failure should be encouraged to keep at or below the recommended 28 units per week for men and 21 for women.

Smoking

Support to stop smoking should be offered. Patients should be advised to have an annual immunization against influenza and against pneumococcal infection every 10 years, to help reduce the risk of chest infections exacerbating their heart failure.

Non-prescription medicines

Advice should be given about over-the-counter medicines, especially the hazards of taking NSAIDs which are best avoided in heart failure. Patients should always be asked if they are taking any herbal or alternative remedies as some of these can interact with prescribed drug treatment or are contraindicated in heart failure. Ephedra (*ma huang*), a Chinese herbal remedy which contains ephedrine, and ginseng are felt by most herbal authorities to be agents to avoid for people with high blood pressure and cardiovascular diseases (Heartpoint 1998).

Exercise

Patients with heart failure frequently complain of fatigue. They should ensure they get adequate rest but the benefits of regular exercise and keeping up with as many of their usual activities as possible should be emphasized. Exercise training programmes for people with heart failure have been shown to improve quality of life as well as increasing functional status (Coats 1993).

Depression

As in many other chronic illnesses, depression is a feature. Symptoms that patients with heart failure experience can be frightening and they may be unable to continue with their employment or other activities they enjoy. Although there is no conclusive evidence that psychological interventions reduce readmission rates for people with heart failure, it is highly likely that the support offered by nurse-led heart failure services achieves a reduction in hospitalizations partly through this mechanism.

PALLIATIVE CARE

For many years people with malignant disease have been supported at the end of life by palliative care teams. Symptoms experienced in end-stage heart failure are similar to those with lung cancer, including breathlessness, pain and fatigue. Therefore in severe heart failure, the benefits of palliative care should be considered for symptom relief and family support (DoH 2000). Although much can now be done to improve the quality of life of patients with heart failure, none of these effect a cure and as patients reach the end of their life they require opportunities to make choices about the care they would like to receive, including resuscitation.

ATRIAL FIBRILLATION

Atrial fibrillation (AF) is a common arrhythmia found in 0.5% of the population aged 50–59, increasing rapidly with age to 8.8% of those over 80 (English & Channer 1999). In the majority of people with AF, it is associated with CHD, heart failure, valvular disease or hypertension but many patients (up to 20%) have otherwise normal hearts.

On developing AF some patients complain of palpitations, tiredness, fatigue or dizziness but many may not notice any definitive symptoms. Hence it is essential that patients at risk of AF should have a pulse check at routine consultations. An irregularly irregular pulse on palpation should be followed up by 12-lead electrocardiography to confirm the diagnosis. On the ECG, AF is shown by the 'replacement of P waves by rapid oscillations of fibrillatory waves that vary in size, shape and timing' (ACC/AHA/ESC 2001). The rate of the ventricular response varies, but it is always irregular.

Once diagnosed, additional tests such as chest X-ray, echocardiogram and blood tests for thyroid function (thyrotoxicosis can cause AF) can aid decisions on how best to treat (ACC/AHA/ESC 2001).

AF is not a benign arrhythmia; it reduces the cardiac output by up to 30%, therefore it can worsen or even cause heart failure. However, its most serious effect is the lack of effective contraction of the atria, which can lead to clot formation in the left atrium, leading to thromboembolism and stroke.

DEFINITIONS OF AF

Some people have paroxysmal or self-terminating AF, which is defined as lasting less than 7 days. However, if they have had two or more such episodes it is termed recurrent (Fig. 11.2) (ACC/AHA/ECS 2001).

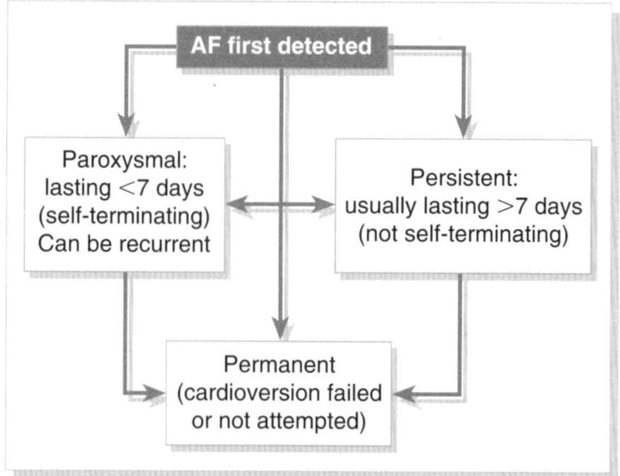

Figure 11.2 Definitions of atrial fibrillation (adapted from ACC/AHA/ESC 2001).

TREATMENT

It may be considered that the treatment of AF is straightforward, yet until recently there existed little consensus as to the best way to treat an arrhythmia which is responsible for causing one in six strokes (ACC/AHA/ESC 2001). There is now an agreed management plan which addresses both persistent and paroxysmal AF (Fig. 11.3).

In persistent AF, ideally an attempt should be made to restore normal sinus rhythm and if it is known that duration of AF has been less than 2 days, electrical DC cardioversion can be attempted immediately. Realistically, in primary care, few patients will come into this category, the time of onset of AF being unknown in the majority of cases. Therefore before electrical cardioversion is attempted anticoagulation with warfarin must be commenced to reduce the risk of stroke, the INR needing to be between 2 and 3 for at least 3 weeks prior to the procedure (Prystowsky 2000). Cardioversion is successful in restoring sinus rhythm in up to 90% of patients but most (70–90%) revert to AF within a year, unless treated with an antiarrhythmic drug (RCPE 1998).

In patients who are not considered suitable for cardioversion or in whom it is unsuccessful, anticoagulation should be commenced (or continued), as it reduces the risk of stroke by 65% (Albers 1994). A rapid heart rate also increases the risk of stroke in AF, so heart rate control is essential. If the patient has heart failure, digoxin is the drug of choice but otherwise a beta-blocker is more effective at controlling rate during exercise and if this is not tolerated (or is contraindicated) a calcium channel blocker such as verapamil can be used (RCPE 1998).

There is much controversy regarding long-term anticoagulation in AF. However, patients at high risk of ischaemic stroke should receive warfarin treatment, unless it is contraindicated (RCPE 1998). High risk factors include:

- previous stroke or transient ischaemic attack
- older than 75 years of age
- hypertension
- diabetes
- coronary artery disease
- heart failure.

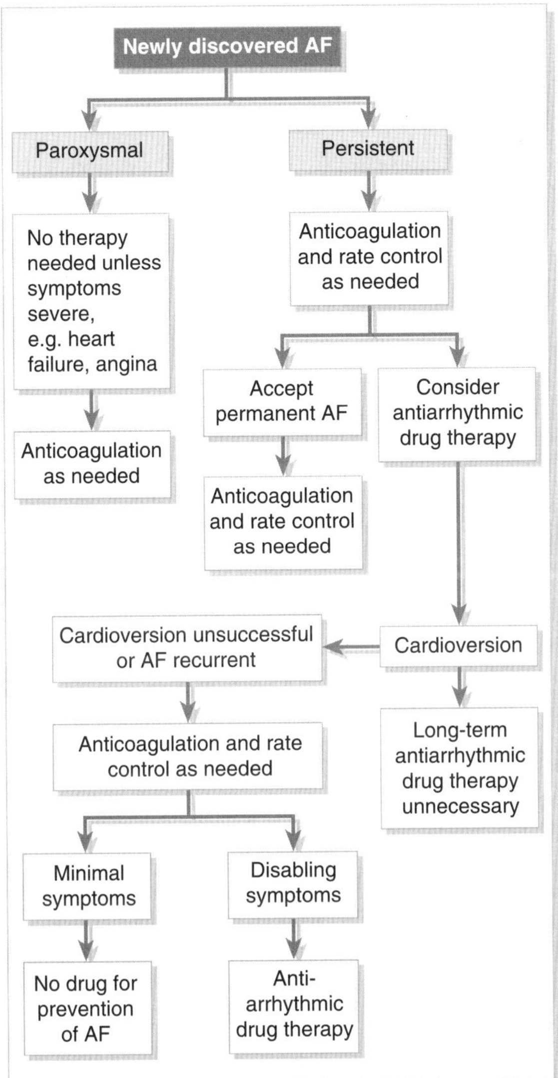

Figure 11.3 Recommended treatment and management of atrial fibrillation (adapted from ACC/AHA/ESC 2001).

Many patients are elderly and at risk of falls, so the decision to anticoagulate is not without risk, even if they have no absolute medical contraindications. Also some patients are unwilling to commence warfarin treatment due to the inconvenience of requiring regular blood tests and the risk of haemorrhage. Studies have shown that fewer than a fifth of patients with AF who are eligible for anticoagulation receive warfarin therapy (Wheeldon et al 1998). Yet it has been shown that patients are more concerned about stroke and less about haemorrhage than their doctors and if they were offered warfarin, would accept the increased risk of bleeding (Devereaux et al 2001, Protheroe et al 2000). It is therefore essential that patients are given clear information and actively involved in the decision to anticoagulate or not. The alternative to warfarin is antiplatelet therapy, but the efficacy of aspirin in preventing stroke in AF is debatable, particularly in those over 75 (Albers 1994), with some suggesting it decreases risk by only 20% against warfarin's 65% (RCPE 1998).

Therefore in order to decrease the serious consequences of AF, routine pulse checks should be undertaken, diagnosis confirmed by ECG and the patient actively involved in treatment decisions, by well-informed healthcare professionals.

CONGENITAL HEART DISEASE

The incidence of congenital heart disease has been estimated at 8–10 per 1000 live births (Moodie 1994). In the early post-war years, 60–70% of children born with congenital heart disease died in infancy or childhood (Somerville 1997a) but due to modern surgical techniques it is estimated that 85% now survive to reach their 16th birthday (Hunter 2000). In the UK these adults with congenital heart disease are known by the acronym GUCH (grown-up congenital heart) and make up a 'new' patient group.

The term 'congenital heart disease' covers a huge variety of lesions, from 'simple' holes in the heart, atrial and ventricular septal defects (ASD and VSD) to very complex conditions involving abnormal connections, absent (atresia) or malformed heart valves and absent (atresia) or malformed major vessels. However, all but the simplest conditions, which can achieve true surgical correction in childhood, will require further interventions later in life. These may include reoperations or treatment for arrhythmias that are common in patients who have had surgery affecting their atria. For this reason it is essential that adults with congenital heart disease receive appropriate lifelong follow-up care (Somerville 1997a).

Children with congenital heart disease receive care in one of 13 paediatric cardiac centres in the UK (BPCA 1999) but difficulties arise when the child becomes an adolescent and adult as there are few specialized GUCH centres. Until recently many adults had their care continued by paediatricians but child health settings are not ideal for adults and there is evidence that the psychological needs of these patients will not be met (Webb et al 1996). Even where a specialized GUCH centre is accessible, the process of transition from child to adult healthcare settings can be fraught with difficulties, which leads to an estimate of less than half of the patients with congenital heart disease successfully transferring, the remainder being lost to optimal follow-up (Reid et al 2001).

The rarity of congenital heart disease in primary care leads to a lack of understanding of the various conditions and can cause inappropriate decisions to be made about the venue for an individual's future care and management (Somerville 1997b). Therefore guidelines have been produced which stratify congenital heart disease into great complexity, moderate severity and simple (Warnes & Liberthson 2001). This enables healthcare professionals to quickly see what level of care an individual requires (Box 11.3).

Box 11.3 Stratification of management required by adults with CHD (Warnes & Liberthson 2001)

Adult patients with CHD of great complexity – should be seen regularly at a specialist GUCH centre
Conduits, valved or not valved
Cyanotic congenital heart disease (all forms)
Double outlet ventricle
Eisenmenger syndrome
Fontan procedure
Mitral atresia
Single ventricle (also called double inlet or outlet, or common)
Pulmonary atresia (all forms)
Pulmonary vascular obstructive disease
Transposition of the great arteries
Tricuspid atresia
Truncus arteriosus

Adult patients with simple CHD – can usually be cared for in the general medical community
Native disease:
- isolated congenital aortic valve disease
- isolated congenital mitral valve disease
- isolated patent foramen ovale of small ASD
- isolated small VSD (with no associated lesions)
- mild pulmonary stenosis

Repaired conditions:
- ligated ductus arteriosus
- repaired secundum ASD without residua
- repaired VSD without residua

Adult patients with CHD of moderate severity – should be seen periodically in a specialist GUCH centre
Aorto-left ventricular fistulae
Anomalous pulmonary venous drainage
Atrioventricular septal defects (AVSD or AV canal)
Coarctation of the aorta
Ebstein's anomaly
Right ventricular outflow tract obstruction of significance
Ostium primum ASD
Patent ductus arteriosus (not closed)
Pulmonary valve regurgitation (moderate to severe)
Pulmonary valve stenosis (moderate to severe)
Sinus of Valsalva fistula/aneurysm
Sinus venosus ASD
Subvalvular or supravalvular aortic stenosis
Tetralogy of Fallot
VSD with:
- absent valve or valves
- aortic regurgitation
- coarctation of the aorta
- mitral valve disease
- right ventricular outflow tract obstruction
- straddling tricuspid/mitral valve
- subaortic stenosis

It may be assumed that adolescents and adults with congenital heart disease, having been under the care of cardiologists all their life, would be well informed about their condition. Yet it appears this is far from the case, with one study showing that 77% of children aged between 7 and 18 could not even name their condition (Veldtman et al 2000). This lack of knowledge can lead individuals to believe they are 'cured' and hence become very resentful, and shocked, when further treatment is needed (Warnes 1995). Therefore it should not be assumed that adults with congenital heart disease are aware of their need for lifelong follow-up or that they are well versed in the effects their condition could have on adult life. These include reproductive issues for women, particularly getting appropriate contraceptive advice and whether they are likely to be able to carry a child to term, and at what risk to themselves (Horner et al 2000).

Health education is as important as in any young adult but should also include strategies to reduce the risk of endocarditis, by ensuring antibiotic prophylaxis is taken prior to dental treatment and also before undergoing tattooing or body piercing (Cetta et al 1999). The risks inherent in using illegal drugs must also be addressed, as even so-called 'recreational drugs' such as ecstasy can cause an increase in heart rate (Ghuran et al 2001) and could trigger serious arrhythmias. Practical help should also be given with the difficulties they may face in gaining insurance and hence a mortgage (Celermeyer 1994). They may also experience difficulty in getting into the workforce, as ill-informed prospective employers fear they will have a high level of sick leave or need time off for hospital appointments (McMurray et al 2001b).

Adults with congenital heart disease will not be seen commonly in primary care, but their numbers are growing and it is essential that the successful surgery they underwent as children is not seen by patients or their primary care team as a once and for all 'cure' and that they receive appropriate lifelong care.

CONCLUSION

Primary care remains the first point of contact with the health service for the majority of people with cardiac symptoms and in the past patients with heart disease have received a varying quality of care in the UK. The NSF has set minimum standards that must be achieved to ensure all patients receive evidence-based care for the prevention and treatment of heart disease. This together with clinical guidelines can ensure that the primary care team refers patients appropriately for specialist advice, but also that they are enabled to offer effective interventions to their patients who do not require secondary care. It is clear that nurses have a very large part to play in the prevention and treatment of heart disease.

References

ACC/AHA/ESC (American College of Cardiology/American Heart Association/European Society For Cardiology) 2001 Guidelines for the management of patients with atrial fibrillation. European Heart Journal 22:1852–1923

Albers G 1994 Atrial fibrillation and stroke. Three new studies, three remaining questions. Archives of Internal Medicine 154:1443–1457

Anderson KM, Wilson PWF, Odell PM, Kannal WB 1991 An updated coronary risk profile. Circulation 83(1):356–362. medicine21.com/heartGP/

Antithrombotic Triallists' Collaboration 2002 Collaborative meta-analysis of randomised trials of antiplatelet therapy for prevention of death, myocardial infarction, and stroke in high risk patients. British Medical Journal 324:71–86

Bandolier 2001 Building on success with a nurse-led hypertension clinic at Bewdley Medical Centre. Bandolier Jan: 11–13. www.jr2.ox.ac.uk/bandolier/ImpAct/imp11/i11-3.html

Bhattacharyya G, Libby P 1997 Atherosclerosis. In: Lilly LS (ed) Pathophysiology of heart disease, 2nd edn. Lippincott, London

BHF 1999 Statistics database. British Heart Foundation, London

BHF 2000 CHD statistics: key facts. British Heart Foundation, London. www.dphpc.ox.ac.uk/bhfhprg/stats/2000/keyfacts/index.html

BHS 2000 Guidelines for the management of hypertension. British Hypertension Society, London. www.hyp.ac.uk/bhs/gl2000.htm

Blue L, Lang E, McMurray J et al 2001 Randomised controlled trial of specialist nurse intervention in heart failure. British Medical Journal 323:715–718

BPCA (British Paediatric Cardiac Association) 1999 Current and potential impact of fetal diagnosis on prevalence and spectrum of serious congenital heart disease at term in the UK. Lancet 354:1242–1247

Celermeyer DS 1994 Employment, insurance and driving. In: Redington A, Shore D, Oldershaw P (eds) Congenital heart disease in adults. A practical guide. WB Saunders, London

Cetta F, Graham LC, Lichtenberg RC, Warnes C 1999 Piercing and tattooing in patients with congenital heart disease: patient and physician perspectives. Journal of Adolescent Health 24(3):160–162

Coats AJS 1993 Exercise rehabilitation in chronic heart failure. Journal of the American College of Cardiology 22:172A–177A

Davis RC, Hobbs FDR, Lip GYH 2000 History and epidemiology of heart failure. British Medical Journal 320:39–40

Devereaux PJ, Anderson DR, Gardner MJ et al 2001 Differences between perspectives of physicians and patients on anticoagulation in patients with atrial fibrillation: observational study. British Medical Journal 323:1218

DLTR 1998 A new deal for transport. Department of Transport, Local Government and Regions, London

DoH 1999a Saving lives: our healthier nation. Department of Health, London. www.official-documents.co.uk/document/cm43/4386/4386.htm

DoH 1999b Making a difference. Department of Health, London. www.doh.gov.uk/nurstrat.htm

DoH 2000 National Service Framework for Coronary Heart Disease. Department of Health, London. www.doh.gov.uk/nsf/coronary.htm#chdnsf

DoH 2001a NHS performance indicators: a consultation. Department of Health, London. www.doh.gov.uk/piconsultation/6011paf.htm

DoH 2001b Smoking: don't give up giving up. Department of Health, London. www.givingupsmoking.co.uk/

DoH 2001c Exercise referral systems: a national quality assurance framework. Department of Health, London. www.doh.gov.uk/exercisereferrals/exercisereferral.pdf

English KM Channer KS 1999 Managing atrial fibrillation in elderly people. British Medical Journal 318:1088–1089

European Society of Cardiology 2001 Guidelines for the diagnosis and treatment of chronic heart failure. European Heart Journal 22:1527–1560

Evangelista LS, Dracup K 2000 A closer look at compliance research in heart failure patients in the last decade. Progress in Cardiovascular Nursing 15(3):97–101

Fidler W, Lambert TW 2001 A prescription for health: a primary care based intervention to maintain the non-smoking status of young people. Tobacco Control 10:23–26

Ghuran A, Van Der Wieken LR, Nolan J 2001 Cardiovascular complications of recreational drugs. British Medical Journal 323:464–466

Heartpoint 1998 Specific herbal remedies. www.heartpoint.com/herbtell.html

Hillsdon M, Thorogood M 1996 A systematic review of exercise promotion strategies. British Journal of Sports Medicine 30:84–89

HLBI 2001 Framingham heart study. Heart, Lung and Blood Institute, Washington. rover.nhlbi.nih.gov/about/framingham/

Hobbs FDR, Davis RC, Lip GYH 2000 Heart failure in general practice. British Medical Journal 320:626

Horner T, Liberthson R, Jellinek MS 2000 Psychosocial profile of adults with complex congenital heart disease. Mayo Clinic Proceedings 75(1):31–36

Humphries SE, Talmud PJ, Hawe E et al 2001 Apolipoprotein E4 and coronary heart disease in middle-aged men who smoke: a prospective study. Lancet 358:115–119

Hunter S 2000 Congenital heart disease in adolescence. Journal of the Royal College of Physicians 34(2):150–152

Jackson G, Gibbs CR, Davis MK, Lip GYH 2000 Pathophysiology of heart failure. British Medical Journal 320:167–171.

Jain D, Fluck D, Sayer JW et al 1997 One-stop chest pain clinic can identify high cardiac risk. Journal of the Royal College of Physicians 31:401–404

Kannal WB, Ho K, Thom T 1994 Changing epidemiological features of cardiac failure. British Heart Journal 72 (suppl):S3–9

Koglin J, Pehlivanli S, Schwaiblmair M et al 2001 Role of brain natriuretic peptide in risk stratification of patients with congestive heart failure. Journal of the American College of Cardiology 38(7):1934–1941

Lowe G 2000 Getting the message across to young drinkers and smokers: brief motivational interventions may help. Health Education 101(1):38–39

Marieb EN 2001 Human anatomy and physiology, 5th edn. Benjamin Cummings, London

McAlister FA, Lawson FME, Teo KK, Armstrong PW 2001 Randomised trials of secondary prevention programmes in coronary heart disease: systematic review. British Medical Journal 323:957–962

McManus RJ, Meulendijks CFM, Salter RA, Pattison HM, Roalfe AK, Hobbs FDR 2000 Comparison of estimates and calculations of risk of coronary heart disease by doctors and nurses using different calculation tools in general practice: cross sectional study. British Medical Journal 324:459–464

McMurray J, Cohen-Solal A, Dietz R et al 2001a Practical recommendations for the use of ACE inhibitors, beta-blockers and spironolactone in heart failure: putting guidelines into practice. European Journal of Heart Failure 3:495–502

McMurray R, Kendall L, Parsons JM et al 2001b A life less ordinary: growing up and coping with congenital heart disease. Coronary Health Care 5:51–57

Moodie DS 1994 Adult congenital heart disease. Current Opinion in Cardiology 9:137–142

Mulvilhill C, Rivers K, Aggleton P 2000 Views of young people towards physical activity: determinants and barriers to involvement. Health Education 100(5):190–199

Neil HAW, Hammond T, Huxley R et al 2000 Extent of underdiagnosis of familial hypercholesterolaemia in routine practice: prospective registry study. British Medical Journal 321:148

NHS Direct 2001 Healthy living. www.nhsdirect.nhs.uk/healthy_living/index.jhtml

O'Connor GT, Buring GE, Yusuf S et al 1989 An overview of randomised trials of rehabilitation with exercise after myocardial infarction. Circulation 80:234–244

Pell J, Morrison C, Blatchford O, Pell A, Dargie H 1996 Retrospective study of influence of deprivation on uptake of cardiac rehabilitation. British Medical Journal 313:267–268

Pocock SJ, McCormack V, Gueyffier F et al 2001 A score for prediction risk of death from cardiovascular disease in adults with raised blood pressure, based on individual patient data from randomised controlled trials. British Medical Journal 323:75–81 www.riskscore.org.uk

Protheroe J, Fahey T, Montgomery AA, Peters TJ 2000 The impact of patients' preferences on the treatment of atrial fibrillation: observational study of patient based decision analysis. British Medical Journal 320:1380–1384

Prystowsky EN 2000 Cardioversion of atrial fibrillation to sinus rhythm: who, when, how and why? American Journal of Cardiology 86:326–327

RCP 2000 International consensus statement on dietary fat, the Mediterranean diet and lifelong good health. Royal College of Physicians, London. europa.eu.int/comm/agriculture/prom/olive/medinfo/uk_ie/consensus/index.htm

RCPE 1998 Consensus conference on atrial fibrillation in hospital and general practice. Royal College of Physicians of Edinburgh, Edinburgh. www.rcpe.ac.uk

Reid GJ, Irvine MJ, McCrindle BW et al 2001 Transition from pediatric to adult health care among a cohort of young adults with congenital heart defects. Poster at 3rd World Congress of Pediatric Cardiology and Cardiac Surgery, 27–29 May. www.pccs2001.com

Rimm EB 1999 Moderate alcohol intake and lower risk of coronary heart disease: meta-analysis of effects on lipids and haemostatic factors. British Medical Journal 319:1523–1528

Sabatine MC, O'Gara PT, Lilly LS 1997 Ischaemic heart disease In: Lilly LS (ed) Pathophysiology of heart disease, 2nd edn. Lippincott, London

Schofield T 1997 Individual interventions and behaviour change. In: Lawrence M et al (eds) Prevention of cardiovascular disease: an evidence-based approach. Oxford University Press, Oxford

Second Joint Task Force of European and other societies 1998 Prevention of coronary heart disease in clinical practice. European Heart Journal 19:1434–1503

Shepherd J, Cobbe SM, Ford I et al 1995 West of Scotland Coronary Prevention Study Group. Prevention of coronary heart disease with pravastatin in men with hypercholesterolaemia. New England Journal of Medicine 333:1301–1307

SIGN (Scottish Intercollegiate Guidelines Network) Secretariat 1999 Diagnosis and treatment of heart failure due to left ventricular systolic dysfunction. Royal College of Physicians of Edinburgh, Edinburgh

Somerville J 1997a Management of adult congenital heart disease. Annual Review of Medicine 48:283–293

Somerville J 1997b Near misses and disasters in the treatment of grown-up congenital heart patients. Journal of the Royal Society of Medicine 90:124–127

Stewart M, Davidson K, Meade D, Hirth A, Makrides L 2000 Myocardial infarction: survivors' and spouses' stress, coping and support. Journal of Advanced Nursing 31(6):1351–1360

Thompson DR, Ersser SJ, Webster RA 1995 The experiences of patients and their partners 1 month after a heart attack. Journal of Advanced Nursing 22(4):707–714

UCL 2001 Whitehall II Study. The Stress and Health Study. University College London. www.ucl.ac.uk/epidemiology/white/white.html

Van Rossum CT, Shipley MJ, Van de Mheen H et al 2000 Employment grade differences in cause specific mortality. A 25 year follow up of civil servants from the first Whitehall study. Journal of Epidemiology and Community Health 54(3):178–184

Veldtman GR, Matley SL, Kendall L et al 2000 Illness understanding in children and adolescents with heart disease. Heart 84:395–397

Wallis EJ, Ramsay LE, Ul Haq I et al 2000 Coronary and cardiovascular risk estimation for primary prevention: validation of a new Sheffield table in the 1995 Scottish health survey population. British Medical Journal 320:671–676

Warnes C 1995 Establishing an adult congenital heart disease clinic. American Journal of Cardiac Imaging 9(1):11–14

Warnes C, Liberthson R 2001 Task Force 1: the changing profile of congenital heart disease in adult life. Journal of the American College of Cardiology 37(5):1170–1175

Webb GD, Harrison DA, Connelly MS 1996 Challenges posed by the adult patient with congenital heart disease. Advances in Internal Medicine 41:437–495

Wheeldon NM, Tayler DI, Anagnotou E, Cook D, Wales C, Oakley GDG 1998 Screening for atrial fibrillation in primary care. Heart 79:50–55

WHO 1993 Needs and action priorities in cardiac rehabilitation and secondary prevention in patients with CHD. WHO Regional Office for Europe, Geneva

Wild S, McKeigue J 1997 Cross-sectional analysis of mortality by country of birth in England and Wales, 1970–92. British Medical Journal 314:705

Resources

British Heart Foundation: www.bhf.org.uk/

Clinical Governance Research and Development Unit: www.le.ac.uk/cgrdu/

European Olive Oil Medical Information Library: europa.eu.int/comm/agriculture/prom/olive/medinfo/uk_ie/index.htm

Grown Up Congenital Heart Patients Association: www.guch.demon.co.uk/

Healthnet fact sheets: www.healthnet.org.uk/new/facts/index.htm

Heart of General Practice. Resources for the management of cardiovascular disease in general practice: medicine21.com/heartGP/

Heart Health Promotion website: www.shef.ac.uk/uni/projects/mshhp/

NHS pregnancy smoking helpline: 0800 169 9 169

Weight Watchers UK: www3.weightwatchers.com/International/uk/

Further reading

Health Education Authority 1999 Helping smokers stop: a new Approach for health professionals. HEA, London

NHS Centre for Reviews and Dissemination 1998 Cardiac rehabilitation. Effective Health Care 4(4):1–11

North of England Evidence Based Guideline Development Project 1999 The primary care management of stable angina. Centre for Health Service Research, Newcastle upon Tyne. www.ncl.ac.uk/chsr/publicn/guide/angina.pdf

Chapter 12

Depression in primary care

Jane Elwood

CHAPTER CONTENTS

INTRODUCTION

The National Service Framework for Mental Health Standard 2 states:

> *Any service user who contacts their primary healthcare team with a common mental health problem should:*
>
> - *have their mental health needs identified and assessed*
> - *be offered effective treatments, including referral to specialist services for further assessment, treatment and care if they require it.* (DoH 1999)

In order to achieve these standards a team approach is essential.

Depression and anxiety are the most common mental illness seen in general practice, with one in five people affected by depression at any one time. This makes it one of the most common conditions seen in primary care. Over 90% of those people with mental health problems are cared for in primary care alone with less than 10% requiring referral on to secondary care.

Depression affects all ages, both genders and those from all backgrounds, yet there remains a reticence in some areas to develop a practice team approach to care for this large cohort of patients. Highlighting awareness, improving recognition and having the ability and skills to open this 'can of worms' can reduce distress and dysfunction and improve the general outcome of patients in our care.

WHAT IS DEPRESSION?

It is important to distinguish between the symptom of feeling unhappy and the diagnosis of depression.

We all have times when we feel unhappy or depressed or, in other words, have a lowering of mood for varying lengths of time. It is not until this symptom is joined by others and continues that a diagnosis of depression may be considered.

Diagnostic features of depression include (WHO 2000):

- low or sad mood
- loss of interest and pleasure

plus at least four of the following symptoms:

- disturbed sleep*
- disturbed appetite*
- guilt or low self-worth*
- pessimism or hopelessness about the future
- decreased libido
- diurnal mood variation
- poor concentration*
- suicidal thoughts or acts*
- loss of self-confidence
- fatigue or loss of energy*
- agitation or slowing of movement or speech.*

Symptoms of anxiety or nervousness are also frequently present.

If the two main symptoms mentioned above plus four marked with an asterisk have been present most of the time for a minimum of 2 weeks this would signify a diagnosis of moderate to major depression requiring medication.

Depression is often described as a continuum (think of a ruler starting at nought and going through to 12) ranging from normal low mood continuing through mild, moderate to severe. Suicidal thinking is common and can occur at any stage of this continuum and should be assessed and reassessed whenever patients are seen.

Explain to patients that as the depression worsens and the symptoms become more severe levels of the neurotransmitters serotonin and noradrenaline decrease. These neurotransmitters are responsible for regulating mood and an imbalance may need to be rectified by the use of antidepressants in order to lift that mood. Relating this imbalance to other similar physical conditions such as diabetes or hypothyroidism sometimes helps to put it in perspective for some patients and normalizes it. Some may find it easier to accept a diagnosis of depression if they can identify a physical cause.

Ask patients to indicate where they feel they are on the continuum right now (use an actual ruler for this). Not yesterday or last week or last month but right now. This suggests the patient's perception of how bad things are for him rather than you making assumptions on the information he has given you.

AWARENESS

Posters and leaflets are available from health promotion units and voluntary groups such as Depression Alliance, Mind, Sane and many others. Displaying these in the waiting room or organizing awareness campaigns within the practice, on Mental Health Day for example, helps to normalize and destigmatize the diagnosis while raising the profile of mental health in the community generally.

Training receptionists to recognize when patients may be uncomfortable and feeling vulnerable at the reception desk is a useful exercise. This is where the 'first consultation' takes place within the practice. Patients may have made and cancelled this appointment several times before eventually attending the practice (or even be noted as a regular non-attender) so one offhand comment from a member of the team may discourage any further consultation.

At most new patient medical appointments, questions are asked about family history or personal history of chronic illness such as asthma, diabetes, glaucoma and coronary heart disease. This is an ideal opportunity to ask about previous, personal or family history of depression. Patients register with a new practice for a variety of reasons. The elderly may have been bereaved or be moving closer to their family, the breadwinner may have been made redundant or be starting a new job, a young mother may have left behind friends and family who used to provide support and simply moving into a new house can be stressful. Recognizing a health professional who is empathetic and prepared to listen may encourage patients to disclose how they feel.

The new patient medical also provides an opportunity to discuss medication, encourage compliance and reduce the possibility of patients stopping too early without being monitored. The possibility of relapse into a further episode of depression is increased if medication is not continued for a minimum of 6 months *after* the patient feels better.

RECOGNITION OF DEPRESSION

Unrecognized, untreated depression can lead to distress, dysfunction and ultimately death through an increased risk of suicide, so there is no excuse for believing this is an area of specialized nursing. All members of the surgery team see these patients on a regular basis and there is no option but to become involved whether we want to or not.

It has often been stated that primary care is not very effective at identifying patients with depression, but recent research has shown that in fact clinicians are successful at recognizing more severe depression and the majority of cases missed were suffering from a milder form of depression.

The way in which patients present is not straightforward. Depressed patients often present at the surgery with physical symptoms. The most common ones include headache, gastrointestinal upset and low back pain. These symptoms do need investigating but where no physical cause is found an emotional cause should be considered. This said, there are certainly ways in which we can improve our recognition skills.

Creating a safe environment where patients feel comfortable to talk without fear of being overheard may give them the freedom and confidence within a consultation to discuss their emotional state and explore the cause. Patients will often actively seek out a nurse within the practice with whom they have built up a relationship to discuss their problems. How often do we hear the following remarks? 'I've come to see you because I don't want to waste the doctor's time' or 'I know I can talk to you without feeling silly.' Practice nurses hold a very privileged position in the eyes of their patients.

The following techniques will improve our consultation skills, leading to better recognition.

- Asking questions with a psychological content early in the consultation.
- Making eye contact.
- Not appearing hurried; this may make people feel there is no time available to discuss their concerns.
- Looking for non-verbal clues.
- Fewer interruptions, allowing an easy flow to develop.
- Encouraging remarks and gestures but *never* saying 'I know how you feel'. You don't.
- Reflecting back to patients what they have said so they can clarify if you have got it wrong.
- Using a combination of open and closed questions.

Patients seen frequently in chronic disease management clinics are at additional risk of depression and practice nurses are in an ideal position to identify any problems. Asking more general questions initially such as:

- How are things since I last saw you?
- What have you been up to recently?
- How's life treating you these days?

may help patients recognize you are interested in them as a person first rather than a 'diabetic' or an 'asthmatic'. If normal good control of their physical condition is no longer being maintained for no easily identifiable reason, explore more deeply and ask questions around emotional and mental well-being.

ASSESSMENT

As with any patient attending general practice, accurate history taking and detailed assessment are crucial to diagnosis, treatment and management. Nurses asking these questions around mental health issues for the first time often feel uncomfortable, not quite sure how to approach it. In fact, the questions are very straightforward and should be asked in exactly the same manner as for any other medical assessment.

Some of the topics explored and the questions asked are very similar to those asked of a patient with asthma, for instance, while some may be less familiar. The more they are used, the more confidence is gained and it soon becomes second nature, helping not only the patient but also the clinician to become more relaxed.

The following are key areas to explore with examples of questions some nurses have found useful.

Severity

- How bad is it?
- Do you feel like this all day, every day?
- Is it worse at any particular time of the day?
- Is there any particular time when you feel better than others?
- If you have felt like this before, does this feel better or worse than last time?

Duration

- How long have you felt like this?
- When did you first start to feel the way you do?
- Did anything in particular happen at that time?

Social network

- Are you still going out as much as you used to?
- Among your friends, do you have one person you feel you can confide in?
- Who do you feel would be supportive if you told them how you feel?

View of self, the world and the future

- How do you feel about yourself?
- Do you feel guilty or worthless?
- What is there in the future you are looking forward to?
- Is there anything you feel excited about?
- How do you feel about the future?

Suicidal thoughts (discussed in more detail under Suicide Risk, p.225)

- Do you ever feel life is not worth living?
- Do you ever wish you wouldn't wake up in the morning?
- Have you ever had suicidal thoughts?

Past history

- Have you ever felt like this before?
- Have you ever attempted to take your own life before?
- How long ago did you feel like that way?
- Did you take any medication at that time?
- What helped you through that time in your life?

Biological symptoms

- How are you sleeping?
- What is your appetite like?
- Have you lost or gained any weight recently?
- Has your concentration level decreased?
- Do you get tired easily?
- Are you as interested in sexual relations as you were before you felt like this?

Other factors

- Are you taking anything else to make you feel better?
- How much alcohol would you normally drink?
- How much are you drinking now?
- Are you using any illegal drugs to improve the way you feel?
- Have you bought anything over the counter to help you?

Other medication

- Are you taking any other medication prescribed by the doctor?
- Have you recently stopped any prescribed medication?
- Have you bought any medication over the counter?

SCREENING TOOLS

Assessment and screening questionnaires may be used as part of an assessment but not instead of one.

The Hospital Anxiety and Depression Scale (HADS) is a well-researched and validated questionnaire for use in primary care. It can be used to aid diagnosis of both anxiety and depression and often helps both the clinician and patient to differentiate between the two, although they frequently coexist. It can be completed quickly by the patient, normally taking no more than 5 minutes to complete the 14-item questionnaire.

The HADS needs to be completed by the patient in the practice, regarding how they have felt over the last 7 days, not thinking about it too much. They should not be given the opportunity to take it home where others may influence how it is completed.

It would not be suitable to use the HADS if patients have literacy problems or difficulty understanding English. Nurses have expressed concern that patients can 'skew' the results to suit their own ends. If this is suspected then it is probably better not to use it as part of the assessment.

The advantages, however, may be any or all of the following.

- Can save time.
- Helps to focus the consultation.
- The language is easy to understand, asking simple straightforward questions.
- Helps patients acknowledge the problem.
- Can be used to aid diagnosis and then repeated to monitor progress.
- A common tool used by other members of the clinical team. (Do remember to record the score in the notes or computer so others can recognize improvement or deterioration.)
- Could be used as an audit tool.
- Helps patients recognize that depression is a common problem.
- May aid in referral by nurse to GP or from GP to community mental health team.

SUICIDE RISK

Any assessment or reassessment of patients with depression must include an assessment of suicidal risk. Approximately 4000 people take their own life annually in England, with the main cause attributed to depression.

Risk of suicide, however, is not dependent entirely on severity of depression alone. As mentioned earlier, suicidal thinking can occur at any stage on the continuum and is very common in the general population.

Nurses often have concerns around discussing suicidal thinking with patients, a common misconception being that asking questions may encourage patients to 'do it'. This is a myth. More often than not, it provides patients with an opportunity to discuss their feelings, thoughts and fears.

In order to carry out a detailed risk assessment the following areas would need to be covered, but not all nurses feel either confident or competent to carry them out. Ultimately any suspicion of suicidal thinking should be referred on to a GP to make a more detailed assessment about treatment and management.

Suicidal ideas:

- Do you feel life is not worth living?
- Do you want to kill yourself?
- Do you have any suicidal thoughts?
- Do you want to top yourself?
- Would you rather not wake up in the morning?

As you can see, there is a very broad range of questioning to elicit suicidal thinking. The question must suit the patient; for example, the last question may be useful when talking with an elderly lady but the previous one may be much more acceptable to young males at a local drop-in centre.

An affirmative answer to any of the above may signal an immediate referral to a GP while those more confident could go on to ask about *intention*.

- Would you act on these thoughts?
- Do you plan to do anything about the way you feel?
- Have you discussed these thoughts with anyone else?

An affirmative answer to the above would lead to asking questions around plans and previous attempts.

- Have you attempted to take your life before?
- How do you plan to carry this out?
- Do you have the means to kill yourself?

Often there is no need to ask about intention or plans as the patient will tell you everything you need to know without any further prompting.

Any patient who expresses intentions and plans requires an urgent referral to psychiatric services while those with suicidal thoughts but no intent still require careful monitoring, especially in the early stages of treatment when motivation may be returning but the mood is still very low.

A small percentage of patients will deny all thoughts of suicide while remaining determined to carry this out. This is not common but it must be remembered it is the patient's choice. Provided the opportunity has been given to the patient to disclose this information by asking appropriate questions, nothing can be done if he does not wish to confide in you.

Suicidal thinking must always be taken seriously. Do not fall into the trap of thinking 'the more people tell you, the less likely they are to do it'. This is not true. It is important to gain information around previous attempts as research shows that of those who attempted to take their own lives in the last year 1% will succeed in the next 12 months and a further 5% will be successful in the next 10 years.

Patients who find it difficult to confide in health professionals may consider speaking anonymously with someone on the phone. The National Samaritan Helpline number should be displayed in the surgery waiting room and mentioned in all written information given to patients with depression. Local branches of the Samaritans are often happy to come to the practice and tell you about their work.

TREATMENT

DRUG THERAPY

Antidepressants have been shown to be beneficial for patients suffering from moderate to major depression but there is no evidence to suggest they are of value in mild depression. This reinforces the need for a detailed and accurate assessment. Patients are sometimes prescribed medication inappropriately and unnecessarily. Those with major depression have an imbalance of the chemicals serotonin and noradrenaline. The majority of antidepressants increase these neurotransmitters, improving mood and restoring the chemical and emotional imbalance.

Patients are often reluctant to take antidepressants, the reason varying from person to person. The following are just a few of the most common reasons expressed.

- Worries about the medication being addictive.
- Unable to recognize they are ill enough to warrant medication.
- Appearing weak or not coping.
- Inability to deal with the side-effects of medication.
- Concerns around the prescription charge.
- Previous bad experience with old-style antidepressants.
- Concerns around the length of time they need to be taken.

Take time to listen to patients' concerns; they are very real and often crucial to concordance. Providing education on why drugs would be beneficial, how they work, how long they need to be taken for, etc. adds to patients' understanding of their condition and treatment. This in turn assists them to make informed choices, thereby sharing in the responsibility of their treatment and ultimately their recovery.

Having background knowledge of the antidepressants most commonly used in the practice provides practice nurses with the ability to recognize when patients have been recently commenced on therapy. Simply acknowledging this with patients and discussing side-effects, as with any other medication, helps to normalize and destigmatize the use of antidepressants. It may also discourage patients from stopping medication due to unpleasant side-effects. Unfortunately, side-effects normally occur before any benefit from the medication takes effect so patients often feel worse before they feel better, leading to discontinuation of medication.

In fact, there is a great deal of information that patients need when starting on antidepressants for the first time. For this reason it is advisable that written information should always be given to patients when providing the first prescription (Fig. 12.1).

This could be given by the GP, the dispensing chemist or, when appropriate, a practice nurse who could go through the information with the patient. A fuller understanding of the way in which drugs work, the length of time patients need to take them and why, together with support and monitoring may lead to better compliance although there is little evidence to date to prove this theory.

The following are the groups of antidepressants most commonly used in primary care. The dosages quoted are the therapeutic doses for patients with depression and it must be remembered that in some cases these medications are given at different doses for other conditions. Patients cared for in secondary care may be prescribed the same medication in higher doses.

Tricyclics

Name	Daily therapeutic dose
Dothiepin (Prothiaden)	75–150 mg
Amitriptyline (Tryptizol)	125–150 mg
Clomipramine (Anafranil)	125–150 mg
Trimipramine (Surmontil)	50–75 mg
Lofepramine (Gamanil)	140–210 mg

Please refer to the *British national formulary* for the most up-to-date information.

Side-effects Anticholinergic effects such as the following: dry mouth, sedation, constipation, headache, urinary retention. May be cardiotoxic.

Advantages Sedation may be both an advantage and a disadvantage but when insomnia is a major symptom of the depression, a good night's sleep may be the first approach to treatment. Tricyclics are also anxiolytic, aiding a reduction in anxiety levels and tension. In comparison with many other antidepressants, they are economical to prescribe. They have been on the market for many years so clinicians are well aware of side-effects and experienced in dealing with them.

Disadvantages Sedation can cause problems for some patients. Young mothers who need to be alert through the night or long-distance lorry drivers needing to concentrate early in the morning would not be appropriate candidates for tricyclic medication.

Unfortunately patients find the anticholinergic side-effects impossible to tolerate if given at therapeutic dose from the outset so the dose requires titration. An acceptable regime may be 50 mg amitryptyline for a week, 100 mg for a further 2 weeks and then the therapeutic dose of 150 mg nocte. This takes time, support and monitoring from practice staff, alongside patience and tolerance of side-effects from the patient.

Because of this rather elongated process patients often discontinue their medication or the therapeutic dose is never actually achieved, with patients remaining on 100 mg for months. If repeat

IMPORTANT ADVICE ABOUT YOUR ANTIDEPRESSANTS

Your doctor has given you a prescription for antidepressants. Before starting them you may find the following information useful.

Depression is COMMON, affecting any age, gender or background, and responds well to treatment.

- Antidepressants are NOT addictive (unlike tranquillizers, which can be).
- **Do not take more or less than your GP has prescribed.** Remember to tell your GP if you are taking anything bought over the counter, have increased your alcohol intake or are taking recreational drugs such as cannabis to help the way you are feeling. Any or all of these affect the action of antidepressants, so your GP will need to be aware of this when prescribing.
- **It can take 3–4 weeks before you feel any improvement** so do keep taking the medication. Just because you do not experience instant improvement in the way you feel does not mean the medication doesn't work. Be patient, give it time.
- Some **side-effects may be experienced** before you feel the benefits. **These usually wear off** after a short period of time.
- The **common side-effects** may be dry mouth, constipation, blurred vision, nausea, headaches or drowsiness.
- These **side-effects can be reduced** by increasing fluid intake, using sugar-free chewing gum, boiled sweets, etc. Increase fibre intake in the form of fresh fruit, vegetables and breakfast cereals.
- Discuss any continuing concerns with your doctor.
- Keep alcohol to a minimum.
- Treatment should be taken **for a minimum of 6 months after you feel better**, to reduce the possibility of your illness returning. Research has shown that patients who take their medication for this length of time have been less likely to suffer further episodes of depression.
- **Do not stop your medication without talking to your doctor.** When stopping, it is advisable to reduce your medication slowly over a period of time with support and monitoring from a member of your surgery team.
- If you require help in addition to your antidepressants, your doctor may discuss with you the possibility of seeing a practice nurse, counsellor or specialist. Many people find **talking therapies**, in addition to taking medication, aid their recovery. The two often go hand in hand.

SAMARITANS HELPLINE TEL 08457 909090

Figure 12.1 Information for patients taking antidepressants.

prescriptions are not given until patients are well established on a therapeutic dose this would help solve this issue.

Tricyclic medication is very toxic in overdose and should never be given to patients expressing suicidal thinking.

Selective serotonin reuptake inhibitors (SSRIs)

Name	Starting daily therapeutic dose
Fluoxetine (Prozac)	20 mg
Paroxetine (Seroxat)	20 mg
Citalopram (Cipramil)	20 mg
Sertraline (Lustral)	50 mg

Side-effects Although the majority of side-effects from all the antidepressants tend to improve with use, some are so bad at the outset that some patients find it difficult to continue. Headaches can sometimes be one of these symptoms. In this circumstance another SSRI may be tried and found to be successful.

Gastrointestinal problems and sweating are often reported alongside increased weight gain or weight loss.

Sexual dysfunction may occur on SSRI medication, but can also be a symptom of depression so care needs to be taken during history taking. If this is already a problem, there is little sense in exacerbating it.

Increased anxiety at the outset of treatment may be intolerable for patients, especially during the night.

Advantages It is possible to commence treatment at the therapeutic dose, with no need for titration. SSRIs are not toxic in overdose, providing a safer option for patients with suicidal ideation. They are non-sedating.

Disadvantages Many of the older SSRIs may now be prescribed generically, which has brought the prescribing cost down, but they are still more expensive than tricyclics.

Although there is no evidence to suggest they are addictive some patients find it very difficult to stop taking some drugs from this group. This problem with discontinuation can be reduced if patients are taken off their medication very slowly over a minimum of 4 weeks and monitored and supported by a health professional during this process.

These are the two most commonly used groups of antidepressants in primary care at the moment but there are other groups now being prescribed.

Serotonin and noradrenaline reuptake inhibitor (SNRI)

Venlafaxine (Efexor): 75–100 mg

Side-effects are similar to SSRIs and tricyclics.

Noradrenaline reuptake inhibitor (NARI)

Reboxetine (Edronax): 4 mg bd

Side-effects include dry mouth, insomnia, constipation and sweating.

Noradrenergic and specific serotonergic antidepressant

Mitazepine (Zispin): 15–45 mg

Side-effects include dizziness and increased appetite.

The three groups of drugs mentioned above would not normally be chosen as first-line therapy in primary care, but patients may be prescribed them as second- or third-line treatment.

Hypericum (St John's wort), which is available to patients over the counter, is often used for the relief of milder symptoms of depression. It has properties similar to some of the other antidepressants so should not be used in combination. Advice from the Committee for Safety of Medicines suggests it should not be taken with some drugs including warfarin, cyclosporin, oral contraceptives, digoxin and theophylline.

Hypericum is prescribed regularly in some European countries but is normally bought over the counter in the UK, making it important to check with patients what other medication they are taking before prescribing.

SELF-HELP AND NON-DRUG APPROACHES

As previously mentioned, there is no evidence to suggest that antidepressants are of benefit in the care of patients with mild depression. This group is more often unrecognized by clinicians and in some cases the depression resolves spontaneously. There are, however, techniques practice nurses can use to improve the mental health of patients and hasten recovery. When used sensitively, patients often acquire new skills and knowledge they can draw on in the future.

Practice nurses are well practised at providing health promotion advice. This area of expertise is useful when helping patients to look at their general lifestyle and helping them recognize how this may impinge on their mental well-being. Routine discussion and advice around healthy diet, smoking habits, alcohol consumption, weight and exercise are all relevant in this client group.

For example, numerous studies have shown that exercise can result in a decrease in clinical depression, improve cognitive function and raise self-esteem. The improvements may be small but they are significant. Lethargy and loss of energy are symptoms of depression and helping patients overcome this through a small increase in exercise, taken regularly and increased slowly, can be beneficial to both physical and emotional well-being.

Alcohol consumption is often increased by patients who are depressed in a misguided attempt to 'cheer themselves up'. Unfortunately, it has the opposite effect by exacerbating depression and making matters worse.

Change in eating habits may also be a symptom of depression, resulting in weight gain or loss. Helping patients to identify what is going on in their lives and encouraging them to address problems may be more helpful than merely providing advice on how to lose weight.

Coping skills

Patients often have their own ways of coping with problems but when they are feeling down they temporarily forget. Asking questions such as 'What activities do you normally enjoy?' 'What activities have you given up that you would normally do?' thus reminding them and 'giving them permission' to enjoy themselves may be useful. It is easy to forget what having fun is all about.

Patients often mention that entertainment is so expensive they have stopped going out as they can no longer afford to enjoy themselves. Encourage activities that are free or inexpensive. Going for a walk with or without a friend, chatting over a cup of coffee, listening to music, reading a book, relaxing in the sunshine, playing with the children, relaxing in a warm bath, a trip to the local recreation ground with the children. Invite friends round for a drink instead of a meal; remember, it is the company they enjoy not necessarily the food! Encourage patients to come up with ideas that are particularly relevant to them rather than imposing your ideas and solutions.

Diary keeping

Keeping a diary as a way of monitoring activities can be useful for some patients. Dividing the diary into activities that provide a sense of achievement and those that provide a sense of pleasure can help patients distinguish between the two but recognize the importance of both. For example, cleaning the house from top to bottom may give a sense of achievement to one person but not a great deal of pleasure, while a chat and a giggle with a friend may provide pleasure but not score a great deal on achievement. Attempting to maintain some sort of balance between the two may be more easily achievable when the patient monitors and reflects back.

A mood diary can be completed in the same way, patients identifying time when they enjoy life as well as times they feel down. This helps patients to monitor their mood swings on a daily basis, identify triggers and find ways for themselves to avoid circumstances that cause anxiety or distress and to increase the things they enjoy or that make them feel better. Encouraging patients to complete these types of tasks as homework saves time in the consultation and passes some of the responsibility back to the patient. Asking them to give themselves an overall score out of 10 on how their mood has been that week enables them to identify improvement or not, as the case may be, in comparison with previous weeks.

Another form of writing therapy is letter writing. This can be particularly useful when there has been some form of conflict or disagreement between the patient and another individual. This provides an opportunity to say all those things one would really love to say but for one reason or another cannot be said. Anything can be written down on paper, no holding back all those nasty thoughts and feelings, but *do not post it*!

Some people rip their letters up, put them on the fire or destroy them in some other way; others go back and change them time and time again until they are structured and written in such a way that they feel they can now post them.

Letter writing is often useful following the loss of someone close when it was impossible to say all the things one would wish to say before it was too late.

Problem solving

This is a useful technique to help patients identify difficulties which may be contributing to their depressed mood and in turn encourage them to find solutions to these difficulties. This technique is only appropriate where there is a realistic solution to a problem.

For example, if part of the problem is that a patient is caring for a terminally ill aunt, nothing could be done to stop the aunt from dying. However, there may well be several issues around the care of the aunt and the well-being of the patient that could be resolved by the use of problem solving.

A randomized controlled trial has shown the technique to be significantly superior to a placebo, not significantly different to amitriptyline at therapeutic dose and acceptable to both patients and appropriately trained primary care workers.

Problem solving is useful on its own for patients with mild depression or can be used alongside antidepressants in patients with moderate to major depression whose motivation is at a level at which they can address their problems and take the relevant steps to solving them.

Steps in problem solving

1. *Identify the problem* – as perceived by the patient, not the nurse. Some patients find this difficult, saying 'I can't be depressed, there is nothing wrong'. Exploring the following issues can be useful: relationships with family and friends, finances, housing, employment or lack of, physical and emotional health, alcohol and smoking habits, sexual difficulties, bereavement or other loss, and support networks. The task of the nurse here is to listen and feed back.
2. *Prioritize* the problems, from what may appear to cause the least concern to the greatest. The patient can do this as 'homework' and bring the list to the next visit.
3. *Choose the problem to work on*. Often better to tackle the least difficult first to increase self-esteem and gain understanding and confidence in the method.

4. *Options*. List all the possible realistic solutions to this particular problem, including ones that may never have been considered before.
5. *Pros and cons*. Look closely at all the advantages and disadvantages of all the options. If the patient would not be able to deal with the worst scenario of an option, this would not be the one to choose.
6. *Choose the solution to work on*. Remember, this is the patient's choice, arrived at with guidance and support from the clinician.
7. *Make a plan*. Decide how, where, when and who might help with this plan. Break it down into small, detailed, manageable steps that are achievable. Remember, what may appear simple and straightforward when fit and well may seem like a mountain to climb when depressed.
8. *Carry out the plan*. Always invite patients back to discuss how thing went. Evaluate success or otherwise. If all went well move onto the next problem; if not, help to explore where and when the solution went wrong and perhaps choose another solution.
9. *Praise success*. No matter how small the success may appear to you, always recognize the achievement of the patient when the plan is successful, encouraging them to move on to the next.

On paper this may appear disjointed but in practice patients find it both useful and rewarding. Having learned the technique and been successful once, they often have the confidence to move on to other areas on their own. It is a coping mechanism that can be used in a variety of situations and used when problems arise in the future.

Cognitive therapy

Cognitive therapy or 'thinking therapy' is an effective treatment for depression aimed at raising the person's awareness of the mistakes in their thinking. Distorted thinking influences the way we feel. When depressed, there are changes in the way we think as well as a lowering of mood. We tend to look on the black side of things, including our view of the future, the world and ourselves in general.

Typical examples might be:

- Nobody phones me any more, nobody likes me.
- I'm useless at my job, that's why I didn't get promoted.
- Why bother going on holiday, I won't enjoy it.
- Life is useless. I just feel awful.

These are often termed negative automatic thoughts. Everybody has them, they are normal, they just pop into our heads and then just as quickly disappear, but when we are depressed they occur much more regularly, don't go away and we start to believe them. This type of thinking alters the way we feel and ultimately the way we behave by making activities seem pointless or unachievable. The more we isolate ourselves and stop socializing, the worse we feel and the more distorted the thinking becomes.

A typical example might be:

- Event – friend doesn't acknowledge you in the street.
- Thought – 'She doesn't like me, nobody does'.
- Feeling – sad, unhappy, hurt, depressed.
- Behaviour – stay at home, don't contact friends.

Cognitive therapy can be broken down into easy steps.

- Highlight the negative thinking and learn to recognize it. Challenge the thoughts. Look for the evidence to prove this thinking is correct.
- Replace the negative thought with facts or more rational thinking.

This may be done using a diary. It is often easier to recognize feelings than thoughts, so when there is a 'bad feeling', *stop* and work out exactly what you were thinking immediately prior to the feeling. When possible, write it down immediately in the diary. This helps to identify how often these thoughts occur in a day. As improvement takes place these thoughts will become fewer and this can be identified in the diary. This may be all patients can cope with to begin with but as they get better at recognizing the thinking behind the feelings they can then start to substitute alternative, more realistic thoughts.

To go back to the event above where your friend didn't acknowledge you in the street.

- Substitute thought may be – 'She didn't see me' or 'She is in a hurry to pick the children up from school'.
- Feeling might be – sad not to have a chat, but knowing you can talk on the phone later.
- Behaviour – phone friend and find out she had a dental appointment and wasn't aware of you.

It takes a long time to become a fully trained cognitive behavioural therapist but there are some skills which can be used in short appointment times by nurses who have received training. CBT is often used by counsellors or community psychiatric nurses. Contact them, arrange a meeting; professionals are normally only too happy to share their knowledge and skills.

It must be remembered that there will be some patients with mild depression who would not present to the practice at all as they may not see the surgery as an appropriate place to discuss emotional issues. Family and friends are often used for support and this should be encouraged. Some may talk with the local vicar or community leader. It doesn't really matter who worries and concerns are shared with as long as there is mutual trust and respect. Simply sharing the problem and saying it out loud may help to put some perspective on the intensity or severity of the problem, thus enabling patients to 'move on'.

KEY TASKS FOR PRACTICE NURSES

- Encourage a team approach to mental health.
- Be aware of the possibility of mental health problems during everyday consultations.
- Recognize there is a need for education around mental health within the primary care team.
- Provide written information to those with a diagnosis of depression.
- Work with other health professionals to improve the care of patients with mental illness, e.g. school nurses, health visitors, community mental health teams and practice counsellors.
- Assist in making the practice 'user friendly', especially to younger men who visit the practice rarely but are at high risk of suicide.
- Help create a 'depression template' so patients with depression can be cared for in exactly the same way as patients with other chronic disease.
- Add a question on depression to the new patient medical.
- Work with GPs and others to develop a protocol on identifying patients at high risk of suicide with appropriate referral criteria.
- Take steps to ensure they are supported and valued themselves within the practice while actively supporting and valuing their colleagues.

CONCLUSION

More and more patients are taking an active interest in their medical conditions, seeking additional information, education and resources from other agencies, including the Internet and voluntary agencies. This is healthy and patients should be signposted to well-established and recognized bodies both locally and nationally (see Resources).

Given the prevalence of depression in those consulting primary care, practice nurses have no option but to get involved. Patients with depression often relapse, with approximately 25% developing a chronic form of the condition. In fact, the WHO estimates it will be the second most common noncommunicable global condition by 2020. Perhaps there is a need to review the way we care for these patients and it has been suggested that the way forward is to provide the same type of monitoring and regular review that is offered to other chronic conditions such as asthma, diabetes or coronary heart disease. Considering the numbers involved, this may be expensive. It must, however, be open to discussion and interested trained practice nurses could play a more proactive role in their management.

References

DOH 1999 National Service Framework for Mental Health: modern standards and service models. Department of Health, London

WHO 2000 WHO guide to mental health in primary care (UK version). Royal Society of Medicine, London

Resources

NFER-Nelson Publishing, Darville House, 2 Oxford Road East, Windsor, Berkshire SL4 1DF. Publishes the Hospital Anxiety and Depression Scale

Depression Alliance, 35 Westminster Bridge Road, London SE1 7JP. Tel: 020 7633 0557. www.depressionalliance.org.uk

Mental Health Foundation, 20–21 Cornwall Street, London NW1 4QL. Tel: 020 7535 7400. www.mentalhealth.org.uk

MIND, Granta House, 15–19 Broadway, Stratford, London E15 4BQ. Tel: 020 8519 2122. www.mind.org.uk

Young Minds Trust, 22a Boston Place, London NW1 6ER. Tel: 020 7336 8445

Talking Life (seminars for nurses), Wendy Lloyd Audio Productions, 1A Grosvenor Road, Hoylake, Wirral CH47 3BS. Tel: 0151 632 0662. Email: wendy@talkinglife.co.uk

Chapter 13

Arthritis

Jane Proctor

CHAPTER CONTENTS

INTRODUCTION

The aim of this chapter is to provide an overview of the presentation and management of arthritic conditions commonly encountered in primary care. Emphasis will be placed on the contribution that practice nurses can make to the holistic care of patients suffering from these conditions.

THE SIZE OF THE PROBLEM

Musculoskeletal diseases are the most common cause of disability in developed countries throughout the world and account for 18.7% of consultations in primary care (Badley 1991).

Changes in the National Health Service (NHS) in the United Kingdom have shifted much of the provision of healthcare to the community (NHS Management Executive 1991). Communication between hospital rheumatology departments and the primary healthcare team is therefore vital if patients are to receive optimal care.

Charlton et al (1995) found that there has been an increase in the incidence of oesteo-arthritis which was probably due to an increase in the elderly population, particularly of women, but also to better surgical techniques and the growth of public expectation regarding treatment (Horbury 1995).

Most of the osteo-arthritis patients presenting in primary care do not require consultant referral but rely on the primary healthcare team for support, education and advice. Much of the monitoring of patients taking disease-modifying drugs for rheumatoid arthritis (RA) is undertaken in primary care by practice nurses who often have little knowledge

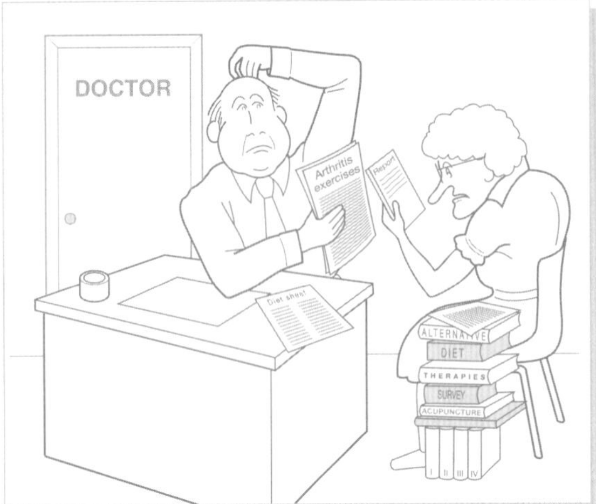

Figure 13.1 Reproduced with kind permission from Dr William Bird.

regarding the potential reactions and side-effects that may be encountered. If doctors and nurses in primary care do not have the necessary skills and knowledge, patients will be denied appropriate treatment and education (Dargie & Proctor 1998).

ANATOMY AND PHYSIOLOGY OF THE MUSCULOSKELETAL SYSTEM

The musculoskeletal system consists of three types of tissue.

- Bones
- Muscle
- Connective tissue

BONES

There are around 200 bones forming the skeleton which are held together with cartilage and ligaments. They provide:

- a framework of support
- protection for organs
- storage for minerals and calcium
- production of red blood cells in the bone marrow.

Bones are composed of collagen fibres made up of crystals of hydroxyapatites which are formed from phosphates of calcium. There are three types of bone cells:

- *osteoblasts* which secrete collagen and become osteocytes
- *osteocytes* which form the matrix of the bone and
- *osteoclasts* which have a phagocytic nature allowing for bone reabsorption.

There are two types of bone.

- *Compact* bone which is dense and hard and forms the shafts of long bones and the surface of flat bones.
- *Trabecular* bone which is spongy in appearance and surrounded by the hard surface of the compact bone.

Haversian canals are a network of tiny canals throughout both types of bone which provide access for blood and lymphatic vessels bringing nutrients to the bone.

Erythrocyte-producing *red bone marrow* is found at the centre of the shafts of long bones and the centre areas of flat bones. The bone is covered by a tough vascular membrane known as the *periosteum*.

The formation and reabsorption of healthy bone require an adequate intake of calcium and vitamin D. It is a continual process which is also affected by the hormones of the pituitary, thyroid and sex glands.

MUSCLES

Skeletal muscles provide the power and movement of the body. They are striated or voluntary muscles composed of bundles of muscle fibres called fasciculi. Groups of fasciculi are covered by a tough fibrous sheath known as the *epimysium*.

Muscles have an ample supply of blood vessels to provide nutrients and remove waste.

Movement of the joints occurs through voluntary contraction of one or more muscles. Grouped in pairs, one muscle acts as an agonist and the other as an antagonist to enable movement in both directions. More complicated muscle groups work together to provide compound movements such as movements of the shoulder joint. These muscle groups are known as synergistic.

CONNECTIVE TISSUE

Connective tissue:

- provides attachment of one bone to another
- provides attachment for muscle to bone
- stabilizes joints.

Muscles are attached to each other and to surrounding structures by *tendons*. These are strong inelastic cords composed of connective tissue which are extensions of the end of the muscles and attach themselves to bone at points of insertion.

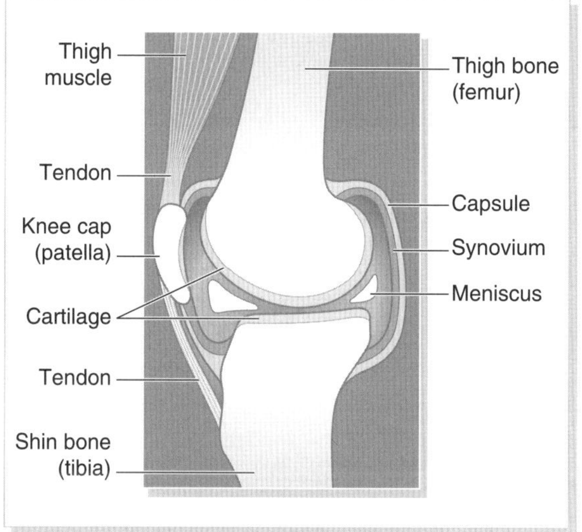

Figure 13.2 A normal knee joint. Reproduced with kind permission from the Arthritis Research Campaign.

Ligaments, whilst similar to tendons, are strong bundles of connective tissue surrounding joints. They provide strength and stability to the joint capsule.

JOINTS

Joints are formed when two or more bones meet. They provide mobility and stabilize the skeleton.

There are three types of joints depending on the range of movement required.

- *Fixed joints* provide little or no movement, such as the sutures of the skull.
- *Cartilaginous joints* permit a limited degree of movement. These would include the intervertebral joints and the symphysis pubis.
- *Synovial* or *diarthrosis joints* occur where a moderate or wide range of movement is required and a space must exist between bones to allow for movement. The bone ends are covered by hyaline cartilage, a firm compressible structure which acts as a cushion between the bone ends. Synovial joints have a joint capsule lined with synovium which has both secretory and macrophage functions. This membrane secretes synovial fluid which fills the joint space and provides lubrication and nutrients to the cartilage.

It is the synovial or diarthrosis joint that is most commonly affected by inflammatory joint disease while the cartilaginous joints are often affected by traumatic and degenerative problems.

THE INFLAMMATORY RESPONSE

Inflammation is a process in which defensive measures are taken by the body in order to remove harmful stimuli from the tissues and to enable restoration of normal structure and function. In joint disease the harmful stimuli within the joint may be caused by:

- bony injury
- bacterial infection
- the presence of crystals
- other unexplained causes which would include most autoimmune diseases such as RA.

Once the inflammatory process begins in a joint, leukotrienes attract white blood cells to the site which cause inflammatory mediators to be released, increasing blood supply to the area and resulting in the signs and symptoms of inflammation.

Box 13.1 Signs and symptoms of inflammation

Redness
Swelling
Pain
Loss of function
Heat

THE COMMON INFLAMMATORY ARTHROPODIES

RHEUMATOID ARTHRITIS

Rheumatoid arthritis is a chronic inflammatory disease affecting not only joints but other organs of the body. The disease activity is characterized by bouts of exacerbation and remission. The morbidity and mortality of RA cause severe pain and distress to both patients and carers and add a huge burden to the economy of the country.

Epidemiology

Rheumatoid arthritis is the most common chronic inflammatory disease. The prevalence of RA in the population is about 3% (Dieppe et al 1985) and it attacks all age groups, with three times more women being affected than men (Lawrence 1994).

Aetiology

The aetiology is unknown but it would appear that people with a genetic disposition who encounter triggering factors develop the disease. These triggering factors are thought to include infection and emotional stresses such as bereavement.

The immune response

The body's immune response is a protective mechanism which recognizes the invasion of a potentially harmful substance such as viruses and bacteria. There are two systems working together.

- Natural immunity is present from birth.
- The adaptive system becomes active when the natural system fails to protect the body and produces a specific response to each invading agent. This provides lifelong immunity should the same agent attack again.

It is thought that certain individuals are susceptible to a stimulus which causes tissue inflammation or abnormal function to occur. The presence of autoantibodies such as the rheumatoid factor is common in patients with RA and indicates that an abnormal immunological activity is occurring (Pisetsky 1994).

Pathology

Rheumatoid arthritis is a disease of the synovium or joint lining. The lining becomes infiltrated with lymphoid cells which cause the synovium to become thickened and inflamed (*synovitis*) with eventual destruction of the articular cartilage causing bone erosion.

The disease activity causes inflammatory markers in the blood to rise so the erythrocyte sedimentation rate (ESR) and the C-reactive protein (CRP) are commonly requested blood tests. The regular monitoring of these tests can give an indication of disease activity. A positive rheumatoid factor may be found in the blood of most patients but some present with normal inflammatory markers and a negative rheumatoid factor (termed seronegative RA). Plain X-ray of affected joints will show bony erosions, confirming the diagnosis.

Clinical presentation

The disease may appear gradually over many years or acutely with severe systemic symptoms. The commonest age of presentation is the fourth and fifth decades although all age groups can be affected. Symmetrical pain and swelling of the peripheral joints of the hands and feet are common early symptoms with the larger weight-bearing joints being affected in more established disease. Early morning stiffness and stiffness following periods of rest may also indicate disease. After years of persistent synovitis the joints become unstable and deformed with subsequent loss of function.

As RA is a systemic disease extraarticular problems frequently arise. General malaise, anaemia of chronic disease and fatigue may also be features.

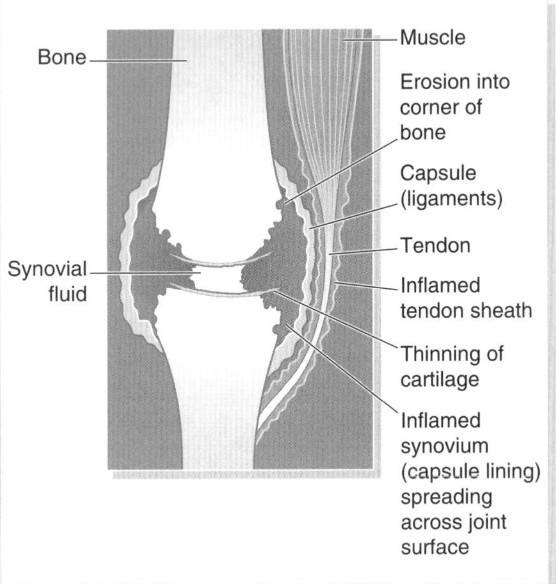

Figure 13.3 A joint badly affected by RA. Reproduced with kind permission from the Arthritis Research Campaign.

Box 13.2 Extraarticular features which may occur in RA

Anaemia
Rheumatoid nodules on the elbows, occiput, Achilles tendon, lungs and myocardium
Sjögren's syndrome (dry eyes and mouth)
Lymphadenopathy
Osteoporosis
Pericarditis
Hepatomegaly caused by amyloid deposits
Pleural effusions
Vasculitis causing nailfold infarcts, leg ulcers and damage to internal organs

Management

Treatment depends on the duration and activity of the disease and careful assessment of the patient and care should be planned to enable the patient to lead as normal a life as possible.

Education of the patient regarding rest, joint protection and pain management is an important nursing intervention with appropriate referral to other members of the healthcare team such as physiotherapy and occupational therapy.

Surgical intervention in the form of joint replacement may be required by some patients to preserve joint function, mobility and to provide relief from pain.

Medication for rheumatoid arthritis

The aims of treatment of RA, as stated by the European Agency for the Evaluation of Medicinal Products, are:

- to relieve pain
- to sustain function
- to decrease inflammation
- to prevent structural damage (Platt 2001).

Nearly every patient with RA relies on some form of analgesia, medication often being a combination of different analgesics. Paracetamol is often the first medication used and is additionally useful in RA flares because of its antipyrexial properties.

Symptom-modifying drugs

Non-steroidal antiinflammatory drugs (NSAIDs) NSAIDs are widely used in RA and if taken on a regular basis have the potential to reduce inflammation as well as providing analgesia. There are many preparations on the market and benefits in pain and function are seen within several days. There is no evidence that NSAIDs affect the course of the disease and damage to joints continues despite improvement in symptoms (Byrne 1998).

There is a large variation in patient response to each NSAID so several drugs may be tried before determining the most effective. Traditional NSAIDs known as cyclooxygenase inhibitors (COX 1 inhibitors) work by inhibiting the production of prostaglandins which have a large role in the inflammatory response. COX 1s are non-selective in inhibiting COX enzymes which are also responsible for maintaining gastrointestinal mucosa, platelet aggregation and renal perfusion. Side-effects associated with this class of drugs include upper gastrointestinal bleeding and perforation and they are estimated to cause 2000 deaths per year in the UK (Platt 2001).

Box 13.3 Side-effects of NSAIDs

- *Gastrointestinal*, including nausea, vomiting, diarrhoea, erosions and peptic ulcers
- *Hepatic*, causing a rise in liver function tests. NSAIDs should be used with caution in patients with hepatic impairment
- *Renal*, may cause renal impairment and should be used with care in patients with real impairment
- *Skin*, causing photosensitivity, urticaria
- *Respiratory*, causing bronchospasm and should not be used in asthmatic patients
- *Central nervous system*, causing headache and drowsiness
- *Hypersensitivity*

The Committee for the Safety of Medicines (CSM) assessed the safety of seven NSAIDs and indicated the following:

- azapropazone has the highest risk of upper gastrointestinal side-effects
- piroxicam, ketoprofen, indomethacin, naproxen and diclofenac have intermediate risks
- ibuprofen has the lowest risk.

Sustained-release preparations may be useful to aid compliance and to help control symptoms at night. Alternative routes of administration, e.g. suppositories and topical preparations, may help to prevent side-effects associated with the gastrointestinal tract but do not prevent systemic side-effects.

Recent years have seen the release of drugs that have a selective inhibition of COX 2 enzymes which reduce inflammation without gastrointestinal side-effects. Rofecoxib and celecoxib are the first in a new generation of NSAIDs although the older drugs meloxicam and etodolac may have some degree of selectivity.

Corticosteroids Corticosteroids have been used to control the inflammatory process in RA for many years. The side-effect profile of this group of drugs when used long term in high dosage has led to a decline in usage by many rheumatologists as the use of newer disease-modifying drugs has increased. When used they can be administered as follows.

- Orally, but then often as a last resort when other medication has failed.

- Intramuscularly to cause remission of an acute flare of RA.
- Intravenous steroids can also be used to induce a remission of symptoms.
- Intraarticular steroids reduce the synovitis of inflamed joints and are often used to relieve pain and improve function in troublesome joints. Only one or two joints should be injected at any one time and normally at intervals of not less than 3 months.

Box 13.4 Side-effects of steroids

- Weight gain
- Thin skin
- Loss of libido
- Bruising
- Predisposition to diabetes
- Increase in body and facial hair
- Acne

Patients taking oral steroids should be closely monitored, should understand the side-effects of therapy and carry a steroid treatment card. The treatment should not be stopped suddenly as an adrenal crisis may result and steroids may need to be increased at times of illness, infection or if requiring hospital or dental procedures.

Disease-modifying antirheumatic drugs (DMARDs) This group of drugs, often known as second-line therapy, includes drugs that modify the natural progression of the disease. These drugs reduce the inflammatory markers and also improve extraarticular manifestations of disease such as vasculitis. DMARDs are initiated by specialists once diagnosis is clear and progression of the disease confirmed. When starting DMARDs little improvement is usually noted for the first 2–3 months of therapy. Some drugs are more potent than others.

Disease-modifying drugs used in RA include the following.

Sodium aurothiomalate (gold) is given by intramuscular injection usually following a test dose. Weekly injections, usually every 4 weeks, with careful monitoring for proteinuria and the development of blood disorders. Rashes may also occur, necessitating discontinuation of treatment. *Auranofin* is an oral preparation but thought to be less effective than IM gold.

Methotrexate has become one of the most widely used DMARDs and is now the first choice of many rheumatologists. Used as a chemotherapy agent, methotrexate inhibits folate action which is required for DNA synthesis. It acts on cells, particularly rapidly dividing cells, making it especially useful in psoriatic arthritis. The drug is taken weekly, usually orally but may also be given intramuscularly. Side-effects of methotrexate include mouth ulcers, nausea and, more seriously, pulmonary toxicity. As methotrexate acts on the folates patients may have a fall in serum folate concentrations, causing an increase in side-effects.

Supplementation with folinic or folic acid may improve symptoms. Monitoring of patients taking methotrexate is paramount and includes blood tests for full blood count and liver function; the frequency of blood tests varies from hospital to hospital and local guidelines should be followed. Before commencing methotrexate patients should have a pretreatment assessment of FBC, U&Es and LFTs and have had a chest X-ray in the preceding year. Reversible oligospermia and the potential for fetal abnormality may limit the use of the drug in younger people. Alcohol should be avoided by patients taking methotrexate.

Penicillamine has a similar action to gold and is particularly beneficial to control extraarticular manifestations of disease such as vasculitis but does not appear to be as effective in seronegative RA. Monitoring includes FBC, urinalysis and U&Es, first 2 weekly and then monthly. Side-effects include thrombocytopenia, leucopenia, aplastic and haemolytic anaemia and proteinuria which may progress to glomerulonephritis. Nausea, vomiting and skin rashes may also occur.

Antimalarials *chloroquine* and *hydroxychloroquine* have a similar action to gold and penicillamine but may be better tolerated. Pretreatment assessment should include U&Es, FBC and creatinine but no blood monitoring is required although patients should have an annual eye check. Side-effects include nausea, vomiting and visual disturbances.

Sulphasalazine is often used when RA has failed to respond to NSAIDs. Many patients experience nausea as a side-effect and the drug should be initiated slowly. Pretreatment assessment includes FBC, LFTs, AST and ALT and blood monitoring should be continued as per local policy. Side-effects other than nausea include leucopenia, aplastic anaemia, thrombocytopenia, proteinuria and nephrotic syndrome. Oligospermia (reversible) may occur.

Cyclosporin is often used in severe disease and in psoriatic arthritis. Taken in daily doses, it is available in tablet or liquid form and may be used in combination with other DMARDs. Pretreatment assessment includes FBC, U&Es and creatinine, LFTs, urinary protein and blood pressure readings. Monitoring should include blood and blood pressure readings, usually at monthly intervals. Side-effects include renal and hepatic dysfunction, hypertension, excess growth of body hair and gastrointestinal disturbances.

Cyclophosphamide may be administered orally or intravenously. It is a potent medication used in refractory RA. Pretreatment assessment should include FBC, LFTs, creatinine and weekly urinalysis for blood as haemorrhagic cystitis is a side-effect. Other side-effects include bone marrow suppression, gastrointestinal upsets, alopecia and hepatic toxicity.

Azathioprine is an immunosuppressant which is given orally. Pretreatment assessment includes FBC, U&Es, LFTs and then regularly as per local guidelines. Side-effects include bone marrow suppression, gastrointestinal upset, arrhythmias, hair loss and a susceptibility to infection.

Leflunamide is the most recently approved DMARD. Evidence shows that it is effective in both early and established disease. Pretreatment assessment should include FBC, LFTs and blood pressure. Regular monitoring, usually 2 weekly for 6 months and then 8 weekly, should include blood pressure recordings. Side-effects include diarrhoea, vomiting, nausea, hypertension, leucopenia, rashes and oral mucosa disorders.

Disease-controlling antirheumatic drugs (DCARTs) The most recently available drugs for RA show evidence of arresting existing structural erosions and the prevention of new erosions and disease progression. These drugs act on the cytokine tumour necrosis factor alpha (TNF-alpha) which is responsible for inflammation within the joints. Two agents have been licensed, known as anti-TNF agents.

Etanercept Given by twice-weekly subcutaneous injection and may be used concurrently with or without methotrexate. The only side-effects reported are injection site reactions.

Infliximab needs to be administered by intravenous infusion and studies have seen rapid improvement in symptoms, C-reactive protein levels and patient well-being. Infliximab is used concurrently with methotrexate. There are reports of infection, particularly of tuberculosis, in patients during trials although generally it is well tolerated.

Both etanercept and infliximab are licensed for use in patients with RA who have not responded to other DMARDs but their use in the UK at present is limited due to cost.

Monitoring of second-line agents Nurses working in primary care are the professionals most often called upon to monitor patients taking second-line agents for RA. Local guidelines and protocols regarding investigations performed, intervals between tests and action to be taken in the event of side-effects may vary and advice should be sought before monitoring commences. The appointment of rheumatology nurse specialists in most rheumatology departments has enabled stronger links between primary and secondary care and effective and cost-effective shared care. The use of shared care monitoring cards and the accessibility of rheumatology nurse specialists should problems arise allow the patient to be monitored effectively without attending hospital, thus avoiding travelling, parking and waiting difficulties and at the same time freeing rheumatology departments to utilize their time more productively.

Educating patients about their medication, the way it works and side-effects that may occur will aid compliance. Verbal information can be reinforced with literature which can be obtained from the British Society of Rheumatology, the Arthritis and Rheumatism Council or local rheumatology departments (see Resources).

CHRONIC JUVENILE ARTHRITIS

Juvenile chronic arthritis is distinct from adult RA and presents rarely in adults.

Epidemiology

Often known as Still's disease, it was first described by Sir George Still in 1897 whilst working at Great Ormond Street Hospital. Usual onset is before the age of 16 years, affecting more boys than girls, most commonly between the ages of 1 and 4 years (Dieppe et al 1985).

Aetiology

The cause is unknown but infection, autoimmunity and heredity may predispose to the disease.

Presentation

Three forms of the disease have been recognized.

- Systemic onset
- Polyarticular
- Monoarticular

Systemic onset disease The child is often acutely ill with pyrexia, rash, generalized lymphadenopathy, with arthritis of multiple joints.

Polyarticular disease Systemic illness is mild and joint symptoms predominate. Joints of the hands and feet are frequently involved. Disturbances of growth with characteristic deformities are common.

Monoarticular disease (pauciarticular) Gradual onset of disease with between one joint and four joints affected. The disease is of gradual onset and systemic features are mild. Girls are more commonly affected than boys with the majority of cases occurring in the under-4s. Eye complications including uveitis are often a feature of the disease.

Management

A multidisciplinary team, often including a paediatrician and ophthalmologist, may be required. NSAIDs, steroids and disease-modifying drugs such as methotrexate are used whilst the disease is active. Physiotherapy is paramount in maintaining joint function and surgery may be required to maintain joint structure. The overall prognosis is good although 30% of children affected will have long-term limitation of activity and 1% will become blind (Dieppe et al 1985). Considerable support for the child and family is required and psychosocial problems are common.

OSTEO-ARTHRITIS

This disease, also known as joint failure, osteoarthrosis, arthrosis or degenerative joint disease, causes inflammation of the joint and bone, destruction of the articular cartilage and an increase in activity of subchondral bone.

Epidemiology

Osteo-arthritis is the most common rheumatic disease and is thought to be present in 80% of the population over the age of 75 (Cooper 1994). It affects more women than men and may vary in severity from causing few problems in some patients to severe pain and disability in others.

Aetiology

Osteo-arthritis can be classified into two groups.

- *Primary osteo-arthritis* for which there appears to be no cause, but may show a genetic tendency.

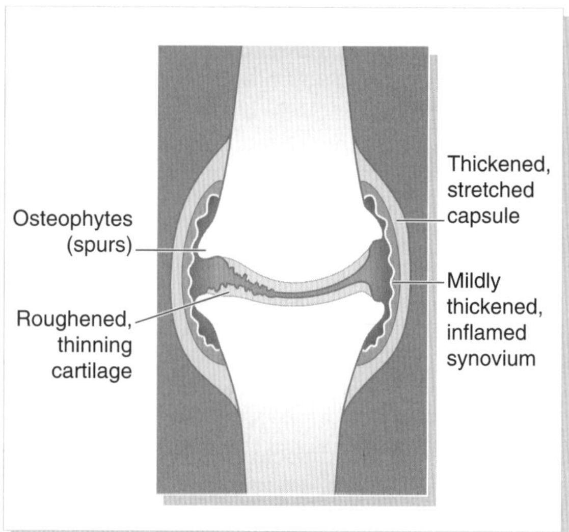

Figure 13.4 A joint with mild osteo-arthritis. Reproduced with kind permission from the Arthritis Research Campaign.

- *Secondary osteo-arthritis* which may be caused by metabolic disease, previous trauma or by occupational hazards; for example, a carpet fitter may develop osteo-arthritis of the knees.

Pathology

Although osteo-arthritis can affect any joint, those most commonly affected are the knees, hips, carpometacarpal joint of the thumb and the distal interphalangeal joints. The disease most commonly starts between the ages of 50 and 60 years. Destruction of the articular cartilage occurs and osteophytes or bony outgrowths form at the joint margins. These outgrowths are visible on X-ray which may also show loss of joint space. The joint capsule may become thickened and there is an increase in synovial fluid. Periarticular soft tissue cysts may also develop.

Clinical presentation

- Pain is usually the main symptom and is worse on using the joint and at the end of the day. It is relieved by rest although may be unremitting in advanced disease.
- Stiffness of the joints noticed in the early morning and after periods of inactivity.
- Restricted range of movement accompanied by pain and crepitus.
- Signs of inflammation may be present – warmth, swelling and tenderness.

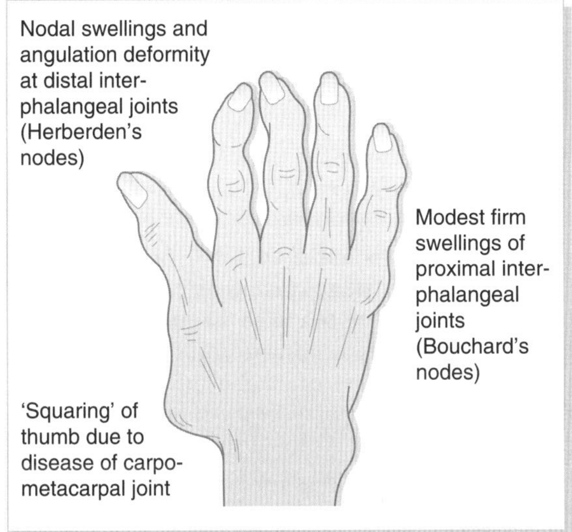

Figure 13.5 The hand in generalized osteo-arthritis. Reproduced with kind permission from Dr Paul Dieppe.

- Heberden's and Bouchard's nodes may be seen in osteo-arthritis affecting the hands (Fig. 13.5). These are caused by swellings over the small joints of the hand and fingers. In severe hand disease function may be severely reduced.

Management

Diagnosis of osteo-arthritis is made on clinical and radiological assessment and a careful history and examination with the help of X-rays should establish the cause of symptoms. There are no specific tests that will help with diagnosis but some may be necessary to exclude other pathology.

- *Education* of the patient and carers regarding the disease process and possible outcomes will provide reassurance and an ability to cope with symptoms. Information on methods of joint protection and alternative methods of pain relief supported by written information may be useful.
- *Control of contributing factors* such as obesity and the correction of deformities by the use of splints and exercise may help relieve symptoms.
- *Exercise* should be encouraged to improve muscle bulk, especially if there is muscle wasting, and referral to a physiotherapist may be helpful.
- *Analgesics* if required will probably be used long term. Therefore 'simple' on-demand medication such as paracetamol should be tried first. NSAIDs are undoubtedly useful in some patients but used long term have a high side-effect profile.
- *Intraarticular steroid injection* and joint aspiration may provide relief, particularly of knee joints where effusions are common and inflammation is often present.
- *Hyaluronan* may be injected intraarticularly to supplement natural hyaluronic acid in the synovial fluid. This procedure is thought to relieve pain for 1–6 months (Dieppe et al 2000). Randomized controlled trials found only slight benefit from the injection compared with placebo.
- *Surgery*, including joint replacement, has transformed the end-stage treatment of the disease, especially of the hips and knees. Elbow and shoulder replacement surgery is becoming more commonplace.

CRYSTAL DEPOSITION DISEASE

This group of diseases is defined by the presence of crystals in the joints which cause joint damage. There are two forms of the disease frequently presenting in general practice – gout and pseudogout.

Gout

Gout is characterized by the presence of monosodium urate crystals in the joint.

Epidemiology Known to occur worldwide, the disease is most frequently seen in males over the age of 40.

Aetiology Hyperuricaemia or high urate levels vary with age, sex and race. The common causes of hyperuricaemia include obesity, high alcohol intake, hyperlipidaemia and taking diuretics. There appears to be a genetic association with the incidence of gout.

Pathology High levels of uric acid in the synovial fluid lead to the formation of needle-shaped crystals in and around the articular cartilage. Persistently high levels of uric acid may lead to the formation of chalky deposits forming most commonly on the ears and hands, known as *tophi*. The disease most frequently affects the first metatarsophalangeal joint and is usually monoarticular. Other joints that may be affected include the ankle, knee and the small joints of the hand, wrist and elbow.

Presentation Usually only one joint is affected and onset is often rapid, the patient presenting with a swollen, hot, red, painful joint. Mild systemic fever may be present. If left untreated, the attack will subside slowly, taking up to 2 weeks for the joint to return to normal. If hyperuricaemia is not treated further attacks of gout may occur, often precipitated by illness or high alcohol intake. Drugs which alter the plasma urate levels, including diuretics and salicylates, may predispose to the occurrence of gout.

Management

- The treatment of *acute* gout is aimed at reducing inflammation and alteration of uric acid levels is best left until the acute phase of the disease has passed. Rest and high doses of NSAIDs used in the short term are effective. Patients unable to take NSAIDs can be treated with colchicine. Joint aspiration may relieve symptoms and examination of joint fluid confirms diagnosis.
- Treatment of *chronic* gout is usually commenced when there are repeated acute episodes, when accompanied by renal disease or when tophi are present. Weight reduction should be encouraged and advice on alcohol consumption given. An alteration in medication may be required in medication-induced gout. Allopurinol is the most commonly used hypouricaemic drug.

Pseudogout

Pseudogout occurs most commonly in the knee and although it may be preceded by injury, usually has no known cause. Elderly women are most commonly affected. More than one joint may be affected at a time and generalized fever may be present. Joints involved become hot, swollen and painful as crystals of pyrophosphate are deposited within the joint. Acute attacks may last for months and the disease becomes chronic with resulting damage to the joint. Treatment includes NSAIDs used carefully in the elderly. Joint aspiration and injection of steroid may be helpful for symptom control and to confirm diagnosis.

SPONDYLOARTHROPATHY

Ankylosing spondylitis

Ankylosing spondylitis is a chronic inflammatory disease of the axial joints. There is enthesopathy or inflammation at the site of insertion of ligaments, tendons and joint capsules to bone.

Epidemiology The disease usually appears in the early 20s, affecting almost three times as many men as women. Around 1% of the white population may be affected with considerable variation in incidence between different racial groups (Dieppe et al 1985).

Aetiology Affected persons appear to demonstrate a genetic predisposition with evidence that the disease may be triggered by an infective agent. The majority of patients have a positive gene and are said to be HLA B27 positive. Blood tests for ESR and CRP are usually elevated and radiological examination shows initial widening of the sacroiliac joints and in later stages fusing of joints with spinal deformity, often referred to as 'bamboo' spine.

Presentation Pain, stiffness and night pain in the lumbosacral area are often the initial complaints, the stiffness being worse in the morning and after periods of inactivity. As the disease progresses hips, knees, shoulders and all axial joints may be affected. Extraarticular disease may occur, including iritis, prostatitis, cardiovascular involvement and pulmonary fibrosis.

Management The aim of treatment is to:

- relieve symptoms and maintain posture and mobility
- educate the patient and family regarding a programme of daily exercise and advice regarding lifestyle changes such as preventing obesity and the use of firm mattresses with only one pillow to ensure a straight spine is maintained
- provide physiotherapy and hydrotherapy to encourage movement.

The use of NSAIDs to provide symptomatic relief will allow exercise programmes to be followed. Agents such as sulphasalazine and methotrexate may be required to control the disease.

Other diseases in this group include Reiter's syndrome and reactive arthritis, psoriatic arthritis and Behçet's syndrome.

BONE DISEASE

OSTEOPOROSIS

A metabolic disease causing loss of bone mass, particularly in postmenopausal women, often leading to fractures of the hip, wrist and spine.

Epidemiology

More women are affected than men with the incidence increasing probably due to an increasing lifespan and a decrease in physical activity (Badley 1991).

Aetiology

Postmenopausal osteoporosis is the most common form of the disease and may be caused by:

- oestrogen deficiency causing an imbalance in the reabsorbing properties of bone
- calcium deficiency due to inadequate diet
- inactivity causing disuse atrophy of the bone, similar to muscle mass loss due to disuse of muscles. Obese women appear to be protected, probably because excess weight places a physical strain on the bones.

Causes of osteoporosis include:

- long-term steroid therapy
- alcoholism
- renal failure
- carcinoma
- previous gastrectomy
- long periods of immobility
- rheumatoid arthritis
- long periods of amenorrhoea and anorexia
- hypogonadism
- smoking.

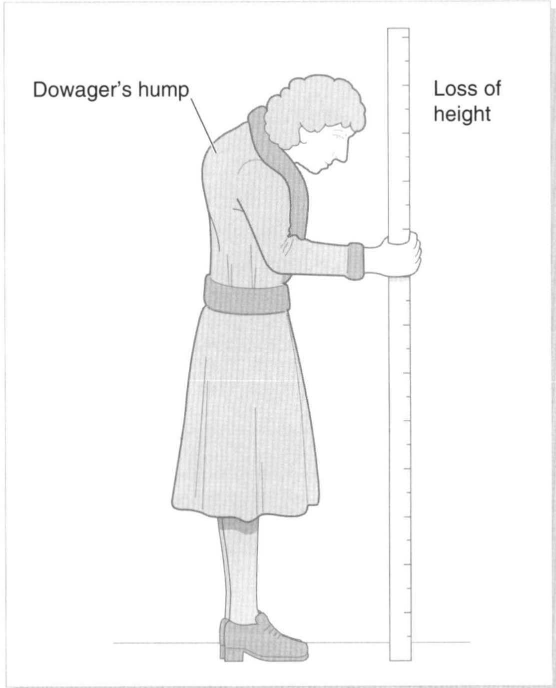

Figure 13.6 Typical patient with senile osteoporosis. Reproduced with kind permission from Dr Paul Dieppe.

Presentation

Fractures, particularly of the vertebrae, distal forearm or hips, may be the first indicator of disease. Gradual weight and height loss in advanced disease causing kyphosis of the spine may occur in a symptomless patient.

Management

As osteoporosis is not painful it is usually diagnosed when a fracture has occurred. Patients at risk of developing the disease and those presenting with fractures may have their bone density measured. Bone density measurements are not likely to alter management and may not be cost effective if ordered routinely. Reduction of risk factors and providing a safer home environment, with education to support exercise programmes, will be beneficial in preventing falls. The overall management of osteoporosis should be geared to prevention.

Drug therapy

Supplements of calcium and vitamin D may be used to prevent further bone loss and hormone replacement therapy (HRT) prescribed for postmenopausal women and those who have undergone hysterectomy.

Other diseases in this group include osteomalacia and Paget's disease.

CONNECTIVE TISSUE DISEASE

This group of chronic inflammatory diseases are found more commonly in women and affect many different organs in the body, giving rise to varied clinical manifestations.

SYSTEMIC LUPUS ERYTHEMATOSUS (SLE)

Epidemiology

A chronic autoimmune disease affecting mainly women and producing symptoms of varying severity. Disease onset is usually between the ages of 16 and 55 with the highest incidence in Afro-Caribbeans who have a worse prognosis than white patients affected by the disease. Thirteen times more women are affected than men.

Aetiology

Genetic factors appear to have an association with the development of the disease and environmental factors such as infection, drugs and exposure to sunlight are also thought to precipitate the disease.

Pathology

Histological changes in the skin include epidermal thinning and degeneration of the epidermal basal layer. Abnormalities of renal tissue may be seen on microscopy.

Presentation and clinical features

- Fatigue, malaise and reduced exercise tolerance
- Fever
- Weight loss
- Peripheral synovitis, generally non-destructive
- Raised macular facial rash which may appear after UV exposure and is usually short-lived
- Discoid lesions of the skin
- Vasculitis
- Alopecia
- Renal abnormalities with proteinuria and glomerulonephritis
- Pulmonary involvement including pleurisy and pneumonia
- Pericarditis and pericardial effusion
- Gastrointestinal symptoms including nausea and vomiting
- Neuropsychiatric abnormalities including depression, psychosis and seizures
- Lymphadenopathy

Management

Treatment is based on symptomatic relief as problems occur. Education and support should be provided for the patient, ensuring adequate rest during periods of active disease and avoidance of sun exposure. Good blood pressure control and urinalysis at frequent intervals to monitor renal function are paramount.

Drug treatment may include:

- NSAIDs
- antimalarial drugs
- local steroid injections
- corticosteroids
- disease-modifying drugs.

Other diseases in this group include systemic sclerosis, poly- and dermatomyositis, polyarteritis nodosa and Sjögren's syndrome.

NON-ARTICULAR DISEASE

This group of diseases affects the muscles, causing pain and weakness without joint involvement.

POLYMYALGIA RHEUMATICA (PMR)

Epidemiology

PMR is rarely seen before the age of 50 with the vast majority of cases occurring between the ages of 60 and 90 years. Women are affected twice as commonly as men and the disease is more common in caucasian populations.

Presentation

Onset of the disease is rapid with patients complaining of pain and stiffness of the shoulders, hips and thighs. Morning stiffness is a feature of the disease, often accompanied by low-grade fever, fatigue and weight loss. The shoulder girdle is most commonly affected and this may give rise to an inaccurate diagnosis of frozen shoulder. The ESR is almost always elevated.

Management

Corticosteroid treatment relieves symptoms dramatically and patients may remain on decreasing doses of steroids for as long as 2 years. Patients may be monitored using symptoms as an indicator of disease and relapses may occur without a rise in the ESR. Prednisolone 10–20 mg daily is the usual starting dose for uncomplicated PMR.

Giant cell arthritis (GCA)

GCA affects the same patient population as PMR and although it may be seen in isolation, is usually a complication of PMR.

Headache is the most common symptom, the pain being severe and localized to the temple region. Visual disturbances can occur and require rapid treatment to prevent blindness. Higher doses of steroids than for PMR are required, usually 40–60 mg of prednisolone. Temporal artery biopsies are often carried out in patients suspected of having GCA to confirm the diagnosis whilst some physicians prefer to use history and examination as evidence of the disease (Hazelman 1996).

FIBROMYALGIA SYNDROME

Fibromyalgia syndrome is a collection of symptoms including muscular pain, severe fatigue and multi-system 'functional' disturbance.

Epidemiology

The condition affects mainly women, most often between the ages of 40 and 50 years. It is most commonly treated in general practice.

Presentation

Widespread musculoskeletal pain and fatigue are accompanied by areas of tenderness at characteristic sites (Fig. 13.7). Patients may also complain of poor concentration and headache and may be weepy. Research in America and Canada in recent years recognized the hyperalgesic tender sites and secondly found an association with sleep disturbance. The exclusion of other pathological conditions is important before a diagnosis is made.

Management

The outlook for a rapid or complete recovery is poor (Sim & Vaghmaria 2001). Sympathy, education and understanding for the patient and family are important. The use of simple analgesics and amitriptyline in small doses to correct sleep pattern disturbances may be of help. Exercise programmes worked out for each individual patient may have a role to play. Self-help groups such as Arthritis Research Campaign and Stiff (UK) may be of benefit in providing educational materials and helpful advice (see Resources).

CARPAL TUNNEL SYNDROME

The symptoms of carpal tunnel syndrome are caused by the compression of the median nerve at the wrist as it runs through the carpal tunnel (Fig. 13.8).

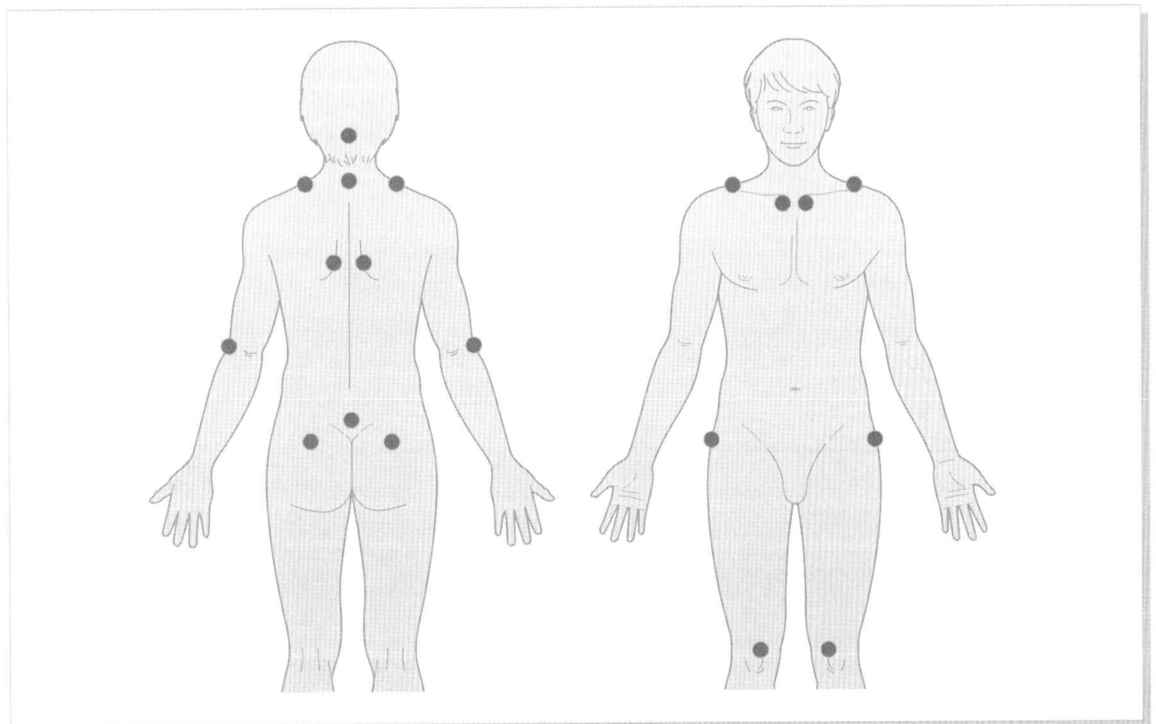

Figure 13.7 Sites of tender points in fibromyalgia. Reproduced with kind permission from the Arthritis Research Campaign.

Aetiology

In most cases no cause is found for the condition but fluid retention, obesity and a history of previous trauma appear to be common. Women are more often affected than men and are typically middle aged (Hawkins et al 1985).

Presentation

Numbness, pain, aching and tingling of the thumb, index and middle fingers are complained of. Sometimes the whole hand is affected and the pain extends up into the forearm. One or both hands may be affected. The symptoms are often worse at night, causing loss of sleep.

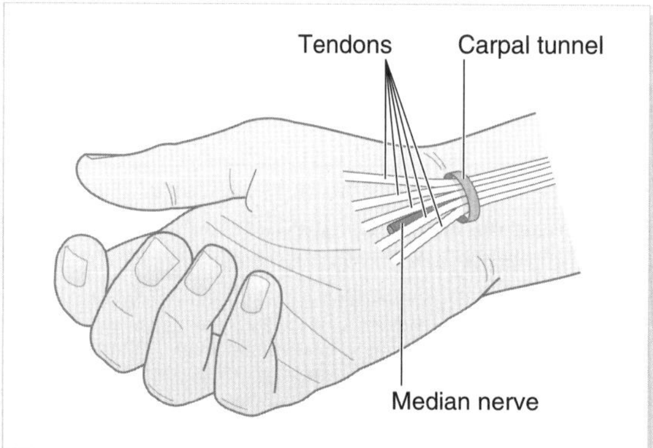

Figure 13.8 The tendons and the median nerve pass through the carpal tunnel in the wrist. Reproduced with kind permission from the Arthritis Research Campaign.

Physical signs include a reproduction of pain on percussion over the nerve at the wrist (Tinel's sign). Full flexion or extension of the wrist may also reproduce pain (Phalen's sign). Wasting of the muscles and loss of power may be present in advanced disease.

Electrodiagnostic studies may be carried out to confirm diagnosis.

Management

- The use of light resting splints worn at night may be all that is required in mild cases.
- Diuretics may be helpful for patients with oedema.
- Local steroid injections into the carpal tunnel are often effective and may provide temporary or permanent relief of symptoms.
- Surgery to reduce the pressure on the median nerve may be required if symptoms persist. The operation is usually carried out under a local anaesthetic.

THE PAINFUL SHOULDER

Van der Windt et al (1998) estimated that 25 out of every 1000 patients presenting in primary care do so with a stiff painful shoulder and that few of these cases are referred to specialists. The shoulder is a complex joint, depending on the surrounding soft tissues for stability and function (Fig. 13.9). Neck

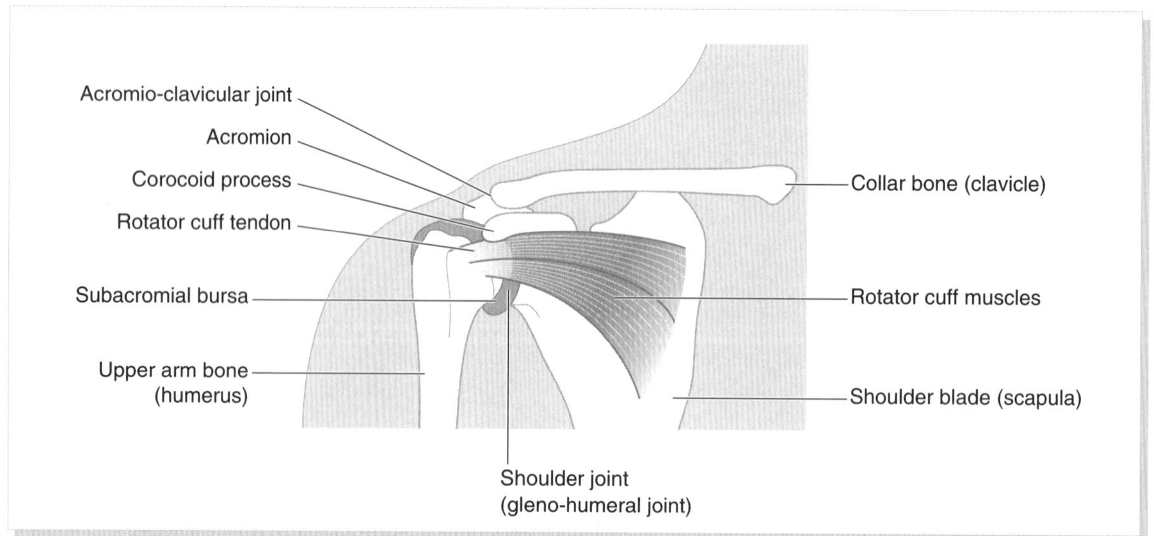

Figure 13.9 Shoulder joint region showing rotator cuff muscles. Reproduced with kind permission from the Arthritis Research Campaign.

disorders may present as shoulder pain and should be excluded before diagnosis is made.

Presentation

Patients suffering from shoulder problems can usually be divided into two groups. A detailed examination is paramount in forming the correct diagnosis.

- *Patients suffering pain on 'passive movement'*. This is movement performed by the examiner who holds and moves the joint through its range of movement with no effort being made by the patient. People with pain and restriction of motion on passive movement are described as suffering from 'intracapsular' problems. Rheumatoid arthritis and frozen shoulder are common reasons for this type of problem.
- *Patients suffering pain on 'active movement'*. When patients move the joint or limb themselves and have no pain on passive movement they are said to be suffering from 'extracapsular' problems or problems with the tendons and bursae around the joint. Tendonitis, tendon ruptures and bursitis are some of the common conditions in this group.

Frozen shoulder (adhesive capsulitis)

This condition may occur spontaneously or may follow trauma. It is commonly seen in patients between the ages of 40 and 60 years. The lining of the joint capsule becomes inflamed and severe pain develops and may last for weeks or months. There is restriction of motion in both active and passive movements and night pain may be a particular problem. It almost always resolves in time.

It is important with frozen shoulder that exercise continues unless pain is severe. Painkillers such as paracetamol or NSAIDs may be used. If pain is severe and continues cortisone (steroid) injections into and around the joint often help to relieve symptoms. Physiotherapy using ultrasound can be of benefit. A few severe cases of the condition may require manipulation under anaesthetic.

Tendonitis

Tears, partial tears and inflammation of the tendons around the shoulder joint (rotator cuff tendons) often present following unaccustomed exercise. Degenerative changes resulting in tendonitis are also prone to occur, particularly in occupations where excessive shoulder movements are necessary (Hazelman 1988). Pain is worst on using the muscles and tendons to move the arm. On examination there is no pain on passive movement. Complete tears of the tendons may occur with resulting weakness of the shoulder. Acute lesions benefit from rest and NSAIDs. Physiotherapy may be prescribed as part of the rehabilitation process. Tendonitis often responds to intraarticular injection of steroid. Occasionally surgery is recommended.

Other conditions in this group include Raynaud's phenomenon, tennis and golfer's elbow, bursitis, repetitive strain injury, chrondromalacia patellae, erythema nodosum and sarcoidosis.

ROLE OF THE PRIMARY HEALTHCARE TEAM

Research has highlighted the need for better, more structured care of rheumatology patients in the community. Davies & Suarez-Almazor (1995) found that NSAIDs were overprescribed and analgesics, joint injections and physiotherapy underused in patients with osteoarthritis. Helliwell & O'Hara (1995) reported that only 65% of patients with RA were receiving ideal monitoring.

The primary healthcare team is well placed to provide early diagnosis, education, treatment and monitoring and is able to anticipate the support a patient will require. The hospital rheumatology team are able to offer specialist knowledge and treatment to patients with more serious conditions.

The employment of increasing numbers of rheumatology nurse specialists has enhanced patient education and provided an opportunity for stronger links between the hospital and community.

SHARED CARE

Shared care is a clinically effective, cost-effective initiative that is acceptable to patients and general practitioners and allows more patients to receive specialist advice (Dargie & Proctor 1994).

Protocols and clinical guidelines can provide details of care to be administered in specific situations and can allow community nurses to maintain continuity of quality care when monitoring, treating and educating patients with rheumatological disease.

The use of shared care cards further improves liaison between the community and the hospital.

Chronic diseases such as diabetes and asthma are now routinely monitored and treated in nurse-led clinics at most general practice surgeries. At Sonning Common Health Centre in Sonning Common near Reading in the south of England, a community-based arthritis clinic has now been running since 1994. A joint protocol was developed following discussion with the hospital consultant and monitoring and education of all RA patients in the practice takes place in the clinic. Patients with other forms of joint disease attend the clinic by referral from other health professionals or by self-referral. The clinic provides an accessible service for patients and strong links have been forged with the rheumatology department at the local hospital, allowing rapid telephone access to sort out problems as they arise. The clinic is jointly run by a practice nurse and a district nurse who work side by side in the clinic, bringing together skills from both specialisms. The primary care trust in which the clinic is situated has allowed both nurses to undergo joint injection training, enabling patients to have rapid treatment without referral.

Case study: monitoring rheumatoid arthritis in primary care using a community-based arthritis clinic

Mary is a 45-year-old woman who has been a patient at the practice for many years. Married with two teenage sons, she rarely comes to see her general practitioner and has no relevant medical history and takes no medication. Mary works as a classroom assistant at a local primary school.

Mary first saw the doctor as she was complaining of painful hands and noticed that she was generally stiff first thing in the morning. The carpometacarpal joints on Mary's hands were swollen and red and gentle examination of the joints found them to be tender. Examination of the rest of the musculoskeletal system was unremarkable although Mary admitted that she had been feeling tired and under the weather of late. There was no history of RA in Mary's family. Blood tests were requested for full blood count, ESR, CRP, thyroid function tests and rheumatoid factor and Mary was advised to take NSAIDs by the doctor and to return for the results of the blood tests the following week.

Mary attended the surgery the following week to be told that her ESR and CRP were raised and that the rheumatoid factor was strongly positive, suggesting a diagnosis of RA. There had been no improvement in Mary's symptoms; in fact, she was having difficulty in using her hands without pain. On the recommendation of the consultant rheumatologist who was contacted by phone, Mary was given 120 mg depo-medrone intramuscularly to settle her symptoms and and an urgent appointment was made for her to be seen at the hospital. When seen by the consultant rheumatologist, Mary was commenced on methotrexate following baseline liver function tests and a chest X-ray.

Mary attended the surgery arthritis clinic where she received help, advice and education backed up with written literature regarding her condition and treatment. She was also counselled regarding side-effects that may occur. Mary continued to attend the clinic for monitoring and continuity of care was maintained using shared care cards for the recording of blood test results and any changes in medication. Monitoring continued using protocols developed with the hospital.

Mary has continued to be seen in the clinic which allows her immediate phone access to the nurses should problems arise. Mary has been well controlled on the methotrexate and her blood tests have remained satisfactory. Problems that do arise can usually be addressed by a phone call to the rheumatology nurse specialist at the hospital with whom strong links have been established since the clinic had been set up.

References

Badley E 1991 Population projections and the effect on rheumatology. Annals of Rheumatic Disease 50:3–6

Byrne J 1998 Medication in rheumatic disease. In: Hill J (ed) Rheumatology nursing. A creative approach. Churchill Livingstone, Edinburgh

Charlton C, Fleming D, McCormick A 1995 Morbidity statistics from general practice. HMSO, London

Cooper C 1994 Osteoarthritis epidemiology. In: Kippel JH, Dieppe PA (eds) Rheumatology. Mosby, St Louis

Dargie L, Proctor J 1994 Setting up an arthritis clinic. Community Outlook 4(7):14–17

Dargie L, Proctor J 1998 Seamless care. In: Hill J (ed) Rheumatology nursing. A creative approach. Churchill Livingstone, Edinburgh

Davies P, Suarez-Almazor M 1995 An assessment of the needs of family physicians for a rheumatology continuing medical education programme: results of a pilot project. Journal of Rheumatology 22(9):1762–1765

Dieppe P, Doherty M, Macfarlane D, Maddison P 1985 Rheumatological medicine. Churchill Livingstone, Edinburgh

Dieppe P, Chard J, Faulkner A, Lohmander S 2000 Osteoarthritis. In: Clinical Evidence. Issue 5. BMJ Publishing, London

Hawkins C, Currey H, Dieppe P 1985 Carpal tunnel syndrome. In: Butler R, Jayson M (eds) Collected reports on rheumatic diseases. Arthritis Research Campaign, Chesterfield

Hazelman B 1988 The painful shoulder. In: Butler R, Jayson M (eds) Collected reports on rheumatic diseases. Arthritis Research Campaign, Chesterfield

Hazelman B 1996 Polymyalgia rheumatica and giant cell arteritis. In: Butler R, Jayson M (eds) Collected reports on rheumatic diseases. Arthritis Research Campaign, Chesterfield

Helliwell P, O'Hara M 1995 Shared care between hospital and general practice: an audit of disease-modifying drug monitoring in rheumatoid arthritis. British Journal of Rheumatology 34:673–663

Horbury J 1995 Bone and joint disorders. In: Bradlow J, Bennet V, Breton S et al (eds) A health strategy for Oxfordshire 1995–2000. Oxfordshire Health, Oxford

Lawrence R 1994 Rheumatoid arthritis: classification and epidemiology. In: Klippel J, Dieppe P (eds) Rheumatology. Mosby, St Louis

NHS Management Executive 1991 Integrating primary and secondary care. Department of Health, London

Pisetsky D 1994 Rheumatic disease etiology: immune mediated inflammation. In: Klippel J, Dieppe P (eds) Rheumatology. Mosby, St Louis

Platt P 2001 The future of rheumatoid arthritis management. Future Prescriber 2(2):6–9

Sim J, Vaghmaria A 2001 How to recognise and treat fibromyalgia. Prescriber 12(8):99–107

Van der Windt D, Koes B, Deville W, Boeke A, Jong B, Bouter L 1998 Effectiveness of corticosteroid injections versus physiotherapy for treatment of painful stiff shoulder in primary care. British Medical Journal 317:1292–1296

Resources

Training

Joint injection training for nurses. Contact the Education Coordinator, Rheumatology Department, Cannock Chase Hospital, Cannock, Staffordshire

Patient information

Arthritis Care, 18 Stephenson Way, London NW1 2HD. Tel: 020 7380 6500. www.arthritiscare.org.uk

Arthritis Research Campaign, St Mary's Court, St Mary's Gate, Chesterfield, Derbyshire S41 7TD. Tel: 01246 558033. info@arc.org.uk

Useful addresses

British League Against Rheumatism, 41 Eagle Street, London WC1R 4AR. Tel: 020 7242 3313

Fibromyalgia Association UK, PO Box 206, Stourbridge, West Midlands DY9 8YL. Tel: 01384 820052. www.ukfibromyalgia.com

Lupus UK, 51 North Street, Romford, Essex RM1 1BA. Tel: 01708 731251

National Osteoporosis Society, PO Box 10, Radstock, Bath BA 3YB. Tel: 01761 471771

Primary Care Rheumatology Society, PO Box 42, Northallerton, North Yorkshire DL7 8YG

Stiff UK, PO Box 1484, Newcastle-under-Lyme, Staffordshire ST5 7UZ. Tel: 01782 562366. www.stiffuk.org

British Society of Rheumatology, 41 Eagle Street, London WC1R 4TL. Tel: 020 7242 3313. bsr@rheumatology.org.uk

Further reading

Arthritis and Rheumatism Council 1991 An introduction to the musculoskeletal system – a handbook for medical students. Arthritis and Rheumatism Council, Chesterfield

Arthritis and Rheumatism Council 1995 Collected reports on the rheumatic diseases. Arthritis Research Campaign, Chesterfield

Dieppe P, Doherty M, Macfarlane D, Maddison P 1985 Rheumatological medicine. Churchill Livingstone, Edinburgh

Ferrari R, Cash J, Maddison P 2000 Rheumatology guidebook. Bios Scientific Publishers, Oxford

Hill J (ed) 1998 Rheumatology nursing. A creative approach. Churchill Livingstone, Edinburgh

Chapter 14

Dermatology in general practice

Mags E Rees

CHAPTER CONTENTS

INTRODUCTION

The skin, the body's largest organ, clothes our features and presents us to the world; it is our protection from the elements and its invaders and covers our internal structures. All of us at some point in our lives will have some dysfunction of the skin. It is obvious and can be devastating when skin function is disturbed.

Skin conditions are often thought to be 'trivial' and 'minor' by those who do not endure them. Skin diseases can be fatal, chronic and disfiguring or at best short-lived but irritating. They are the reason for many consultations in general practice; a 6-month audit of a nurse practitioner's workload in one inner-city practice revealed that 15% of the consultations related to skin disorders (Rees 2000).

A rash may be a common reason for a consultation in general practice but recognizing that rash and knowing what to do about it is often a struggle. This chapter seeks to describe the common skin conditions presenting in primary care and how these are identified and managed and the particular contribution made by nurses in this process.

ANATOMY AND PHYSIOLOGY

The skin is a large organ containing over a million nerve endings. It consists of two layers, the epidermis and the dermis, and also the skin appendages – sweat glands, sebaceous glands, nails and hair. The skin varies in thickness, being thicker over the palms, back and soles and thin around the eyes.

The outer covering, the epidermis (stratified squamous epithelium), consists of five distinct layers.

The horny outermost layer of the epidermis, the stratum corneum, consists of flattened dead cells or corneocytes. A mixture of lipids and proteins is found between the corneocytes which provides the main barrier to water loss. Cell production in the basal layer allows a constant renewing of the epidermis. The main cell structure is the keratinocyte but there are also melanocytes which are responsible for the production of melanin, the pigment which determines skin colour. The epidermis has no direct blood supply and is nourished by the dermis.

The supportive dermis consists mainly of connective tissue which gives it its strength and elasticity. It consists of a highly vascular papillary layer and the reticular layer of collagen fibres which contains the sweat glands, hair follicles, nerves, adipose tissue and blood vessels. The nails and hair are skin appendages.

Sebaceous glands are associated with the hair follicles and they vary in numbers and size according to site, larger ones being found on the face, upper chest and neck. They are under androgenic influence, becoming more active at puberty. They secrete sebum, a lipid-rich substance which oils the skin and hair and has a bactericidal effect. When sebum accumulates and blocks a pore, a whitehead is formed; if the sebum then dries and oxidizes it forms a blackhead.

Sweat glands are numerous (2–3 million) and vary in size according to site, e.g. larger in the palms, soles and forehead. There are two kinds of sweat glands.

- *Eccrine*, which open directly on the skin surface as a pore and produce and secrete sweat.
- *Apocrine*, which are usually associated with the hair follicles and produce sweat and protein and fatty substances. Modified apocrine glands include the cerumous glands in the ear canal.

THE FUNCTION OF THE SKIN

The skin is a slightly permeable barrier that has several distinct functions (Fig. 14.1).

- *Protection from trauma and infection*. The skin constitutes a physical barrier against microorganisms. Normal skin commensals protect against endogenous pathogenic activity; sweat also has antibacterial properties. The immune function of the skin allows it to recognize and deal with harmful substances;

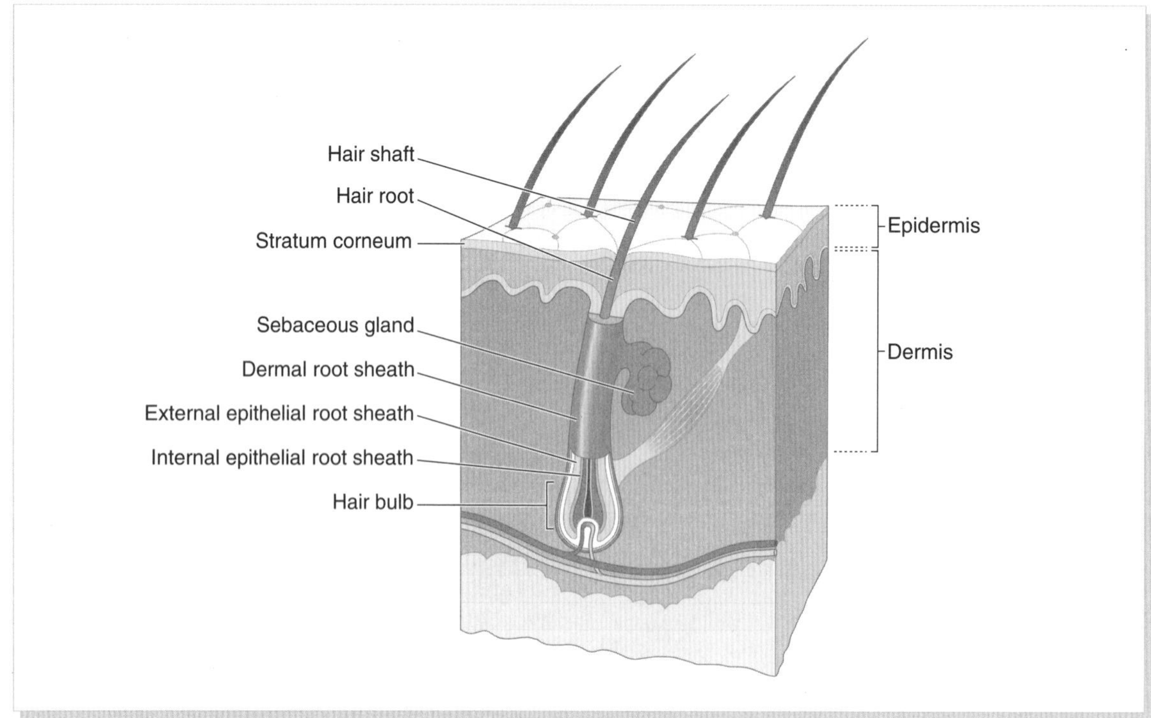

Figure 14.1 The epidermis and dermis and how the hair follicle relates to these.

however, hypersensitivity resulting from the immune system working against the body can cause problems, most commonly seen as an allergic response. Melanin protects the epidermal cells from the harmful effects of ultraviolet radiation (UVR).

- *Protection from dehydration* by preventing loss of essential body fluids. The structure of the outer horny layer of the skin makes it both tough and pliable and gives it the capacity to absorb three times its weight in water. It is when this layer dries out that this elasticity can fail (Gawkrodger 1997a).
- *Temperature regulation*. The subcutaneous fat provides a cushioning effect for underlying tissues and also protects from cold. Evaporation of sweat also aids temperature regulation.
- *Sensation*. The millions of nerve endings in the skin alert us to dangers from heat and cold, as well as aiding sensation and touch.
- *Endocrine*. On being exposed to sunlight the skin produces the precursor of vitamin D.
- *Psychosocial/sexual*. Skin plays a part aesthetically in social interaction and sexual attraction.

DERMATOLOGICAL TERMINOLOGY

Much of the mystique that surrounds dermatological consultations lies in its descriptive vocabulary. While it is useful to have a universal terminology it is acceptable to use your own words and to describe just what you see. Many dermatological texts will give you a glossary of words – one of the most useful for general practice is that given by Poyner (2000). It is important to describe and record what you see as this will aid diagnosis and allow comparisons to be made at later consultations. There are also helpful guides to doing this (Ashton 1998).

ASSESSMENT

Time is limited for both the practitioner and the patient in a general practice consultation but this should not detract from a thorough assessment of the presentation. The diagnosis may not be obvious when you first see a rash. 'The skin tells its own story but often takes its time to reveal itself' (Hughes & Van Onselen 2001). Ask patients to return as often as you need to review and treat. Putting patients at their ease is essential, especially as there is potential for embarrassment. Rapport is something that needs to be quickly established in the brief general practice consultation.

Listen

- When the patient explains why they have come
- To what their concerns are
- To what they think might be the cause or their anxieties about what it might be

Ask

Take a good history, remembering that skin symptoms can be an indication of systemic disease.

- Where/when/how did the rash start?
- Where did it spread?
- How does it feel – sore/itchy/hot?
- Does it weep?
- Has it changed?
- What treatments have been used and how were they applied?
- Medication?
- Does anything make it better or worse?
- What is bothersome about it?
- Are there any other systemic symptoms?
- Personal and family history including allergies?
- Has anyone else in the household got it?
- Occupation/hobbies?
- Lifestyle?
- Recent foreign travel?

Look

- Where
- Pattern/distribution/symmetry
- Appearance – is it scaly, wet, dry, inflamed?
- Is there evidence of excoriation?
- It is worthwhile examining the whole of the skin rather than just the part the patient offers (Peters 1998). Check nails and mucosa too
- Use a good light and a magnifying glass – it is surprising what a help this is not only for small lesions but also for defining the margins of a lesion and is particularly useful for looking at a potential skin malignancy
- Compare the sun-exposed areas with other parts
- Colour

Feel

- It is often worth feeling a lesion or an area where nothing much is visible to assess dryness/rough skin

- Is the lesion hard/soft or fluid filled?
- Scratching the surface may also tell you something – is it scaly?
- Palpating an acne can detect if there are deep nodules
- Stretching the skin over a lesion can also reveal clues, e.g. it may make more obvious the pearly appearance of a basal cell carcinoma
- Does it blanch with pressure?

EXAMINATION OF CHILDREN

This will naturally be different although it will include much of the same assessment. There is even more need to establish a good rapport with the child to ease the process and in a young child you will be depending on the parents' observations. The history should include additional information such as birth history, feeding and use of supplements, developmental history, sleep pattern, nursery/school routine and immunization history.

INVESTIGATIONS

Taking samples for laboratory investigation will aid diagnosis and avoid inappropriate treatment. Swabs and skin scrapings and urinalysis to rule out diabetes are simple tests that can be done in a practice consultation.

Skin swabs, for culture and sensitivity, should be done with a swab moistened with normal saline or transport medium, firmly rotating the swab in a zigzag motion over the whole of the surface of the lesion.

Skin scrapings should be taken by using a blunt scalpel or the blunt side of a stitch cutter. Scrapings should be taken from the scaliest part of the lesion and preferably from the active edge and transported on black filter paper. These are sent for culture, microscopy and mycology (Winsor 2000).

The patient may also be referred for other tests such as blood tests, especially where there is unexplained itch, or patch testing for contact allergic dermatitis.

PSYCHOLOGICAL ASPECTS

More than in any other aspect of bodily dysfunction, the psychology of skin dysfunction is of paramount importance.

> *The skin is the window into the patient's inner feelings, which are also often reflected through their facial expressions before they first speak.*
>
> (Mairis 1992)

Disruption of the normal skin function will be obvious in most skin conditions to a lesser or greater degree. Skin dysfunction has wide-ranging effects that are both physical and psychological. Pain and irritation are an obvious cause of upset but the psychological effect on self-image is often more difficult to bear. Embarrassment, pain and disability can lead to poor self-image and low self-esteem affecting both social interaction and job prospects (Chu 1993, Cunliffe 1986). The physical restrictions that skin conditions can impose and the time-consuming nature of treating with topical applications can be frustrating. The effect on the family in terms of time spent in using treatments, financial implications of medications, e.g. special clothing and bedding for parents coping with a child with eczema (Lawson 1998), are difficult to quantify but nevertheless real issues.

Recognition that the impact of a skin condition can be profound is increasingly accepted by clinicians. Research undertaken with patients who suffer skin conditions gives us an idea of what it is to live with them (Cotterill & Cunliffe 1997, Finlay 1997). A person's response to skin dysfunction is very subjective. Minor conditions can cause major misery for some people while others adapt well to extensive disease. Therefore any quality of life measures need to be independent of physical impairment (Lewis-Jones 2000). Tools to assess the effect on quality of life have been developed (Finlay & Khan 1994). Nurses have long understood that physical disease has a psychological effect and the importance of caring for patients in a way that embraces their whole life context (Adams 2000, Hughes & Van Onselen 2001, Popadopoulos & Bor 1999). These texts include eloquent examples from patients of what it is really like to experience a visible skin disease.

Patients may present in a variety of ways. They may be direct and come specifically with a symptom or concern about their skin. Patients may underestimate symptoms. They may consult for a completely different medical reason and yet it is obvious that there is a skin problem, e.g. a teenager with acne or an elderly person with a basal cell carcinoma. We need therefore to be alert to skin lesions and to signs and symptoms which may be serious. Developing a sensitive approach is also a prerequisite for skin consultations.

COMMON SKIN CONDITIONS

ACNE VULGARIS (Plate 1)

Acne is a common condition predominantly occurring in the teenage years but it can affect any age group. It starts at the age of 11–14, reaching peak severity between 17 and 21. It often occurs and peaks earlier in females because of earlier puberty and usually resolves by the age of 25, although it can affect older age groups. It has been said that 80% of people will experience some degree of spottiness (Graham-Brown & Burns 1996).

Hormonal changes can trigger acne, which usually starts at puberty when androgen levels surge in males. Androgens produced by the adrenal glands and ovaries also affect females – 70% of women report a premenstrual flare between 2 and 7 days before a period (Cunliffe 1981). However, acne is not a condition solely of teenage years and some women may develop perimenopausal acne.

Acne is characterized by spots, which range from comedones (blackheads) to nodulocystic lesions. The aetiology of the condition is not fully understood but involves the overproduction of sebum under androgenic stimulation, the blockage of the pilosebaceous duct and the action of bacteria, *Propionibacterium acnes*, and inflammation. The main sites for acne are the face, neck, back and upper chest.

Acne is as severe as the subjective view of the sufferer. However, clinically, acne is graded as being:

- mild – blackheads, small papules, pustules and non-inflamed lesions
- moderate – more extensive inflamed lesions, possible scarring
- severe – many lesions and significant scarring.

Managing the acne consultation

Acne, a common condition, causes much misery. Increasing understanding of the effect of acne on the psyche has led to a more systematic approach to treatment. Most patients with acne can be treated in general practice. Patients may consult directly because of the acne or they may offer other reasons for consulting, too embarrassed to mention their acne, particularly teenagers, and it takes some sensitivity to bring up the subject. It is, however, essential to give them information and management options.

Dispelling myths of acne aetiology is important – diet, hygiene and greasy hair are still propounded as causes. Time spent in explaining the causes and course of the condition will not only gain benefits for compliance with treatment but also ease the psychological burden of being 'unclean' for the patient.

Treatment options

The main emphasis in treatment is to avoid scarring. Treatment options will depend on the severity and site of the condition and the patient's wishes. Generally topical treatments are used initially for mild to moderate acne with review of these after 2 months, adding in systemic antibiotics if acne is not 50% improved (Chu et al 2000).

Topical therapy Benzoyl peroxide, e.g. Brevoxyl. Start with the lowest strength and apply for an hour intially and if tolerated, gradually increase the time with subsequent applications. It works by providing oxygen, thus killing *P. acnes*, which is an anaerobe. It is likely to cause irritation and can bleach hair and clothing. Using an emollient will help with the drying effect.

Topical antibiotics kill the bacteria which cause infection and also have an antiinflammatory effect, e.g. clindamycin (Dalacin T lotion). Applied twice daily, these are effective and acceptable to patients. Bacterial resistance is a problem and avoiding a different concomitant oral antibiotic can reduce this, as can combining it with benzoyl peroxide or zinc. Combination treatments are available.

Topical retinoids, e.g. Retin A gel or cream, Isotrex gel (topical isotretinoin), remove debris from the follicular canal to prevent blackheads. These are the favoured option of dermatologists because of the rapidly developing resistance to antibiotics of *P. acnes*, though they must be avoided in pregnancy. They may cause mild skin irritation, especially in the sun.

Adapalene is a retinoid-like drug which may be less irritant than other topical retinoids.

Oral therapy *Antibiotics* Oxytetracycline 500 mg bd is commonly used; it should be taken half an hour before food and dairy products need to be avoided. Compliance can be poor in teenagers who often eat erratically. It can cause gastrointestinal upset and vaginal thrush is common. It should not be given to children under 12 or pregnant women (causes tooth staining in the unborn). Erythromycin 500 mg bd is an alternative though bacterial resistance is a problem. Minocycline 100 mg od is well tolerated but there have been concerns regarding its side-effects (Garner et al 2001). Oral antibiotics should be given for at least 6 months; if there is no improvement after 3 months bacterial resistance may be the cause so a change in antibiotic is recommended. Using concomitant benzoyl peroxide topical application, 5-day courses every 6–8 weeks, may also prevent an overgrowth of antibiotic-resistant strains of *P. acnes* (Eady 1999).

Antibiotics potentially reduce the efficacy of the pill so women on oral contraception should be advised to use additional contraception for the first month of long-term antibiotic treatment and again if any diarrhoea develops.

Hormonal treatment for women Ethinyl oestradiol 35 μg/cyproterone acetate 2 mg (Dianette) can be effective on its own or in combination with antibiotics or topical therapy. It may also be prescribed with isotretinoin (Roaccutane).

Retinoids Moderate to severe acne or even mild acne where there is significant psychological distress will require referral to a dermatologist. Isotretinoin (Roaccutane) works by inhibiting sebum production and comedo formation and reduces inflammation and the number of *P. acnes*. It is given usually over a 4-month period. Isotretinoin is a potent drug that is teratogenic and women must be advised to avoid pregnancy while on treatment and for a month after. It can also alter the liver function. It is worth commencing an oral contraception such as Dianette prior to referral and take blood for LFTs and fasting lipids, all of which will be helpful in speeding up the initiation of therapy for the patient.

Side-effects of the treatment are sore, dry lips, skin and nasal passages and regular use of emollients will help. Patients should be advised to use mild soaps or a soap substitute and a moisturizer to counteract the drying effects of treatment.

Whatever treatment option is prescribed, monitoring of therapy and supporting the patient during the course lead to a more positive outcome. Side-effects can be a problem and good information about what might be expected at the start of treatment and a regular monthly review with advice on how to deal with side-effects can improve compliance. Patients should be experiencing at least a 50% improvement in the first 2 months; if this is not so then treatment needs modifying (Chu et al 2000).

ROSACEA (Plate 2)

A chronic, distressing condition, rosacea (Plate 2) is characterized by an erythematous, spotty, symmetrical eruption of the nose and cheeks. It tends to be progressive with exacerbations and remissions. More common in women than in men, it usually occurs between the ages of 30 and 50. Its aetiology is unknown but aggravating factors are the vasodilating effect of alcohol and other stimulant drinks, heat and sun and some foods, especially spicy ones.

Discussing with the patient the effect of the condition and how to adapt lifestyle is essential. Advice centres on limiting the aggravating factors such as extremes of temperature, stimulant and hot drinks, using gentle cleansing and make-up regimes, avoiding sunlight and using sunblock (Chalmers 1997).

Treatment is as follows.

- Mild – topical metronidazole cream
- Moderate – add oral antibiotic, e.g. oxytetracycline or erythromycin 500 mg bd, minocycline, doxycycline
- Severe – consider oral isotretinoin

ECZEMA/DERMATITIS

Eczema and dermatitis are interchangeable terms. Eczema accounts for a large number of dermatology consultations in general practice. There are two types:

- exogenous eczema – contact irritant and contact allergic dermatitis
- endogenous – atopic eczema, seborrhoeic eczema, discoid eczema, gravitational eczema, pompholyx eczema.

The range of eczematous conditions exhibit similar symptoms which are:

- inflammation
- dry skin
- itch.

Acute eczema will also include vesicle formation and these often rupture to form wet patches and crusting. Chronic eczema will include features of lichenification or thickened skin and scaling.

Contact dermatitis (Plate 3)

This is caused by an external agent, either an irritant such as a chemical, repeated wetting and drying of the skin or allergic, e.g. response to nickel in jewellery (Plate 3). An allergic contact dermatitis can be exacerbated by ultraviolet light. It can have employment implications, e.g. a hairdresser may have contact with particular chemicals. Referral to a dermatologist is necessary if there are continuing employment implications.

Management includes:

- history to determine cause
- patch testing to identify allergen in suspected contact allergic eczema
- exclusion or avoidance of irritant or allergen
- protection to avoid contact, e.g. wearing gloves
- regular use of emollients and a topical steroid if necessary.

Atopic eczema (Plate 4)

Twenty percent of children by the age of 7 will have developed some degree of eczema (Plate 4). The usual age of onset is under 1 year of age. By teenage years about 75% will be clear although there is a tendency for recurrence later in life. Aetiology is not fully understood but it is probable that the immune function is disturbed (Gawkrodger 1997a). The classic distribution of eczema is facial and flexural, particularly knees and elbows, although any part of the skin can be affected.

Atopic eczema is a distressing disease, which has disruptive effects on sleep and behaviour and therefore affects the sufferer and the family as a whole. It requires much time and effort in assessing, informing, teaching and supporting the patient and parent through treatment. Patients appreciate an explanation of the condition and guidance on the use of treatments (Long et al 1993). This is where efforts should be made to work collaboratively with doctors and with paediatric nurse specialists to give comprehensive, consistent advice to parents.

A careful assessment is necessary to determine the impact of the disease for the patient. This should include a physical examination to see the extent and severity of the disease and discussion of lifestyle issues and the impact of the disease on the patient and family.

Management There are several aspects to the management of atopic eczema, each of which has equal importance.

Avoidance of irritants

- Soap is very drying
- Wearing cotton rather than wool or synthetic clothing

Addition of moisture The use of emollients is a mainstay of treating dry skin; they provide a lipid surface to the skin to prevent further dehydration, reducing dryness and itching. A well-hydrated skin allows better absorption of topical medicaments such as corticosteroids (Hanifin et al 1998) and emollients themselves have an antiinflammatory effect.

There are several emollient preparations, each one made up of varying proportions of water and oil. Choosing an emollient will depend on the condition of the skin and patient preference – ointments are thicker and greasier and creams and lotions are lighter and often more acceptable to patients. Patients often find that using creams in the day and an ointment at night is acceptable. Some preparations are combined with an antibacterial, with an antipruritic to treat very itchy skin or with urea, a hydrating agent useful in scaly conditions which also enhances the penetration of other topical applications. Advice on keeping nails short will also limit the damage from scratching.

Most patients will benefit from a regime of bath oil, soap substitute and direct application of emollient to the skin. Teaching patients the importance of emollients is essential. Applying an emollient after a bath will aid its absorption. During the day frequent application, at least every time the skin feels dry, will necessitate carrying small daily quantities of emollient. It is therefore important to avoid giving the wrong message by prescribing small tubes of applications, e.g. a child with moderately severe eczema would need 500 g of emollient every two weeks and an adult 500 g every week (Kerrigan et al 2001).

An emollient should be applied thinly, in the direction of the hair growth so the skin glistens. It should neither be rubbed in, as this can block the hair follicles, nor applied thickly, which traps heat (Burr 2000). There is a potential for bacterial contamination of pots of emollients if regularly dipped into by hand so patients should be advised to decant a daily amount using a clean spoon into smaller pots (Hughes & Van Onselen 2001).

Dealing with infection Skin infection is often a complicating factor. *Staph. aureus* is found on normal healthy skin in 10% of the population and in the nose and perineum in about 35% of the population. However, in the atopic population almost all eczematous lesions are colonized with *Staph. aureus* which can also be isolated from other parts of their skin (McFadden 1999).

Skin infection is suspected if there is a deterioration in the eczema lesions or failure to respond to topical corticosteroids. Skin and nose swabs should be taken to identify the bacteria and treated with a topical or systemic antibiotic. Topical antimicrobial/corticosteroid combinations are useful only in localized eruptions of clinically infected eczema. A systemic antibiotic such as flucloxacillin will be necessary for more extensive or severe infections. Flucloxacillin on its own will not clear nasal *Staph. aureus* so a concomitant nasal application (mupirocin or neomycin ointment) is necessary. In repeated infected eczema, the use of an antiseptic moisturizer such as Oilatum Plus in the bath or Dermol 500 on the skin is advised and swabs should be taken from the patient's family to determine carriers of *Staph. aureus*.

Eczematous patients are more prone to other infections. Infection with the herpes virus causing eczema herpeticum is a serious condition requiring urgent antiviral treatment.

Topical corticosteroids Most atopic eczema exacerbations will require a topical corticosteroid at some point. These are synthetic corticosteroids, which have antiinflammatory, immunosuppressive, vasoconstrictive and antimitotic effects. They are available in different strengths; the most commonly used in general practice are weak and moderately potent steroids, e.g. hydrocortisone 0.5–1% (weak) and clobetasone (moderately potent).

Side-effects such as thinning of the skin are only a problem when potent topical steroids are used for a prolonged time. Corticosteroids are effective in improving eczema and are safe in the short term (applied twice daily for 2–4 weeks) (Charman 2000). It is more effective to use a more potent steroid for a short period than a weak one for a longer time. Steroid strength should be stepped down as stopping a steroid abruptly can cause a rebound effect. Aim to use the least potent steroid for the shortest amount of time to clear the inflammation. Ointment is the vehicle of choice here as it is greasier and does not contain preservatives which can cause hypersensitivity but patients need guidance on how to use it.

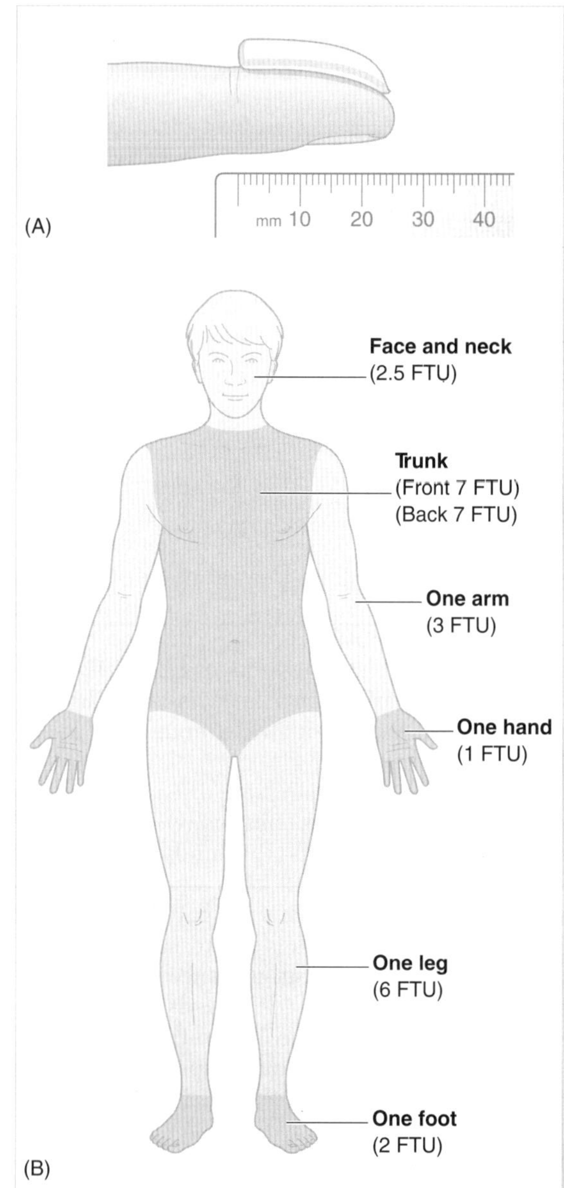

Figure 14.2 A: One fingertip unit. B: Number of fingertip units required to treat various anatomical sites once. Mean for both sexes (to nearest half FTU) (adapted from Long & Finlay 1991).

- Apply thinly.
- Apply twice a day (there are some once-a-day preparations).
- The exact amount required is measured in fingertip units (FTU) which is the amount of cream or ointment squeezed along the index finger from the tip to the first joint; 1 FTU = ½ gram. Use a diagram (Fig. 14.2) showing the divisions of the body to indicate to the patient how many FTUs are needed to cover a particular area. There are specific body diagrams for adults and children (Long & Finlay 1991).
- Current best practice suggests application 30 minutes after an emollient has been applied to allow even distribution.

Environmental House dust mite excrement plays a part in atopic eczema. There is some evidence that reducing house dust mites has some beneficial effect. Damp dusting, avoiding too many soft toys and washing them frequently, keeping the house well ventilated and if possible using hard flooring may all help. However, using special pillow and mattress covers is the most effective measure (Charman 1999).

Some patients experience a flare-up of eczema in the presence of animals. Here the wisest course of action is to discourage the introduction of a pet but avoid the stress of getting rid of an established, much-loved pet.

Wet wraps Occlusive bandaging in the form of impregnated bandages or wet wraps aims to maximize hydration and the effect of topical applications, additionally providing a barrier against scratching, and can be very effective for children with extensive eczema.

Wet wraps are usually tubular bandages soaked in emollient and/or water, covered by a second layer of dry bandaging. Occlusive bandaging should only be used where there is no infection. The skin is usually treated first with an emollient with a low potent topical corticosteroid on the affected areas. It is possible to guide parents on their use in general practice but time and much parental effort are required and referral to a specialist nurse is useful.

Antihistamine May be used in the short term where there is severe itching and where sleep is disturbed. It is unclear whether histamine is the cause of all itches (Beltrani 1999).

Gammalinoleic acid (evening primrose oil) This is licensed for prescription for eczema but there is little to support its effectiveness and it is costly.

Diet Some patients will ask about dietary triggers such as dairy produce allergies. There is insufficient evidence that dietary manipulation in children or adults reduces the severity of symptoms (Charman 1999).

Alternative therapies The evidence for the effectiveness of alternative therapies is lacking. Chinese herbal remedies are prescribed by dermatologists although their effectiveness is unclear and liver toxicity can occur (Sidbury & Hanifin 2000).

Other eczemas

Seborrhoeic dermatitis

- *Infantile* (cradle cap). This is a scaly, inflammatory condition of the scalp which can extend to the face. It is self limiting and is treated with a tar shampoo.
- *Adult*. More common in men, this causes mild erythema, scaling and pruritus in the scalp, hairline and areas around the eyes, nose and ears. Often a recurrent condition, it is thought to be associated with pityrosporum yeasts.

Treatment consists of tar shampoos, some containing salicylic acid and coconut. Anti-yeast products are also effective, e.g. ketoconazole shampoo (Nizoral) which should be used twice weekly for 2–4 weeks until the condition clears, then every few weeks prophylactically. Hydrocortisone 1% ointment bd may be used for the face.

Discoid eczema This presents as coin-shaped lesions of raised red skin with scaly, itchy plaques, usually on shins, calves and arms. It can occur in patients with no previous history or patients with atopic eczema can present with a discoid pattern. Management is the same as for atopic eczema.

Varicose eczema This is the dry inflamed irritated skin associated with venous insufficiency and leg ulcers and patients should be advised to:

- use emollients
- avoid irritants such as soap
- wear support hosiery
- mobilize to improve circulation
- use topical steroids if necessary and prescribed for inflamed areas.

Pompholyx eczema Usually on hands or feet. Of unknown cause, it is characterized by severe itching and an eruption of blisters, often leading to peeling of the skin and the potential for infection. It is treated with emollients and topical steroids in the early stages and may need more aggressive treatment if more severe.

PSORIASIS

This is a chronic condition affecting men and women equally at any age and characterized by inflammatory, raised, very scaly, discoid plaques which have a well-defined margin. The lesions affect any part of the body and can affect the nails and joints – some 7% of all psoriasis sufferers have psoriatic arthropathy. A disfiguring condition, it has a profound impact on life.

Its aetiology is poorly understood. The erythema is caused by dilation of the blood capillaries in the dermis and greatly increased proliferation of skin cells leads to scaling and thickened skin. The whole skin is affected so plaques can appear anywhere on the skin surface. Although the cause is unknown familial and immune factors are known to play a part (Griffiths & Kirby 1999). It may be triggered and aggravated by infection, skin trauma, medication (e.g. beta-blockers, antimalarials, lithium) and stress. Sun exposure aggravates it in only 10% of sufferers; the majority find sun beneficial. Hormonal factors also play a part; the condition usually peaks at puberty and menopause and may improve in pregnancy.

Scalp and *plaque* psoriasis are common but there are other manifestations.

- *Guttate* – common in children and often preceded by a streptococcal sore throat infection. Characterized by small drop-like spots all over the body (Plate 5) and may take 2–3 months to clear. While an emollient or tar therapy may help, there is currently no firm evidence to guide treatment (Chalmers et al 2001).
- *Flexural* – red smooth plaques often confused with a fungal infection.
- *Localized pustular* – found on the palms or soles of feet.
- *Generalized pustular* and *erythrodermic psoriasis* are acute, rapidly developing dermatological emergencies and require immediate referral.

Assessment

Determining the patient's knowledge and experience of the condition should be the starting point. Patients may have had many encounters over the years with clinicians and may have lost heart with management. Taking a history to include the patient's feelings about the condition, how it is affecting daily life and past experience with treatments will help assess current motivation to use treatments. Patients often have an anxiety about relapse of their disease. Supporting the patient and encouraging perseverance with treatment regimes is a valuable part of care.

Management

Plaque psoriasis (Plate 6) Emollients are an essential part of treatment and should be used at least once daily to remove scale and previous treatments and to soothe skin in preparation for topical therapies (see emollient use in eczema section).

In addition to emollients, a range of topical preparations are used to treat psoriasis (Plate 6).

Vitamin D analogues Vitamin D analogues, e.g. calcipotriol (Dovonex), tacalcitol (Curatoderm), normalize skin proliferation. They are applied twice or once daily to the plaques and gently rubbed in. Treatment is effective and acceptable to patients (Ashcroft et al 2000). Patients should be advised that a slight irritant reaction is normal. Encouraging perseverance with treatment is also important as they may take 8 weeks to be fully effective.

Dithranol Dithranol, e.g. Dithrocream 0.1–2%, is applied in graduated strength and for 30 minutes daily. Patients are advised to shower to remove the treatment. Necessitates precise application and protection of the skin adjacent to the plaques since it causes irritation and staining of skin and clothing. Often used with ultraviolet light (UVB) therapy in hospital.

Coal tar preparations The exact action of coal tar is unknown but it is thought to inhibit DNA synthesis. Still used in many bath preparations, creams and shampoos, it is effective although recent concerns regarding the carcinogenicity of coal tar may limit its use in the future. It may not be acceptable to patients because preparations can be smelly and messy.

Topical retinoids The action of these preparations, e.g. Tazarotene gel, is unclear but thought to normalize epidermal differentiation and to limit hyperproliferation and inflammation.

Topical steroids These treat the inflammatory process but not the hyperproliferation. Mild to moderate steroids should only be used for short periods in specific sites (face, scalp, genitals and in flexural psoriasis). The British Dermatology Association has issued guidelines for the use of topical steroids in psoriasis (Gawkrodger 1997b).

Phototherapy Ultraviolet radiation (UVA or UVB) is used three times a week for 6–8 weeks in patients who do not respond to topical treatments alone. The addition of oral psoralen, a light-sensitive chemical, can potentiate the action of UVA.

Scalp psoriasis Affects 50% of all those with psoriasis. Mild conditions can be treated with a tar shampoo, e.g. Alphosyl, and massaging with an oil will help to descale and improve dandruff. When there are thicker plaques an emollient with a keratolytic is necessary to remove scale, e.g. Cocois ointment.

Lifestyle advice

- General skin care – use of emollients.
- Correct application of treatments – it is useful to supply patients with written advice to reinforce this.

- Avoidance of aggravating factors.
- Keep home cool and well ventilated.
- Wearing light-coloured clothing can avoid the scaly patches and dandruff appearing so obvious.

Psychological effects of psoriasis

The condition is a particularly distressing one with major effects on self-image and social function. It has been shown to have a greater life effect than other chronic diseases (Finlay & Coles 1995).

Regular review of how patients are coping and effectiveness of treatments will be helpful. Providing a place to discuss their feelings and the stress of bearing the condition is important and helping them to explain the condition to other people when the need arises may be useful, e.g. it's not infectious, it's a common condition, it's a nuisance and difficult to treat as well as being unsightly. Long-term support will be necessary and patients should be advised to consult whenever they have concerns and at the earliest sign of a flare-up so that they can be referred on quickly. The Psoriasis Association is a useful source of information for the patient (see Resources).

INFECTIONS

When skin is damaged its barrier function is breached by microorganisms either bacterial, fungal or viral. Many of the most common skin infections are seen and treated in the primary care setting.

BACTERIAL

Impetigo (Plate 7)

The causative organisms are *Staph. aureus* or a streptococcus. Often this starts as a small spot or graze which rapidly enlarges and may exhibit superficial blistering and crusting, usually on the face or neck but can spread elsewhere. It also occurs as a secondary infection in patients with eczema or scabies. It is highly infectious and patients should be advised on hygiene and avoid sharing towels, etc. Children should be excluded from school until treated.

Treatment is with topical antibiotic for small lesions and oral antibiotic for more extensive or multiple lesions. The treatment of choice is neomycin (Cicatrin) or fusidic acid (Fucidin) though resistance is seen in some areas. Mupirocin (Bactroban) is an alternative but is an effective treatment for MRSA and should be reserved for this use.

Folliculitis

A *Staph. aureus* infection of the superficial hair follicles causing inflammation and irritation, mainly in the beard area in men. This is treated with a topical antibacterial or a systemic antibiotic if there is an extensive eruption.

Boils

An infection of the hair follicle caused by *Staph. aureus*, resulting in a hard, inflamed, tender nodule which sometimes comes to a head, discharging pus. A swab will confirm infection and a systemic antibiotic is usually necessary. If boils are recurrent swabs should be taken to detect nasal carriage of *Staph. aureus* and a urinalysis to rule out diabetes. Prevention measures such as using an emollient/antibacterial combination may be helpful.

Cellulitis/erysipelas (Plate 8)

An infection of the dermis and subcutaneous tissues, the causative organisms are *Streptococcus pyogenes* or *Staph. aureus*. Commonly occurring on the lower legs, oedema is a predisposing factor. It is characterized by a well-demarcated, unilateral area of inflammation, which is often oedematous and painful and sometimes blisters. The portal of entry is often through fissures in the webs caused by fungal infections. Treatment is with systemic high-dose antibiotic. Patients who are systemically ill need hospitalization.

FUNGAL

Fifteen percent of the population have a fungal infection of the skin or nails at any one time (Hart et al 1999). There are two types of organisms: dermatophytes which cause the tinea (ringworm) infections and yeasts, e.g. *Candida albicans*.

Tinea

Tinea infections are usually named according to their location, e.g. tinea pedis (fungal infection of the foot). Infection occurs usually after contact with skin debris containing fungal hyphae. It is vital to get a correct diagnosis of a rash since inappropriate treatment with a topical steroid will mask the symptoms. The steroid will deal with the inflammation but change the appearance of the lesion; the scaly edge will disappear, making subsequent management protracted. If the rash is asymmetrical and scaly and not obviously psoriasis or eczema, then tinea should be considered and skin scrapings taken for culture.

Tinea corporis (ringworm) This manifests itself as single or many scaly plaques (Plate 9) that clear centrally as they enlarge, giving the typical ringworm appearance.

Treatment consists of topical antifungals, e.g. Canesten/Daktarin applied twice daily for 2–4 weeks and for 1 week after clearance. Combining this with an oral antifungal may be necessary. Combination preparations of antifungal and topical steroid may also improve the response time. Advice regarding hygiene should be given and using emollients to keep the skin hydrated and potentiate topical medicines will also help. Encouraging perseverance with treatment will avoid recurrence.

Tinea pedis (athlete's foot) (Plate 10) Common in adults, this causes smelly maceration of the skin between the toes and can be complicated by bacterial or candida infection.

Topical antifungals are successful in curing this condition (Crawford et al 2000), the cheaper azoles being the first choice (Hart et al 1999), e.g. clotrimazole (Canesten) 2–3 times a day and for 14 days after lesions have healed or terbinafine (Lamisil) 1–2 times daily for one week. Combination antifungal/antibacterial preparations may be helpful. The patient should be advised to wash and dry the feet thoroughly daily, avoid communal bathing and sharing towels, wear cotton socks and non-restrictive footwear and to use an antifungal powder as a means of prevention.

Yeast infection

Candida albicans is a normal commensal of the digestive tract that multiplies and becomes pathogenic in warm, moist areas where skin is in close contact, causing:

- intertrigo, candida (thrush) of skinfolds, e.g. submammary, nappy area and groin
- chronic paronychia
- balanitis/vulvovaginitis
- buccal mucosal candida.

Characteristically skin becomes inflamed, sore and itchy with maceration and bleeding if it is not treated.

The appearance of a candida infection is very typical but if in doubt a skin swab will confirm infection. It is treated with a topical antifungal imidazole preparation, e.g. clotrimazole (Canesten) or miconazole (Daktarin), or combined with a steroid if severe. In the case of genital candida the sexual partner should also be treated. Urinalysis should be done to rule out diabetes. The patient should be advised to wash and dry the affected area daily and expose the area if possible.

Pityriasis versicolor

This is a common condition in young people caused by a yeast-like organism, which is a commensal that becomes pathogenic. It is seen as light brown, slightly scaly patches, usually on the trunk and arms, causing no symptoms. Skin scrapings will confirm diagnosis and it is treated with a selenium sulphide shampoo (Selsun) on the affected skin for a few minutes daily for 2–3 weeks and may also require a topical antifungal. It can recur, in which case treatment is repeated.

VIRAL

Warts

Warts (Plate 11) are a common presentation in primary care. Caused by human papillomavirus (HPV), transmission is by direct contact – touch, sexual contact or indirect contact such as from swimming pool sides. Thirty to 50% of common warts will resolve spontaneously, especially in children (Gawkrodger 1997a), but can take up to 2 years to do so. Painful and ugly, they can be the cause of much social distress.

Treatment Although there is a lack of evidence on which to base local treatment of warts, what evidence there is suggests that simple topical treatments containing salicylic acid have a therapeutic effect (Gibbs et al 2001). These can be bought over the counter. Patients need to be encouraged to protect the normal skin around the area to be treated and persevere with treatment long term (up to 100 treatment days) to effect a cure. An initial irritation will settle if treatment is stopped for a few days. Use of a pumice stone prior to treatment will help maximize the topical treatment.

Cryotherapy, which freezes the wart with liquid nitrogen, is used but is painful and therefore not suitable for children. There is no evidence that cryotherapy is any more effective than topical treatment (Gibbs et al 2001). Genital warts are usually treated with cryotherapy or topical application of podophylline (which should not be used in pregnancy). Women with genital warts or those who have partners with genital warts should be referred to the genitourinary clinic for assessment and have annual cervical cytology since HPV is associated with cervical cancer.

Molluscum contagiosum (Plate 12)

A DNA pox virus which causes tiny, pearly, umbilicated papules, usually on the face or trunk. Transmission is by direct contact and it is most common amongst the 2–5 year age group, particularly those with eczema or who are immunosuppressed. It is benign and will resolve spontaneously, although this may take several months.

Patients should be given information about the cause and course of the spots and advised to avoid sharing towels, etc.

Herpes simplex (cold sores)

Painful blistering sores around lips or genitals, these are highly contagious, transferred by direct contact. After the primary infection the virus lies dormant in the nerve, awaiting reactivation. Advice therefore centres on avoiding contact in the active phase. Sunscreens are useful to prevent further attacks. Topical aciclovir (Zovirax) five times daily for 5 days is prescribed in the acute phase and should be used as early as symptoms are noticed. Oral aciclovir can be used for more severe attacks.

Herpes simplex can be a serious complication for the immunocompromised or someone with eczema, causing the widespread eruption of eczema herpeticum.

Herpes zoster (shingles) (Plate 13)

An acute painful self-limiting eruption, usually presenting with pain and paraesthesia before anything is visible on the skin, followed by erythema and vesicles lasting 7–10 days. It occurs in people who have previously had chickenpox and can cause serious illness in the immunocompromised. The diagnosis can be unclear when the patient presents early with pain before a rash is visible.

Mild eruptions can be treated conservatively. When the face is affected prompt treatment is essential. The more severe cases, if presenting in the first 48 hours, should be treated with systemic aciclovir (Zovirax) or famciclovir (Famvir). There is some evidence that treating with aciclovir reduces the risk of postherpetic neuralgia (Jackson et al 1997). An analgesic is often necessary.

The patient will need information on the cause and course of the condition. Most people will need to know that shingles cannot be caught but since the virus is in the fluid of the vesicles, chickenpox can be contracted by someone who has never had chickenpox.

INFESTATION

SCABIES (Plate 14)

This is caused by the mite *Sarcoptes scabei* which burrows into the stratum corneum and lays eggs there, causing the host to start itching within 4–6 weeks of initial contact as a result of hypersensitivity to the mite. Burrows are classically seen between the fingers, in the axillae, periumbilical area, buttocks, penis and in the nipples of the female. In the elderly a truncal eruption may be seen and in children the face, scalp, palms and soles are often affected. Excoriation can cause secondary bacterial infection and an eczema-type appearance which can confuse the picture. Occasionally crusted (Norwegian) scabies occurs, particularly in the immunocompromised, which is resistant to routine treatment.

Management consists of application of a scabicide, of which there are several. Permethrin is the most effective with a 90% cure rate (Walker & Johnstone 1999); others include crotamiton, malathion and benzylbenzoate. All close contacts, irrespective of their symptoms, must be treated and this must be done on the same day to prevent reinfection.

Clear advice reinforced with written instructions should be given. Correct application is essential; the scabicide should be applied to cool dry skin (not after a hot bath which potentiates systemic absorption away from its area of action on the skin) and after the set time for treatment, should be washed off in plain water. Clean towels and bed linen should be used after treatment. Patients should be advised that itching may persist for at least 2 weeks post treatment. The outcome of treatment should be reviewed in 28–30 days as this is the time it takes for lesions to heal and for any eggs or mites to reach maturity if treatment has failed.

HEAD LICE (PEDICULIS HUMANUS CAPITIS)

Head lice (Plate 15) are most commonly found in children aged 4–11, girls more than boys and are a cause of much angst among parents. Considered now to be a community issue and not one for schools alone, a multidisciplinary approach to eradication is necessary.

Lice are found close to the scalp, the eggs closely adherent to the hair. Lice excrete faeces which is sometimes seen as black particles on brushing hair. Itching is caused by an allergic reaction due to the louse saliva.

Head lice are transmitted by prolonged head-to-head contact; the head louse is unable to fly.

Management

Treatment with insecticide should only be done where there is visible evidence of active lice – empty eggshells are not enough. Parents can be taught to detect lice themselves by wet combing onto white paper. Contact tracing is vital and treatment should be commenced if lice are detected (Aston et al 1998). Physical treatments such as wet combing have been shown to be ineffective (Dodd 2001).

Chemical treatment involves the use of permethrin (Lyclear), phenothrin (Full Marks) or malathion (Derbac-M); the latter two are not recommended for use in children with asthma or severe eczema. Treatment should be used according to the manufacturer's instructions as an initial treatment and again in 7 days. The recommendation of rotational use of insecticides has been superseded by a 'structured mosaic' approach, i.e. if live head lice are still present after the second treatment another preparation should be used. There is no evidence that any one insecticide is more effective than another so the choice should depend on local resistance patterns (Dodd 2001). Carbaryl is reserved as a third-line treatment since there are no published reports of its resistance.

There is no evidence for the effectiveness of alternative therapies such as herbal treatments.

Preventive measures after treatment consist of applying conditioner after washing and combing with a fine-toothed comb for early detection of recurrence.

CHILDHOOD INFECTIOUS DISEASES INVOLVING A RASH

Although most childhood infectious illnesses are regarded as a natural part of childhood, national immunization programmes have significantly reduced the numbers of some of these illnesses seen in the community. Consequently identification can be more difficult as many of us have not seen them before and also the few cases in non-immunized children have the potential to be more serious.

Assessment involves how long the rash has been present, how unwell the child is, the immunization history and sibling/maternal issues (Table 14.1).

SKIN TUMOURS

Growths on the skin are a common presentation in general practice. Most are benign but it is essential to be able to recognize possible malignancies. Many skin tumours are associated with the depletion of the stratospheric ozone layer and consequent risk of overexposure to ultraviolet radiation (UVR) from sun. The effect is enhanced with proximity to the equator and at high altitude where the sun's rays are strongest. Even in the UK, UVR is strongest between 11am and 3pm. The effect of UVA/UVB radiation on the skin is to cause sunburn and thickening of the epidermis, leading to decreased elasticity with consequent wrinkling and tanning. There is a link between excessive UVR exposure and skin cancer (Mackie 1989). Short, intense episodes of exposure and sunburn are more likely to cause skin damage (Austoker 1994).

PREVENTION

Primary prevention by educating patients about safe sun practices and actively encouraging social change in attitudes towards tanning is a nursing responsibility. Large-scale screening of the population is not practical but nurses with the knowledge and skill to recognize suspicious lesions are in a good position to integrate 'mole watching' into their assessments (Buchanan 2001).

Parents need to be particularly vigilant for their children. Motivating sun-related behaviour change is a challenge and should be done in a positive way, helping people to understand the dangers and consequences of sun exposure while still enjoying the benefits of leisure in the sun.

The following are the things that need to be achieved.

- Help patients assess their skin type.
- Limit exposure between 11am and 3pm and seek shade.

Table 14.1 Childhood infectious diseases involving a rash

	Incubation	Symptoms of prodrome	Rash	Complications	Infection period
Measles (Plate 16)	9–11 days	Coryza Conjunctivitis Fever	Koplik's spots on buccal mucosa Maculopapular red rash starting on face Older lesions become more blotchy Begins to disappear after 3–4 days	Conjunctivitis Otitis media Febrile convulsion Encephalitis	From 1 day before to 5 days after onset of rash
Rubella	14–21 days	Mild fever occasionally	Widespread fine discrete macular rash on face and trunk May not be present in up to 25% of cases	Risk to fetus	From 7 days before to 5 days after onset of rash
Chickenpox (Plate 17)	14–21 days	Mild fever	A progression of macular-papular – vesicle – pustule Spots on trunk and face appearing in crops can extend to whole of skin and mucosal areas	Secondary bacterial infection Rarely pneumonia Encephalitis	From 2 days before spots appear until all vesicles have dried
Parvovirus B19 (slapped cheek) (Plate 18)	5–7 days	Mild systemic symptoms	Intensely red raised rash on cheeks with circumoral pallor	Arthralgia can cause fetal death in <10% of cases if contracted in pregnancy	During the incubation period only
Coxsackie A virus (hand, foot and mouth disease)	5–14 days	Fever	Crops of small vesicles in mouth, on palms and soles of feet	Nil	From 2 days before to 7 days after the onset of spots

- Advise about sun avoidance measures. Cover up and wear loose, dark, closely woven clothing which gives most sun protection. Wearing a hat is also helpful. Several companies now manufacture clothing which has a sun protection factor.
- With children aim never to allow the skin to redden or burn.
- Advise on the use of suncreams to avoid burning in the sun. The SPF is the amount of time it takes from exposure before reddening occurs compared with untreated skin so using a factor 15 suncream means that it should take 15 times longer to cause burning; this is an arbitrary figure as other factors are involved such as the thickness of the application, rubbing off with movement. Sunscreens should block both UVA and UVB radiation and a factor of 15 or above is necessary. Sunscreen should be applied 20 minutes before exposure and should be reapplied every 2 hours and after swimming and exercise.
- Advise patients to regularly examine the skin for changes or new moles.
- Examine the skin, especially the face, as part of a routine health check.

BENIGN EPIDERMAL TUMOURS

Seborrhoeic keratosis (basal cell papilloma)

A benign, usually pigmented, uniformly round or oval, warty tumour caused by proliferation of basal keratinocytes. More common now with an ageing population, they occur in multiple numbers on the trunk or face.

Treated with curettage or shave biopsy, cryotherapy (liquid nitrogen) is also used if it is certain that it is not melanoma.

Actinic (solar) keratosis

These are hyperkeratotic, red, scaly papules in sun-exposed sites, especially the backs of hands, face and bald scalps (Plate 19). They may progress to squamous cell carcinoma. If malignancy is not suspected, cryotherapy can be used or otherwise an excision biopsy. Further sun exposure should be avoided.

Bowen's disease

A common squamous cell carcinoma in situ occurring typically on the lower leg of elderly women. It consists of pink, sometimes lightly pigmented, well-demarcated, thickened scaly plaques, single or multiple (Plate 20). They are related to solar damage, are slow growing and rarely invasive. They can present as an ulcerated lesion and should be considered as a possible diagnosis in a leg ulcer that fails to heal.

Treatment is by cryotherapy, excision or curettage.

Basal cell carcinoma (BCC) (rodent ulcer) (Plate 21)

This is the most common form of skin cancer and is usually found in middle-aged or elderly people, on sun-exposed sites on the upper face, around the nose, eyes or temple. Local destruction of tissues can occur but they hardly ever metastasize. Early recognition will limit the extent and scarring of treatment. The appearance is a small, skin-coloured papule, which typically has a rolled pearly edge with telangiectasia or, less commonly, a cystic or superficial plaque-like tumour.

Surgical excision is the treatment of choice. Patients should be reviewed for any new lesions and advised to report any other lesions that may appear and fail to heal. Elderly people with a history of skin cancer should avoid excessive sun exposure.

MALIGNANT TUMOURS

Squamous cell carcinoma

A malignant tumour arising from an area of damaged skin which can metastasize, usually found in men more than women and over the age of 55. It is a rapidly growing, fleshy nodule (Plate 22), which can ulcerate and is faster growing and more aggressive than a BCC. It is usually found in sun-exposed sites, e.g. face, neck or forearm, and in these areas it rarely metastasizes. It can also occur at sites of skin damage such as ulcers, burn scars or irradiated areas. Squamous cell carcinoma on sun-exposed areas has a higher risk of metastasis.

Treatment is by wide surgical excision and large defects may need skin grafting. Early detection allows less radical treatment and better prognosis. Advice should include protection against further sun damage and follow-up to check for recurrence, further lesions and lymph involvement.

Malignant melanoma (Plate 23)

A rare but dangerous skin cancer which affects the melanin-producing cells in the epidermis. It is increasing in incidence, accounting for 2% of all cancers in the UK (CRC 1997), doubling in numbers every decade and there is a causal relationship with UVR. It metastasizes and is the most common cancer in women aged between 25 and 29 and second only to breast cancer in the 30–50 age group (Marks 1992).

Malignant melanoma can arise from a new mole or a preexisting mole that undergoes a change. Prognosis depends on the anatomical site, the size, spread and most significantly the microscopic thickness of the tumour.

It is vital to be aware of a change in a preexisting mole or the appearance of a new mole. Early detection and treatment means a better prognosis.

Signs of melanoma

Asymmetry – one half of the mole different from the other half
Bleeding
Colour – variation across the mole
Diameter – larger than 7 mm
Edges irregular
Feeling – is it itchy, painful?
Growth – is it getting bigger?

If any of these signs are present an urgent referral to dermatology is necessary. To confirm the diagnosis, the mole is excised completely and once histology confirms the diagnosis a second wider excision is done. Patients will require support as they undergo treatment and advice regarding sun protection and inspection of other moles.

CONCLUSION

To be effective, clinical care must be based on current knowledge of best practice. Access to education and evidence-based information is increasingly available. Nurses must acquire the skill not only of accessing such knowledge and critically assessing the quality of the findings but also of finding ways of implementing the findings in their current practice.

The culture in general practice, where autonomy in decision making may be outside the nurse's role, is one which can militate against nurse-led change of practice (Dickson & Morrison 1999). However, there are encouraging signs of change in some practices where collaborative work between nurses and doctors has established advances in evidence-based care. One area where there is little specific general practice research and development is in the dermatological field and it is therefore an ideal area for collaborative work in developing evidence-based practice and even in developing the evidence itself.

Acknowledgement

The author would like to acknowledge Dr Peter Holt, Consultant Dermatologist University Hospital of Wales, Sr Ann Davies, Dermatology Nurse Specialist UHW, and Mrs Lynette Stride (patient) for their help in preparing this chapter.

References

Adams T 2000 Beyond the skin. British Journal of Dermatology Nursing 4(4):16–17

Ashcroft D, Po A, Williams H, Griffiths C 2000 Systematic review of comparative efficacy and tolerability of calcipotriol in treating chronic plaque psoriasis. British Medical Journal 320:963–967

Ashton R 1998 The art of describing skin lesions. Part 2. Dermatology in Practice 16(3):9–13

Aston R, Duggal H, Simpson J 1998 Head lice: report for consultants in communicable disease control. Public Health Medicine Environmental Group Executive Committee. HMSO, London

Austoker J 1994 Melanoma prevention and early diagnosis. British Medical Journal 308:1682–1686

Beltrani V 1999 Managing atopic eczema. Dermatology Nursing 11(3):171–185

Buchanan P 2001 Skin cancer. Nursing Standard 15(45):45–52

Burr S 2000 Using emollients. Nursing Times Plus 96(27):15

Chalmers DA 1997 Rosacea: recognition and management for the primary care provider. Nurse Practitioner 22(10):18–30

Chalmers RJG, O'Sullivan T, Owen CM, Griffiths CEM 2001 Interventions for guttate psoriasis (Cochrane Review). Cochrane Library 2. Update Software, Oxford

Charman C 1999 Clinical review: atopic eczema. British Medical Journal 318:1600–1604

Charman C 2000 Atopic eczema. Clinical Evidence 3:797–808

Chu A 1993 Acne in women. Well Woman Team Issue 11. Medicom UK, London

Chu A, Poyner T, Rose A 2000 Acne – the challenge in general practice. A&M Publishing, Surrey

Cotterill JA, Cunliffe WJ 1997 Suicide in dermatological patients. British Journal of Dermatology 137(2):246–250

Crawford F, Hart R, Bell-Syer S, Torgerson D, Young P, Russell I 2000 Topical treatments for fungal infections of the skin and nails of the foot. Cochrane Library 1. Update Software, Oxford

CRC 1997 Cancer statistics. Office for National Statistics, London

Cunliffe WJ 1981 Acne. Update Postgraduate Centre Series. Update Publications, London

Cunliffe WJ 1986 Acne and unemployment. British Journal of Dermatology 115(3):386

Dickson R, Morrison C 1999 Nursing and evidence-based practice: a world away from evidence-based health. In: Gabbay M (ed) The evidence-based primary care handbook. Royal Society of Medicine Press, London

Dodd C 2001 Interventions for treating head lice (Cochrane Review). Cochrane Library 3. Update Software, Oxford

Eady EA 1999 Treating acne: what is the role of benzoyl peroxide? Medicine Matters in General Practice 1:1–4

Finlay AY 1997 Quality of life measurement in dermatology: a practical guide. British Journal of Dermatology 136(3):305–314

Finlay AY, Coles EC 1995 The effect of severe psoriasis on the quality of life of 369 patients. British Journal of Dermatology 132:236–244

Finlay AY, Khan GK 1994 Dermatology Life Quality Index (DLQI): a simple practical measure for routine clinical use. Clinical and Experimental Dermatology 19(3):210–216

Garner SE , Eady EA, Popescu C, Newton J, Li Wan Po A 2001 Minocycline for acne vulgaris: efficacy and safety (Cochrane Review) Cochrane Library 2. Update Software, Oxford

Gawkrodger D 1997a Dermatology: an illustrated colour text, 2nd edn. Churchill Livingstone, London

Gawkrodger DJ 1997b Current management of psoriasis. Journal of Dermatological Treatment 8:27–55

Gibbs S, Harvey I, Sterling J, Stark R 2001 Local treatments for cutaneous warts (Cochrane review). Cochrane Library 2. Update Software, Oxford

Graham-Brown R, Burns T 1996 Lecture notes on dermatology, 7th edn. Blackwell Science, Oxford

Griffiths CEM, Kirby B 1999 Psoriasis. Martin Dunitz, London

Hanifin JM, Herbert AA, Mays SR et al 1998 Effects of a low potency corticosteroid lotion plus a moisturising regimen in the treatment of atopic dermatitis. Current Therapy Research 59:227–233

Hart R, Bell-Syer SE, Crawford F et al 1999 Systematic review of topical treatments for fungal infections of the skin and nails of the feet. British Medical Journal 319:79–82

Hughes E, Van Onselen J 2001 Dermatology nursing: a practical guide. Churchill Livingstone, London

Jackson JL, Gibbons R, Meyer G et al 1997 The effect of treating herpes zoster with oral aciclovir in preventing post herpetic neuralgia. A meta analysis. Archives of Internal Medicine 157:909–912

Kerrigan P, Hale C, Lowe J, Newton-Bishop J 2001 The value and use of emollients in eczema. Practitioner 245:1–4

Lawson V 1998 The family impact of childhood atopic dermatitis: the Dermatitis Family Impact Questionnaire. British Journal of Dermatology 138(1):107–113

Lewis-Jones S 2000 The psychological impact of skin disease. Nursing Times Plus (Skin Care) 96(27):2–4

Long CC, Finlay A 1991 The finger tip unit – a new practical measure. Clinical and Experimental Dermatology 16(6):444–447

Long CC, Funnell CM, Collard R, Finlay AY 1993 What do members of the National Eczema Society really want? Clinical and Experimental Dermatology 18:516–522

Mackie RM 1989 Skin cancer. Martin Dunitz, London

Mairis E 1992 Four senses for a full skin assessment: observation and assessment of the skin. Professional Nurse 7(6):376–380

McFadden J 1999 What is the role of Staphylococcus aureus in atopic eczema? CME Bulletin of Dermatology 2:4–6

Peters J 1998 Assessment of patients with a skin condition. Practice Nurse 15(9):525–530

Popadopoulos L, Bor R 1999 Psychological approaches to dermatology. BPS Books, Leicester

Poyner TF 2000 Common skin diseases. Blackwell, Oxford

Rees ME 2000 Self-audit of a nurse practitioner's workload over six months (personal)

Sidbury R, Hanifin JM 2000 Old, new and emerging therapies for atopic dermatitis. Dermatology Clinics 18(1):1–11

Walker GJA, Johnstone PW 1999 Treating scabies. Cochrane Library 4. Update Software, Oxford

Winsor A 2000 Sampling techniques. Nursing Times Plus 96(27):12–13

Resources

Training for nurses

Diploma in Dermatology Nursing, UWCM/Royal Gwent Hospital. Contact the Course Administrator on 01633 238561

Acne Distance Learning Programme for Nurses, Acne Support Group (see below for address)

Useful addresses

British Dermatological Nursing Group, affiliated to the British Association of Dermatologists. Membership, including excellent quarterly journal, £15. Primary care nurses are encouraged to become members. Tel: 020 7383 0266. Email: admin@bad.org.uk

National Eczema Society and Skin Care Campaign. Tel: 020 7388 4097. Information line: 020 7388 3444. www.eczema.org/www.skincarecampaign.org

Acne Support Group. Tel: 020 8561 6868. www.stopspots.org.uk/www.m2w3.com/acne

Psoriasis Association. Tel: 01604 711129. Email: mail@psoriasis.demon.co.uk

Useful websites

University of York Centre for Evidence-Based Nursing: www.york.ac.uk/evidence. Part of the UK national network of centres for evidence-based practice

Teaching/learning resource for EBP: www.mdx.ac.uk/www.rctsh/ebp/main.htm. A site to aid learning in evidence-based practice

Nursing and Health Care Resources on the Net – Netting the Evidence: www.shef.ac.uk. Web links to evidence-based sites

Skin Care Campaign: www.skincarecampaign.org

Bandolier – NHS Directorate: www.jr2.ox.ac.uk/bandolier. Contains bullet points of evidence-based medicine

TRIP database: www.tripdatabase.com. Turning Research into Practice – a site with relevance to general practice

Further reading

Hughes E, Van Onselen J 2001 Dermatology nursing: a practical guide. Churchill Livingstone, London

Poyner TF 2000 Common skin diseases. Blackwell, Oxford

Chapter 15

Anticoagulation monitoring

Nancye Carr

CHAPTER CONTENTS

INTRODUCTION

Few drugs can claim the notoriety that is attributed to the anticoagulant warfarin sodium. Nor can many drugs boast being the focus for the Nobel Prize or the subject of an international standard, the international normalized ratio (INR). Warfarin, an acronym from the first letters of the Wisconsin Alumni Research Foundation, went on to become the anticoagulant of choice in Britain and worldwide, a position it still holds today.

Over recent years the number of people taking warfarin has more than doubled, with each person requiring regular INR blood monitoring at intervals of 1–12 weeks. This can be attributed to the growing body of evidence that demonstrates that anticoagulant therapy prevents strokes in patients with non-rheumatic atrial fibrillation and reduces the risks of mortality and cardiovascular morbidity after an acute myocardial infarction (MI) (ASPECT Research Group 1994, EAF Study Group 1993, 1995).

It has been estimated that we now have one INR being done to every six full blood counts (Bevan 2000). The increase in demand for anticoagulant monitoring has resulted in a greater proportion of services being moved into primary care.

This chapter aims to provide the nurse working in primary care with the physiology, pharmacokinetics and management knowledge required to lead an anticoagulation service that adheres to clinical governance standards of care.

UNDERSTANDING WARFARIN SODIUM

Warfarin is an oral coumarin anticoagulant given once a day in a dose tailored to the individual patient's response and anticoagulant requirements. It is most commonly prescribed because of its predictable onset, low incidence of side-effects and excellent bio-availability (Reynolds 1996).

So why is warfarin management, unlike other drugs, the focus of so much attention? The differentiating factor is that warfarin has a very high risk/benefit profile (Ansell 1997).

- *It has a narrow therapeutic index.* Relatively small changes in systemic warfarin concentration can lead to excessive anticoagulation and haemorrhage or to inadequate anticoagulation and a thrombotic event. Even in the presence of a stable concentration warfarin can display a pharmacodyamic response to certain factors (Ansell 1997, 1998).
- *Its action is affected by numerous concomitant factors.* There is a positive correlation between specific patient characteristics and co-morbidities and resultant adverse events (Ansell 1997, 1998).

Based on this evidence it is clear that to ensure safe effective management of patients, prescribing warfarin requires a clinical and theoretical knowledge that accounts for all influencing factors.

PHARMACOLOGY

Warfarin acts by inhibiting the synthesis of vitamin K-dependent clotting factors II, VII, IX, X and the naturally occurring endogenous proteins C and S. The degree of anticoagulant inhibition is dependent upon the dose administered and occurs primarily in the liver (Hirsh 1991, Reynolds 1996). The antagonistic effect of warfarin upon vitamin K reduces the rate at which these factors and proteins are produced and produces a state of anticoagulation (Horton & Bushwick 1999, PIENO 2002). This results in a prolongation of bleeding time that is measured as an international standard, the INR. It follows that a transfusion of vitamin K and plasma protein will overcome the effect of warfarin.

Warfarin has a narrow therapeutic margin between the therapeutic and the toxic dose.

Pharmacokinetic interactions

Pharmacokinetic interactions influence the dose response to warfarin by causing a difference in its absorption, distribution or metabolic clearance.

Absorption Warfarin is taken orally and is readily absorbed from the stomach and small intestine and can also be absorbed through the skin. It has no effect on existing thrombi and its anticoagulant properties occur following the clearance of circulating coagulation factors. Each factor has a different half-life, with factor II (prothrombin) taking up to 5 days to be eliminated (BMA/RPS 2002, Carr 1998, Horton & Bushwick 1999, PIENO 2002). This means that with normal hepatic function the effect of warfarin will not be detected until 24–36 hours after the first dose, with the maximum anticoagulation effect reached in 72–96 hours. Thus the warfarin tablet taken on day one exerts its maximum effect on day 2–3 and is still exerting its effect on day 5.

Distribution 97% to 99% of warfarin is rendered inactive because it is bound to plasma protein,

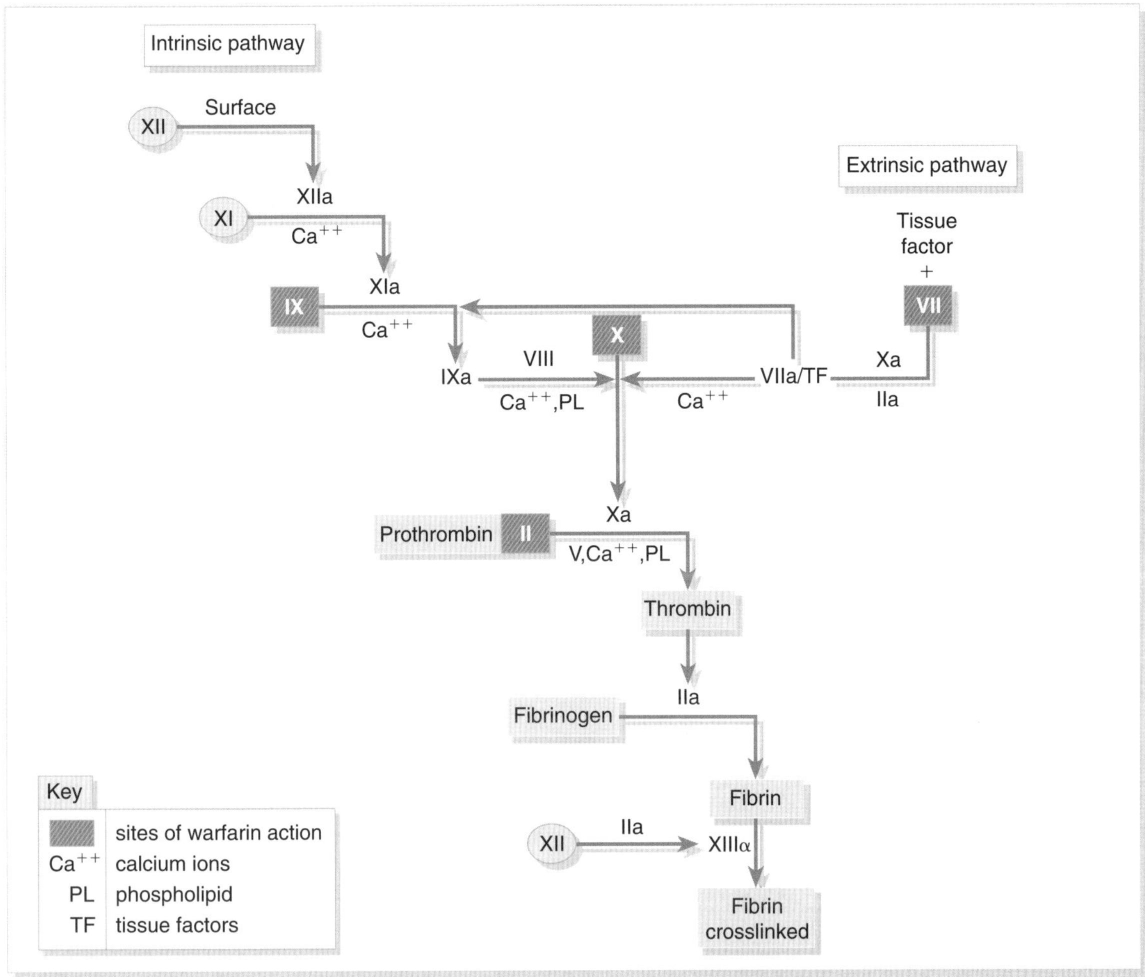

Figure 15.1 Network of interaction: sites of warfarin action. Modified from Ansell E, Oertel LB 1997 *Managing oral anticoagulation therapy.*

primarily albumin; it is only the remaining free unbound drug that actively exerts its effect on coagulation factors (Carr 1998, Horton & Bushwick 1999, PIENO 2002, Wittowsky 1997). It is important to note that this protein-bound aspect of warfarin pharmacokinetics has, in certain circumstances, the ability to increase and decrease with a corresponding increase or decrease in anticoagulation.

Warfarin is distributed to the liver, lungs, spleen and kidneys (PIENO 2002). It crosses the placenta barrier and is a major teratogen and can cause fetal haemorrhage particularly in the first and third trimesters, but it is not thought to affect breast milk (BMA/RPS 2002, Kearon & Hirsh 1997).

Metabolism Warfarin is metabolized in the liver by hepatic microsomal enzymes to produce metabolites.

Elimination These metabolites have negligible or no anticoagulation activity and are excreted in the urine following reabsorption from the bile (Reynolds 1996).

Pharmacodynamic interactions

Pharmacodynamic interaction occurs when the effects of another substance cause a difference in the haemostatic response to a given concentration of warfarin (National Prescribing Centre 1999). All interactions can increase the risk of a thromboembolic or haemorrhagic event.

Drug interactions are most likely to occur when an interacting drug is started, the dose is adjusted or the drug is stopped (Carr 1998). The time course of the interaction can vary depending upon the dosage,

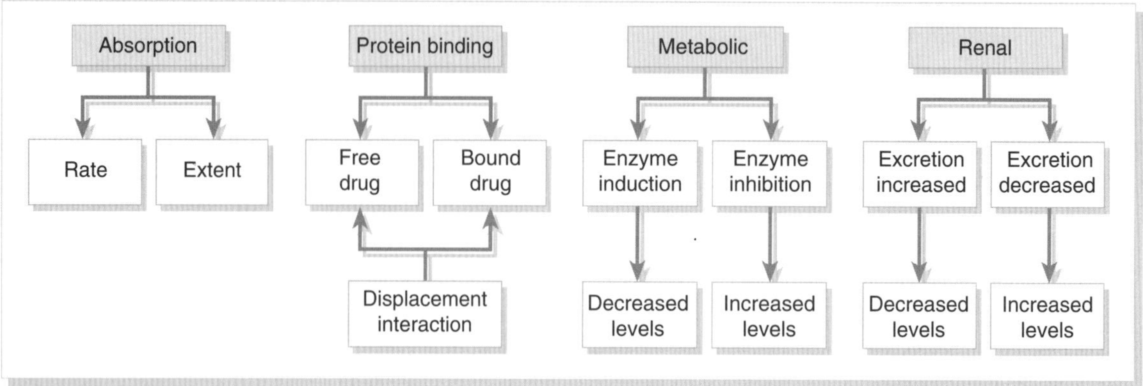

Figure 15.2 Pharmacokinetic interactions. From MeRec bulletin 1999, with permission of the National Prescribing Centre.

route of administration, importance of active metabolites and the half-lives of the drugs involved.

Not all drug interactions are clinically significant. Some are theoretical, while others require either avoidance of a combination of drugs or careful monitoring. Variability in dose response can also be attributed to technical and human failure, inaccuracies of testing equipment, poor communication between all parties concerned and poor patient concordance. Over-the-counter preparations and herbal products could also have the potential to interact with prescribed medication.

Potentially harmful drug interaction is also dependent upon individual client characteristics. The elderly and the frail may be at increased risk of drug interaction as they are likely to be taking multiple drugs and may have impaired renal or hepatic function. The disease requiring anticoagulation and any concomitant disease can influence drug reaction. It is important to be aware of the patient's preexisting clinical condition and concurrent medication.

Avoid the combination If the potential hazards of adding an interacting drug outweigh the benefits, an alternative drug should be chosen. However, if there is no alternative to the new drug then the existing anticoagulant may need to be changed.

Adjust the dose If the net effect of an interaction is to antagonize or potentiate the anticoagulant, then modification of the dose of one or both drugs may compensate for this.

Monitor the patient If an interacting combination of drugs is used, then additional monitoring will be required until stabilization is achieved. Additional monitoring will also be necessary if the drug is stopped or changed. This must be done in partnership with the patient who should be made aware of possible signs and symptoms caused by the drug interaction.

Continue medication as before If an interaction is not clinically significant or if the interacting drugs are optimal therapy for the condition, the patient's therapy may be continued unchanged and require additional monitoring. An alternative anticoagulant could be prescribed.

Food interactions

Dietary changes that increase or reduce vitamin K (phylloquinone) can lead to changes in the intensity of anticoagulation. High concentrations are commonly found in green leafy vegetables.

Patients should be advised not to make changes in their level of consumption of these foods, as stopping, starting or changing will produce a pharmacokinetic interaction, as will vitamin E and fish oil supplements. Their interaction will be one of potentiation so they should be excluded from the diet (Mason 1995).

Alcohol interactions

Alcohol has a variable effect upon anticoagulant stability.

- Moderate consumption of less than 14 units, spread throughout the week, is usually not problematic.
- Regular heavy intake of more than 24 units a week may antagonize anticoagulants.
- Acute intake may potentiate anticoagulants.

An INR reading taken following alcoholic binge drinking may be inaccurate. The INR should be

Box 15.1 Drugs that interact with warfarin

Gastrointestinal tract

Potentiating drugs	Antagonistic drugs
Antacids	Cholestyramine
Cimetidine	Colestipol
Liquid paraffin & other laxatives	Vitamin K

Cardiovascular system

Potentiating drugs
Amiodarone
Fibrates
Dextrothyroxine
Diazoxide
Dipyridamole
Ethacrynic acid
Quinidine
Simvastatin
Sulphinpyrazone

Central nervous system

Potentiating drugs	Antagonistic drugs
Chloral hydrate & related compounds	Barbiturates
Chlorpromazine	Carbamazepine
Dextropropoxyphene	Dichloralphenazonelate
Diflunisal	
Tricyclic antidepressants	

Respiratory system

Potentiating drug
Antihistamines

Infections

Potentiating drugs	Antagonistic drugs
Aminoglycosides	Griseofulvin
Antimalarials	Rifampicin
Erythromycin	
Gentamicin	
Influenza vaccine	
Kanamycin	
Neomycin	
Streptomycin	
Tetracyclines	
Trimethoprim	

Endocrine system

Potentiating drugs	Antagonistic drugs
Anabolic steroids	Oral contraceptives
Chloropropamide	Oestrogen
Corticosteroids	Progestogens
Danzol	
Glucagon	
Metoclopramide	
Propythiouracil	
Sulphonylurea	
Thyroxin	
Tolbutamide	

Malignant disease and immunosuppressants

Potentiating drugs	
Cyclophosphamide	Methotrexate
Mercaptopurine	Tamoxifen

Musculoskeletal and joint disease

Potentiating drugs			
Allopurinol	Fenclofenac	Indomethacin	Paracetamol (high daily doses, with dextropropoxyphene)
Aspirin & the salicylates	Fenoprofen	Ketoprofen	Distalgesic/coproxamol
Azapropazone	Flufenamic acid	Mefenamic acid	
Diflunisal	Flurbiprofen	Naproxen	

NB: This list is not exhaustive

Box 15.2 Managing drug interaction

Avoid the combination. *Choose an alternative drug*
Adjust the dose. *When stopping, starting, changing*
Monitor the client. *As required*
Continue medication as before.

Box 15.3 Foods that interact with warfarin

Foods that antagonize

Avocado	Collards
Broccoli	Endives
Brussels sprouts	Kale
Cabbage, fresh, boiled or raw green	Watercress
Lettuce, dark green or red	Soya bean products
Spinach	Swiss hard cheese
Ice cream in large quantities	

Foods that potentiate
Fish oil supplement
Vitamin E supplement

NB: This list is not exhaustive

repeated after one week to reestablish stability (Carr 1998, Kearon & Hirsh 1997).

Concomitant disease interaction

The condition that requires warfarin treatment, and any concomitant disease, can influence the pharmacokinetic response to warfarin. It is accepted that the dose–response relationship of anticoagulants differs among healthy subjects, so it follows that this dose response can vary to an even greater extent among the sick.

Fever The hypermetabolic state produced by pyrexia increases the catabolism of vitamin K-dependent coagulation factors, thereby potentiating the effect of warfarin. If sick patients, who already have an inadequate vitamin K intake, are treated with antibiotics and IV fluids without vitamin K supplementation, this will potentiate the effect of warfarin. Nutritional fluid supplements rich in vitamin K given to the same patient will result in antagonizing the effect of warfarin (Hirsh et al 1995).

Diarrhoea This is defined as more than four very loose or watery stools in one day. It will cause a raised INR as it is thought that diarrhoea impairs the absorption of vitamin K from food and impairs the bowel's ability to synthesize vitamin K. This can be problematic for patients with irritable bowel disease.

Liver function Oral anticoagulants are mainly metabolized in the liver. Primary or secondary hepatic dysfunction impairs synthesis of coagulation factors and has a potentiating effect. Severe liver disease impairs coagulation by decreased synthesis of vitamin K-dependent clotting factors. As these patients do not respond to vitamin K, which is given for an excessively high INR, the risk of haemorrhage is increased (Wieland 1997).

Cardiac failure A potentiating response to anticoagulants has been reported in patients with congestive heart failure. It is thought that this is due to congestion of the liver (Killip & Payne 1960).

Renal disease The kidneys excrete the metabolites of warfarin, this having only a minimal anticoagulation effect. Only severe renal disease will interfere with anticoagulation.

Hyper/hypothyroidism Hyperthyroidism causes an increase in the rate at which vitamin K-dependent clotting factors are excreted. This may only become apparent if a patient develops hyperthyroidism or commences treatment for hypothyroidism.

Box 15.4 Concomitant disease interaction with warfarin

Potentiating	*Antagonistic*
Hyperthyrotoxicosis	Hypothyrotoxicosis
Cardiac failure	Diabetes mellitus
Renal failure	Oedema
Liver failure	Hyperlipidaemia
Biliary obstruction	Visceral carcinoma
Diarrhoea	
Fever	
Infectious diseases	
Malnutrition/weight loss	
Carcinoma	
Radiation therapy	
Menstrual disorders	

NB: This list is not exhaustive

Because the dose response of warfarin is dependent upon physical well-being, it is accepted that variation will occur during the course of therapy. Occasionally the exact cause of variability in dose response will be unidentified because there will always be the individual who deviates from the norm because of the non-specific nature of the condition associated with the need for warfarin. During such times anticoagulant dosage must be closely monitored to prevent overdosing or underdosing. Increasing or decreasing the warfarin dose should not be undertaken without monitoring the INR.

INDICATIONS FOR ORAL ANTICOAGULATION

The aim of warfarin therapy is to reduce the risk of a thromboembolic event or the extension of an existing event, by maintaining patients at the optimal level of anticoagulation without producing an unacceptable risk of haemorrhage (BMA/RPS 2002).

Anticoagulants are indicated in situations where a patient is at increased risk of a thromboembolic event that may result from abnormalities of the blood vessels or blood flow or the constituents of the clotting mechanism (National Prescribing Centre 1997).

INTERNATIONAL NORMALIZED RATIO

The degree of anticoagulation is measured by comparing the patient's prothrombin time to an international standard. The ratio is expressed as the INR and is the recommended method for monitoring patients maintained on an oral anticoagulant (Haemostasis and Thrombosis Task Force 1998).

Target INR

It has been normal practice for patients to be maintained within an INR range of, for example, 2.0–3.0 (target 2.5), this allowing a deviation of 0.5 above or below the target INR. A patient within this range was said to be 'within ratio'. Research evidence has shown that when using this range only 50% of INRs were within range at any one time (Haemostasis and Thrombosis Task Force 1998, Rose 1996). When this range was increased to 0.75 above or below target, 80% of INRs were within range at any one time. Due to these results, and the increased use of computer decision support software which regulates dose adjustment for a target, the guidelines now give recommended INR targets.

VENOUS THROMBOSIS (NON-PREGNANT PATIENTS)

The initial anticoagulation with heparin and the period of anticoagulation, minimum 6 weeks, is dependent on the patient's individual thrombus, its size, whether it was triggered by a precipitating

Table 15.1 Indications for oral anticoagulation (with permission from Haemostasis and Thrombosis Task Force 1998)

Indication	Target INR	Duration
Pulmonary embolus	2.5	6 months
Proximal deep vein thrombosis	2.5	6 months
Calf venous thrombosis, non-surgical, no persistent risk factors	2.5	3 months
Calf venous thrombosis, postoperative, no persistent risk factors	2.5	6 weeks
Continued treatment should be considered if risk factors are persistent		
Recurrence of venous thrombosis, following discontinuation of therapy	2.5	
Recurrence of venous thrombosis, whilst on therapy	3.5	
Requires a further episode of therapy or alternative therapy and further investigations		
Symptomatic inherited thrombophilia	2.5	Variable
Antiphospholipid syndrome	2.5 or 3.5	Not clarified
Non-rheumatic atrial fibrillation and one risk factor	2.5	Prolonged
Atrial fibrillation:		
rheumatic heart disease	2.5	Prolonged
thyrotoxicosis	2.5	Prolonged
Cardioversion	2.5	3 wks before, 4 wks after
Mural thrombus	2.5	3 months
Cardiomyopathy	2.5	Prolonged
Mechanical prosthetic heart valve	3.5	Prolonged

event, for example surgery and on the patient's existing risk factors for recurrence.

Recurrence of venous thrombosis

If this occurs after warfarin has been discontinued further warfarin therapy at the same target will be required. Recurrence whilst taking warfarin requires consideration of higher intensity of therapy or alternative anticoagulation therapy and evaluation of any underlying factors.

INHERITED THROMBOPHILIA

Although these patients are usually monitored in the acute sector it is important to note that a positive family history of thrombosis can be found in 24–40% of thrombosis patients and they often present within primary care. They include deficiencies of antithrombin, protein C, protein S and the factor V Leiden mutation (Zoller & Dahlback 1997). Thrombotic events require initial treatment with heparin followed by oral anticoagulation therapy.

ATRIAL FIBRILLATION

This is a heart arrhythmia with complete absence of coordinated atrial systole.

Non-rheumatic atrial fibrillation

Patients with non-rheumatic atrial fibrillation have an increased risk of a thromboembolic event, especially cardioembolic. Warfarin, while being effective as a prophylactic, has a higher risk of bleeding than aspirin. Patients are divided into high risk and low risk.

- *High risk: warfarin.* Non-rheumatic atrial fibrillation and at least one risk factor.
- *Low risk: aspirin.* Non-rheumatic atrial fibrillation and no risk factor.

Box 15.5 Non-rheumatic atrial fibrillation

High risk	*Low risk*
Previous thromboembolism	No transient ischaemic attack
Hypertension	No previous stroke
Heart failure	Non-diabetic
Abnormal left ventricular function on echocardiography	Under 65 years

All patients require regular assessment of their medication and risk/benefit status which can change with increasing age and concomitant factors.

CARDIOVERSION

A thromboembolic event may follow cardioversion, due to either dislodgement of a thrombus or stasis in the left atrium caused by the cardioversion (O'Kane & Jackson 2000). Acute atrial fibrillation patients are usually considered for cardioversion. If cardioversion takes place within 48 hours of the onset of atrial fibrillation, anticoagulation is not usually required. Cardioversion beyond 48 hours requires the patient to be anticoagulated.

HEART VALVE PROSTHESES

Certain factors influence the risk of a thrombotic event.

- The position of the prosthesis
- The age of the prosthesis
- Any past history of atrial fibrillation
- Any previous thromboembolic event

Mechanical prosthetic valves

Evidence shows there is a clear relationship between anticoagulant-related bleeding events, thromboembolic events and INR stability (Cannegieter et al 1995).

- There is a rise in embolism with an INR <2.5.
- There is a rise in haemorrhage with an INR >5.0.

Bioprosthetic valves

Lifelong warfarin is not required for patients with bioprosthetic valves in the absence of atrial fibrillation and any risk factors. Patients not anticoagulated should be considered for antiplatelet therapy, e.g. aspirin.

ISCHAEMIC STROKE

Aspirin should be considered as secondary prophylaxis. Anticoagulants are given to reduce the risk of stroke in patients with:

- atrial fibrillation
- transient ischaemic attacks without atrial fibrillation, to prevent the evolution of stroke and a complete stroke.

PROCEDURE FOR AN UNACCEPTABLY HIGH INR

This may be an indication of an unidentified problem or it may be an isolated event. All incidents must be evaluated to identify the cause and referred for further investigation when necessary. Bleeding events increase significantly with an INR >5 and should be recorded and included in an audit.

It is important to exclude factors that may be responsible for the rise.

- Concomitant drug therapy
- Additional potentiating factors
- Underlying medical condition

A decision on the medical intervention required to lower the INR to an acceptable level is dependent upon the INR, the presence of minor or major bleeding and individual patient characteristics.

Box 15.6 Recommendations for an unacceptably high INR (modified from Haemostasis and Thrombosis Task Force 1998)

Target INR 2.5, INR of between 3.0 and 5.9

- If INR is at lower end reduce warfarin dose
- If INR is at upper end omit 2 days' warfarin therapy and check INR prior to recommencing
- Reduce dose by 1 mg if the client is taking concomitant potentiating medication
- Check INR in one week

Target INR 3.5, INR of between 4.0 and 5.9

- If INR is at lower end reduce warfarin dose
- If INR is at upper end omit 2 days' warfarin therapy and recommence when INR is below 5.0
- Reduce dose by 1 mg if the client is taking concomitant potentiating medication
- Check INR in one week

INR of between 6.0 and 7.9 with no associated bleeding or minor bleeding

- Omit warfarin for 2–3 days and check INR prior to recommencing when INR is below 5.0
- Reduce dose by 1 mg if the client is taking concomitant potentiating medication
- Check INR in one week

INR of above 8.0 with no associated bleeding or minor bleeding

- Omit warfarin therapy
- After assessment: 1. Recommence warfarin when INR is below 5.0; 2. If other risk factors for bleeding give 0.5–2.5 mg of oral vitamin K
- Check INR after 3 days, then 1 week if stable

INR of greater than 10.0 with or without associated bleeding

- Omit warfarin therapy
- Admit the patient to hospital
- After assessment: 1. Prothrombin complex concentrate 50 units/kg; 2. or transfusion with fresh frozen plasma 15 ml/kg; 3.5 mg of oral or IV vitamin K
- Warfarin restarted after reassessment; check INR day 1, 2 and 3 then 1 week if stable

ANTICOAGULANT-RELATED BLEEDING

Warfarin has a narrow risk/benefit profile. In deciding whether to commence anticoagulation therapy, the benefits have to outweigh the risks. Bleeding events diminish the benefits and may lead physicians to avoid anticoagulants. We have a growing elderly population, amongst whom are those who most often have indications for therapy. Consequently the incidence of bleeding may increase.

Bleeding is influenced by:

- the intensity of therapy
- the patient's clinical condition
- concomitant factors, such as pharmacokinetic and pharmacodynamic interaction (Landefeld & Beyth 1993).

Each medical or surgical condition which indicates the need for anticoagulation therapy brings with it its own risk of bleeding, and forms part of the equation in deciding the duration and intensity of therapy.

Bleeding most often occurs in the nasopharynx, gastrointestinal tract, soft tissue and urinary tract (Landefeld & Beyth 1993). This can be a consequence of therapy and may not be the result of a raised INR. The indication to discontinue therapy must be judged by the bleeding's severity, its ongoing consequences and its acceptability to individual patients.

RISK OF BLEEDING

Secondary and primary care

Incidents of bleeding differ due to several factors. Heparin is more widely used in hospitals and

Box 15.7 Haemorrhagic risk factors (Haemostasis and Thrombosis Task Force 1998)

Co-morbid factors	*Patient factors*
Serious cardiac condition	Poor compliance
Liver dysfunction	Alcoholism
Renal insufficiency	Medication errors
Severe anaemia	Drug interaction
Poor general condition	Recent surgery
History of cerebrovascular accident	Length of therapy
History of gastrointestinal bleeding	Intensity of therapy
Hypertension	
Cancer	
Radiation therapy	

commonly associated with soft tissue bleeding related to wounds and trauma and often the patient's general condition is poor due to their indication for hospitalization. This risk has been reduced with the introduction of low molecular weight heparin that is as good as unfractionated heparin in preventing peroperative deep venous thrombosis and thromboembolism, with a lower risk of bleeding.

In primary care there can be up to 12 weeks between clinic visits and the risk of haemorrhage due to individual patient factors can be higher.

Age

The issue of whether the frequency of bleeding increases with age, over 65 years, remains controversial. Some studies found the frequency of bleeding increased with age, others did not and some that the risk increased above 40 years (Landefeld & Goldman 1989, O'Kane & Jackson 2000, Van Der Meer et al 1993).

Length of anticoagulant therapy

Anticoagulants incur a cumulative risk of bleeding that is directly related to the length of therapy. The risk of bleeding is greatest in the first month of therapy, then decreases during the remainder of the first year (Landefeld & Goldman 1989). There is a cumulative risk of major bleeding of approximately 10% at 1 year, increasing to 25% at 4 years (Landefeld & Goldman 1989, Petiti et al 1986).

Long-term bleeding

There is a small percentage of patients who will continually bleed but who unquestionably need anticoagulation, for example those with mechanical heart valves and atrial fibrillation. Investigations to identify and reverse the cause of bleeding should be instigated and the possibility of lowering the intensity of the anticoagulant effect explored (Hirsh et al 1995).

Aspirin could be added to low-intensity warfarin therapy, for example target INR 1.5. Replacing warfarin therapy with aspirin could be considered in patients with atrial fibrillation. This is not an option for patients with mechanical valves, where there is no evidence that antiplatelet therapy is effective (Becker & Spencer 1997).

Intensity of therapy

There is a relationship between the intensity of anticoagulant therapy and the risk of bleeding. Managing a patient with a target of 4.0 compared to one with a target of 2.5 increases the risk of bleeding by approximately threefold (Landefeld & Beyth 1993).

It is important to remember that in a third of all bleeding events investigation leads to identification of previously unknown lesions, even when the INR is elevated (Landefeld & Beyth 1993). The presence of such factors need not be regarded as a contraindication to anticoagulant therapy, but as an indication for increased vigilance in clinical assessment.

INITIATING ORAL ANTICOAGULATION

The goal of anticoagulation therapy is to stabilize the patient on the lowest possible dose of therapy required to maintain a target INR that prevents a bleeding event or thrombosis.

A full risk assessment is required to ensure the patient's medical and mental suitability for warfarin therapy. This should include blood samples taken for:

- prothrombin time
- activated partial thromboplastin time (when haparin is also commenced)
- full blood count (haemoglobin, platelet count)
- liver function test.

Modifications to the loading dose may be necessary if these baseline coagulation results are abnormal. It should also be remembered that some patients are particularly sensitive to warfarin, namely:

- the elderly
- those with high risk factors, e.g. congestive cardiac failure
- liver failure
- various cancers
- potentiating drug therapy.

Where immediate anticoagulation is required, warfarin can commence on day 1 with heparin. Heparin is given for at least 4 days and should not be discontinued until the INR has been in the therapeutic range for 2 consecutive days (Haemostasis and Thrombosis Task Force 1998).

Following the initial administration of warfarin therapy, an observed anticoagulant effect is delayed until newly synthesized dysfunctional vitamin K-dependent clotting factors replace the normal clotting factors and the latter are cleared from the system (Haemostasis and Thrombosis Task Force 1998, Hirsh et al 1995). The delay may range from 2 to 7 days.

LOADING DOSE

This is the subject of much discussion. Clearance of prothrombin to an effective antithrombotic level may take up to 5 days. For this reason it has been suggested that loading doses are of limited value and may potentiate a bleeding event due to the rapid reduction in factor VII production (Harrison et al 1997, Hirsh et al 1995, Horton & Bushwick 1999). It has also been postulated that the initiation of therapy is associated with a procoagulant state due to the rapid depletion of protein C, with the possible consequences of thrombosis (Haemostasis and Thrombosis Task Force 1998). A safer approach of 5 mg daily, which should result in an INR of 2.0 in about 4–5 days, may be employed (Harrison et al 1997, Hirsh et al 1995).

In an emergency situation where an anticoagulant state is required quickly, heparin is concurrently prescribed.

For initiation of therapy within the community a low loading dose regimen is recommended, with an initial dose of 2 mg daily and the INR checked weekly. The dose is increased slowly until the target INR is achieved.

HOSPITAL DISCHARGE

Prior to the patient's discharge from hospital an appointment for INR monitoring must be made, this not to be in excess of 7 days. Once stable, the recall period for INR monitoring should not exceed 12 weeks.

DISCONTINUING ORAL ANTICOAGULANTS

The British Committee for Standards in Haematology *Guidelines on oral anticoagulants* do not give specific recommendation for the discontinuation of warfarin therapy. Clinicians vary in their approach, using a reducing dose regime over several weeks for patients who have been on long-term warfarin and complete withdrawal for patients on short-term therapy.

Complete sudden discontinuation of warfarin therapy may result in rebound hypercoagulability that may predispose to thrombosis (National Prescribing Centre 1997).

TEMPORARY DISCONTINUATION OF ORAL ANTICOAGULANT

The aim in temporary discontinuation of anticoagulants is to minimize any associated bleeding that may occur during the procedure to be undertaken, without compromising the condition which necessitates anticoagulation. It can be initiated in secondary or primary care.

Surgical treatment

The type and extent of surgery are the governing factors in anticoagulation management during surgical procedures. Each patient requires individual assessment to achieve a balance between the risk of a thromboembolic event and the risk of haemorrhage.

Major surgery Anticoagulation may be stopped or surgery performed with an INR <2.5. The European Society of Cardiology also suggests that the INR should be 2.0 or less for a major surgical procedure. Emergency surgery will require therapeutic reversal of anticoagulation.

Minor surgery For minor surgical procedures a target INR of 2.0 on the day of surgery is required.

- Stop warfarin or adjust dose prior to surgery.
- Preoperatively check INR.

- <2.5 – proceed to surgery.
- >2.5 – surgeon and haematologist decide if safe to proceed.

Dental treatment

Extraction Patients requiring tooth extraction should be referred to the dental hospital for specialist management and where their INR can be monitored prior to treatment.

Guidelines vary between haematologists and the patient's condition requiring anticoagulation. The dilemma is that withdrawing therapy increases the risk of a thromboembolic event and maintaining levels above 2.5 may prolong bleeding from the extraction site.

Valvular heart disease patients should have an INR of 2.0–2.5 on the day of treatment. This may involve withdrawing warfarin for 1–3 days prior to the procedure and resuming therapy on its completion (Gohlke-Barwolf et al 1993, Haemostasis and Thrombosis Task Force 1998).

Other forms of treatment For tooth filling or cleaning, the patient should have an INR within ratio. Valvular heart disease patients are prescribed 1 g antibiotic powder to be taken on the morning of treatment to ensure its rapid absorption at the appropriate time. Subsequent treatments are at 1-month intervals.

Reinstating of anticoagulation

The reinstating of oral anticoagulants is dependent upon the risk of postoperative haemorrhage and the 48–72 hour delay to achieve anticoagulation. They may be commenced as soon as the patient has an oral intake. To achieve an INR of 1.5 will take about 4 days (Haemostasis and Thrombosis Task Force 1998).

CONCOMITANT CONDITIONS THAT REQUIRE REFERRAL

Anticoagulation cannot be viewed in isolation from the condition initiating anticoagulation or any other developing medical or social issue. If clinicians are unable to deal with a problem they should ensure that the patient is referred appropriately.

NON-URGENT REFERRAL

Anaemia

A reduction in the concentration of haemoglobin in the circulating blood increases the risk of haemorrhage in anticoagulated patients. Due to the nature of anticoagulation it is possible that, over a period of time, minor undetected bleeding can result in anaemia.

Any presenting anaemia may have an underlying pathophysiological or morphological cause and as clinical signs of anaemia only increase with its severity, it can be difficult to identify. Complaints of tiredness and lethargy can easily be attributed to the patient's medical condition requiring anticoagulation, but should not be ignored.

A full blood count should be included in the initial assessment before initiation of anticoagulants. This can be measured against a repeated specimen in an identified time period. Values outside the normal or a drop of more than 2 g/dl should be investigated.

A haemoglobin higher or lower than the patient's normal will have an effect upon the INR result.

Hypertension

Hypertension is a persistently raised arterial pressure and is the most common condition requiring lifelong therapy in the Western world and, if left untreated, it will affect the entire circulatory system (Jordon 2000). Treating hypertension in patients who experience transient ischaemic attacks reduces the incidence of stroke by 15% and the risk of having a stroke in any hypertensive patient by 40% (Macwalter 1997).

Uncontrolled hypertension is a contraindication to anticoagulation and, if present, increases the risk of intracranial bleeding (Laupacis et al 1994, Levine et al 1995). Blood pressure should be monitored in accordance with hypertension guidelines.

URGENT REFERRAL

Unexplained signs and symptoms may be masking an undiagnosed condition and may be the first indication of a life-threatening situation. Haemorrhagic complications may be manifested by signs or symptoms that do not indicate obvious bleeding. Any unexplained symptoms, even in the presence of a normal INR, should be investigated. Almost any organ in the body can be involved. It is important therefore to investigate any unexplained condition for underlying haemorrhage and/or co-morbid condition.

Box 15.8 Unexplained signs and symptoms

- Headaches
- Pains in the chest
- Pains in the abdomen and joints
- Swelling
- Shortness of breath
- Confusion, memory loss
- Pallor
- Any unexplained symptoms

Pregnancy

Pregnancy increases the risk of thromboembolic disease due to venous stasis and hypercoagulability.

Oral anticoagulants are major teratogens and therefore it is not advisable for women to become pregnant while taking warfarin. Oral anticoagulants cross the placenta barrier, causing the risk of placental and fetal haemorrhage, especially in the immature fetal liver and particularly in the first and third trimesters (BMA/RPS 2002, Haemostasis and Thrombosis Task Force 1998, Kearon & Hirsh 1997). Organogenesis occurs during week 6–12 of gestation and can produce a characteristic embryopathy (Hirsh 1991).

Heparin may be substituted for warfarin as it lessens the likelihood of teratogenicity and fetal haemorrhage associated with early and late warfarin use, but heparin can cause maternal osteoporosis and thrombocytopenia. It will need to be used during the first trimester and for 2–3 weeks before delivery. Neither is heparin thought to be as effective in patients with mechanical heart valves where there is a high risk of embolism. In situations where loss of anticoagulation control would be considered life-threatening, warfarin would be continued throughout pregnancy (Haemostasis and Thrombosis Task Force 1998, Hirsh 1991).

Premenopausal females taking warfarin therapy should be made aware that there is a risk associated with becoming pregnant and they should be referred to a specialist if they are, or wish to be, pregnant.

There is not thought to be any contraindication to breastfeeding after recommencing warfarin therapy following the birth (Kearon & Hirsh 1997).

Malignancy

The association of coagulation abnormalities with cancer and the predisposition to a thromboembolic event has long been acknowledged. In some cases the first indication of a malignancy is when the patient presents with a DVT, which when investigated leads to identification of a cancer.

Certain malignant cells express tissue factor from their surface, thereby facilitating the contact of powerful procoagulant substances with circulating blood, this having the potential to cause the formation of a thrombus. If the disease process is progressive, malignant cells invade the blood vessels and damage the endothelium, causing tissue factor VIIa complexes to form, which may result in the generation of thrombin and this also has the potential to cause the formation of thrombus (Goodnight 1997, Hickey et al 1997).

HEREDITARY RESISTANCE AND ACQUIRED RESISTANCE TO ANTICOAGULANTS

A hereditary resistance to warfarin can result in a patient requiring a warfarin dose from five to twenty times higher than the norm. It is thought that this is caused by an altered affinity of the receptor for warfarin since the plasma warfarin levels required to achieve anticoagulation are much higher than average (Hirsh et al 1995, O'Reilly et al 1993).

It is believed that some patients metabolize warfarin slowly which may or may not be associated with increasing age. This results in rapidly achieved stability and a maintenance dose that is relatively low. The opposite effect holds for the patient who metabolizes warfarin quickly and takes a longer period of time to reach the therapeutic INR (Harton & Bushwick 1999).

ANTICOAGULATION CLINIC

Starting a clinic for the first time requires the identification of policies and procedures agreed by the primary healthcare team and the secondary care service.

AIM OF THE CLINIC

To maintain patients at the optimal level of anticoagulation that reduces their risk of a thromboembolic event or an extension of an existing event without producing an unacceptable risk of haemorrhage (BMA/RPS 2002).

Objectives

- To facilitate a service that encourages patient and carer involvement in their management.
- To manage warfarin therapy by evaluating the INR and advising on dosage and appointment recall.
- To assess for co-morbidities.
- To provide education and support for anticoagulation patients and carers.
- To support communication network between disciplines and secondary and primary care.

POLICIES AND PROCEDURES

First of all, define your service. A structured systematic approach will aid the introduction of a clinic and minimize potential problem situations and identify a framework of the elements you wish, or are able, to provide. This is dependent upon factors such as cohort, geographical area, transport and the available resources and finance.

The following is an example of what should be included, though this is not an exhaustive list.

Step 1. Identify your clients

- Initiate a computer search for all patients taking warfarin.
- Initiate a patient survey for all patients identified, including details of proposed service.

Step 2. Involve the primary healthcare teams

- Identify a lead doctor, nurse, receptionist.
- Identify community procedure, recall procedure.
- Identify documentation procedure.

Step 3. Involve secondary care

- Identify an integrated pathway of care between hospital wards, hospital INR service, pathology, haematologist.

Step 4. Monitoring and blood testing facilities

- Decide on near patient testing (NPT) or intravenous blood samples.
- Decide if you are going to use computer decision support software (CDSS) with guidelines.

Step 5. Referral systems

- Identify procedure for an unacceptably high INR with secondary care.
- Identify procedure and information required for referral into community clinic.
  a) Indication for warfarin therapy
  b) Duration of therapy
  c) Recommended target INR
  d) Past three INR readings
  e) Any antagonistic or potentiating factors
  f) Date of follow-up appointment
  g) Name of doctor initiating therapy

Step 6. Audit

- Identify patient questionnaires and surveys.
- Identify clinical audit in accordance with the Haemostasis and Thrombosis Task Force of the British Committee for Standards in Haematology, e.g.:
  a) % patients within 0.5 units of target
  b) % patients within 0.75 units of target
  c) % patients above/below target ratio
  d) adverse events, bleeds, thrombosis
  e) deaths and cause
  f) patient quality of life issues.

Step 7. Quality control

- Identify internal procedure and external quality assessment scheme for INR NPT.
- Adhere to manufacturer's recommendations for NPT machine calibration.

Step 8. Education and training

A minimum competency standard should be defined for both the patient and the providers of the service.

- Patient and carer.
- Patient who self monitors.
- Clinicians, qualified and unqualified.

GUIDELINES

In conjunction with a doctor, pharmacist and patient group, guidelines should be developed and endorsed by the primary care trust (NHS Executive 2000, NHS Scottish Executive 2001).

Guidelines are about setting specific standards for high-quality clinical effectiveness. It is an opportunity for clinicians, whilst abiding by governing bodies' guidelines, to establish and incorporate their own standards. Guidelines should be developed following discussion with the whole team responsible for the service and should incorporate every aspect of anticoagulation management. Upon completion, they should be endorsed by all the team and include the date of authorization and the review date.

Box 15.9 Guideline requirements

- A standard
- Clinical guidelines, medication
- Referral procedure
- Emergency procedure
- Appointments/non-compliance with therapy/appointments procedure
- Management of triage, therapy-related and unrelated problems
- Audit/qualitative research
- Quality control
- Clinicians responsible for the service
- The medical overseer
- Laboratory support
- Communication procedure, primary to secondary care and vice versa
- Patient education

STANDARD

Your standard should be the team's identified principles that define the appropriate environment, process and procedures necessary for quality medical care and optimal health outcomes (Clark & Kinney 1992). It should be a reproducible framework that provides the multidisciplinary team with a mechanism that fulfils their identified standard.

CLINICAL GUIDELINES

Directing principles agreed by a professional body and based on the medical condition and patient-specific information.

REFERRAL PROCEDURE

What you need to know about patients before undertaking their anticoagulation management and what information needs to accompany patients if they are referred elsewhere.

EMERGENCY PROCEDURE

In the event of an emergency, where and to whom you refer.

APPOINTMENTS/NON-COMPLIANCE/ NON-ATTENDANCE PROCEDURE

Process that identifies and tracks the regular monitoring of any patient prescribed warfarin.

MANAGEMENT OF TRIAGE, THERAPY-RELATED AND UNRELATED PROBLEMS

Concomitant complications do not always correlate with the INR, nor with clinic time. Patients therefore need a point of reference to contact should a problem situation occur.

QUALITY CONTROL

To ensure safe monitoring, this should include the following:

- *Which clinicians are responsible for the service.* Identification and ownership of roles.
- *Who is the medical overseer.* The physician, who should be an integrated part of the team but may not be an active participator, with ultimate responsibility for therapeutic decisions.
- *Laboratory support.* Suboptimal INR results and routine blood tests require laboratory processing. This requires a different procedure for retrieval, communication of results and next appointment.
- *Communication procedure between primary and secondary care.* Poor communication results in poor patient care. Effective anticoagulation management requires interaction between all participants. All interaction should be documented.
- *Patient education.* Desired goals and objectives of verbal and written information.

THE PATIENT

PATIENT ASSESSMENT

As therapeutic outcomes of anticoagulation are affected by medical and concomitant lifestyle factors, a patient assessment is an integral part of management. This assessment should include their beliefs and expectation of anticoagulation and their presenting condition.

Box 15.10 Patient assessment for anticoagulation therapy

- Medical condition requiring anticoagulation
- Co-morbid conditions
- Concomitant medication
- Dietary and lifestyle history
- Level of understanding and literacy
- Health beliefs and attitudes
- Compliance
- Motivation for self-care, empowerment
- Socio-economic factors

PATIENT AGREEMENT

Although not a written agreement, it is important that patient and carer are aware that the prescribing of warfarin therapy brings with it a commitment on their part to adhere to certain guidelines.

Box 15.11 Warfarin patient agreement

- The patient must agree to take their medication as indicated by their blood result.
- The patient must agree to attend a clinic for regular blood monitoring.
- The patient must agree to report to the clinic, their GP or the hospital any signs of bleeding or concerns regarding their therapy or health.
- The patient must acknowledge that failure to comply with the patient agreement may result in termination of warfarin therapy.

PATIENT NON-PARTICIPATION PROCEDURE

Situations do occur where patients are unable to manage their own therapy. Systems must then come into play to assist them. This could be in the form of a daily dosing box or support from a family member. Only when all alternative methods of safe anticoagulation dispensing have been exhausted should therapy be discontinued.

Box 15.12 Patient non-participation procedure

The patient is responsible for rescheduling clinic appointments if they are unable to attend and if they have missed an appointment.

It is important to identify if a missed appointment is the result of hospital admission or sudden ill health or death.

1st missed appointment
- Patient contacted (that day) by telephone or letter
- Appointment given for same day or next clinic
- Situation documented, written/database

2nd missed appointment
- Patient contacted (that day) by telephone and letter
- Appointment given for same day or next clinic
- Situation deocumented, written/database

3rd missed appointment
- A letter is sent to the patient (that day) stressing the importance of attending clinic
- Appointment given for next clinic
- Situation documented, written/database
- Lead clinician informed

4th missed appointment
- A letter is sent to the patient (that day) stressing the importance of attending clinic and stating that therapy cannot be continued if there is not an agreement to have regular blood monitoring and that failure to respond to this letter could result in termination of therapy
- A reference to this will be placed on the repeat prescription database
- Appointment given for next clinic
- Situation documented, written/database
- Lead clinician/referring physician informed
- Placed on the agenda for the next team meeting

If the patient has not contacted the clinic within 7 working days
- Lead clinician and referring physician informed
- Multidisciplinary team decision made, whether to terminate therapy
- Letter sent by recorded delivery of decision
- Situation documented, written/database, copy to secondary/primary care

PATIENT EDUCATION

The aim of anticoagulation patient education is to provide information about warfarin and its associated factors to produce the degree of knowledge required in order to foster adherence to therapy and to promote self-care (Oertel 1997). There is a diversity of education levels, life experiences and social background in patients receiving anticoagulants and education must be tailored to the individual in order to accommodate this.

Basic patient information

There is a minimum level of anticoagulation knowledge that is required to ensure the safety of patients taking warfarin.

- *What is warfarin?* Why they are taking it. How long they have to take it. The different colours and strengths.
- *What the blood test is.* Why it is necessary. How often it is done. What it means if it is too high or too low. How it would alter their medication. What their target is.
- *What interferes with warfarin*, e.g. drugs, diet, alcohol, illness.
- *What to do if a dose is missed or late.*
- *What the signs of bleeding are and what they would do about it.*
- *What the procedure is when buying over-the-counter medication.*
- *What the procedure is for dental and surgical treatment.*
- *That it is not advisable for women to become pregnant and why.*

Anticoagulation education is reinforced and extended at each clinic visit. It is clear that to facilitate patient education and empowerment, a vast amount of information has to be presented. Initially this can have an overwhelming effect upon the patient. There is no endpoint in the education and it is a continual reinforcement process. It is only through continual conversation with the patient and the carer that the provider can ascertain what knowledge has been assimilated and thereby identify the areas that need to be readdressed.

Patient's questions and answers

General knowledge

- *What is it?* It is an oral anticoagulant, which means it slows down your blood-clotting ability.
- *Why am I taking it?* To prevent blood clots forming in your blood vessels/new valve/graft.
- *How long will I take it?* Short term can be for 3–6 months, long term can be for life. This should still be regularly reviewed.
- *Are there any side-effects?* As your clotting is slower, if you cut yourself it will take longer to stop bleeding. A knock can result in a larger bruise than normal. A small percentage of people may have a bleed, e.g. nose bleed or blood in urine. Rarely more serious bleeding problems can occur, despite good control.
- *How is it monitored?* By taking a sample of blood; this can be a fingerprick sample or from a vein in your arm. The test measures the speed at which your blood clots, called the international normalized ratio, known as INR for short.
- *What alters my target?* A wide variety of things: medication, food, being unwell. Remember the key, Stopping, Starting or Changing.
- *How do I take it?* By tablet, once a day, at the same time each day. Always check that you are taking the right colour and strength.
- *What happens if I forget?* If you remember within 6 hours take your warfarin as normal. If over 6 hours, do **not** take your warfarin. Never take a double dose. Record this in your dosing diary.
- *What do I have to do?* Understand your warfarin treatment. If there is something you don't understand then ask. Attend your warfarin clinic regularly; if you can't attend, then telephone. Always ensure that you have a follow-up appointment.

Problem knowledge

- *Bleeding.* If you have any bleeding or excessive bruising without knocking yourself, seek medical advice.
- *Diarrhoea, fever, sickness or not eating.* This will affect your blood readings, your INR. You must seek medical advice, saying that you are taking warfarin.
- *Doctor's appointment.* Remind your doctor that you are taking warfarin, especially when stopping, starting, changing medication.
- *Dentist appointments.* Remind your dentist that you are taking warfarin, before you have your teeth cleaned or have treatment. You may need an antibiotic before treatment.
- *Chemist.* Do not buy over-the-counter medication; this includes herbal remedies and

supplements. Ask the pharmacist's advice and say that you are taking warfarin.

Lifestyle knowledge

- *No smoking*. The best thing you can do is stop. Breaking the habit is hard but the rewards are high. Your taste buds will revive and you will enjoy your food more. It will reduce the chance of health problems. Enlist the help of a friend.
- *A varied balanced diet*. A Mediterranean diet is recommended but remember stopping, starting, changing, especially greens, for example broccoli, sprouts.
- *Maintain a healthy weight*. This is more about healthy eating not how much you weigh.
- *Moderate alcohol intake*. Enjoy a drink now and then. Moderate consumption of 14 standard units, spread throughout the week.
- *Regular exercise*. This is according to your age, level of activity and physical limitations. 30 minutes a day 5 days a week. This need not be a chore; you could take a brisk walk, go swimming, gardening, dancing. Choose something you enjoy. Contact sports are best avoided.
- *Reduce stress*. Most of us feel stress at some time, so discover your own 'chilling out' strategy. It could be going for a walk, listening to some music, a chat with a friend. It is important that you don't let your stress levels build up.
- *Holidays*. Prepare well for your health requirements and remember to take adequate supplies of all your medication.

  Countries inside the European Economic Area: obtain an E111 form from your Post Office. This will provide free or reduced cost emergency medical cover.

  Countries outside the European Economic Area: you are advised to take out full medical insurance cover. It is a good idea to carry a first aid kit.

  Remember that you will be affected more than other people if you are unwell, so take extra care when eating and drinking; this includes water.
- *Emergency INR monitoring*. Remember that the INR is the international normalized ratio, which means that it can be monitored by the same standards internationally, so if you are unwell or away for a prolonged length of time you can have your INR taken at a local hospital. Take your warfarin diary and any additional medical information with you.

PATIENT EMPOWERMENT

Today's health agenda supports the decentralization of management and the role of the autonomous and independent specialist practitioner, which in turn facilitates patient empowerment.

Some patients are unable to participate in their own management and others may not wish to be part of the decision making but this must not be used as a reason to exclude them from the empowerment concept (Chavasse 1992, Dennis 1990). Everyone can be involved at their own level of understanding.

Elements that support patient empowerment

Information leaflets The giving of a leaflet is not an end in itself and has been shown to be of minimal use when not supported by other information-giving strategies (Gloucestershire Primary Care Clinical Audit Group 1999). All verbal information given to the client should reflect and support information leaflets.

Newsletter Produced quarterly, it should be friendly, informal, easily understood and made available to everyone who is prescribed warfarin. It should contain information about the clinic, the staff, the service and any proposed changes and be written in such a way as to confirm client ownership of the services. An invitation should be included for clients to suggest any changes that they think might benefit the service. It is also a vehicle to reinforce seasonal information, e.g. summer holidays, influenza vaccine.

Patient-held records Patients need to have their ownership of the clinic confirmed. By holding their own records it is seen that no information is withheld from them and they have the freedom to peruse them at their leisure.

Emergency card An anticoagulant patient identification emergency card can be issued to all patients to be carried at all times. This incorporates the patient's computer number so that in an emergency their anticoagulant record can be accessed.

Database A regional database for all anticoagulant patients would be a major step forward to prevent the problems associated with emergency admissions and patients who are treated at more than one hospital.

Telephone helpline This must reliable. If no one is available to take a call, a message must be taken and left in a designated way. Patients must be made aware of the hours within which this service operates. A telephone helpline can both reduce nurse and doctor appointments and increase the ability for patients to become involved in their own management (Mackie 1996).

POTENTIAL SOURCES OF ERROR

With the consequences of an INR outside a target range being, at one end of the scale, haemorrhage and potential death and at the other end thrombosis and potential death, it is important to be aware of areas where there is the potential for error.

INR stability is focused on prescribing the correct dose of warfarin, receiving the correct dose of warfarin and taking the correct dose of warfarin. When factors come into play that cause a deviation from this pathway, stability is lost.

- Pharmaceutical: prescribing, dosing, taking
- Concomitant factors: drugs, food, alcohol, illness
- Communication problems
- Patient concordance

PHARMACEUTICAL

Warfarin in Britain is produced in different strengths, each with a different colour. Prescribing is usually initiated in a hospital setting and patients are discharged with a supply of all strengths. Prescribing is then undertaken by the GP with warfarin being put on the repeat prescription database system.

Prescribing

As there is no consistent dose of warfarin it is not under the same repeat prescription control as other medications. Patients should be encouraged to use the same pharmacist. Some pharmacists have a prescribing record on database and are able to identify any major deviation in prescribing. They are also able to advise on over-the-counter medication and prevent inadvertent drug interaction.

Dosing

The different colours and strengths of warfarin can give rise to a variety of problems. If possible, prescribe only one strength of warfarin and avoid using the 0.5 mg strength. If more than one strength is given, emphasize the importance of reading the strength on the label. With each clinic visit patients should be asked what colour and strength they are taking as a way of confirming they are taking the correct dose.

CONCOMITANT FACTORS: DRUGS, FOOD, ALCOHOL AND ILLNESS

Add any one of these factors to anticoagulation management and the result could be either subtherapeutic or excessive anticoagulation. Increasing the patient's knowledge through education is a significant step towards combating this.

COMMUNICATION PROBLEMS

The majority of problems that occur in services are those of communication. We need to be extravagant communicators. This is not an easy task for we each have different perceptions, values and priorities. Patients are on lifelong therapy and may attend different hospitals under the care of different physicians, even in different countries. We need to ensure that information goes *with* the patient as following the patient can be too late.

PATIENT CONCORDANCE

This can be due to non-participation which results in breaking of the patient agreement.

Not all patients can read and may be too embarrassed to say and this would not necessarily be documented. There may be some cognitive or physical impairment, which is not always obvious. Or they may just make a mistake.

CONCLUSION

The criteria for today's health agenda are to give a cost-effective service, delivered locally that meets patient-identified needs. The most important goal is to improve patient care. In anticoagulation management, clinicians have to play their part in assuring that the consequences of therapy do not outweigh the benefits and to do this new approaches are required.

The approach to anticoagulant management suggested in this chapter, that looks at the total needs of the patient and not solely INR monitoring, fulfils these criteria.

References

Ansell JA 1997 The value of an anticoagulation management service. In: Ansell JA, Oertel LB, Wittkowsky AK (eds) Managing oral anticoagulation therapy: clinical and operational guidelines. Aspen, Gaithersburg, Maryland

Ansell JA 1998 Anticoagulation management as a risk factor for adverse events: grounds for improvement. Journal of Thrombosis and Thrombolysis 5:s7–s11

ASPECT (Anticoagulants in the Secondary Prevention of Events in Coronary Thrombosis) Research Group 1994 Effects of long-term oral anticoagulant treatment on mortality and cardiovascular morbidity after myocardial infarct. Lancet 343:499–503

Becker CR, Spencer F 1997 Cardiovascular indications for oral anticoagulation therapy. In: Ansell JE, Oertel LB, Wittkowsky AK (eds) Managing oral anticoagulation therapy: clinical and operational guidelines. Aspen, Gaithersburg, Maryland

Bevan D 2000 The union of clinical chemistry and haemostasis laboratories: for better or for worse? Presentation at UK NEQAS for Blood Coagulation Annual Meeting, 8 March, University of Sheffield

British Medical Association and the Royal Pharmaceutical Society of Great Britain 2002 British national formulary. BMA/RPS, London

Cannegieter S, Rosendaal F et al 1995 Optimal oral anticoagulant therapy in patients with mechanical heart valves. New England Journal of Medicine 333:11–17

Carr N 1998 Nurse-led oral anticoagulation management: a teaching pack. RCN Publishing, London

Chavasse J 1992 Guest editorial. New dimensions of empowerment in nursing – and challenges. Journal of Advanced Nursing 17:1–2

Clark CM, Kinney ED 1992 Standard for the care of diabetes: origins, uses and implications for third-party payment. Diabetes Care 15(1):10–14

Dennis KE 1990 Patient control and the information imperative: clarification and confirmation. Nursing Research 39(3):162–166

European Atrial Fibrillation Study Group 1993 Secondary prevention in non-rheumatic atrial fibrillation after transient ischaemic attack or minor stroke. Lancet ii:1255–1262

European Atrial Fibrillation Study Group 1995 Optimal oral anticoagulant therapy in patients with nonrheumatic atrial fibrillation and recent cerebral ischaemia. New England Journal of Medicine 333:5–10

Gloucestershire Primary Care Clinical Audit Group 1999 Atrial fibrillation and anticoagulation. Results from a countywide audit, 1998–99. Gloucestershire Primary Care Group, Gloucester

Gohlke-Barwolf C, Acar J, Burckhardt D et al 1993 Committee of the Working Group on Valvular Heart Disease, European Society of Cardiology. Guidelines for the prevention of thrombolic events in valvular heart disease. Journal of Heart Disease 2:398–410

Goodnight SH 1997 Thrombogenesis and hypercoagulable states. In: Ansell E, Oertel LB, Wittkowsky AK (eds) Managing oral anticoagulation therapy. Aspen, Gaithersburg, Maryland

Haemostasis and Thrombosis Task Force for the British Committee for Standards in Haematology 1998 Guidelines on oral anticoagulation: third edition. British Journal of Haematology 101:374–387

Harrison L, Johnson M, Massicotte M et al 1997 Comparison of 5-mg and 10-mg loading doses in initiation of warfarin therapy. Annals of Internal Medicine 116:133–136

Hickey AD, Wallace DM, Bona R 1997 Managing the patient with cancer. In: Ansell E, Oertel LB, Wittkowsky AK (eds) Managing oral anticoagulation therapy. Aspen, Gaithersburg, Maryland

Hirsh J 1991 Oral anticoagulant drugs. New England Journal of Medicine 324:1865–1875

Hirsh J, Dalen JE, Deykin D et al 1995 Oral anticoagulants: mechanism of action, clinical effectiveness, and optimal therapeutic range. Chest 108:231–241

Horton JD, Bushwick BM 1999 Warfarin therapy: evolving strategies in anticoagulation. www.aafp.org/afp/990201ap/635.html

Jordon S 2000 Hypertension. Nursing Times. Symptoms and Diseases supplement:5–8

Kearon C, Hirsh J 1997 Changing indications for warfarin therapy. In: Pollard L, Ludlam CA (eds) Recent advances in blood coagulation. Churchill Livingstone, Edinburgh

Killip T, Payne MA 1960 High serum transaminase activity in heart disease. Circulation 21:646–660

Landefeld CS, Goldman L 1989 Major bleeding in outpatients treated with warfarin: incidence and prediction by factors known at the start of outpatient therapy. American Journal of Medicine 87:144–152

Landefeld CS, Beyth RJ 1993 Anticoagulant related bleeding: epidemiology, prediction and prevention. American Journal of Medicine 95:315–328

Laupacis A, Boysen G, Connolly S et al 1994 Analysis of pooled data from five randomized controlled trials. Archives of Internal Medicine 154:1149–1157

Levine MN, Raskob G, Hirsh J 1995 Haemorrhagic complications of anticoagulant treatment. Fourth ACCP Consensus Conference on Antithrombic Therapy. Chest 108:277–290

Mackie C 1996 Nurse practitioners managing anticoagulation clinics. Nursing Times 92(1):25–26

Macwalter RS 1997 Managing TIAs. Cardiology Update 54:368–374

Mason P 1995 Diet and drug interaction. Pharmaceutical Journal 225:94–97

National Prescribing Centre 1997 MeRec bulletin no. 8.

National Prescribing Centre 1999 MeRec bulletin no. 10.

NHS Executive 2000 Patient group directions. HMSO, London

NHS Scottish Executive 2001 Patient group directions. NHS Scottish Executive, Edinburgh

O'Kane P, Jackson G 2000 Cardiology: the cutting edge. Atrial fibrillation: an update. Update 241–249

O'Reilly RA, Aggeler PM, Hoag M 1993 Hereditary transmission of exceptional resistance to coumarin anticoagulation drugs. New England Journal of Medicine 308:1229–1230

Oertel LB 1997 Education curriculum for patients and teaching methods. In: Ansell E, Oertel LB, Wittkowsky AK (eds) Managing oral anticoagulation therapy. Aspen, Gaithersburg, Maryland

Petiti O, Strom B, Melmon K 1986 Duration of warfarin anticoagulant therapy and the probabilities of recurrent thromboembolism and hemorrhage. American Journal of Medicine 81:255–259

PIENO 2002 Parkinson's list drug database. Warfarin/coumadin, anticoagulation. www.parkinsons-information-exchange-network-online.com/drugdb/138.html

Reynolds JEF 1996 Martindale. The extra pharmacopoeia, 31st edn. Royal Pharmaceutical Society, London

Rose P 1996 Audit of anticoagulation therapy. Journal of Clinical Pathology 49:5–9

Van Der Meer FJ, Rosendaal FR, Briet E 1993 Bleeding complication of anticoagulant therapy: an analysis of risk factors. Archives of Internal Medicine 153:1557–1562

Wieland KA 1997 Initiation of therapy and estimation of maintenance dose. In: Ansell JE, Oertel LB, Wittkowsky AK (eds) Managing oral anticoagulation therapy: clinical and operational guidelines. Aspen, Gaithersburg, Maryland

Wittkowsky AK 1997 Warfarin pharmacology. In: Ansell JA, Oertel LB, Wittkowsky AK (eds) Managing oral anticoagulation therapy; clinical and operational guidelines. Aspen, Gaithersburg, Maryland

Zoller B, Dahlback B 1997 Inherited resistance to activated protein C as a pathogenic risk factor for venous thrombosis. In: Pollard L, Ludlam CA (eds) Recent advances in blood coagulation. Churchill Livingstone, London

Resources

Journals for clinicians

Thrombus. Circulated quarterly to requesting healthcare professionals who are involved in the management of DVTs as part of their everyday practice. Hayward Medical Communications, Rosemary House, Lanwades Park, Kentford, Newmarket, Suffolk CB8 7PW.

Journal of Thrombosis and Thrombolysis. An international journal for clinicians and scientists. Kluwer Academic Publishers, Distribution Center, PO Box 322, 3300 AH Dordrecht, The Netherlands.

Journal for patients

INReview. Information publication for users of warfarin and other oral anticoagulation drugs, circulated quarterly. Anticoagulation Europe, PO Box 405, Bromley, Kent BR2 9WP.

Accredited courses

The University of Northumbria at Newcastle is in the process of developing a unit focusing on 'The Principles and Practice of Anticoagulation Management'. This unit will carry 20 points of academic credit at either Diploma or Degree level and will be facilitated via electronic delivery, with a possible alternative form using paper-based materials.

Chapter 16

User involvement in primary care

Linda Drake

CHAPTER CONTENTS

INTRODUCTION

The past decade has seen patients changing from passive recipients to active consumers of healthcare services. The new NHS places the patient firmly in the centre of healthcare delivery, with the government promoting a more equal relationship between professionals and their patients. User involvement has a role in the planning, delivery and monitoring of health services.

This chapter will set the context for user involvement in health and social policy and outline the levels at which participation may occur. Opportunities for involving patients in the primary care setting will be outlined, with the emphasis on methods which may facilitate the implementation of National Service Frameworks. The use of patient participation groups in general practice will be described in detail.

WHAT IS USER INVOLVEMENT?

In this chapter, the term 'user' refers to anyone who is using, has used or may use the services provided by the organization. Users will primarily be patients, carers and relatives but can also refer to the local community, representatives from local patients groups and voluntary organizations.

A review of the literature on user involvement reveals no agreement on its definition and little evaluation of the way in which it may lead to health gain or improved decision making or how such benefits can be measured. Definitions of levels or intensity of involvement are often described as a spectrum, ranging from information giving at one end of the continuum to genuine power sharing at the other (Arnstein 1969).

A distinction can be made between individual and collective involvement. Individual involvement is that which occurs during the clinical encounter between healthcare professionals and patients. Collective involvement includes initiatives which either seek to improve the quality of services by making them more responsive or to extend the capacity of users to participate in service design, management and monitoring.

The paternalistic approach to decision making in the healthcare encounter, which has dominated for many years, is gradually being replaced by the realization that there are benefits in involving patients more closely in treatment decisions and giving them more information about their conditions. The debate on genuine informed consent is beyond the scope of this chapter but it is important to note that courts in England have adopted a more patient-centred standard for the information that professionals should give their patients – that which a reasonable patient might expect to receive rather than what a reasonable body of professionals might think to provide (Skene & Smallwood 2002).

Practice nurses have been at the forefront of developing partnership approaches to patient care and education, especially in the area of chronic disease management. However, there is a real lack of suitable patient educational materials to support such work: patient access to the Internet and the development of decision support software should prove helpful.

The 'Expert Patient Programme' creates a relationship where health professionals and patients are genuine partners, seeking the best solutions together. It is based on developing the confidence and motivation of patients, in order to use their own skills and knowledge to take effective control over life with a chronic disease.

Opportunities for collective participation in the NHS have been extended through the government's modernization strategy by the development of primary care trusts (PCTs), which have a lay majority on their boards. A multiplicity of new structures, overseen by the Commission for Patient and Public Involvement in Health, will be responsible for ensuring public involvement in all aspects of primary and community care and the purchase of secondary services.

WHY IS USER INVOLVEMENT IN HEALTHCARE IMPORTANT?

The government's ambition is for a patient-centred NHS, in which the voices of patients, their carers and the public are heard through every level of the service, acting as a powerful lever for change and improvement. A sense of 'ownership' by the public is vital for the success of the modernization agenda, as outlined in *Shifting the balance of power within the NHS* (DoH 2001a).

Commentators agree that involvement in health and social policy is important to legitimate decisions, enhance local accountability and respond to local needs (Winkler 1996). Participation is considered intrinsically good, especially in a climate where the electorate appear reluctant to engage in national politics. Alternative forms of civil engagement are emerging, such as self-help, environmental, charitable and voluntary groups. The alternative is fragmenting social networks, leading to the breakdown of the community (Puttnam 2000). Public involvement could be expected to contribute to social capital and thus to the community's ability to regenerate itself.

Unprecedented media attention followed the inquiry at the Bristol Royal Infirmary, and the Kennedy Report (BRI Public Inquiry 2001) outlined the need for transparency, honesty and openness in a relationship where patients and healthcare professionals are equal partners in care. A more mature relationship must evolve, one in which patients are perceived as a valuable resource in their own care, with the doctor no longer being seen as the infallible fount of all knowledge.

Following the announcement of the abolition of community health councils, a discussion document and listening exercise, *Involving the patients and the public in healthcare* (DoH 2001b), proposed the creation of a Commission for Patient and Public Involvement in Health. Its role will be to oversee the new arrangements for involving patients, including patients' forums, patient advice and liaison services and the availability of independent complaints and advocacy services in every trust. The Commission will also support local citizens and community groups to become involved in health issues. Widespread resistance to the abolition of community health councils was provoked by the perception that the new structures lacked independence and it remains to be seen whether these new structures can effect real changes in organizational culture.

For the first time in 25 years, local authority overview and scrutiny committees will have the powers to inspect local health services and to call NHS managers to account, thus remedying the present democratic deficit between local government and health services.

The challenge for the nurse in general practice is to translate health and social policy into meaningful participation for patients in order to enhance primary care provision.

HOW CAN USERS BECOME INVOLVED IN GENERAL PRACTICE?

User involvement toolkits describe a wide variety of approaches to participation (see Resources section). The following examples from the spectrum of participation may be suitable for use in the primary care setting.

INFORMATION GIVING

Traditionally practices have used written information to inform and educate their patients and this may be the initial method used to raise patients' awareness of how to get involved. Increasingly alternative sources such as audio and video cassettes and interactive computer programs are becoming available. Health promotion units will advise on producing accessible material. Public meetings may also be used, at practice or PCT level, to inform and consult users.

INFORMATION GATHERING

Questionnaires are often used to gauge the satisfaction of the practice population, although response rates tend to be poor. Good questionnaire design, which is essential to obtain meaningful results, requires skill and experience and help should be available from medical audit advisory groups or academic institutions. Alternative approaches include focus groups or semi-structured interviews, which are useful when specific information or views are required. They are labour intensive if the results are to be documented and analysed and again require skilled design.

EXPERT PATIENT APPROACHES

'Expert patient programmes' are based on developing the confidence and motivation of groups of patients, to enable them to use their own skill and knowledge to take effective control over life with chronic diseases. The evidence for lay-led self-management approaches clearly demonstrates both health gain and an improved sense of well-being for patients with chronic disease and they have been used successfully for patients with arthritis, CHD, diabetes, neurological disorders and mental health problems. The courses are delivered by patients who themselves have undergone training (DoH 2001c).

PATIENT PARTICIPATION GROUPS

Patient participation groups (PPGs) can take many forms and may incorporate some of the above functions. The practice nurse is ideally placed to initiate the formation of a PPG within the practice or locality and the method adapts readily to a variety of levels of participation. The establishment and maintenance of such a group will be described below.

COMMUNITY DEVELOPMENT

Community development recognizes the social, economic and environmental causes of ill health and links user involvement and commissioning to improve health and reduce inequalities. It involves a process of working in collaboration with community members, first to assess the collective needs and desires for health change and second to address those needs through a combination of utilization of local talent, resource development and management. Community development approaches require sustained input and are resource intensive but there is good evidence that they can be protective of people's health (Fisher et al 1999). Increased opportunities for multi-agency working and partnerships with the voluntary sector can be used to bid for resources for such work, especially in areas attracting funding for health improvement or regeneration.

PATIENT PARTICIPATION GROUPS

The first PPGs were part of a grassroots movement by GPs in the early 1970s and appear mainly to have focused on raising funds to provide equipment and amenities for practices or to legitimate decisions on local funding priorities. Very few PPGs exist in inner-city areas with relatively high levels of socio-economic deprivation. However, the National Association for Patient Participation Groups reports an increase in enquiries and the formation of new groups coinciding with the formation of PCG/Ts and the government's agenda for patient participation.

THE ROLE AND FUNCTIONS OF PPGs

PPGs aim to involve users in the planning, management or monitoring of services provided in the practice or community or commissioned by the practice or PCT (Chambers 2001, Salford CHC 1998). They can take many forms and may perform some of the following roles:

- making services more responsive to local need through feeding back patients' needs, concerns and interests
- involving patients in improving service quality through gathering their views on services provided and advising the practice/PCT on the priorities for service development
- involving the public as citizens in health and health service decision making, thus increasing a sense of local ownership and understanding of how local services need to be changed and developed
- promoting the needs of traditionally excluded groups such as people from black and ethnic minority groups or those with disabilities
- liaising with voluntary sector organizations, including local branches of national organizations
- enabling patients to become more informed about their treatment and care and to make informed decisions and choices
- encouraging health promotion and preventive care for patients within both the practice and the local community
- providing opportunities for self-help and peer support for patients
- influencing local and national health policy through lobbying
- raising funds to purchase equipment or amenities for the practice.

SETTING UP A PPG IN GENERAL PRACTICE

A prerequisite for a successful PPG is a practice which is committed to high-quality, patient-centred care, genuine dialogue between professionals and patients, openness in clinical practice and a willingness to adapt to change. The method is versatile, readily adapting to a variety of levels of participation. A member of the team who is prepared to take the role of 'champion' for user involvement is required to support the project, with other members of the primary healthcare team and patients joining in as they become convinced of the benefits to both patients and staff. The practice nurse is often ideally placed to assume this role and may initiate the formation of a PPG within the practice or locality.

Planning

A planning group is established at the start of the project. Members could include a colleague from the practice, such as the practice manager or a GP, a representative from an organization which can provide support such as the National Association for Patient Participation Groups (NAPPG) or a member of a local voluntary sector organization and at least two patients (if a single patient attends, he or she may initially feel overwhelmed by professionals). The following factors need consideration.

- The purpose of the group must be clear and agreed by the members and the practice. The aims may be amended as the group develops.
- Will the group be open for all patients to join or focused on certain patient or population groups such as older people, women, patients with CHD or other chronic disease?
- Recruitment methods include advertising broadly within the practice or local community, written invitations available at reception or by post, telephone calls. Specific patient groups can be targeted through disease registers, repeat prescriptions or personally during consultations.
- Location may be a problem for practices without a meeting room, although the waiting area may be suitable out of surgery hours. Local community organizations may be prepared to lend or rent a room.
- Timing should be suitable for those attending, i.e. evening meetings for those in employment or before dark for older people.
- Facilitation by someone with experience of group work may be helpful for the first few meetings.
- Resources will be required for room hire and refreshments. The issue of remunerating for participation is being negotiated nationally;

however, the practice should at least consider refunding out-of-pocket expenses for guest speakers.

The first meeting

Meetings are held approximately 3 monthly and last for about 2 hours. Whilst staff should not dominate, representation from the practice is important to indicate to the participants that their views will be fed back to the staff. The facilitator or chairperson invites all members to introduce themselves, saying why they have attended and what their hopes/aspirations for the group are. An open discussion allows the opportunity to review and amend the aims of the group and to suggest topics for future meetings. Issues such as the appointment of officers, possible affiliation to a national organization (e.g. NAPPG), formulation of a code of conduct or constitution may be discussed at the first or subsequent meeting, depending on the readiness of the participants to commit to the group.

Maintaining the group

Maintaining the momentum of the group requires effort and commitment. A successful group may become semi-autonomous relatively quickly, with clearly defined channels of communication with the practice. The following suggestions may enhance chances of success (Salford CHC 1998).

- Start with a 'quick win' where the group can work towards a modest, achievable goal.
- Keep recruiting new members who will bring fresh ideas and enthusiasm to the group.
- Ensure the practice/PCT responds constructively, not defensively, to comments raised.
- Network with other local and national groups.
- Consider producing a regular newsletter to keep all practice patients and staff informed of the group's activity.
- Evaluation should be planned from the start and it is important that the success criteria are defined by group members. The group may periodically choose to review its progress against its aims using both process and outcome measures to evaluate success.

BARRIERS TO USER INVOLVEMENT

Placing user involvement high on the national agenda will not ensure its universal acceptance or implementation and so far minimal resources have been made available to facilitate participation. Barriers include the following.

- Lack of capacity of certain groups or individuals may result in participants not reflecting the make-up of the local community. Community development approaches may be required at the start of a project to enable traditionally excluded groups to participate. PPGs may be more likely to succeed if they are targeted at specific patient or population groups, such as those with coronary heart disease or from a specific minority ethnic community. If the significance of representativeness is ignored, there is a risk of developing inappropriate strategies and perpetuating inequalities in health (Agass et al 1991).
- Many healthcare professionals find the concept of increased patient participation threatening or an unnecessary additional burden in an already overstretched practice. Concerns include falsely raising patients' expectations, unrealistic suggestions or increasing complaints. In fact, participants in PPGs appear to have a clear understanding of many of the constraints of the NHS and take a constructive approach to problem solving.
- Feedback to users about the effect of their involvement is vital if participants are not to become disillusioned. Increasingly public organizations are consulting their users on the services they provide but users will only continue to be engaged if they feel that their contribution makes a difference. Participants have realistic expectations of the ways in which their suggestions will be incorporated, valuing openness and transparency in the process (Staley 2001).
- Well-intentioned attempts to engage users can fail because equal access has not been ensured. Points to consider include physical access, language and literacy barriers, cultural diversity, appropriate timing of events, childcare facilities or provision for carers, impaired hearing or vision and learning difficulties.
- Resources for user involvement are rarely included in practice budgets but the mainstreaming of such activity may result in associated funding. Opportunities for joint working with community or voluntary organizations may allow applications to a wider range of non-NHS sources. PPGs may become registered charities to support their activities.

CONCLUSION

Effective user involvement will inevitably change the balance of power within the healthcare arena and this may be challenging to both healthcare professionals and patients. Practice nurses must reflect on their own values and understanding of the implications of increasing patient empowerment and may need to facilitate such reflection within the primary healthcare team. Peter Pritchard (1981), a pioneer of patient participation groups, suggested:

> *Bringing the patient into the team increases his power, and also that of the doctor. This implies an overall increase of power at primary care level rather than a transfer of power. There is no certainty that there is only a limited quantum of power which must be shared.*

Case study

A practice nurse in a deprived urban area decided to establish a patient participation group, in response to comments from patients regarding lack of resources on how to prevent and live with coronary heart disease (CHD). The practice managers and partners were reluctant to involve patients in a general participation group, fearing unrealistic demands and an increase in complaints, but they were prepared to host a group focusing on CHD. A stakeholder group, including two patients and the area representative of the NAPP, met to plan the first meeting. A community development worker from a local voluntary sector organization offered to facilitate the group.

Eighteen patients attended the first meeting, expressing a commitment to support and extend the group. Topics for future meetings were suggested, with all participants agreeing that a visit from a cardiologist, who could answer questions in a relaxed environment, would be very popular, although they felt it unlikely that it would be possible to persuade one to attend a small local meeting! In fact, the local cardiologist was happy to speak and claimed he had gained a unique insight from hearing the patients describe their experiences.

One patient suggested the topic and speaker for the fourth meeting and another offered to prepare the publicity material. The group is conscious that, although it is growing, it is not fully representative of the local community and is considering ways to address this.

The practice is establishing patient participation groups for older people and those with diabetes, in line with the National Service Frameworks. Some Personal Medical Services monies have been used to appoint a parttime patient involvement and voluntary sector liaison officer to support user involvement and, although the practice nurse attends the CHD group, she is no longer administering it.

Now a neighbouring practice is at the planning stage for a group focusing on women's health issues, with liaison between the respective practice nurses.

References

Agass M, Coulter A, Mant D, Fuller A 1991 Patient participation in general practice: who participates? British Journal of General Practice 41:198–201

Arnstein SR 1969 A ladder of citizen participation. Journal of the American Institute of Planners 35(4):216–224

Bristol Royal Infirmary Public Inquiry 2001 The report of the public inquiry into children's heart surgery at the Bristol Royal Infirmary 1984–1995: learning from Bristol. The Stationery Office, London

Chambers R 2001 User involvement. Practice Nurse 22(10):15–19

DoH 2001a Shifting the balance of power within the NHS: securing delivery. Department of Health, London

DoH 2001b Involving patients and the public in healthcare. A discussion document. Department of Health, London

DoH 2001c The expert patient: a new approach to chronic disease management for the 21st century. Department of Health, London

Fisher B, Neve H, Heritage Z 1999 Community development, user involvement and primary health care. British Medical Journal 318:749–750

Pritchard P 1981 Patient participation in primary care. Royal College of General Practitioners, London

Puttnam R 2000 Bowling alone: the collapse and revival of American community. Simon and Schuster, New York

Salford CHC 1998 Developing patient participation groups in primary care. A brief guide. Salford Community Health Council, Salford

Skene L, Smallwood R 2002 Informed consent: lessons from Australia. British Medical Journal 324:39–41

Staley K 2001 Voices, values and health. Involving the public in moral decisions. King's Fund, London

Winkler F 1996 Involving patients. In: Meads G (ed) A primary care-led NHS. FT Healthcare, London

Resources

Organizations

National Association for Patient Participation. PO Box 999, Nuneaton, Warwickshire CV11 5ZD. www.napp.org.uk
NAPP is a registered national charity that exists to encourage the establishment and continuation of patients' groups in general practice.

The Patients' Forum. River Bank House, 1 Putney Bridge Approach, London SW6 3JD. Tel: 020 7736 7903. www.thepatientsforum.org.uk
The Patients' Forum is a network of national and regional organizations concerned with the healthcare interests of patients, their families and carers. It provides a wide range of information relating to the patients' movement in the UK.

Preparing Professionals for Partnership with the Public. Regional Education Support Unit, Third Floor, Courtfield House, London W10 6DZ. Tel: 020 8962 4552. kcyrus@londondeanery.ac.uk
A development programme to enable people who work in primary care to explore through facilitated learning what public involvement means to them, review what they are doing already and build on their strengths.

The Long-term Medical Conditions Alliance (LMCA). Unit 212, 16 Baldwins Gardens, London EC1N 7RJ. Tel: 020 7813 3637. www.lmca.org.uk
The LMCA can provide information about the Living with Long-term Illness (LiLL) project and other self-management initiatives.

Toolkits and manuals

Barker J, Bullen M, de Ville J 1999 Reference manual for public involvement, 2nd edn. Bromley Health, West Kent Health Authority and Lambeth, Southwark and Lewisham Health Authority, London

Southwark Action for Voluntary Organizations (SAVO) and the Office for Public Management 2000 Toolkit for community development. London Borough of Southwark, London

NHSE Northern and Yorkshire 2000 Primary care groups public engagement toolkit. NHSE, Leeds

Department of Health publications

DoH 1997 The new NHS: modern, dependable. Department of Health, London

DoH 1999 Patient and public involvement in the new NHS. Department of Health, London

DoH 2000 The NHS Plan. A plan for investment, a plan for reform. Department of Health, London

DoH 2001 The expert patient: a new approach to chronic disease management for the 21st century. Department of Health, London

NHSE 1998a Patient partnership: building a collaborative strategy. Department of Health, London

NHSE 1998b Involving patients: examples of good practice. Department of Health, London

Books and journal articles

Anderson W, Florin D 2000 Involving the public – one of many priorities. King's Fund, London

British Medical Journal 1999 Embracing patient partnership. Theme issue, no. 7212, dedicated to patient participation

Farrell C, Gilbert H 1996 Health care partnerships. King's Fund, London

Hanley B, Bradburn J, Gorin S et al 2000 Involving consumers in research and development in the NHS: briefing notes for researchers. Consumers in NHS Research Support Unit, Winchester

NEF 1999 Participation works! New Economics Foundation, London

New B 2000 Resurrecting the notion of the active citizen. King's Fund, London

Pietroni P, Pietroni C 1996 Innovation in community care and primary health. Churchill Livingstone, Edinburgh

Pritchard P 1993 Partnership with patients: a practical guide to starting a patient participation group, 3rd edn. Royal College of General Practitioners, London

Roberts E 2000 Improving services for older people: what are the issues for PCGs? King's Fund, London

Seargeant J, Steele J 1998 Consulting the public: guidelines and good practice. Policy Studies Institute, London

Shepherd B 2000 A voice for Londoners in the doctor's surgery. Age Concern, London

Stevenson J 1999 Involving older people in health developments. King's Fund, London

SECTION **3**

Health maintenance and clinical procedures

SECTION CONTENTS

Chapter 17

Minor illness

Claire Pratt

CHAPTER CONTENTS

INTRODUCTION

In 1996 the government published two documents (NHSE 1996, Secretary of State for Health 1996) which encourage a primary care-led NHS with flexibility of resources in primary healthcare teams, followed by the DoH publications *The new NHS* (DoH 1997) and *Making a difference* (DoH 1999). As a result we have seen new ways of working and delivering healthcare, including NHS Direct, walk-in centres, minor injury units and open access nurse practitioner clinics. Primary medical service (PMS) pilots are an exciting and innovative way of delivering primary healthcare which enable nurse practitioners and practice nurses to take on new roles to deal with minor illness (DoH 1999, Walker 1997).

One of the fundamental requirements of diagnosing and treating minor illness is the ability to exclude urgent or major pathology. As with all areas of clinical nursing practice, any new or additional role undertaken by qualified nurses must be done with full knowledge of their nursing regulatory body guidelines for professional practice (NMC 2002a,b). It is therefore essential that nurses moving into this field of healthcare undertake the necessary education and training to ensure the promotion of safe clinical care and prevent poor practice (UKCC 2001).

THE CONSULTATION AND THE CLINICAL ASSESSMENT

Nurses can now provide an alternative first point of contact for the examination, diagnosis and treatment of minor complaints (Chambers 1998). Nurse prescribing has been shown to meet the needs of the patient (Brooks et al 2001). One study demonstrates that fewer patients are demanding antibiotics (Clinical 2001) and parents find a delayed approach to commencing antibiotics for their children with otitis media acceptable (Little 2001).

THE CONSULTATION

> *An effective consultation is one that brings about desired outcomes, including the successful operation of the cycle of care.* (Pendleton et al 1991)

Much has been written about face-to-face consultation styles and techniques, ranging from biomedical to biopsychosocial (holistic) models of healthcare. The most important thing to remember is how appropriate the model is to the needs of the patient at the time of consultation.

Those attending with life-threatening conditions require someone to take control and provide an immediate decision (biomedical approach). A consultation involving minor illness may take a broader approach (holistic model), including health education on self-care measures and lifestyle changes. However, serious pathology must be excluded, requiring the nurse to consider differential diagnoses.

With the increase in workload of health professionals the importance of self-care and self-medication for minor ailments is gathering increasing interest (Kendall 2001). Nurses involved in minor illness clinics can help patients become more empowered and knowledgeable regarding appropriate independent action.

There are a number of theoretical models that analyse the consultation process. Pendleton's model (Pendleton et al 1991) described seven tasks of the consultation.

1. Define the reason for the patient's attendance, including:
   - the nature and history of the problems
   - the aetiology
   - the patient's ideas, concerns and expectations
   - the effects of the problem.
2. Consider other problems, including:
   - continuing factors
   - at-risk factors.
3. Choose, with the patient, an appropriate action for each problem.
4. Achieve a shared understanding of the problem with the patient.
5. Involve the patient in the management and encourage him to accept appropriate responsibility.
6. Appropriate use of time and resources:
   - in the consultation
   - in the long term.
7. Establish or maintain a relationship with the patient which helps to achieve the other tasks.

Neighbour's model of the consultation (Neighbour 1992) focuses on what is happening outwardly between the professional and the patient, plus the internal dialogue of the professional during the consultation. Neighbour breaks the consultation down into five milestones and pictorially represents each point as one finger on your hand, making it easy to remember in clinical practice.

1. *Connect with the patient.* Greeting and communicating on a level where both parties understand each other.
2. *Summarize the problem.* The professional reflects the scenario back to the patient, thus letting the patient know he has been heard and understood.
3. *Hand over responsibility for management.* Options are discussed regarding the direction in which the patient could move forward. Choices are made with informed consent.
4. *Safety netting, contingency planning.* Here the professional thinks of differential diagnoses, the worst case or most probable scenarios, and questions whether she has thought of all aspects to the presenting problem.
5. *Housekeeping.* The professional needs to wrap up and complete the consultation before seeing the next patient to ensure another effective consultation can take place.

Telephone consultation

As with face-to-face consultation, the nursing and medical literature provide numerous papers on telephone consultation. This method of consultation is not a new phenomenon. Since 1879 the telephone has assisted in healthcare provision, with 94% of the UK households now having one.

In the current climate of improving access to healthcare for patients, the management of some minor illness is being dealt with over the telephone, i.e. by telephone triage. Nurses providing this type of consultation are still accountable for their practice, as in any other clinical setting.

Effective telephone consultation requires the nurse to have highly developed listening skills. She needs to know when to interrupt and when to hold back, when and how to prompt the caller. These skills will enable her to gain the relevant information for a safe and full analysis of the presenting situation.

During the telephone consultation the nurse needs to be able to build and develop a rapid rapport with the caller, interpret their symptoms and be able to recognize life-threatening problems. In addition, she must apply clinical reasoning, reflect, summarize the history and assessment, explain and gain agreement regarding follow-up and initiate, engage in and apply audit outcomes in future practice.

These are skills that need to be taught. Telephone consultation should no longer be regarded as an unstructured, ad hoc assessment option. Computer software systems exist (i.e. CAS AXA) and are being used nationally by NHS Direct and NHS walk-in centres. Such systems provide a framework for nurses to operate independently with the confidence that they are working within their clinical, professional and legal accountability (Moore 2001). Moore (2001) discusses Peplau's theoretical model in relation to its appropriateness for analysing the telephone consultation.

However, computerized clinical assessment systems are not going to find their way into general practice overnight and their relevance to other clinical environments needs to be debated. Therefore alternative safe methods for assessing the patient, recording the consultation (see Appendix 1), auditing and assessing patient outcomes must be developed by those professionals involved. Introducing new ways of working will affect the whole primary healthcare team and need to be planned, led and managed thoughtfully (Richards & Tawfik 2000).

CLINICAL ASSESSMENT

The clinical assessment can be divided into three components: history taking, examination (if indicated) and appropriate investigations, which may be commenced depending on the information gained during the history taking and examination process.

History taking

History taking has to be both general and focused in nature (Bickley 2000, Munro & Edwards 1995).

General history taking includes:

- previous medical history (i.e. serious illness or operations)
- drug history (i.e. prescribed and OTC medication)
- allergies
- family history
- social history (i.e. occupation)
- systematic review of other systems (if necessary).

Focused history taking includes:

- the present concern (allow patient to express/describe symptoms)
- the history of the present concern:
  - focused history on relevant system
  - location, quality, quantity or severity
  - timing (onset, duration, frequency)
  - aggravated/relieved by.

Use good communication skills, ascertain the patient's perception of the cause and confirm each other's meanings.

An alphabetical checklist technique can be used during the history taking to help develop critical thinking about the presenting problem.

Normal: information about patient's baseline function
Onset: gradual, sudden, new, recurrent
Provocation/palliation: activity, food, cold, stress, medication
Quality/quantity: sharp, dull, stabbing, 1–10 pain scale
Region/radiation: location, site, e.g. referred pain
S associated Symptoms: e.g. fever, nausea, cough
Timing: frequency, duration, time of day
Underlying disorders: previous disease, risk factors, immunocompromised
Verification: physical examination, investigation

However, the whole point of collecting information and data is to help reach a diagnosis about the presenting condition. The nurse must be able to understand the clinical significance of the questions and answers and interpret accordingly.

Physical examination

Following the history taking, a physical examination might be required to either confirm or exclude a diagnosis. The principles of examination require the professional to:

- be systematic
- explain and be sensitive
- work from the right
- work from head to toe
- work from external to internal
- work from normal to abnormal
- use symmetry.

The time-honoured sequence of physical examination includes:

- inspection
- palpation
- percussion
- auscultation.

However, this pattern can be altered according to the patients and their presenting problem, so that the experience is less tiring for the patient.

The aetiology of illness falls into three broad categories:

- physical (either congenital or acquired)
- psychological
- social.

Acronyms can be used to help develop critical thinking to identify the possible cause of a physical disease, such as the word VINDICATE.

V vascular
I inflammatory
N neoplastic
D deficiency
I iatrogenic
C chemical
A autoimmune
T trauma
E endocrine

During the final stages of the consultation a clinical management plan will be formulated with the patient. This plan could consist of conservative measures, health education (including possible self-care advice), therapeutic intervention (including self-medication advice), referrals to other healthcare professionals, undertaking initial (or referral for) investigations, plus advice on any follow-up care.

CLINICAL GUIDELINES AND PATIENT GROUP DIRECTIONS

Developing clinical guidelines (CG) and patient group directions (PGD) requires a formal structure to meet both legal and professional standards (see Chapter 22). The ability to use the Internet is now an essential skill that nurses need to acquire and will assist them in developing evidence-based CG and PGD, giving advice on OTC medications and accessing patient information leaflets. The ability to evaluate the resources found on the Internet is essential. Computer and Internet skills can be developed through specific computer books (Bessant 2000), journal articles (Ward 2001) and courses. Nurses need to seriously consider these courses in addition to accessing the traditional clinical-based programmes. Workforce development confederations, managers and nurse leaders must also understand the relevance of such courses for nurses needing to develop these new professional skills.

The following section provides:

- a format for developing minor illness CG
- seven CG for specific minor illness commonly seen in nurse-led minor illness clinics
- examples of PGD (supplied by kind permission of innovative primary healthcare teams in the West Country: Appendix 2).

Box 17.1 Format for minor illness clinical guidelines

- Overview of the minor illness
- Symptoms may be described as
- Should be investigated if
- Differential diagnosis
- Specific history should include
- Examination
- Tests
- Action for minor illness
- Complications
- Refer to GP immediately if

CLINICAL GUIDELINES FOR THE MANAGEMENT OF SORE THROAT, SEVERE ACUTE TONSILLITIS, PHARYNGITIS

OVERVIEW OF ILLNESS

- Acute inflammation of the pharynx, tonsils or both
- Caused by environmental irritants, viruses or bacteria

- May be part of a more generalized respiratory infection
- Sore throat is usually due to viral infection
- Group A beta-haemolytic streptococcal is the most common bacterial infection

SYMPTOMS MAY BE DESCRIBED AS

Raw feeling in throat causing discomfort, especially when swallowing. Loss of voice, swollen glands, hoarse voice, sore throat, difficulty and/or pain with swallowing. Plus fever, rash, stiff neck, coryza, malaise, earache, halitosis.

SHOULD BE INVESTIGATED IF

Duration >7 days. However, throat swabs are not worth taking routinely as they cannot differentiate between infection and carriage.

DIFFERENTIAL DIAGNOSIS

Cold, influenza, streptococcal infection, infectious mononucleosis (glandular fever), epiglottitis, quinsy, meningitis, scarlet fever, sexually transmitted infection, neutropenia (e.g. ensure patient is not on carbimazole).

SPECIFIC HISTORY SHOULD INCLUDE

- Duration of illness
- What self-care measures have been taken
- Fever, malaise
- Is this a recurrent problem?
- Altered immunity due to illness or medication

EXAMINATION

DO NOT examine if there is drooling, breathing difficulties, stridor or unable to swallow (epiglottitis is an ENT emergency).

- Observe for signs of systemic illness
- Examine body for rash:
  - non-blanching purpuric rash (consider meningitis)
  - macular rash (small red patches, not raised) (consider streptococcal infection)
  - papular rash (sandpaper texture), strawberry tongue (consider scarlet fever)
- Examination of throat and ears
- Use tongue depressor if throat not visible
- Examine neck for enlarged lymph nodes
- Take temperature (if <37°C and mild sore throat, probably viral infection)

TESTS

- FBC, Paul Bunnell and Monospot test if glandular fever suspected (i.e. tonsillitis >7 days)

ACTION FOR MINOR ILLNESS

- Rest until temperature returns to normal, rest voice, increase fluids, increase room humidity, discourage smoking, avoid irritants
- No antibiotic prescription is required in most patients (viral infections > bacterial). They offer minimal benefit and reduce illness time by 8 hours
- OTC paracetamol and/or soluble aspirin to control pain and fever
- OTC throat lozenges to relieve discomfort
- Consider antibiotics (including liquid option) if severe inflammation, high fever, painful enlarged lymph nodes, tonsillar exudate, recurrent tonsillitis, macular rash
- Prescribe as per local PGD (possible antibiotics include penicillin V or erythromycin when history of penicillin allergy. In children <10 years old amoxicillin suspension may be preferable to penicillin V due to taste)

COMPLICATIONS

- Peritonsillar abscess (quinsy): a large swelling around one tonsil and shift of uvula
- Otitis media
- Sinusitis
- Suppurative cervical adenopathy
- Rare complications: rheumatic fever and post-streptococcal glomerulonephritis

REFER TO GP IMMEDIATELY IF

- Non-blanching purpuric rash
- Peritonsillar abscess (quinsy)
- Epiglottitis
- Child is very sick

Box 17.2 Taunton & Area Primary Care Group Nurse Practitioner Open Access Service, Crossway Centre, Halcon. Patient group direction for the supply/administration of phenoxymethylpenicillin (penicillin V)

The master document for this protocol is held by the Pharmaceutical Advisor

1. Clinical condition

Define situation/condition	Severe acute tonsillitis/pharyngitis
Criteria for inclusion	As per clinical guideline for sore throat
Criteria for exclusion	Sensitivity to penicillins or cephalosporins Children under 1 year old
Caution	Patients may be unaware/unclear about drug names. If there is a history of hypersensitivity to any drug consider withholding treatment until medical records can be checked
Action if excluded or patient declines	If sensitive/allergic to penicillin refer to PGD for erythromycin Otherwise refer to GP
When healthcare professional should seek further medical advice	Patients with renal impairment Pregnancy Breastfeeding mothers (due to risk of sensitization) Patients taking probenecid (this drug is now only available on a named-patient basis)

2. Description of treatment

Name of medicine	Phenoxymethylpenicillin tablets 250 mg, oral solution 125 mg/5 ml or 250 mg/5 ml
POM/P/GSL	POM
Black Triangle status	No
Route/method	Oral
Dose	*Adult*: 500 mg (as two 250 mg tablets) *Child 1–5 years*: 125 mg (given as 5 ml of 125 mg/5 ml strength solution) *Child 6–12 years*: 250 mg (given as 5 ml of 250 mg/5 ml strength solution)
Frequency	Four times a day
Duration	Seven days
Total dose/number	*Adult*: 56 tablets (2 packs of 28) *Child 1–5 years*: 140 ml oral solution strength 125 mg/5 ml *Child 6–12 years*: 140 ml oral solution strength 250 mg/5 ml
Written/verbal advice for patient/carer	Patients should be told to: • Always complete the course • Take the medicine on an empty stomach (i.e. 1 hour before food or 2 hours after food) • Store oral solution in a refrigerator and shake before each dose • Take the medicine at regular intervals • Contact their GP if side-effects occur • Contact their GP if symptoms do not improve after 3–4 days • Discard (or ideally return to a pharmacy) any unused medicine
Arrangements for follow-up	None

Side-effects	Hypersensitivity reactions: patients should be warned to seek immediate medical assistance if they experience any severe hypersensitivity reaction Nausea, diarrhoea, skin rashes
Specific method of recording supply/administration sufficient to include audit trail and significant events	As per Crossway Centre policy

3. Characteristics of staff

Qualifications required	• First-level registered nurse • A specific course of study of at least first-degree level • Nurse practitioner diploma (accredited)
Additional requirements	Training session organized by Taunton & Area PCG on the administration and supply of medicines under PGDs
Continued training requirements	Maintains own level of updating with evidence of continued professional development (PREP requirements)

4. Management of patient group directions

Date of 1st issue: 18th June 2001
Next review date: 31st March 2002

5. Signatories

	Name	Signature	Date
Taunton & Area PCG Pharmaceutical Advisor			
Crossway Centre Medical Advisor/Taunton & Area PCG Chairman			
Director of Service Provision, Somerset Coast PCT			
Consultant Microbiologist, Public Health Laboratory Service, Musgrove Park Hospital, Taunton (antimicrobials)			

NB. All antimicrobial PGDs are subject to approval by the Somerset Health Economy County Prescribing Group.

The PGD is to be read, agreed to and signed by all the healthcare professionals to whom it applies. One copy is given to the healthcare professional, another to the manager and the original is retained by the Pharmaceutical Advisor of the PCG.

I have read the PGD and agree to use it only in accordance with the criteria described.

Name: .... Signature ....

Designation: ....

Date: ....

CLINICAL GUIDELINES FOR THE MANAGEMENT OF EARACHE

OVERVIEW OF ILLNESS

Most common causes of earache are infections in the middle ear (otitis media) and outer ear (otitis externa) caused by common germs such as streptococcus, staphylococcus and *Haemophilus influenzae.* Other causes of ear pain could include symptoms due to foreign bodies, impacted wax, injuries, air travel, underwater diving or blunt trauma.

SYMPTOMS MAY BE DESCRIBED AS

Pain or discomfort in or around the ear(s). Pain may be dull and throbbing or sharp and stabbing. Other symptoms may include fever, dizziness, discharge, itch, coryza, swelling, hearing loss, loss of appetite, irritability (may be only indication in infants).

SHOULD BE INVESTIGATED IF

Severe pain, discharging, possibility of foreign body, febrile or irritable infant.

DIFFERENTIAL DIAGNOSIS

Dental abscess, impacted ear wax, localized otitis externa (furunculosis), postauricular adenitis, inflammation of temporomandibular joint, herpetic lesion of ear, mastoid abscess, cervical arthritis, tumour.

SPECIFIC HISTORY SHOULD INCLUDE

- Duration of this occurrence and previous episodes
- What self-care measures have been taken
- Fever, deafness, discharge
- Recent swimming

EXAMINATION

DO NOT examine ear if history of head trauma.

- Assess for systemic illness
- Examine both pinna/canals for inflammation, discharge, swelling, tenderness
- Look at both eardrums: colour, perforation, bulging/retracted drum, fluid level
- Palpate temporomandibular joint
- Inspect neck and palpate lymph nodes
- Throat

TESTS

Ear swab (be careful not to perforate drum) if recent history of swimming, copious discharge or patient is not responding to initial treatment.

ACTION FOR MINOR ILLNESS

OTC analgesic advice, e.g. paracetamol, aspirin or ibuprofen.

ACUTE BACTERIAL OTITIS MEDIA

Signs and symptoms include: pain >24 hours, deafness, fever >37°C, vomiting, loss of balance, red eardrum (often unilateral), bulging, possible discharge. Antibiotics are not indicated in the majority of cases – approximately 80% will resolve within 3 days without antibiotic. Prescribe as per local PGD (possible antibiotics include amoxicillin, erythromycin, trimethroprim).

Give self-help advice.

- Explain, reassure and advise on symptomatic treatment
- OTC analgesia, e.g. paracetamol and/or ibuprofen (refer to local PGD)
- Advise rest until temperature returns to normal, increase fluids, local warmth may ease pain and avoid air travel
- Return to clinic if in pain or hearing still impaired 10–14 days later
- Do not use OTC eardrops

OTITIS EXTERNA

Signs and symptoms include: itchy discomfort rather than pain, canal red, moist, possible discharge or scaling skin, sometimes hearing loss.

Take ear swab for culture if history of treatment failure or chronic infection.

Give self-help advice.

- Explain, reassure and advise on symptomatic treatment
- Advise to clear ear canal of discharge by dry mopping (not to occlude with cotton wool, not to scratch or clean with cotton buds)

- Recommend cotton wool and Vaseline to keep water out of inflamed ears while showering or washing hair
- Recommend avoidance of swimming while ear is inflamed
- Prescribe as per local PGD (i.e. Otosporin eardrops or antibiotic ciprofloxacin)

Complications

Abscess, spreading cellulitis, mastoiditis, malignant otitis externa.

Refer to GP immediately if

Systemically unwell or evidence of spreading infection.

LOCALIZED OTITIS EXTERNA (FURUNCULOSIS)

- Red swelling in canal, often with severe pain. Can be very painful on pressing tragus nerve or when inserting auriscope
- Warn patient ear may discharge
- Prescribe as per local PGD (e.g. flucloxacillin or erythromycin)

Differential diagnosis

Foreign body, otitis media, cholesteatoma, mastoiditis, bullous myringitis, malignant otitis externa (rare, mainly immunocompromised or diabetic), referred pain (from sphenoid sinus, teeth, neck, throat).

EUSTACHIAN CATARRH

- Impaired hearing, ear discomfort
- Drum normal, retracted or bulging
- Fluid level may be seen behind drum which is not inflamed
- Give explanation. Encourage 'popping', steam inhalations
- Prescribe as per local PGD (e.g. pseudoephedrine)

Complications

Glue ear, perforation of eardrum (usually heals within a few weeks).

Refer to GP immediately if

Mastoid abscess, paraesthesia of jaw line, immunocompromised or if pain persists after course of antibiotics or chronic infection.

Box 17.3 Exeter Primary Care Trust, Exeter NHS Walk-In Centre. Patient group direction for the supply/administration of amoxicillin

Written 11/2000	Review date 11/2002
NAME OF DRUG:	**Amoxicillin**
Definition of condition/situation:	Otitis media, chest infection and sinusitis Urinary tract sensitive to trimethoprim
Criteria for confirmation:	As per protocol for earache, chest infection, sinusitis and urinary symptoms Need for antibiotic has been established
Criteria for exclusion:	Known sensitivity to amoxicillin, its ingredients or related compounds Risk of glandular fever Patients with chronic lymphatic leukaemia, human immunodeficiency virus or lymphoma Child under the age of 1 year
Action to be taken for patients excluded from Patient Group Direction:	Contact GP Refer to Patient Group Direction for trimethoprim. If sensitive to trimethoprim, see GP
When nurse should seek further advice from GP:	Children under 5 years Patients with history of atopic allergies or renal impairment Pregnancy Women who are breastfeeding Patients taking allopurinol, warfarin, phenindione or probenecid

Action to be taken for patients who do not wish to receive or adhere to care under this Patient Group Direction:	Refer to GP
Patient advice to be given:	Always complete the course even if you feel better. The original infection may still be present and reoccur if treatment is stopped too soon Take medication at regular intervals Increase daily fluid intake whilst taking amoxicillin Possible side-effects: nausea, diarrhoea, rash. If these occur speak to GP before next dose Women on the pill should be advised on use of extra precautions, reasons and duration If symptoms do not improve in 4 days contact GP Warn patients who need to test their urine that they may not be accurate whilst taking amoxicillin
	TREATMENT AVAILABLE
Names of all medicines or appliances to be supplied or administered via this Patient Group Direction:	Amoxicillin capsules 250 mg Amoxicillin suspension 125 mg/5 ml
Legal status of drug:	Prescription-only medicines
Doses to be used (including criteria for use of differing doses):	Adult: 250 mg tds Child 1–10 years: 125 mg tds Child over 10 years: 250 mg tds
Method or route of administration:	Oral
Frequency of doses:	tds, 8 hourly
Total dose and number of times drug to be given (including timeframe):	tds for 5 days Capsules: 15 × 250 mg capsules Suspension: 100 ml
Warnings and advice re adverse reactions:	If you experience any breathing difficulty, swelling of mouth/tongue, severe rash, joint pain/swelling after taking this medication, SEEK IMMEDIATE MEDICAL ASSISTANCE

METHOD OF RECORDING

Nursing notes, including name, dose and route of administration of drug along with time and date of administration

Local recording policy in agreement with pharmacy

STAFF AUTHORIZED TO USE THIS PATIENT GROUP DIRECTION

Registered nurses Grade F and above working in Exeter NHS Walk-in Centre employed by Exeter & District Community Health Service Trust. Registered nurses below Grade F must be supervised by a senior Grade nurse

And practising within the limits of: The Code of Professional Conduct, The Scope of Professional Practice, The Standards for the Administration of Medicines, Guidelines for Professional Practice, Health Service Circular 026/2000

who have completed the Exeter NHS Walk-In Centre approved education programme and met competencies laid out within said scheme

APPROVED EDUCATION PROGRAMME

Details of the education programme will incorporate the following:

- a preset curriculum
- clinical placements to facilitate experiential learning
- details of which professionals from which specialism will be involved in the education programme
- the procedure for assessment of student competence by the medical directors, using multi-choice questionnaires and viva
- system for reviewing competence to include six monthly patient notes and illness prescribing audits

RECORDING OF ERRORS AND ADVERSE INCIDENTS

Reporting via internal reporting procedure and incident forms, reporting to medical directors yellow cards and general practitioner follow-up

CLINICAL GUIDELINES FOR THE MANAGEMENT OF COUGH

OVERVIEW OF ILLNESS

Cough is the most common symptom of respiratory disease. Cough is a reflex action to clear the airways. Most coughs are viral, some are due to secondary infection. It may occur with infection, irritation or obstruction. Cough may also occur with heart disease or as a side-effect of medication, e.g. ACE inhibitors. Expectoration of mucus may accompany the cough.

SYMPTOMS MAY BE DESCRIBED AS

Dry, productive, short of breath, wheeze, rattle, tight, congested, hacking.

SHOULD BE INVESTIGATED IF

Persistent for >7 days, produces coloured phlegm, immunocompromised patient, short of breath, wheeze, pyrexia, recently commenced new medication.

DIFFERENTIAL DIAGNOSIS

Asthma, congestive cardiac failure, tuberculosis, cancer, chemical irritation, habit, stress, iatrogenic cause.

SPECIFIC HISTORY SHOULD INCLUDE

- Duration
- Dry/productive/wheeze
- Colour of sputum
- Fever
- Chest pain
- Breathlessness
- Previous similar episode
- Known chest problems
- Smoking history
- Medication

EXAMINATION

- Pallor/cyanosis
- Confusion
- Fever
- Respiratory rate
- Crackles in chest

TESTS

- Peak flow if asthmatic or asthma suspected in adults or children over 5 years
- Sputum sample for microscopy if abnormal colour

ACTION FOR MINOR ILLNESS

- Increase fluids, including apple juice to relieve cough symptoms
- Steam inhalations 2–3 times a day
- Antibiotics (amoxicillin (Box 17.3) or erythromycin (Box 17.4) if penicillin sensitive) indicated if: sputum brown, bloodstained or green/yellow. Malaise, sweats, persistent fever, crackles or wheezes in chest, history of co-existing illness, e.g. diabetes, COPD, CCF

- Health education, e.g. antibiotics not indicated for viral coughs, smoking cessation advice

REFER TO GP IMMEDIATELY IF

- Cyanosed
- Confused, unwell or distressed
- One-sided chest pain worse with coughing or deep inspiration (consider pleurisy, pneumonia or pulmonary embolism)

Make GP appointment if cough persistent or recurrent (consider cancer, tuberculosis).

Box 17.4 Taunton & Area Primary Care Group Nurse Practitioner Open Access Service, Crossway Centre, Halcon. Patient group direction for the supply/administration of erythromycin

The master document for this protocol is held by the Pharmaceutical Advisor

1. Clinical Condition

Define situation/condition	Treatment of the following conditions in penicillin-sensitive patients: Severe acute tonsillitis/pharyngitis Boils/cellulitis/furunculosis Impetigo Otitis media Bronchitis
Criteria for inclusion	As per clinical guidelines for sore throat, boils/cellulitis, impetigo, otitis media and bronchitis
Criteria for exclusion	Sensitivity to erythromycin Children under 1 year old Patients with hepatic impairment Patients with myasthenia gravis Patients with porphyria Patients taking ergotamine, mizolastine, pimozide, reboxetine, simvastatin, terfenadine and tolterodine
Caution	
Action if excluded or patient declines	Refer to GP
When healthcare professional should seek further medical advice	Patients with renal impairment Pregnancy Patients taking carbamazepine, cyclosporin, clozapine, disopyramide, rifabutin, sildenafil, tacrolimus, theophylline valproate, warfarin, zopiclone

2. Description of Treatment

Name of medicine	Erythromycin tablets e/c 250 mg Erythromycin ethyl succinate oral suspension 125 mg/5 ml or 250 mg/5 ml
POM/P/GSL	POM
Black Triangle status	No
Route/method	Oral

Dose	*Adult*: 250 mg (250–500 mg for cellulitis/impetigo depending on severity) *Child under 2*: 125 mg (given as 5 ml of 125 mg/5 ml strength suspension) *Child 2–8 years*: 250 mg (given as 5 ml of 250 mg/5 ml strength suspension)
Frequency	Four times a day
Duration	Otitis media, bronchitis: 5 days Tonsillitis/pharyngitis, boils, cellulitis, furunculosis, impetigo: 7 days
Total dose/number	**Otitis media, chest infection** *Adult*: 20 tablets *Child under 2 years*: 100 ml suspension (strength 125 mg/5 ml) *Child 2–8 years*: 100 ml suspension (strength 250 mg/5 ml) *Child over 8 years*: 20 tablets or 100 ml suspension (strength 250 mg/5 ml) **Tonsillitis/pharyngitis** *Adult*: 28 tablets *Child under 2 years*: 140 ml suspension (strength 125 mg/5 ml) *Child 2–8 years*: 140 ml suspension (strength 250 mg/5 ml) *Child over 8 years*: 28 tablets or 140 ml suspension (strength 250 mg/5 ml) **Boils, cellulitis, furunculosis, impetigo** *Adult*: 28 or 56 tablets depending on severity *Child under 2 years*: 140 ml suspension (strength 125 mg/5 ml) *Child 2–8 years*: 140 ml suspension (strength 250 mg/5 ml) *Child over 8 years*: 28 tablets or 140 ml suspension (strength 250 mg/5 ml)
Written/verbal advice for patient/carer	Patients should be told to: • Always complete the course • Swallow the tablets whole and don't take them at the same time as indigestion remedies • Store oral solution in a refrigerator and shake before each dose • Take the medicine at regular intervals • Contact their GP if side-effects occur • Contact their GP if symptoms do not improve after 3–4 days • Discard (or ideally return to a pharmacy) any unused medicine
Arrangements for follow-up	Patients with furunculosis should be referred to their GP for follow-up within 72 hours
Side-effects	Nausea, vomiting, diarrhoea, abdominal discomfort Skin reactions ranging from mild eruptions to serious conditions have rarely been reported Symptoms of hepatitis and/or hepatic dysfunction may occur Cardiac arrhythmias have been very rarely reported Allergic reactions are rare and mild but patients should be warned to seek immediate medical assistance if they experience any severe hypersensitivity reaction
Specific method of recording supply/ administration sufficient to include audit trail and significant events	As per Crossway Centre policy

CLINICAL GUIDELINES FOR THE MANAGEMENT OF FEVER

OVERVIEW OF ILLNESS

Fever is a symptom, not a disease, and may be due to viral or bacterial infections such as the common cold, influenza, chest infection, urinary tract infection, food poisoning or tonsillitis. Pyrexia has been shown to be beneficial by increasing the body's defence response and is defined as:

- oral temperature >37.5°C
- rectal temperature >38°C
- axillary temperature >37.2°C.

SYMPTOMS MAY BE DESCRIBED AS

Chills, cold sweats, fever, flushed, sweating.

SHOULD BE INVESTIGATED IF

- Oral temperature >38.6°C (or >38.1°C in immunocompromised patient)
- Persistent
- Other symptoms are present
- There is a preexisting disease

DIFFERENTIAL DIAGNOSIS

Consider other more serious viral or bacterial infections, e.g. meningitis, malaria.

SPECIFIC HISTORY SHOULD INCLUDE

- Duration
- What self-care measures have been taken
- Are there any other symptoms, e.g. specific pain (i.e. abdominal, sinuses, breasts in lactating women), pain on bending neck, headache, vomiting, photophobia, rash, shortness of breath, cough/phlegm, vomiting/diarrhoea, sore throat/cold, dysuria/frequency, severe back pain, recent foreign travel

EXAMINATION

As suggested by symptoms above.

TESTS

Dependent on accompanying symptoms.

- Test urine for protein and blood if cause for fever is not obvious
- Send MSU if Multistix GP test is positive or patient is symptomatic

ACTION FOR MINOR ILLNESS

Common cold, flu-like symptoms, mild headache, mild sore throat.

- Rest until temperature returns to normal
- Increase fluids

Box 17.5 Taunton & Area Primary Care Group Nurse Practitioner Open Access Service, Crossway Centre, Halcon. Patient group direction for the supply/administration of paracetamol

The master document for this protocol is held by the Pharmaceutical Advisor

1. Clinical Condition

Define situation/condition	Mild to moderate pain relief, pyrexia
Criteria for inclusion	*For adults and children over 12*: immediate pain relief for headache, migraine, musculoskeletal pain or trauma, soft tissue injuries such as wounds, sprains and strains, dysmenorrhoea, toothache, sore throat; treatment of pyrexia *For children from 3 months to 12 years*: immediate pain relief for headache, sore throat, otitis media, soft tissue injuries such as wounds, sprains and strains; treatment of pyrexia
Criteria for exclusion	Children under 3 months old Sensitivity to paracetamol

Caution	The maximum total daily dose must not be exceeded (see later). Patients may be taking other paracetamol-containing preparations and it is frequently included in cold and cough remedies. If there are any doubts about exceeding the total daily dose then treatment must be withheld
Action if excluded or patient declines	If sensitive to paracetamol or already taking paracetamol-containing medicines refer to PGD for ibuprofen Otherwise refer to GP
When healthcare professional should seek further medical advice	History of drug abuse, liver disease, alcohol dependency or previous paracetamol overdose Renal impairment

2. Description of Treatment

Name of medicine	Paracetamol 500 mg tablets Paracetamol 250 mg/5 ml suspension Paracetamol 120 mg/5 ml suspension
POM/P/GSL	P (paracetamol 500 mg tablets are GSL in pack sizes up to 16)
Black Triangle status	No
Route/method	Oral
Dose	*Adults and children over 12*: 1 g (two tablets of 500 mg) *Child 3 months to 1 year*: 60–120 mg (given by oral syringe as 2.5–5 ml of 120 mg/5 ml suspension) *Child 1–5 years*: 120–240 mg (given as 5–10 ml of 120 mg/5 ml suspension) *Child 6–12 years*: 250–500 mg (given as 5–10 ml of 250 mg/5 ml suspension)
Frequency	Every 4–6 hours up to a **maximum of four doses in 24 hours**
Duration	Do not use for more than 3 days without consulting a doctor
Total dose/number	*Adults and children over 12*: 16 tablets *Child 3 months to 1 year*: 70 ml of 120 mg/5 ml suspension *Child 1–5 years*: 70 ml of 120 mg/5 ml suspension *Child 6–12 years*: 100 ml of 250 mg/5 ml suspension
Written/verbal advice for patient/carer	Do not take more than four doses in 24 hours and do not repeat doses more frequently than 4 hourly The suspension should be shaken thoroughly before use Patients should be told to contact their own GP if side-effects occur
Arrangements for follow-up	None
Side-effects	These are rare at usual recommended doses. Skin rashes may occur infrequently Most cases of adverse reactions relate to overdose
Specific method of recording supply/administration sufficient to include audit trail and significant events	As per Crossway Centre policy

- To relieve sore throat try throat lozenges, salt water gargles
- Increase room humidity and/or advise steam inhalation
- For pain and fever consider paracetamol, ibuprofen, or aspirin (but not <16 years old) as per local PGD
- Referral to pharmacist for OTC analgesia is an alternative

REFER TO GP IMMEDIATELY IF

- >1 week duration
- Photophobic, neck stiffness, drowsiness, petechial rash
- Appears unwell
- Recent travel to tropical region

CLINICAL GUIDELINES FOR THE MANAGEMENT OF DIARRHOEA

OVERVIEW OF ILLNESS

Diarrhoea is a symptom of a disease, not the disease itself. May be caused by stress, food poisoning, infections, poor absorption, overeating, increased alcohol consumption, nicotine addiction, abuse of laxatives, bowel disease. Diarrhoea caused by staphylococcus may occur within 1 hour of contracting the infection, whereas campylobacter infections may take 2–5 days to manifest.

SYMPTOMS MAY BE DESCRIBED AS

Frequent passing of loose, watery or unformed stool. Diarrhoea may be accompanied by additional symptoms such as cramps just before or with bowel action, thirst, nausea, vomiting, flu-like symptoms, blood or mucus in stool.

SHOULD BE INVESTIGATED IF

Altered bowel pattern and age >45.

DIFFERENTIAL DIAGNOSIS

Diverticulitis, irritable bowel, tumours, obstruction.

SPECIFIC HISTORY SHOULD INCLUDE

- Duration and severity
- What is the stool like?
- What self-care measures have been taken
- Fever
- Contacts with similar symptoms
- Does the stool contain blood or mucus?
- Are symptoms related to commencing new medication?
- Family history
- Occupational history, i.e. food handler
- Recent suspected meals or foreign travel

EXAMINATION

- Assess for dehydration (particularly in very young or elderly)
- Record temperature

TESTS

Send stool culture if food poisoning suspected, blood in motion, recent foreign travel, symptoms >5 days or food handler.

ACTION FOR MINOR ILLNESS

- If no vomiting eat soft, bland carbohydrate diet
- If vomiting, sips of clear fluid only for 12 hours (consider OTC oral rehydration salts, i.e. Dioralyte)
- Resume normal diet within 2–3 days
- Food handlers should not go to work until stool microbiology result known
- If food poisoning suspected complete form from Notification of Infectious Disease Book. Advise patient that Public Health Department may contact them
- Avoid foods associated with possible food poisoning for 48 hours
- Use of anti-diarrhoea drugs is often inappropriate
- Antibiotics (severe cases only) as per local PGD (e.g. metronidazole)

REFER TO GP IMMEDIATELY IF

- Continuous severe abdominal pain for >1 hour

- Patient suffers with diabetes, ulcerative colitis, Crohn's disease, diverticulitis
- Severely ill/dehydrated or if blood in vomit or stool
- Diarrhoea has lasted >48 hours
- Symptoms are due to side-effects of a prescribed medication

Box 17.6 PatientWise: medical and health information for patients

12.11 GASTROENTERITIS

* What is it?

Gastroenteritis is a very common cause of illness in the Western world. It is usually produced by an infection of the gut. The infection will mainly cause you to have vomiting or diarrhoea. The diarrhoea may be watery or contain blood with mucus. Other symptoms include nausea, shivering, headache, griping abdominal pain and fever. The cause of the infection is often not very obvious. Gastroenteritis usually does not last for more than a few days. However, longer infections may occur. The infections can usually be managed at home but more severe symptoms, especially in infants and the elderly, may need hospital care. This is because the very young and the very old are more likely to suffer from the effects of dehydration. Diarrhoea can be caused by the direct effect of the virus or bacterium. Some germs, however, produce a chemical (called a toxin) which is the agent causing food poisoning and irritation to the stomach or bowel. The time between 'catching' the infection and getting the first symptom (incubation period) varies from an hour (germs like staphylococcus) to 2–5 days (germs like campylobacter).

* How does it occur?

Agents causing gastroenteritis are usually transmitted through contaminated food or water. Meat, poultry, dairy products, shellfish, parboiled rice are often the culprits. Inadequate reheating of frozen or chilled foods often allows the germs to flourish. The irritation of the stomach or bowel causes a loss of fluid into the cavity of the bowel. The same irritation causes the muscle in the wall of the gut to contract. This causes vomiting (if mainly a gastritis) or diarrhoea (if mainly affecting the lower bowel).

* Why does it occur?

Poor nutrition and certain chronic illnesses make it much more likely for some people to get these infections. There is nothing to suggest a hereditary factor. Poor personal hygiene and food preparation are the biggest problems. The breaking of *basic rules* leads to most big outbreaks: food *must* be cooled and heated thoroughly; frozen food *must* be thawed completely before cooking (especially meat and poultry); food *must* be eaten within one hour of cooking; recently cooked food *should* be cooled and stored (at less than 4°C) within 90 minutes; cooked and raw foods *should* be prepared and stored in different areas and sections of the refrigerator. Hands should be washed before cooking.

Traveller's diarrhoea (a form of gastroenteritis) occurs because food is casually chosen; for example, water that is not sterilized or non-sealed bottled drinks.

* What does treatment/management involve?

A stool sample is usually sent to the laboratory for analysis only if the condition is bad enough to justify hospital admission or if the problem does not settle within a week. Because dehydration can be a serious problem, it is important that you maintain fluid intake. This is even more important in the very young and old. Fluid should be given often and in small amounts. The best way of correcting dehydration is with a preparation called Dioralyte. This is available on prescription and over the counter at chemists. One sachet of Dioralyte (which is a glucose and mineral mixture) is dissolved in 200 ml of water. In young children, one sachet is given for each kilogram of body weight per 24 hours. An alternative to Dioralyte is flat Coca-cola, which may be more acceptable. If fluids cannot be maintained it may be necessary to be admitted to hospital so that fluids can be given (by drip into a vein). Anti-diarrhoea drugs are not usually given to children but may be given to adults if symptoms are bad. Codeine, kaolin and morphine, and loperamide are often used. Sometimes anti-vomiting and anti-spasm drugs may be given. Antibiotics are only used rarely for severe infections. For traveller's diarrhoea abroad, try to ensure that food and water come from reliable sources, and that food is freshly and thoroughly cooked. Do not eat food bought in the street. Avoid buffets which will have been handled in preparation then displayed at room temperature. When buying drinks, ensure that bottles of water and even cap-top bottles have not been opened and refilled. Always wash fruit in water which has been sterilized with tablets, or peel it.

*** What to watch out for during treatment**
Gastroenteritis due to most bacterial and virus infections improves in a few days. In some infections, abdominal pain, disturbed bowel habit, and general ill health may continue for 2–3 weeks. Hospital admission is occasionally needed if dehydration occurs. Contact the doctor if the diarrhoea or vomiting is uncontrollable. The doctor also needs to know if the treatment is not helping to control the symptoms or if the diarrhoea lasts more than 7 days. Careful hygiene is essential to avoid infecting other people.

*** What to watch out for after treatment**
Most attacks of gastroenteritis do not recur. However, if diarrhoea returns, or if weight loss or pale floating stools occur, then further tests may be needed. Any unusual symptoms not mentioned above are a reason for letting the doctor know immediately.

*** What would happen if the condition was not treated?**
Most attacks of gastroenteritis will get better by themselves with no treatment other than plenty of fluids and rest.

*** What is involved for family and friends?**
Their main concern should be to avoid getting infected themselves. Hygiene is all-important for them as well. If they prepare food, it is their responsibility to be sure that the basic rules of safe food preparation are followed.

12.11 This sheet describes a medical condition or surgical procedure. It has been given to you because it relates to your condition and may help you understand it better. It does not necessarily describe your problem exactly. If you have any questions, please ask your doctor.

CLINICAL GUIDELINES FOR THE MANAGEMENT OF URINARY TRACT INFECTION

OVERVIEW OF ILLNESS

It is important to differentiate increased frequency of urine due to, for example, diabetes, diuretics or increased alcohol levels from frequent small amounts of urine being passed due to infection or irritation. Some women may confuse the symptoms of thrush and cystitis, plus chlamydia infections may also cause dysuria.

SYMPTOMS MAY BE DESCRIBED AS

Dysuria, frequency, nocturia, urgency, suprapubic pain, cloudy offensive urine, haematuria.

SHOULD BE INVESTIGATED IF

- Child under 16
- Women with severe/persistent symptoms
- Patients with loin pain
- Men

DIFFERENTIAL DIAGNOSIS

- Urethral syndrome
- Bladder or other urinary tract irritative lesion, e.g. calculi, tumour
- Candidal infection
- Chlamydia or other sexually transmitted disease
- Urethritis
- Drug-induced cystitis (e.g. cyclophosphamide, allopurinol, danazol, tiaprofenic acid and possibly other NSAIDs)

SPECIFIC HISTORY SHOULD INCLUDE

- Duration of illness and specific symptoms, e.g. dysuria, frequency, obvious haematuria
- Associated symptoms, e.g. back ache, fever, low abdominal pain, vaginal or penile symptoms
- Previous history of renal stones or pyelonephritis
- Current medical history, including possibility of pregnancy
- Sexual history, e.g. new sexual partner, sexual orientation, contraceptive history

EXAMINATION

Dependent on symptoms, e.g. genital examination may be required.

TESTS

- Urinalysis – use Multistix GP. If positive for blood and protein, take MSU.
- Take high vaginal and cervical swabs for culture and chlamydia test if required
- If sexually transmitted infection suspected refer to genitourinary clinic

ACTION FOR MINOR ILLNESS

- High fluid intake
- Cranberry juice may relieve symptoms
- Hot water bottle against the abdomen may ease any pain
- Prescribe antibiotic as per local PGD, e.g. uncomplicated UTI – trimethoprim

COMPLICATIONS

- Ascending infection
- UTI of pregnancy
- Recurrent infection

REFER TO GP IMMEDIATELY IF

- High fever and severe pain/malaise
- History of kidney stones or pyelonephritis
- Pregnant women
- Immunosuppression

Box 17.7 Exeter Primary Care Trust, Exeter NHS Walk-In Centre. Patient group direction for the supply/administration of trimethoprim

Written 11/2000	Review date 11/2002
NAME OF DRUG:	Trimethoprim
Definition of condition/situation:	Urinary tract infection and as an alternative in penicillin-sensitive patients with otitis media and respiratory tract infection
Criteria for confirmation:	• As per protocol for earache, urine infection and respiratory tract infection • Always send MSU in patients with UTI if starting therapy • Need for antibiotic has been established
Criteria for exclusion:	Known sensitivity to trimethoprim, its ingredients or related compounds Child under the age of 1 year Pregnancy Patients with known renal impairment or folate deficiency Patients known to have porphyria Patients with known blood disorders
Action to be taken for patients excluded from Patient Group Direction:	Contact GP
When nurse should seek further advice from GP:	Children under 5 years Patients taking cyclosporin, warfarin, procainamide, antimalarials, rifampicin, phenytoin and digoxin Women who are breastfeeding Patients over 70 years
Action to be taken for patients who do not wish to receive or adhere to care under this Patient Group Direction:	Refer to GP
Patient advice to be given:	Always complete the course even if you feel better. The original infection may still be present and reoccur if treatment is stopped too soon. Take tablets with plenty of water Take medication at regular intervals

	• Possible side-effects: nausea, diarrhoea, itching or rash. If experienced, speak to GP before next dose • Suspension should be shaken before each use If symptoms not resolved on completing course contact GP
	TREATMENT AVAILABLE
Names of all medicines or appliances to be supplied or administered via this Patient Group Direction:	Trimethoprim 200 mg tablets Trimethoprim suspension 50 mg/5 ml
Legal status of drug:	Prescription-only medicines
Doses to be used (including criteria for use of differing doses):	Adult: 200 mg bd Child 1–5 years: 50 mg/5 ml bd Child 6–12 years: 100 mg/10 ml bd
Method or route of administration:	Oral
Frequency of doses:	bd, 12 hourly
Course length, quantity and dosage:	**Otitis media**: bd for 5 days Tablets: 10 × 200 mg tablets Suspension: 50 mg/5 ml *Child 1–5 years*: 5 ml bd (50 ml) *Child 6–12 years*: 10 ml bd (100 ml) **Chest infection**: bd for 5 days Tablets: 10 × 200 mg tablets Suspension: *Child 1–5 years*: 5 ml bd (50 ml) *Child 6–12 years*: 10 ml bd (100 ml) **Urinary tract infection**: *Women*: bd for 3 days *Men and children*: bd for 7 days Tablets: *Women*: 6 × 200 mg tablets *Men*: 14 × 200 mg tablets Suspension: *Child 1–5 years*: 5 ml bd (70 ml) *Child 6–12 years*: 10 ml bd (140 ml) **Pyelonephritis**: bd for 14 days Tablets: 28 × 200 mg tablets
Warnings and advice re adverse reactions:	If you experience any breathing difficulty, swelling of mouth/tongue, severe rash, joint pain/swelling after taking this medication, SEEK IMMEDIATE MEDICAL ASSISTANCE

CLINICAL GUIDELINES FOR THE MANAGEMENT OF CONJUNCTIVITIS

OVERVIEW OF ILLNESS

Conjunctivitis can be acute or chronic, caused by infection (viral or bacterial), an allergic reaction (e.g. grass or pollen), as a result of trauma (e.g. chemical) or due to degenerative changes (e.g. dry eyes).

SYMPTOMS MAY BE DESCRIBED AS

In infectious conjunctivitis: red, sore gritty eye(s), sticky discharge, gummed-up eyelids on waking, sometimes swollen eyelids.

In allergic conjunctivitis: watery, itchy eyes, swelling of the white of the eye.

SHOULD BE INVESTIGATED IF

Photophobic, reduced visual acuity and/or pain.

DIFFERENTIAL DIAGNOSIS

Uveitis, iritis, chlamydia, herpes, subconjunctival haemorrhage.

SPECIFIC HISTORY SHOULD INCLUDE

- Symptoms and their duration
- What self-care measures have been taken
- Associated symptoms (e.g. upper respiratory tract infections, siblings with symptoms)
- Visual disturbance
- Use of contact lenses
- Occupation

EXAMINATION

- Check both eyes for: pupil size, discharge, inflammation, visual acuity, foreign body
- Stain eye with fluorescein if history of foreign body, trauma or use of power tools
- Check conjunctiva in lower fornix and evert upper lid

TESTS

- Swab eye(s) if persistent or recurrent symptoms or if chlamydia is suspected
- FBC and rheumatoid factor if acute uveitis is suspected

ACTION FOR MINOR ILLNESS

Infectious conjunctivitis

Consider need for chloramphenicol eyedrops 0.5%. In severe cases chloramphenicol ointment 1% may be administered at night also.

- Remove contact lenses, clean and do not reuse until infection has settled
- Conjunctivitis is contagious so use separate towels and flannels
- Avoid school/nursery until condition settled

Allergic conjunctivitis

Consider need for sodium cromoglycate 2% eyedrops.

- Avoid triggers (e.g. make-up)
- Cold compress over eyelids may ease symptoms

Dry eyes

Consider need for artificial tears (Hypomellos 0.3% eyedrops).

Box 17.8 Taunton & Area Primary Care Group Nurse Practitioner Open Access Service, Crossway Centre, Halcon. Patient group direction for the supply/administration of chloramphenicol eyedrops 0.5%, chloramphenicol eye ointment 1%

The master document for this protocol is held by the Pharmaceutical Advisor

1. Clinical Condition

Define situation/condition	Treatment of superficial eye infections
Criteria for inclusion	Adults and children with the following superficial eye infections: Conjunctivitis (NB: refer to clinical guideline for bacterial conjunctivitis) Blepharitis Stye Infected meibomian cyst
Criteria for exclusion	Sensitivity to chloramphenicol Severe/recurrent conjunctivitis as per clinical guideline History of blood disorders

Caution	
Action if excluded or patient declines	Refer to GP
When healthcare professional should seek further medical advice	Pregnancy Breastfeeding mothers

2. Description of Treatment

Name of medicine	Chloramphenicol eyedrops 0.5% Chloramphenicol eye ointment 1%
POM/P/GSL	POM
Black Triangle status	No
Route/method	Use either eyedrops or ointment depending on type of condition and patient/carer preference Apply topically to eye – instil in lower conjunctival sac For blepharitis apply ointment to lid margins as appropriate
Dose	*Eyedrops* Adults: Instil one or two drops in affected eye Children: Instil one drop in affected eye *Eye ointment* Adults and children: Apply small amount to affected eye
Frequency	*Eyedrops* Every 2 hours at first, reducing to four times a day as infection is controlled *Eye ointment* Three to four times a day
Duration	Use until the condition returns to normal and for a further 48 hours (maximum of 7 days)
Total dose/number	Eyedrops – 10 ml vial Eye ointment – 4 g tube
Written/verbal advice for patient/carer	Temporary blurring may occur immediately after use; do not drive until vision is clear The eyedrops should be stored between 2° and 8°C (i.e. in a fridge but not a freezer) Contact lenses should not be worn when using the medicine Use the medicine at regular intervals Contact GP if side-effects occur Contact GP if symptoms do not improve after 3–4 days Discard (or ideally return to a pharmacy) any unused medicine
Arrangements for follow-up	If swab taken send result and refer patient to GP
Side-effects	Short-term irritation, burning, stinging and itching may occur after application
Specific method of recording supply/administration sufficient to include audit trail and significant events	As per Crossway Centre policy

COMPLICATIONS

Ulceration.

REFER TO GP IMMEDIATELY IF

- History of eye disease (e.g. uveitis, glaucoma or iritis)
- Reduced acuity, abnormal shape or pupil reaction, foreign body present, severe inflammation, recurrent problem, shingles suspected, fluorescein staining uptake

EVALUATION AND AUDIT

Audit is a cycle of activity that can be used to scrutinize practice, identify problems, develop solutions, implement change and review the scenario again (Jones 2000).

In 1991 (NHS Management Executive 1991) a framework for auditing nursing services was developed and provided a structure for audit to be undertaken at a number of levels within any healthcare organization.

In the current healthcare arena audit is seen as a crucial component of clinical governance (RCN 1998), evidence-based practice (Le May 1999) and significant event audit (Hamer 2000) where audit is part of a multiprofessional process to improve the quality of patient care, to safeguard standards and reduce risks.

In addition to this, audit can be used during clinical supervision as part of peer review, encouraging professional reflection, where each nurse can build upon his or her knowledge of accountability for maintaining and improving standards of patient care (Hamer 2000).

This chapter has highlighted a number of clinical and professional issues that are suitable for auditing and evaluating practice. Evaluation can be undertaken using a variety of media such as audiotapes, video, peer review and written documentation. However, do not forget to consider the Data Protection Act or the need for patient consent to allow other professionals to review the consultation with you.

Acknowledgements

I would like to express my appreciation to the Nurse Practitioner Open Access Clinic, Crossway Centre, Halcon, Taunton and the Taunton PCG (Somerset), the Exeter NHS Walk-In Centre and the Exeter PCT (Devon) for allowing me to reproduce their Patient Group Directions for the purpose of this chapter. And to PatientWise for the use of their patient medical and health information sheets.

Finally a special thank you to Mrs Cheryl White, Nurse Practitioner, Taunton.

References

Bessant A 2000 Learning to pass the European Computer Driving Licence – using Office 2000. Heinemann, Oxford

Bickley LS 2000 Bates pocket guide to physical examination and history taking, 3rd edn. Lippincott, Williams and Wilkins, Philadelphia

Brooks N, Otway C, Rashid C 2001 Nurse prescribing: what do patients think? Nursing Standard 15(17):33–38

Chambers N 1998 Nurse practitioners in primary care. Radcliffe Medical Press, Oxford

Clinical 2001 Patient demand for antibiotics is decreasing, survey finds. Pharmaceutical Journal 266(7135):211

DoH 1997 The new NHS: modern, dependable. HMSO, London

DoH 1999 Making a difference: strengthening the nursing, midwifery and health visiting contribution of health and healthcare. Department of Health, London

Hamer S 2000 Clinical governance. Nursing Times clinical monographs. Emap Healthcare Ltd, London

Jones A 2000 In: Carey L (ed) Practice Nursing. Baillière Tindall, London

Kendall L 2001 The future patient. Institute of Public Policy Research, London

Le May A 1999 Evidence-based practice. Nursing Times clinical monographs. Emap Healthcare Ltd, London

Little P 2001 Pragmatic randomised control trial of two prescribing strategies for childhood acute otitis media. British Medical Journal 322(7282):336–342

Moore R 2001 A framework for telephone nursing. Nursing Times 97(16):36–37

Munro C, Edwards C 1995 Macleod's clinical examination, 9th edn. Churchill Livingstone, London

Neighbour R 1992 The inner consultation. Kluwer Academic, London

NHS Executive 1996 Primary care: the future. Department of Health, Leeds

NHS Management Executive 1991 Framework for Audit of Nursing Services. HMSO, London

NMC 2002a Code of professional conduct. Nursing and Midwifery Council, London
NMC 2002b Guidelines for records and record keeping. Nursing and Midwifery Council, London
Pendleton D, Schofield D, Tate P, Havelock P 1991 The consultation: an approach to learning and teaching. Oxford University Press, Oxford
RCN 1998 Guidance for nurses on clinical governance. Royal College of Nursing, London
Richards D, Tawfik J 2000 Introducing nurse telephone triage into primary care. Nursing Standard 15(10):42–45
Secretary of State for Health 1996 Choice and opportunity. Department of Health, London
UKCC 2001 Accountability in practice. United Kingdom Central Council for Nursing, Midwifery and Health Visiting, London
Walker J 1997 It's urgent: can I see a nurse? Primary Care 7(7):10–14
Ward R 2001 Internet skills for nurses. Nursing Standard 15(12):47–53

Resources

Education/courses available

- RCN Nurse Practitioner Diploma (e.g. Southbank University)
- Autonomous Practice (e.g. Bournemouth University)
- Minor Illness module (e.g. Plymouth University)
- Telephone Consultation and Triage module (e.g. Bournemouth University)
- Computer courses (e.g. European Computer Driving Licence)

Details and availability will vary across the United Kingdom. It is therefore suggested you to contact your local university or Adult Education centre or use the following points of reference.

NHS Careers Line (England). Tel: 0845 606 0655
Nursing and Midwifery Council (www.nmc-uk.org)
UK Nurse Practitioner website (www.nursepractitioner.org.uk)
RCN Direct. Tel: 0845 772 6100

Websites

www.prodigy.nhs.uk (clinical guidelines)
www.eguidelines.co.uk (clinical guidelines)
www.doctoronline.nhs.uk
www.groupprotocol.org.uk
www.medicinechestonline.co.uk (PAGB OTC Directory)
www.rcn.org.uk (section on patient group directions)
www.nhsdirect.nhs.uk
www.doh.gov.uk/nhsinfo/index.htm
www.nice.org.uk

APPENDIX 1 TELEPHONE CONSULTATION FORM

DATE and TIME CALL RECEIVED

....

NAME of CALLER

....

RELATIONSHIP TO PATIENT (e.g. mother, father, neighbour)

....

NAME of PATIENT .... Date of Birth .... Gender M/F

ADDRESS ....

....

....

.... Tel No ....

Name of Patient's GP Dr ....

BRIEF REASON FOR CALL (condition, severity, duration) ....

....

....

GENERAL HEALTH HISTORY ....

....

....

CURRENT MEDICATION ....

....

ALLERGIES ....

....

CONTRACEPTION/LAST MENSTRUAL PERIOD ....

FOCUSED HISTORY AND ASSESSMENT

....

....

....

....

....

....

....

....

....

MANAGEMENT (tick appropriate box and comment)

- A+E ....
- Referral to GP (name/date/time) ....

- Referral to NP/PN/HV/DN/midwife (name/date/time) ....
- Other referral ....
- OTC medication recommended ....
- Self-care advice ....
- Information call only ....

Health education/advice given ....

....

....

....

....

....

TELEPHONE CONSULTATION CLOSURE STATEMENTS

Caller/patient understands instructions/advice

..........YES/NO

Caller/patient agrees to follow advice

..........YES/NO

Caller/patient advised to call back if symptoms do not improve or worsen

..........YES/NO

Signature of nurse

....

Time call completed

....

APPENDIX 2 PGD DISCLAIMER STATEMENTS

1. **Nurse Practitioner Open Access Clinic, Halcon, Taunton** cannot accept responsibility for the use of the enclosed Patient Group Directions as they have been developed in conjunction with the Nurse Practitioner Open Access Clinic Clinical Guidelines.
2. **Exeter NHS Walk-In Centre, 34–36 Bedford Street, Exeter EX11JT.** The enclosed protocols and patient group directions have been developed for use by nurses working within the Exeter NHS Walk-In Centres after a supportive training programme and assessment of competencies.

Members of a designated ratifying committee, supported by the Exeter Primary Care Trust, have approved them for use in the Walk-in Centres.

Whilst we are happy to share this information with our professional colleagues, responsibility cannot be accepted by any member of the ratifying committee or the Walk-in Centres management board for the use of these protocols or patient group directions outside the Exeter NHS Walk-In Centres.

Dr Adrian Harris	Dr Ben Leger	Sue Vining
Medical Director	Medical Director	Lead Nurse

Chapter 18

A new approach to ear care

Atie Fox

CHAPTER CONTENTS

INTRODUCTION

Ear care is an important area of work in general practice as it is thought that one in four people in the United Kingdom experiences some degree of hearing impairment and ear problems (Davis 1995). Although these are seldom life threatening, they can cause pain, discomfort, social isolation and embarrassment to many people.

It is evident from the literature that there appears to be a gap in education and training in ear care in general practice, which may have lead to the perception of ear care as synonymous with ear syringing and based on tradition rather than knowledge and evidence (Harkin & Vaz 2001, Rodgers 1997, Sharp et al 1990).

With the expansion of the practice nurse's role to include nurse-led services in general practice, it is important for patients to be comprehensively assessed, a differential diagnosis considered and treatment commenced based on evidence. The latter might be dependent on the practice nurse's competence but all health professionals in primary care can participate in patient education as many ear conditions can be prevented.

ANATOMY AND PHYSIOLOGY (Fig. 18.1)

The ear consists of three parts: the outer, middle and inner ear.

THE OUTER EAR

Considering the structures from the outer ear inwards, remember that the pinna consists of elastic

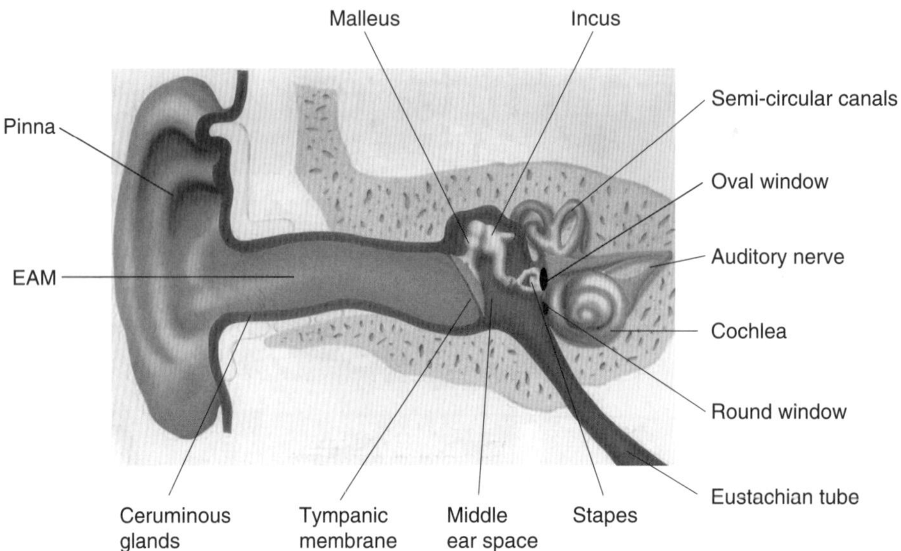

Figure 18.1 Anatomy of the ear. Reproduced with permission from the Primary Ear Care Centre, Rotherham PCT.

cartilage, which continues to the outer one-third of the external auditory meatus. In adults the external canal tends to slope slightly down from the tympanic membrane. In children the reverse is the case. Before any procedure on the ear is carried out, therefore, the pinna should be pulled back and up in adults and back and down in children in order to maximize visibility of the tympanic membrane.

The external auditory meatus is lined by epidermis, which forms a protein-based barrier between the internal and external environments and is composed of squamous epithelial tissue.

At the entrance to the auditory meatus are the ceruminous glands, the function of which are to produce cerumen. This substance, when combined with squamous epithelium, dust and secretions of the sebaceous glands, forms earwax. Its main function is to protect this very sensitive lining; earwax is thought to be fungicidal and bactericidal and acts like a flytrap, yet most patients (and health professionals) spend considerable time trying to remove it! The glands are similar to the apocrine sweat glands and are stimulated by touch and emotional stimuli. Frequent touch (including ear irrigation) and vibration is therefore likely to contribute to the build-up of wax in the ear. Excessive earwax can be the cause of considerable discomfort and hearing problems and will be discussed in more detail later.

The inner two-thirds of the meatus is tightly stretched over the temporal bone, the lowest portion of which is palpable behind the pinna as the mastoid process. This part of the canal is therefore more sensitive and easily traumatized by touch – a point to remember when you examine the ear. The ample blood supply can cause a small blood blister or bleeding when touched. One must be especially careful with patients who take anticoagulant medicine.

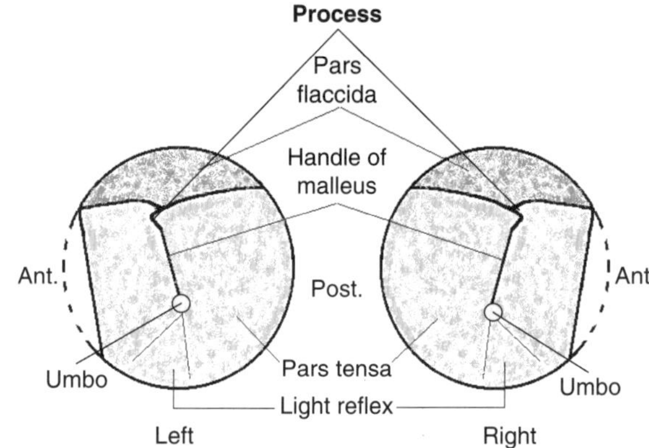

Figure 18.2 Normal tympanic membrane. Reproduced with permission from the Primary Ear Care Centre, Rotherham PCT.

The canal is 2.5 cm long and at its end lies the tympanic membrane (eardrum), which amplifies sound received by the pinna and external auditory meatus to the three tiny ossicles in the middle ear. The tympanic membrane consists of three layers: the epidermal, fibrous and mucous layers. The epidermal layer is responsible for the continuous migration of keratin from the umbo outwards (Fig. 18.2). It is through this process that keratin and excessive wax are expelled from the ear canal – thus the ear is thought to be self cleansing.

Box 18.1 Points for patient education

- Wax is wonderful – it protects the ear
- Poking will only push wax deeper in the canal and cause problems
- The ear is self cleansing and does not need poking with flannels and direct streams from showerheads!

A small side branch of the vagus nerve whose main branch sends impulses down through the chest to the lungs and heart is sometimes activated when touching the inside of the ear canal. This can provoke a vagus reflex in the form of violent coughing fits and nausea. In a few cases the heart rhythm is affected, causing it to slow down.

The eardrum is an oblique membrane held inward at its centre by one of its ossicles, the malleus. The handle and the short process of the malleus are the two chief landmarks when examining the tympanic membrane with the auriscope. Following the handle down to the umbo, a light reflection called the cone of light (or the light reflex) should be present if the tympanic membrane is healthy. A second ossicle, the incus, can sometimes be seen through the eardrum. The pars tensa is tightly stretched from the process down and across. Superior to the short process, the membrane is much less tense and folds back and is then called the pars flaccida. Here the chordi tympani, the ending of the facial nerve, is sometimes visible. The handle of the malleus is held in place in the middle ear by some muscles, the strongest of which lies at the top and the back of the tympanic membrane. This part of the eardrum is therefore the strongest and should be the part to aim for when irrigating the ear.

Box 18.2 Points to remember when irrigating ears

- Aim the waterjet to the top and posterior part of the tympanic membrane
- Advise patients to tell you if they feel adverse effects and stop immediately. Watch for vasovagal attacks

THE MIDDLE EAR

The middle ear is an air-filled cavity containing the ossicles which, through a plunging action of the stapes on the oval window, transmits sound into the inner ear. The middle ear is lined by mucous membrane and inflammation or infection can therefore lead to a collection of fluid in the middle ear, changing the appearance of the tympanic membrane and causing reduction in hearing. A copious amount of fluid in the middle ear creates pressure on the membrane, causing severe pain in the ear and possible perforation of the tympanic membrane.

Leading from the middle ear cavity to the pharynx is the eustachian tube which is responsible for equalizing air pressure, so that the tympanic membrane can follow the vibrations of sound. Normally, the pharyngeal opening is sealed but under certain conditions, such as changes in atmospheric pressures (i.e. flying and diving), this pressure may become negative and draw the eardrum inwards (retract), causing pain and loss of hearing. This seal is opened by yawning and swallowing which will therefore relieve the pressure. As the eustachian tube leads from the pharynx, any obstruction at this end will also produce negative pressure. A common cause for this is a collection of fluid (such as catarrh) in the postnasal space.

Negative pressure in the middle ear, through infection or trauma (flying, diving or assault or, indeed, syringing), can result in perforation of the tympanic membrane.

Perforations

Perforations occur when all three layers of the tympanic membrane have been ruptured. In uncomplicated perforations, the epithelial and mucous layers will heal in 10–12 weeks but the fibrous layer, which gives the tympanic membrane its strength, does not regenerate properly so a healed perforation will be much weaker. As a precautionary measure, irrigating healed perforations should be carried out as a last resort only and with the lowest possible power.

If on examination a perforation has been identified, it is helpful to describe its exact location. A perforation surrounded by tympanic membrane and in the pars tensa is usually considered safe, as keratinous debris is unlikely to fall into the middle ear but will be extruded naturally. A perforation on the margin of the eardrum or, more commonly, in the pars flaccida is often caused by a retraction pocket, created by negative pressure. These perforations can lead to a cholesteatoma, which is dangerous. These are therefore called unsafe perforations. As the retraction pocket gets deeper, keratinous debris is unable to migrate out and builds up, starts to decompose and becomes chronically infected. This infection can cause a perforation and the keratinous debris will collect in a pouch, continuing to build up layers of debris in the middle ear. The principal danger of a cholesteatoma is that this chronic infection can lead to erosion through the surrounding bone and the vital structures beyond.

The main feature of a cholesteatoma is a chronic or recurrent, extremely offensive discharge from the ear. As the cholesteatoma erodes through the ossicular chain, conductive deafness will ensue. Pain is not usually acute as there is no severe tension on the tympanic membrane due to the perforation, but patients may complain of a headache. Rarely the cholesteatoma may erode into the semicircular canal which will lead to vertigo.

Box 18.3 Points for assessment

- If a copious amount of discharge is found in the ear, especially preceded by pain, perforation of the tympanic membrane is likely
- *Always ask* about previous infections of the ear prior to irrigation as you cannot see what is behind the wax!
- *Never* assume the perforation has healed – some do not!
- *If discharge is present and you are unable to visualize the eardrum*, invite the patient for a follow-up appointment for identification of possible safe/unsafe perforations
- *Beware* patients with a history of recurrent discharge from the ear. This may be caused by a cholesteatoma

THE INNER EAR

This is responsible for both hearing and balance. The inner ear consists of a complex set of tiny tubes and chambers embedded in the temporal bone. The bony labyrinth has three parts: the cochlea, which is a closed ended tube, coiled like a snail's shell, the vestibule and semicircular canal. The cochlea contains a cavity, which consists of three channels (Fig. 18.3):

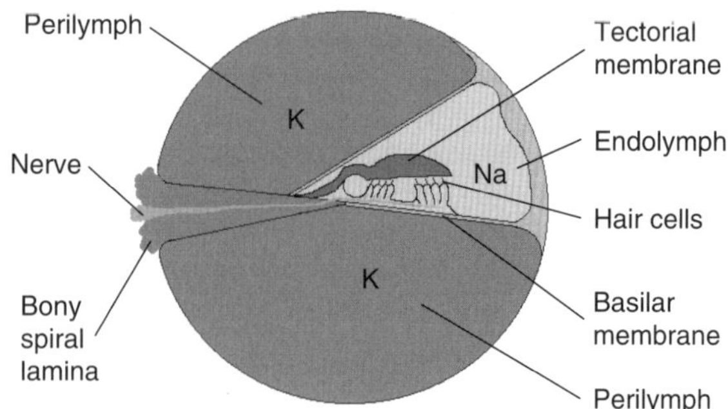

Figure 18.3 Section through cochlea. Reproduced with permission from the Primary Ear Care Centre, Rotherham PCT.

- upper channel (scala vestibuli)
- middle channel (scala medial)
- lower channel (scala tympani).

Separating the middle and lower channels is the basilar membrane, which supports the tectorial membrane and the organ of Corti.

The scala vestibuli and scala tympani are filled with perilymph, which contains potassium. Within the perilymph floats a complex and delicate structure – the membranous labyrinth or middle channel, which is distended with endolymph (like the inner and outer tubes of a bicycle tyre). The composition of endolymph (sodium) and perilymph (potassium) must be kept constant and is normally in equilibrium with the blood. Disturbance of this equilibrium can produce a change in the electrolyte balance and destroy the very sensitive nerve receptors. Abnormal accumulation or increased pressure of endolymph is thought to be the cause of Ménière's disease. Nerve receptors are located within the wall of the membranous labyrinth. In the cochlea, this consists of the organ of Corti and contains sound receptors. In the vestibule are the receptors for position sense and in the semicircular canal those of the sense of rotation. Therefore disturbance or injury of the inner ear can cause deafness as well as a sense of rotation (vertigo).

TRANSMISSION OF SOUND

Sound waves are received by the external auditory meatus and amplified by the tympanic membrane. This is then propagated through the ossicles and the oval window into the inner ear. The plunging action of the stapes transmits vibrations to the perilymph

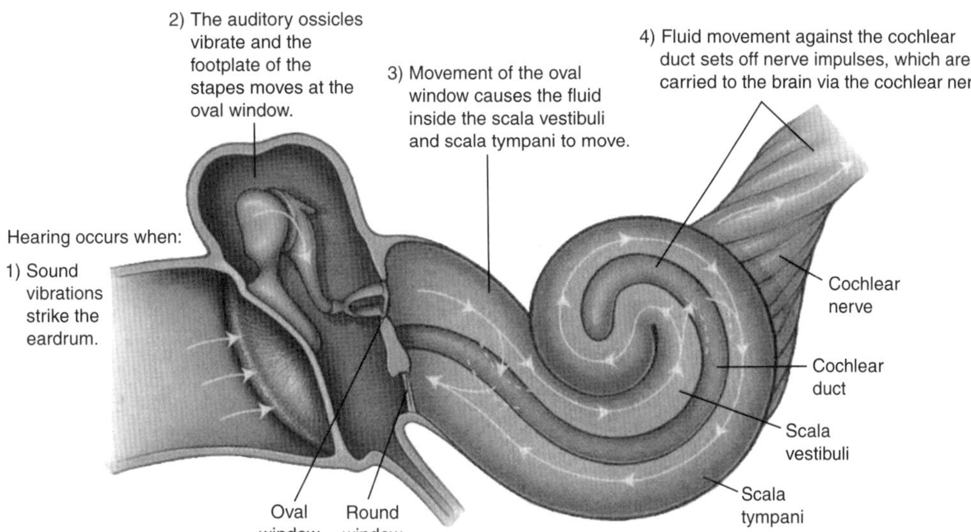

Figure 18.4 Mechanism of sound conduction.

upwards in the scala vestibuli, then to the endolymph in the cochlear duct and continues through the basilar membrane to the scala tympani, where they pass downwards through the round window. In the cochlear duct, the hair cells on the basilar membrane are activated, sending vibrations to be interpreted in the brain via the cochlear branch of the auditory nerve (VIII cranial nerve). These hair cells can be damaged or reduced in number by increased volume, altered biochemical content of the endolymph or vascular insufficiency, causing hearing loss.

Hearing loss can be divided into two classes: conductive hearing loss and sensorineural hearing loss, though some patients will have a mixture of the two.

Causes of conductive hearing loss

1. Obstruction of the external canal by:
   - otitis externa
   - wax
   - foreign bodies
   - tumours
   - congenital malformation
2. Damage to the drum by:
   - trauma
   - mastoiditis
   - adhesions
   - destruction of ossicles
   - cholesteatoma
3. Eustachian tube dysfunction:
   - middle ear pathology such as otitis media, serous otitis
   - nasopharyngeal pathology, e.g. adenoids, rhinitis
   - pressure changes, e.g. barotrauma
4. Otosclerosis through fusion of the ossicles
5. Tumours of the middle ear and mastoid

Causes of sensorineural hearing loss

1. Interference with blood supply:
   - vascular spasm
   - thrombosis of vessels to the ear
   - senile changes causing presbyacusis
   - excessive noise
2. Trauma from:
   - direct injuries – skull fracture
   - indirect injuries – blast wave
3. Infections:
   - viral infections such as labyrinthitis
4. Drugs:
   - streptomycin, quinine, Aspirin, gentamicin destroying cells in the cochlea
5. Congenital non-formation of inner ear
6. Ménière's disease
7. Pathological lesions of the acoustic nerve within the skull, e.g. acoustic neuroma, basal meningitis

IMPLICATIONS OF HEARING LOSS

Hearing loss obviously interferes with communication and therefore the level of social functioning.

This may lead to social and emotional isolation, which can be experienced even when living within a community/family/residential home. Any real exchange of news, views, opinions and feelings can become too much effort (usually for those with hearing). Gradually the skill of listening is lost and with it much personal responsibility.

There is the embarrassment of misunderstanding, the humiliation of being thought stupid, the inability to enjoy jokes or quick passing comments. Lack of information from which to select, particularly where visual impairment is also present, may become the norm. Decisions affecting the patient's well-being may be made by others, without involvement or consent, resulting in a situation where the patient feels powerless.

All health professionals need to be aware of their communication skills when consulting with hearing-impaired patients. A recent survey by the Royal Institute for the Deaf found that one in four patients leaves a doctor's appointment without knowing what is wrong with them (Robins & Mangan 1999). Specific skills for communicating include the following.

- Attract attention
- Always face the person, with the light on your face and at the same height, without encroaching on their personal space. Keep your mouth visible at all times
- Try not to distract with excessive hand/body movements
- Speak normally – do not exaggerate
- Do not shout – it contorts your face and makes it look aggressive
- Use short sentences and do not talk too quickly
- If understanding has not taken place, rephrase your sentence – do not just repeat it
- Write it down on a piece of paper if necessary
- Avoid any background noise
- Never say: 'It does not matter'
- Avoid speaking through a third person
- Be patient, calm and interested

If hearing loss is not recognized, it can be mistaken for indifference, bad manners, lack of cooperation or even mental confusion, which may lead to unjustified labelling. When it is recognized the speaker may shout, feel inadequate, embarrassed or angry or decide not to bother. To the deaf person, others can look extremely furtive when talking about quite trivial matters. If their voices cannot be heard and understood, a false and adverse impression can be given. When a deaf person asks what has been said, often the reply is 'It does not matter' or 'It is not worth repeating – it was not important'. What seems a passing comment when heard may seem tantalizingly important when it is missed.

Practice nurses have an important contribution to make in identifying people who are having difficulty hearing and encouraging them to ask to be referred for hearing aid assessment. Many patients attend for repeated removal of wax, as the obstruction takes them past the point where they can hear comfortably. Many are unwilling to seek help because they fear that a diagnosis of hearing loss will label them as 'ageing'. In some patients hearing loss may be due to an underlying pathology that needs urgent attention.

HEARING ASSESSMENT

Patients who have a suspected hearing loss can be assessed by asking the following questions.

- Do you have difficulty hearing other people's voices when there is background noise?
- Do you find other people's TV or radio too quiet?
- Do you sometimes misunderstand what people are saying?
- Do family and friends comment on your hearing?
- Do you often have to ask others to repeat what they have said to you?

Patients identified with hearing loss should be referred to the GP who may in turn refer on to an ENT specialist or audiologist, depending on local guidelines. **Any sudden and/or unilateral hearing loss should be referred immediately.** Some patients are not aware of the equipment now available to improve their quality of life and should be referred to the social worker for the hearing impaired.

The most common cause for a reduction in hearing, however, is the accumulation of wax.

WAX ACCUMULATION

As already discussed, in normal circumstances, wax protects the ear from foreign bodies and infection. The most common cause of wax accumulation is poking in the ears with cotton wool buds, hair clips or pencils, causing the wax to be pushed deep into the canal. However, there are groups of individuals who seem to be particularly prone to wax build-up.

AGE

Possibly due to a reduction in activity of the ceruminous glands in later years, cerumen can become drier and cannot be expelled from the ear canal. Obstruction of hearing aids and the increasing size and coarseness of hairs can also cause wax retention at the entrance to the external auditory meatus (EAM), especially in men.

GENETICS

Some individuals seem to produce an excessive amount of wax, which the migration of the epithelial cells is unable to cope with. Others appear to have abnormalities of epithelial migration or separation, causing long sheets of keratin to build up in concertina-like fashion in the EAM, thus predisposing these people to accumulation and impaction.

ANATOMY

A tortuous or narrow canal may lead to failure to dislodge the wax produced (Hanger & Muller 1992).

LEARNING DISABILITIES

In a study of 117 adults with learning disabilities, researchers found that this group showed an individual propensity for excessive cerumen production that may be anatomical or physiological (Crandell & Roeser 1993). The specific reason for this appears to be unknown. As this group sometimes have difficulty in communicating and hearing anyway, regular otoscopy and management of excessive wax is needed for this group.

Prior to removal of any wax, a history needs to be taken from the patient and both ears should be examined thoroughly in order to assess consistency of the wax, amount, location and identification of any abnormalities present.

GUIDANCE FOR EAR EXAMINATION (NHS 2002)

1. Before careful physical examination of the ear, listen to the patient, elicit symptoms and take a careful history. Explain each step of any procedure of examination and ensure that the patient understands and gives consent. Ensure that both you and the patient are seated comfortably, at the same level, and that you have privacy.

2. Examine the pinna, outer meatus and adjacent scalp. Check for previous surgery incision scars, infection, discharge, swelling and signs of skin lesions or defects. Decide on the most appropriate-sized speculum that will fit comfortably into the ear and place it on the auriscope.

3. Gently pull the pinna upwards and outwards to straighten the ear canal (directly down and back in children). Localized infection or inflammation will cause this procedure to be painful so do not continue in this situation.

4. Hold the auriscope like a pen and rest the small digit on the patient's head as a monitor for any unexpected head movement (Fig. 18.5). Use the light to observe the direction of the ear canal and the tympanic membrane. There is improved visualization of the eardrum by using the left hand for the left ear and the right hand for the right ear but you must assess your own ability. Insert the speculum gently into the meatus to pass through the hairs at the entrance to the canal.

5. Looking through the auriscope, check the ear canal and tympanic membrane. Adjust your head

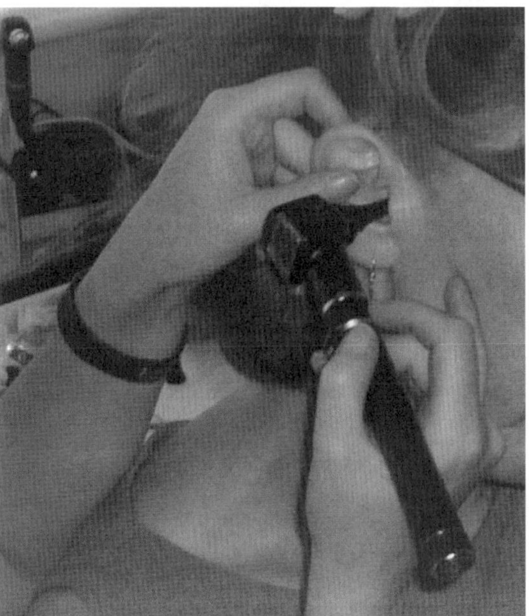

Figure 18.5 Sit down when examining the ear, holding the auriscope like a pen. Reproduced with kind permission from the Primary Ear Care Centre, Rotherham PCT.

and the auriscope to view all of the tympanic membrane. The ear cannot be judged to be normal until all areas of the membrane are viewed: the light reflex, handle of malleus, pars flaccida, pars tensa and anterior recess.

6. If the patient has had mastoid surgery, methodically inspect all parts of the cavity, tympanic membrane or drum remnant by adjusting your head and the auriscope. The mastoid cavity cannot be judged to be completely free of ear disease until the entire cavity and tympanic membrane or drum remnant have been seen.

7. The normal appearance of the membrane or mastoid cavity varies and can only be learned by practice. Practice will lead to recognition of abnormalities.

8. Carefully check the condition of the skin in the ear canal as you withdraw the auriscope. If there is doubt about the patient's hearing an audiological assessment should be made. Providing they meet certain criteria stated in local referral guidelines, older adults with a bilateral hearing loss can be referred directly to the audiology department.

9. Document what was seen in both ears, the procedure carried out, the condition of the tympanic membrane and external auditory meatus and treatment given. Findings should be documented following the NMC guidelines on record keeping and accountability. If any abnormality is found a referral should be made to the ENT outpatient department following local policy.

Common problems when examining the ear

- If you cannot see properly, check your light is adequate and the battery is fully charged. You may need to reassess if your auriscope is of good quality – a poor auriscope will not allow an accurate assessment of the tympanic membrane.
- If you cannot identify any structures but just see a red drum you may be looking at the posterior canal wall. Try directing the auriscope forwards and upwards or straighten the canal by pulling the pinna further.
- If you are not sure what structures you can see, identify the lateral process first, as other structures may have been destroyed. Once you have identified the process, orientation gets easier.
- If you are unsure whether you can see a perforation or not, look for blood vessels in the middle ear mucosa.

PREVENTION OF WAX BUILD-UP

Rather than wait for wax accumulation and impaction, wax can be removed from the external canal by instrumentation under direct vision (Fig. 18.6), provided that training and supervision, such as provided by the Primary Ear Care Centre, has taken place. Patients would need to initially attend the surgery at short intervals, e.g. 3–6 months, but this is likely to lead to less friction than irrigation, avoid stimulation of the ceruminous glands and reduce discomfort to the patient.

Where accumulation of wax is thought to be due to dryness, it can be useful for the patient to insert drops of olive oil once a week to encourage the wax to be expelled from the EAM.

Use of ear drops to soften wax

Correct technique and frequency of insertion of olive oil drops, as these are the least astringent, is likely to lead to easier removal of wax and therefore cause less friction and trauma. Several studies have compared different earwax solvents, sodium bicarbonate and water (Browning 2001). Water seemed to be the most efficient medium to expel wax, with no statistical difference between pharmaceutical agents. However, water is likely to cause maceration of the epithelium and astringent drops can cause contact sensitivities, leading to otitis externa if left in the ear for any length of time. Very few patients, however, are allergic to olive oil and these are therefore the drops of choice.

As patients tend to remember only about 20% of advice given, developing a handout would be useful. Receptionists can distribute these when an

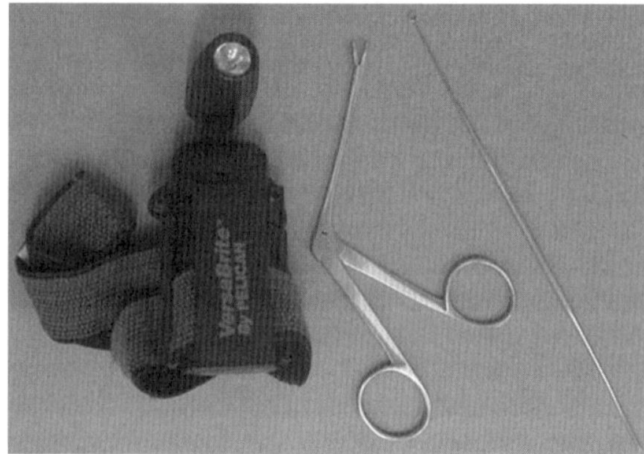

Figure 18.6 A headlight, Hanckle forceps and Jobson Horn are essential tools for carrying out ear care.

appointment is made for ear care. Ideally, the patient should be instructed to insert oil for a minimum of 3 days and a maximum of 2 weeks. However, impacted wax can be extremely uncomfortable and a minimum of 3 days is sufficient, providing oil has been inserted 2–3 times a day.

Box 18.4 Installation of ear drops: patient instructions

1. Obtain some olive oil and preferably a dropper bottle (your chemist may sell this).
2. Lie down on your side with the affected ear uppermost.
3. Pull your ear back and up to straighten your canal.
4. Drop 2–3 drops of oil, at room temperature, into the ear canal and massage the front of the ear to enable the oil to run down the ear canal.
5. Stay lying on your side with your ear uppermost for **at least 5 minutes.**
6. Do not leave cotton wool at the entrance to your ear.
7. Have a tissue ready to wipe excess oil away when you get up.

Sodium bicarbonate drops can be used as a second line to break up hard wax but as with other cerumenolytic agents, the elderly and those prone to recurrent otitis externa may react badly to their use.

Removal of wax by instrumentation

As described in the prevention of wax build-up, it is sometimes useful to remove wax with instruments under direct vision, provided the appropriate training has been undertaken. The following guidelines for this have been developed by the Primary Ear Care Centre.

- Examine the ear to discern the type of wax to be removed. Ask yourself is this healthy wax or may it be bacterial debris of wax-like appearance? Is it dry and crumbly wax related to seborrhoeic dermatitis?
- Excessive soft wax or crumbly wax and debris can be wiped out with cotton wool wound onto a Jobson Horn probe (especially useful to wipe wax off coarse hairs in the canal) (see p.334).
- Hard, crusty wax can sometimes be removed with a Jobson Horn or Henckle forceps under direct vision. Prepare your patient to tell you if this causes discomfort/pain and stop immediately if this is the case. The patient will have symptoms long before any real damage has occurred. Instruct the patient to insert olive oil for up to one week and ask him to return for ear irrigation.

EAR IRRIGATION

Ear irrigation is an invasive procedure. This means that a thorough risk assessment should be carried out in order to demonstrate that minimum harm will be caused to the patient. This includes ensuring that the safest equipment is used and that professionals have had education and training, including regular updating of new skills and new equipment.

There is evidence that ear care and irrigation are perceived by some as a simple task with little training and education necessary. Sharp et al (1990), Harkin & Vaz (2001) and Price (1997) have all demonstrated the problems that exist. Sharp found in his survey that health professionals appeared to be unaware of potential hazards and that incidents could be greatly reduced by a more careful selection of patients. Price (1997), in a 5-year review of complaints from patients to the MDU, found that ear syringing accounted for 19% of the total general practice procedure claims settled and was the third highest of all claims. In this review, 92% used a metal syringe, 68% kept incomplete or inadequate records and 38% had a previous history of perforation of the tympanic membrane. Harkin & Vaz (2001) conclude that the choice of who carries out ear syringing appears to be based not on whether the practice nurse is trained but on tradition or GP/nurse preference. This has implications for practice nurses, their employers and patients, especially in the current litigious climate.

CHOICE OF EQUIPMENT

Metal syringes produce the highest pressure (median 240 mmHg) in the external auditory meatus, when compared to other types of equipment. Mean rupture pressure for atrophic tympanic membranes is 456 mmHg (range 228–608 mmHg). Existing metal syringes are also often old, rusty, can be difficult to handle sensitively and accurately due to the large endpiece and may therefore be potentially harmful (Thurgood & Thurgood 1995). Rodgers (1997) concurs that metal syringes can also have problems because of stiff action.

The Steering Board of Action on ENT (see guidelines below), the MDA and the Primary Ear Care Centre recommend the use of electronic irrigators provided staff are properly trained in their use. The new electronic syringes meet the standards of the MDA (beware old Propulse models – safety notice MDA SN 9807 Feb 1998). Other reported benefits include controllable and reduced water pressure, ease of use and improved vision into the meatus. Although the reduced water pressure could potentially lead to inability to remove wax, provided the patient has been thoroughly educated and has complied with advice, this should not be a problem.

CONSENT

As discussed, this procedure is invasive and therefore the professional is responsible for the assessment. Traditionally, general practitioners have perceived that, because of vicarious liability, they themselves would be responsible for this assessment. However, this ignores the nurse's accountability under the Nursing and Midwifery Council's *Professional Code of Conduct*. Nurses should ensure that information related to consent is accessible, understandable, and informative. Consent in writing is preferable to verbal.

In view of the above, a written protocol demonstrating authorization of the policy and procedure would be sensible. This should include:

- specifics of education and training for the procedure to be carried out, including updates required
- assessment of patient and recording
- how informed consent is obtained (attach leaflet)
- equipment to be used
- guidelines for ear irrigation (include diagram of correct angle)
- cleaning guidelines
- when to refer.

The protocol should be dated (and review date set) and signed by all professionals involved.

GUIDANCE FOR EAR IRRIGATION USING THE ELECTRONIC IRRIGATOR

The following guidelines were launched in September 2002 by the Action on ENT Steering Board. They have been endorsed by the Royal College of General Practitioners and the Royal College of Nursing. Copies are available from the NHS Modernization Agency.

This procedure is only to be carried out by a trained doctor, nurse or audiologist.

Principles

Irrigating the ear is carried out in order to:

- facilitate the removal of cerumen and foreign bodies which are not hydroscopic from the external auditory meatus. Hydroscopic matter (such as peas, polystyrene and lentils) will absorb the water and expand, making removal more difficult
- remove discharge, keratin or debris from the external auditory meatus.

An individual assessment should be made of every patient to ensure that it is appropriate for ear irrigation to be carried out.

Reasons for using this procedure

- Correctly treat otitis externa where the meatus is obscured by debris
- Improve conduction of sound to the tympanic membrane when it is blocked by wax
- Examine the external auditory meatus and the tympanic membrane

Contraindications

Irrigation should not be carried out when:

- the patient has previously experienced complications following this procedure in the past
- there is a history of a middle ear infection in the last 6 weeks
- the patient has undergone *any* form of ear surgery (apart from grommets that have extruded at least 18 months previously and the patient has been discharged from the ENT department
- the patient has a perforation or there is a history of a mucous discharge in the last year
- the patient has a cleft palate (repaired or not).

Equipment

- Auriscope
- Head mirror and light or headlight and spare batteries
- Electronic irrigator
- Jug containing tap water heated to 40°C

- Noots trough/receiver
- Jobson Horne probe and cotton wool
- Tissues and receivers for dirty swabs and instruments
- Waterproof cape and towel

Procedure

This procedure should be carried out with both participants seated and under direct vision, using a headlight or head mirror and light source, throughout the procedure.

1. Informed consent should be obtained prior to proceeding.
2. Examine both ears by first inspecting the pinna, outer meatus (ear canal) and adjacent scalp by direct light. Check for previous surgery incision scars or skin defects, then inspect the external ear with the auriscope.
3. Check whether the patient has had his ears irrigated previously or if there are any contraindications to irrigation.
4. Explain the procedure to the patient and ask him to sit in an examination chair with his head tilted towards the affected ear. (A child could sit on an adult's knee with the child's head held steady.)
5. Place the protective cape and towel on the patient's shoulder and under the ear to be irrigated. Ask the patient to hold the receiver under the same ear.
6. Check your headlight is in place and the light is directed down the ear canal. Check that the temperature of the water is approximately 40°C and fill the reservoir of the irrigator. Set the pressure at minimum.
7. Connect a clean jet tip applicator to the tubing of the machine with a firm push/twist action. Push until a 'click' is felt.
8. Direct the irrigator tip into the Noots receiver and switch on the machine for 10–20 seconds in order to circulate the water through the system and eliminate any trapped air or cold water. This offers the opportunity for the patient to become accustomed to the noise of the machine. The initial flow of water is discarded, thus removing any static water remaining in the tube.
9. Twist the jet tip so that the water can be aimed along the posterior wall of the ear canal (towards the back of the patient's head) (Fig. 18.7).
10. Gently pull the pinna upwards and outwards to straighten the ear canal (directly backward in children).

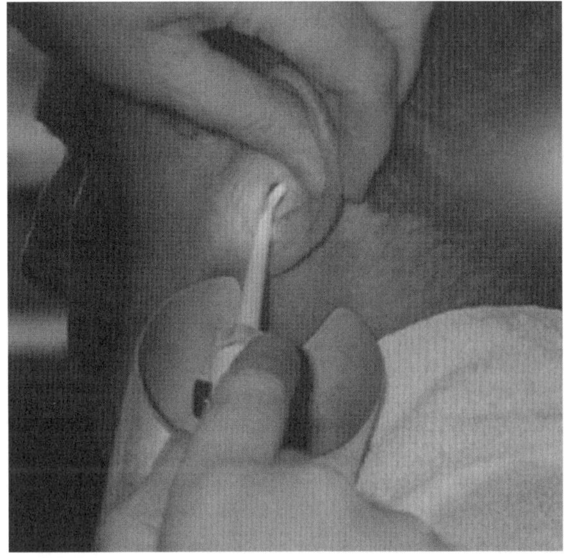

Figure 18.7 Twist the jet tip to the superior and posterior part of the ear canal.

11. Warn the patient that you are about to start irrigating and that the procedure will be stopped if he feels dizzy or has any pain. Place the tip of the nozzle into the ear canal entrance and using the foot control, direct the stream of water along the roof of the ear canal and towards the posterior canal wall (directed towards the back of the patient's head). If you consider the entrance to the ear canal as a clock face you would direct the water at 11 o'clock on the right ear and 1 o'clock on the left ear. Increase the pressure control gradually if there is difficulty removing the wax. It is advisable that a maximum of two reservoirs of water are used in any one irrigating procedure.
12. If you have not managed to remove the wax within 5 minutes of irrigating it may be worthwhile moving onto the other ear as the introduction of water via the irrigating procedure will soften the wax and you can retry irrigation after about 15 minutes.
13. Periodically inspect the ear canal with the auriscope and inspect the solution running into the receiver.
14. After removal of wax or debris, *dry mop excess water from meatus under direct vision using the Jobson Horne probe and best-quality cotton wool.* Stagnation of water and any abrasion of the skin during the procedure predisposes to infection. Removing the water with the cotton wool-tipped probe reduces the risk of infection.

15. Examine ear, both meatus and tympanic membrane, and treat as required following specific guidelines or refer to doctor if necessary.

16. Give advice regarding ear care and any relevant information.

17. Document what was seen in both ears, the procedure carried out, the condition of the tympanic membrane and external auditory meatus and treatment given. Nurses should record all findings and treatments according to NMC guidelines on record keeping and accountability.

Cautions

- Irrigation should *never* cause pain. If the patient complains of pain, stop immediately.
- Always use a clean speculum, jet tip applicator and probe for each patient.

Cleaning

It is recommended that you follow the manufacturer's guidelines for cleaning and disinfecting the irrigator and its components. The Primary Ear Care Centre, however, has developed the following cleaning guidelines for the Propulse electronic syringe.

Propulse

Stage 1. Each day before use, the Propulse must be disinfected using a solution of sodium dichloroisocyanurate 1% (NaDCC). Use Chlor-clean tablets, or similar, according to manufacturer's instructions to get a solution which provides 1000 parts NaDCC per million (0.1%).

- Fill the water tank with NaDCC solution.
- Run the Propulse for a few seconds to allow the solution to fill the pump and flexible tubing.
- Leave to stand for 10 minutes. Empty the tank and rinse the system through with tap water before use.

Stage 2. At the end of the day (or end of ear irrigation session), disinfect the Propulse for 10 minutes using the NaDCC solution.

Rinse the machine by running sterile/boiled water through and dry it prior to leaving it overnight.

After each individual patient treatment, items of equipment should be disinfected as follows.

Jet tip applicator

- Remove from tubing and place in a detergent solution (dilute washing up liquid) to remove wax.
- Wash under hot water to remove debris.
- Soak for 10 minutes in the NaDCC solution prepared as in stage 1.
- Rinse and dry thoroughly.

Speculum for auriscope

- Same procedure as for jet tip applicators.

Jobson Horn probe, Henckle forceps, Gruber speculae

- Place in detergent solution to remove wax.
- Rinse under hot water.
- Dry thoroughly.
- After initial cleaning these should be sterilized in an autoclave. They must be allowed to cool completely before using.

Nootes ear tank

- Clean with detergent solution.
- Rinse under hot water. Dry thoroughly.

Any NaDCC solution prepared for disinfecting equipment must be discarded at the end of each session/day. Following cleaning *all* equipment must be stored dry. Please remember that aural care and ear irrigation procedures are 'clean', not 'sterile' procedures. However, you must ensure that *all* items of equipment used have been thoroughly disinfected before use.

Chlor-clean tablets may be obtained from Guest Medical, a pharmacy or through the Primary Ear Care Centre. These items should be added to your computerized pharmacy request form.

EAR CARE IN GENERAL PRACTICE

Ear care forms a large part of the practice nurse's workload. With the increasing demand from the DoH to provide direct access appointments and nurse triage, it would be very beneficial to expand present knowledge to include common ear care presentations and their treatment. Furthermore, research has shown that nurse-led ear care (provided by nurses trained in ear care) significantly reduced GP consultations and treatment costs.

Earache is a common presentation in general practice. It can present in all ages but particularly in children under the age of 5 as they are prone to upper respiratory infections and the eustachian tube is much shorter and straighter than in adults, allowing infections to spread to the middle ear space. A substantive history needs to be taken to arrive at a differential diagnosis. The following questions have been found to be useful:

- How long has the pain been present?
- Where is it?
- Is it constant, sharp, aching or dull – does it radiate?
- Has there been any discharge?
- Has hearing been affected?
- Worse when moving pinna?
- Any recent trauma – poking in ears or ear syringing?
- Recently been swimming, diving, flying?
- Recent cold or sore throat?
- Pyrexia, vomiting, anorexia?
- Especially in children: interested in surroundings, responsive to verbal cues?
- Allergies?
- Previous medical history and medication

A good history should give you an idea of what you might be dealing with and enables you to concentrate on the appropriate examination to be carried out.

- Observe/palpate the external ears for size, symmetry and colour.
- Palpate the tragus and move the pinna.
- Observe/palpate the mastoid area and neck for tenderness, swelling, redness and warmth.
- Observe for signs of skin disorders such as eczema and shingles.

Inspect/examine:

- the outer ear with an auriscope for debris, wax, discharge, foreign bodies, scaliness, swelling, inflammation
- the tympanic membrane for signs of perforation, bulging, inflammation, retraction, movement of tympanic membrane
- urine for signs of chronic infection.

Apart from wax, the most common painful ear presentations in general practice are likely to be:

- acute otitis media
- acute otitis externa
- eustachian tube dysfunction.

Occasionally, earache can be due to:

- temporomandibular joint dysfunction
- dental problems, such as abscess or impacted molar
- trigeminal neuralgia.

ACUTE OTITIS MEDIA

Acute otitis media is an acute inflammation of the mucosa of the middle ear. The history usually includes a painful ear, which may be of sudden onset or gradually getting worse, following an upper respiratory tract infection. An acute bacterial infection will manifest with marked pyrexia and a bulging, acutely inflamed tympanic membrane whereas a viral infection will present with a mild pyrexia and an erythematous flush or redness of the tympanic membrane only.

Treatment

The treatment of otitis media remains controversial. The latest research, carried out on children aged 6 months to 10 years, suggests that in most children with otitis media without fever and vomiting, antibiotic treatment has little benefit and is unlikely to prevent complications. Those with fever or vomiting may benefit from a delayed prescription to prevent these. Most children with otitis media will settle without antibiotics anyway, so it is still reasonable to wait 24–48 hours before considering antibiotic treatment. However, it is a distressing condition and advice on the management, monitoring of symptoms and when to return is most important. Advice should include the following.

- Pain and fever control. Recommend appropriate dose of paracetamol and ibuprofen to be given regularly for first 24 hours. Sit the child up to relieve pressure on the eardrum. Cold or hot flannels over the ear can also be helpful. Antibiotics will not reduce pain in the first 24 hours.
- Majority of ear infections will settle in the first 48 hours. The child may get side-effects and become resistant to antibiotics if taken when not needed.
- Encourage fluids and monitor micturition to avoid dehydration.
- Avoid water entering the ear when having a bath, shower or during swimming for 2 weeks until after infection has cleared.
- Do not poke – nothing smaller than your elbow in the ear!
- Symptoms should begin to improve in 48 hours. If not or if symptoms get worse, get medical attention.
- Do not worry if the child continues to have symptoms of hearing loss. This should settle

after a month or two. If not, make an appointment.

- Invite for check-up appointment when symptoms have settled, if unable to visualize the tympanic membrane.
- If prescribing antibiotics, inform patient of the side-effects and that the drug will take 48 hours to have an effect.

Children with symptoms of dehydration, abnormal drowsiness, vomiting, not responding to treatments, tenderness and inflammation behind ear, and aged below 6 months should be referred to a general practitioner immediately.

As treatment is still controversial a policy for treatment within the practice – if not your PCT – would be desirable to avoid confusion of staff and patients.

Treatment of choice Amoxicillin syrup 125 μg tds for 5 days up to the age of 10

Amoxicillin 250 μg tds for 5 days for adults

If allergic to penicillin Erythromycin syrup 125 μg qds for 7 days up to the age of 2

Erythromycin 250 μg qds for 7 days age 2–8

Erythromycin 250–500 μg qds for 7 days aged 8 years and over

Side-effects Nausea, diarrhoea (especially with erythromycin), rashes. For details see BNF.

OTITIS EXTERNA

Otitis externa is dermatitis of the external auditory canal, which sometimes involves the pinna. It is usually an acute condition, with trauma being the single most common cause for infection of the external meatus: initial itching usually leads to scratching of the ear with fingernail, paperclip or hairpin, resulting in inflammation, causing more itching and scratching, setting up a vicious cycle. The trauma caused allows for microbial invasion and the resultant infection will cause symptoms of pain (especially when pulling the pinna) and dullness in hearing. On examination, oedema and inflammation of the canal lining, debris and a watery discharge are frequently visible in the meatus.

Otitis externa often affects both ears simultaneously. Patients often have eczema or have an allergy to shampoos, hairspray or chemicals. It is thought that otitis externa is on the increase as a result of swimming, particularly in hot, humid climates or frequent swimming in recreational fresh water.

Treatment

There is a consensus of opinion in the literature and from otology experts that aural toilet followed by instillation of a topical preparation should be standard treatment for otitis externa. However, it is rarely carried out in general practice and access to ENT departments is limited. The ear can be irrigated, providing the canal is not too painful to do so and the ear is dried after this procedure. However, tapwater contains *Pseudomonas aeruginosa*, so the dry removal of debris is preferable wherever possible. As discussed, this is a skill which should be developed under supervision following suitable training.

For mild otitis externa, aural toilet may be all that is needed. Nurses trained in ear care, however, are able to apply topical ointments directly to the external meatus and insert wicks for more severe otitis externa under patient group direction. For information see www.earcarecentre.com.

Aural toilet consists of the use of instruments and wicks to clean the ear of debris and discharge and needs education and training under supervision to develop these skills safely. It is recommended that a minimum of the 5-day ear care course provided by the Primary Ear Care Centre and Bournemouth University is completed before providing this service (see Resources).

The Primary Ear Care Centre has developed the following guidelines for safe practice.

Aural toilet Aural toilet is used to clear the aural meatus of debris, discharge, soft wax or excess fluid following irrigation. **This procedure is only to be carried out by a trained nurse or doctor.**

1. Examine the ear.
2. Dry mop, using a Jobson Horne probe and a small piece of fluffed-up cotton wool, the size of a postage stamp, applied to the probe. Under direct vision (with headlight or headmirror and light) and pulling the pinna to straighten the canal, clean the ear with a gentle rotary action of the probe. Do not touch the tympanic membrane.
3. Replace the cotton wool directly it becomes soiled. Pay particular attention to the anteroinferior recess which harbours debris.
4. Reexamine the meatus intermittently, using the auriscope, during cleaning to check for any debris/discharge/crusts which remain in the meatus at awkward angles.
5. If an infection is present, treatment should follow the guidelines below or as dictated by the result of a swab culture and sensitivities.

Box 18.5 Aural treatment regime recommended by the Primary Ear Care Centre

ALWAYS FIRST: Thorough aural toilet

Minor or secondary infection or perforated tympanic membrane or prevention of returning infection
Application of Betnovate C ointment and/or prescription for Locorten-Vioform drops

Itchy or dry flaky ears
Application of Betnovate C ointment or hydrocortisone 1% ointment

Oedematous painful meatus (furuncle)
Wick containing glycerine + ichthammol

Antibiotic/antiinflammatory
Application of wick containing nystatin ointment with prescription for Otomize spray/Betnesol-N, etc. or other neomycin-based drops

Other treatments
Aurecort ointment or Gentisone HC drops or Sofradex ointment with Sofradex drops

Fungal element
Canesten HC cream* or Nystaform HC cream

*Canesten drops are available over the counter for self-care

It is important that treatment with an antibiotic ointment, if followed up by self-care with drops, uses the drop containing the same antibiotic as in the ointment.

Patients (and health professionals!) may perceive this condition as a minor problem and can be reluctant to seek medical advice. *All* health professionals, though, should give clear advice on the treatment and prevention of otitis externa. Chronic or recurrent otitis externa, though seldom life threatening, can severely affect quality of life.

Advice given should include the following.

- Keep your ears dry when showering, bathing, swimming, shampooing hair. This can be achieved by well-fitted earplugs or cotton wool dipped in Vaseline to create a waterproof plug.
- Avoid all known allergies.
- Do not poke in your ears (nothing smaller than your elbow).
- Obtain glacial acetic acid (Earcalm) spray (available OTC) for use at first sign of itching to reduce irritation.
- Hearing aids
  - Check earpiece for rough surface.
  - Clean earpiece according to instructions from audiology department.
  - Leave hearing aid out whenever possible to allow air to circulate.
  - If recurrent episodes occur, return to the audiology department for assessment for an alternative hearing aid (may need referral).
- Medication
  - Advice on insertion of drops (as for olive oil).
  - If pain increases following insertion of drops stop use and contact surgery (may have developed a sensitivity to ear drops).
  - Continue for at least 2 days after symptoms have resolved.
  - If not resolved in 7–10 days return to surgery for further assessment and swab to be sent for culture, sensitivity and fungi and tuberculosis from affected ear(s). If topical antibiotics are used for longer than this period, a fungal infection can occur.

Box 18.6 Key points

- Profuse discharge implies middle ear disease – not otitis externa
- Persistent unilateral 'otitis externa' equals otitis media until proven otherwise
- Treatment of otitis externa depends on satisfactory aural toilet
- Beware otitis externa in diabetic (or any immunosuppressed) patients

NECROTIZING ('MALIGNANT') OTITIS EXTERNA

Otitis externa can become more destructive, especially in an immunosuppressed individual or elderly diabetic. Periostitis can develop and, if uncontrolled, can spread to the mastoid bone and affect some lower cranial nerves, causing facial palsies. Pain is usually severe.

EUSTACHIAN TUBE DYSFUNCTION

Eustachian tube dysfunction is a condition where the tympanic membrane is retracted due to negative pressure in the eustachian tube. This can be due to a variety of problems and it is therefore particularly important to take the previous history into account. Allergies such as hayfever, recent colds or nasal airways problems, adenoid enlargement and barotrauma can be responsible. The patient often complains of his ear feeling blocked and a reduction in hearing.

Apart from the examination already stated, further investigation is necessary.

- Check that process and malleus are in the normal position; in a retraction the malleus is usually more horizontal.
- Check the colour of the tympanic membrane and look for fluid levels.
- Check the movement of the tympanic membrane by asking the patient to swallow or gently blow through his nose while closing the mouth and pinching the nose. Use a tympanometer if available.
- Check nasal airway patency by asking the patient to blow through each nostril separately.
- Use headlight to examine the mucous membrane lining of the nose for rhinitis, foreign bodies, nasal polyps. Check for nasal deviation.
- Check for hearing loss with tuning fork or audiometer if available.

Always refer unilateral symptoms – these may be due to tumours and need to be investigated.

If a retraction pocket is present, the tympanic membrane has collapsed onto the ossicles or symptoms are not clearing, it is important to ask the patient to have his ears checked in about 2 months. (This situation may lead to cholesteatoma, as discussed on pp.329–330, or the tympanic membrane can become adherent to the ossicles.)

Treatment

Treat the cause.

- If due to allergy, consider antihistamines, steroid drops/sprays.
- Remove any foreign body.
- Refer to ENT specialist if due to polyps, nasal septum deviation, persistent problems, chronic otitis media.
- If due to nasal catarrh, advise on the inhalation of steam at least twice daily. Combined with blowing the nose following this procedure, this may prevent the development of glue ear in children.
- If appropriate, advise on stopping smoking.

CONCLUSION

Ear problems are a large part of the practice nurse's workload. Education and training to deal with these has been lacking in the past which has lead to many complaints from patients to the MDU. The increasing emphasis on direct access and triage necessitate updates, training and education to improve quality of care and quality of life for patients with ear problems. Nurse-led ear care by trained nurses leads to improved access and reductions in costs and referrals to secondary care.

References

Browning G 2001 Wax in ear. In: Clinical evidence. BMJ Books, London

Crandell CC, Roeser RJ 1993 Incidence of excessive/impacted cerumen in mentally retarded individuals. American Journal of Mental Retardation 97:568–574

Davis A 1995 Hearing in adults. Whurr, London

Hanger H, Muller G 1992 Cerumen: its fascination and clinical importance. Journal of the Royal Society of Medicine 8:346–349

Harkin H, Vaz F 2001 Provision of ear care in the primary care setting. Primary Health Care 10(10):30–33

NHS Modernization Agency 2002 Action on ENT. Department of Health, London

Price J 1997 Problems of ear syringing. Practice Nurse 14:126–128

Robins J, Mangan M 1999 Seen and not heard. Nursing Times 95(37):30–32

Rodgers R 1997 How safe is your ear syringing? Community Nurse June:28–29

Sharp JF, Wilson J, Barr-Hamilton R et al 1990 Ear wax removal: a survey of current practice. British Medical Journal 90(301):1251–1252

Thurgood K, Thurgood G 1995 Earwax removal: a survey of current practice. British Journal of Nursing 12:682–686

Resources

Helplines

RNID: www.rnid.org.uk
Helpline: 0870 6050 123
Textphone: 0870 6033 007

Hearing Concern (advice for deaf people and their families)
Tel: 01245 344600
Fax: 01245 280747

Education and training

The Primary Ear Care Centre provides a 1-day study day and a 5-day course at Diploma level for more in-depth development of clinical practice in ear care. The 1-day study day is also available through a network of trainers throughout the UK. For details contact:
The Primary Ear Care Centre
c/o Kiveton Park Primary Care Centre
Chapel Way
Kiveton Park
Sheffield
South Yorkshire S26 6QU
Tel: 01909 772746
www.earcarecentre.com

One-day and 5-day courses are also available from Bournemouth University; for further information contact:
Angy Forsey
Programmes Administrator
IHCS Bournemouth University
Royal London House
Christchurch Road
Bournemouth BH1 3LT
Tel: 01202 464782
or afox@bournemouth.ac.uk at the same address.

Further reading

Coley K, Kay N 1998 ENT Practice for Primary Care. Churchill Livingstone, Edinburgh

Coopey S 2001 Ear syringing – a case for clinical governance. Journal of Community Nursing 15(1):20–22

Corbridge R, Hellier W 1998 Essential ENT practice. Arnold, London

Fall M, Read S, Walters S 1997 An evaluation of a nurse led care service in primary care: benefits and costs. British Journal of General Practice 47:699–703

Little P, Gould C, Moore M 2002 Predictors of poor outcome and benefits from antibiotics in children with acute otitis media: pragmatic randomised trial. British Medical Journal 325:22

Robson L 2002 Hearing. Practice Nurse 23(4):18–22

Roesser R, Ballachanda B 1997 Physiology, pathophysiology and anthropology/epidemiology of human earcanal secretions. Journal of the American Academy of Audiology 8:391–400

Wormwald PJ, Browning GG 1996 Otoscopy: a structured approach. Arnold, London

Chapter 19

Wound management

Janette Swift Julia Lucas

CHAPTER CONTENTS

Management of wounds is a complex process, which requires knowledge, skill and experience. All too often wounds are treated inappropriately, which results in delays in the healing process, at a cost to both the patient and the service, in terms of resources, time and discomfort.

If quality is to be realized as being central to all care delivered by the health service, it would seem appropriate to write this chapter within a clinical governance framework, which is described as:

> *A framework through which NHS organisations are accountable for continuously improving the quality of their services and safeguarding high standards of care by creating an environment in which excellence in clinical care will flourish.* (DoH 1998)

In terms of wound management, there are several issues that need to be considered in the provision and delivery of appropriate and effective wound care. The most important of these is about the patient and the development of a holistic approach towards wound management. Patient involvement in the delivery of wound care is undoubtedly a key component in achieving rapid effective healing. Practically, this involves a wound assessment that considers a patient's medical and social history in conjunction with a full examination of the wound to identify the stage of healing.

Any factors that may have an adverse effect upon the healing process should be documented at the time of assessment and the information utilized to enable the practitioner to select the most appropriate treatment. This will not only include the selection of dressing but will allow the practitioner to provide health education advice that may support compliance with the treatment and thus enhance healing.

In discussing compliance with any treatment, altered body image should be considered, as this may be important to patients for a variety of reasons. For example, the exudate from the wound may be offensive and have an effect on the patient's social activity or the dressing may be bulky and not allow the patient to mobilize. There will also be those patients who do not like the aesthetic appearance of a specific type of dressing.

Wound care should be evidence based and it is in this area that conflict often occurs for the nurse. Developments in wound care are evolving and the choice of treatments available is becoming wider than ever before. It is therefore important that nurses keep up to date with current research and are able to appraise it objectively. Access to guidance from the National Institute of Clinical Excellence (NICE) and medical databases should be available to all nurses, to enable them to make an objective assessment of treatments available. This is particularly important because nurses working in primary care are often bombarded with research findings from the commercial sector, which may or may not carry a bias towards the product being marketed. It is probably worth mentioning that the development of nurse prescribing will make targeting of nurses by the commercial sector more attractive as traditionally nurses tend to be given autonomy in the provision of wound care.

Equally, for clinical effectiveness it is important for nurses to be able to assimilate information in research papers and apply it in practice, if appropriate.

Given that the aim of wound management is to provide an optimum healing environment, while treating the patient holistically, it would seem that the fundamental element upon which the delivery of high-quality care is based is an in-depth knowledge of the healing process and it is for this reason that the following information is described.

THE WOUND HEALING PROCESS

There are several factors that can affect the healing process in each individual. To enable practitioners to treat each wound appropriately it is important that the nurse understands the normal physiological process of healing. There are two reasons why this is important:

- by understanding the normal process, nurses are able to identify stages of wound healing and provide the most appropriate care required at each stage
- by recognizing the normal physiology a nurse is able to identify abnormal signs and symptoms that are delaying the healing process.

There is some debate as to how many stages are involved within the healing process. Some suggest five (Eckersley & Dudley 1998), some three (Casey 2000), whilst the majority state four (Dealey 1999). For the purpose of explaining this according to the consensus opinion, we will talk about the following stages of the wound healing process:

1. inflammatory stage
2. destructive stage

3. proliferative stage
4. maturation stage.

INFLAMMATORY STAGE

This occurs immediately and can last up to 3 days and may be prolonged in very traumatic wounds or if a patient is on steroids or anticoagulants.

Following injury to the skin there is a local reaction, the affected area becomes red, swollen and hot and the patient may experience some degree of pain.

Initially vasoconstriction occurs followed by a release of platelets that clump together and release growth factors and fibronectin. Growth factors are naturally occurring proteins that are secreted by the cells and are induced as a result of a challenge, i.e. a wound. The growth factors are mediators of cutaneous repair and work by attaching themselves to specific receptors on the surface membrane of target cells within the wound environment. The binding of a growth factor to a specific receptor activates a chain of events that starts the healing process.

Damage to tissue activates two systems: the complement system and the kinin system. The complement system is made up of plasma proteins, which arrive at the wound initially, as the capillaries and arterioles vasoconstrict. The plasma proteins act as precursors that, when activated, cause the release of histamine from the mast cells, which ultimately results in vasodilation of the capillaries and arterioles, thereby increasing the capillary permeability.

As the capillaries dilate, fluid flows from the capillaries into the tissues and swelling occurs. This fluid becomes what is known as the inflammatory exudate, containing plasma proteins, antibodies, red and white blood cells and platelets. It also contains antibodies to neutralize any foreign materials in the wound and precursors to fibrin which is laid down in the wound bed initially.

This effect is enhanced by the kinin system, which activates kininogen to kinins. Kinins have many effects: for example, they attract neutrophils to the wound bed and enhance the process of phagocytosis.

Apart from being involved in clot formation, platelets also release growth factors and fibronectin.

The first leucocyte to arrive at the wound site is the neutrophil. This is attracted to the wound bed by fibronectin and will be present within the wound from as soon as 1 hour after injury. Neutrophils arrive in large numbers and their primary function is to begin the process of phagocytosis by engulfing bacteria.

Growth factors from the platelets attract monocytes to the wound; once these have reached the tissues they become macrophages.

The huge number of processes taking place during the inflammatory phase requires both energy and nutritional resources, namely vitamins C and B. Very often wounds break down as a result of poor nutrition or continued irritation, i.e. infection or foreign body, and this can cause a delay in the healing process.

DESTRUCTIVE STAGE

This phase occurs between 2 and 5 days following injury. Polymorphs and macrophages are present in the wound and they begin to attract neutrophils. Because macrophages are larger than neutrophils they are able to phagocytose larger particles and bacteria. Neutrophils eventually die and are ingested by the macrophages.

PROLIFERATIVE STAGE (EPITHELIALIZATION)

The first part of reepithelialization is the migration of epithelial cells across the wound surface. Following this a basement membrane is laid down under the new epithelial covering. The tissue is pink/white in colour and in large wounds may begin to appear in isolated clusters or islets.

MATURATION STAGE

During maturation collagen is converted and reorganized. Cellular activity and blood supply reduce. Dermal healing forms scar tissue.

ASSESSMENT

The aim of accurate wound assessment is to ensure that appropriate wound management is carried out. To enable this the wound must first be classified and it may be helpful at this point to define what a wound is.

> *A wound may be defined as a defect or break in the skin that results from physical, mechanical or thermal damage, or that develops as a result of underlying medical or physiological disorder.*

Given the above definition, wounds can be classified within the following areas.

- *Abrasions* (grazes): these are usually confined to the outer layers of the skin, caused by friction.
- *Lacerations* (tears): more severe than abrasions, involve the skin and underlying tissue.
- *Penetrating wounds* (caused by knives and bullets): internal damage can be considerable, but may look minor on the outside.
- *Bites* (animal or human): can become infected by pathogenic organisms if left untreated.
- *Surgical*: this is classified as a specific type of mechanical injury.
- *Burns and chemical injuries*: there are several different types of burn:
  - thermal
  - chemical
  - electrical
  - radiation
- *Ulcerative wounds*: ulcers can be divided into different types depending upon their underlying cause:
  - decubitus (pressure sore)
  - leg ulcers
  - systemic infection induced
  - caused by radiotherapy
  - resulting from malignant disease.

METHOD OF HEALING

Wounds heal by one of four methods.

Primary closure

Where there is no skin missing and the wound is clean, sutures, clips or retaining products such as glue or Steristrips may be used.

Open granulation

Where skin is missing, for example a leg ulcer, and the wound has to heal from the base upwards.

Delayed or secondary closure

Where skin is not missing, but the wound cannot be closed due to infection or a foreign body.

Graft or flap formation

Where skin is missing and a skin graft is used to aid healing. This is most frequently used for patients presenting with burns.

Having classified the wound, the next stage is to examine the physiological factors. Wounds require measurement and observation at regular intervals, to enable a practitioner to select an appropriate wound dressing. This should ideally be chosen depending on the shape and depth of the wound, type of wound tissue present, amount of exudate and presence of odour. Documentation of the above will enable the practitioner to monitor progress and will also facilitate involvement of the patient as a method of evaluation.

WOUND DEPTH

Used most frequently to assess burns or pressure sores, this methodology is described in terms of tissue damage. For example, a superficial burn would indicate that just the epidermis had been destroyed, whereas a full-thickness wound would indicate that the wound had penetrated both the dermis and epidermis.

SHAPE AND SIZE OF THE WOUND

This alters during the healing process and can often be an indicator as to wound type/category.

The simplest measure is in terms of centimetres and consists of length by breadth. It is most frequently applied where wounds are regular in shape. The only problem with this type of measurement is that different people measuring the wound will not measure it in the same way and monitored progress can become distorted. Additionally, in wounds that are necrotic to start with, the practitioner may see an increase in the size of the wound as it improves, due to exposure of the true wound surface underneath the slough and necrotic tissue.

Wound mapping is an alternative measure that is far more robust in recording the shape and size of the wound. There are several products available which generally have some form of acetate base that is placed over the wound, allowing the practitioner to draw around the wound area, the tracing is then placed upon a grid of squared centimetres thus allowing the practitioner to measure more accurately the area of the wound. Wound maps are useful for filing in patient notes and can be repeated to demonstrate progress.

Wound mapping: a step-by-step approach

1. Ensure that the area around the wound is clean and dry before mapping.

2. Thoroughly wash hands.
3. Cover the wound with a suitable transparent material to protect the chart from contamination.
4. Place the wound-mapping chart over the covered wound.
5. Trace the outline of the wound margin using a permanent fibre-tip pen.
6. Remove and dispose of the contact layer, leaving the uncontaminated grid behind to be filed in the patient's notes.
7. Count up the number of complete squares (usually measured in 1 cm^2 squares). The remaining squares that fall outside the wound perimeter and whose area is equal to or greater than ½ cm^2 are counted as ½ cm^2. Adding these two figures together gives an approximate wound surface area in centimetres squared.
8. Where possible, it is desirable for the same practitioner to repeat this procedure, which can demonstrate the progression or deterioration of the wound.

Mapping charts are available from:

> Consumer and Professional Health Care
> 3M Health Care Ltd
> 3M House
> Morley Street
> Loughborough
> Leicestershire LE11 0BR

The only other way of determining the size and shape of a wound that is currently likely to be used in the community would be photography. Polaroid cameras with special film allow nurses to measure the length and width of a wound with a fair amount of accuracy, if the camera is held at the same angle and distance on each occasion. The only drawback is that this methodology is expensive to maintain in comparison with wound mapping, although pictures do have the advantage of being able to demonstrate progress of wound management more effectively.

Other measures include computer imaging and stereophotogrammetry although these would most likely not be used in primary care.

The depth of a wound is usually measured using a probe and this is recorded in the patient's notes. Although there are alternative methods of measuring depth, such as by computer imaging, this is not available to nurses working in the community at present.

WOUND EXUDATE

The amount of exudate varies throughout the healing process and is usually more productive during the inflammatory phase and less productive during the maturation phase of wound healing. Large amounts of exudate indicate a prolonged inflammatory phase, which is often indicative of a wound infection, or an underlying physiological problem. The colour of the exudate and the odour will also be good indicators of infection.

Dressing selection is often determined by the amount of exudate.

POSITION OF THE WOUND

The position of the wound would indicate potential problems, for example risk of contamination, ease of maintaining the position of the dressing. It may also have an impact upon the dressing selection as one dressing may sit comfortably on the stomach but would not perhaps stay in situ on the sacrum. Additionally, other problems such as the ability to mobilize may be encountered with wounds to the feet or lower limbs. It should also be remembered that in a wound such as a leg ulcer, the position of the wound may indicate whether it is arterial or venous, thus contributing towards the diagnosis of ulcer type.

WOUND APPEARANCE

Wound appearance will indicate the stage of the healing process that the wound has reached and can be classified as:

- necrotic
- infected
- sloughy
- granulating
- epithelializing.

Necrotic

Necrotic areas present as an eschar or scab and are black or brown in colour. Occasionally necrotic tissue presents as thick slough that is greyish in colour. In these types of wound it is of value to remember that eschar or slough can mask the true size of the wound and it is generally more extensive than it looks. Necrotic tissue must always be removed as failure to do so will mean that the wound will continue to increase in size.

Infected

This is normally indicated by signs of local erythema/redness. It can be localized or spread throughout the wound.

Cellulitis may be apparent in the adjacent tissue and this will become obvious by an increase in skin temperature. Oedema may also be present.

The colour of the exudate, which will be increased if infection is present, is dictated by the nature of the bacteria causing the infection. This also applies to the odour of the wound.

Sloughy

Usually a white/yellow colour, that forms a patch-like appearance on the wound surface. It is made up of dead cells. In the most suitable environment for wound healing, the macrophages usually remove all of the slough.

Granulating

The colour of the wound is red and it takes on a granular appearance as the capillary loops emerge. The walls of the new capillary loops are very thin and will bleed easily if traumatized. At this stage the wound will demonstrate signs of inward contraction.

Epithelializing

The wound margin becomes raised and is pink in colour. As epithelial tissue spreads over the wound surface the wound margins become flat. New epithelial tissue presents as islands of pink/white tissue in large flat wounds. The process of epithelialization can be monitored easily as the new cells are different in colour from the surrounding tissue.

In completing a wound assessment all of the above elements will need to be considered. This will obviously take time but, in terms of risk management, will ensure that patients are treated with the most appropriate medication/dressing for their individual wounds. It should be remembered that prescribable items are issued on a named patient basis only and as such, should only be used on the patient for whom they were prescribed.

NUTRITION

The aim of nutritional assessment in relation to a patient with a wound is to establish and evaluate the recent nutrient intake, to identify which individuals are likely to require support to promote healing. According to Rollins (1997), nutrition has a vital role in the management of surgical wounds, ulcers and pressure sores.

McClaren (1992) suggested that the impact of an acute or chronic wound could affect the nutritional status of a patient as wounds like this were likely to lead to depletion in protein reserves. Severe tissue injury and infection would initiate a metabolic response which could alter the nutritional requirements of an individual dramatically. Therefore, patients with chronic unhealed wounds may be malnourished and require several dietary supplements to improve healing.

Individuals with energy and protein depletion will have reduced fat stores and are therefore more prone to pressure damage. As a result, these patients will have a tendency to use protein stores for energy rather than tissue regeneration.

In protein depletion, maturation of connective tissue is delayed and wound healing is compromised. A large wound can lose up to 100 g protein in one day.

Where possible all patients should be encouraged to have nutritionally balanced regular meals, including foods from each of the four main food groups daily. For those that are unable to consume food normally, supplements should be advised.

In patients who are not obese but have large chronic wounds it is important to ensure that enough calories are taken in to support the increased metabolic rate. In this instance high-calorie foods, which include sweets, etc., may be advised.

Vitamin C is essential for wound healing (Utley 1992), as it is required for the synthesis of collagen. Lack of vitamin C will cause a reduction in the tensile strength of the wound and impairs angiogenesis and will result in capillary fragility (McClaren 1992). Despite this, large doses of Vitamin C are not recommended as studies to date have demonstrated efficacy only in cases of severe depletion. Patients with wounds should aim for an intake of 60 mg/day.

Vitamin A promotes the epithelial proliferation and enables granulation of healing wounds. Usually dietary intake is adequate, although the exception would be in patients with burns when a decrease in vitamin occurs.

Zinc deficiency inhibits wound healing and supplementation has been shown to promote healing in individuals who are biochemically zinc deficient

Table 19.1 Essential vitamins and minerals required at each stage of the healing process

Stage	Vitamins and minerals	Activity
Haemostasis	Vitamin K	Clotting
Inflammatory	Essential fatty acids Vitamin C	Produce histamine and prostaglandins
	Vitamin B	Release of polymorphs and macrophages (WBC formation)
Destructive	Vitamin C	Encourages fibroblasts and promotes angiogenesis Essential for the hydroxylation of proline and lysine before their formation into collagen
	Vitamin A	An essential co-factor for collagen crosslinkage Supports epithelial proliferation and migration
	Copper	Adds strength to collagen strands
	Manganese	Triggers chemical reaction to form collagen
Epithelialization	Vitamins A & C	Stimulate migration of epithelial cells
	Zinc	Promotes epithelialization
Maturation	Calcium	Required for wound contraction

(Andrews & Gallagher-Allred 1999). Zinc is essential to the activity of over 200 enzymes concerned in protein and nucleic acid synthesis, carbohydrate and lipid metabolism and as such, deficiency can have a considerable impact on all stages of the wound healing process.

Table 19.1 demonstrates the essential vitamins and minerals required at each stage of the healing process.

WOUND CLEANSING

The aim of wound cleansing is to create optimal local conditions at the wound site to enhance the healing process. This is achieved locally by aiding the removal of debris, necrotic and sloughy tissue prior to the application of an appropriate dressing. It also reduces the risk of cross-infection and the spread of microorganisms.

When cleansing wounds, there are several key points that need to be considered.

- Irrigation is the preferred method of cleansing.
- Bleeding wounds and wounds with exposed nerve endings should not be irrigated.
- The pressure of irrigation needs to be gentle as high pressure may cause injury.
- With the exception of diabetic wounds, all chronic wounds can be washed in warm tap water.
- Only non-woven gauze should be used to clean wounds if irrigation is inappropriate.
- Cotton wool should be avoided as this tends to leave fibres within the wound bed.
- Disposable gloves should be worn when treating wounds, to ensure that cross-infection does not occur.

CLEANSING SOLUTIONS

Not all wounds require cleansing. Cleansing a clean wound can delay the healing process, as this often involves the wound bed being disturbed. Wounds should only be cleansed if necessary using an appropriate technique, as described above. The solutions used for cleansing have in the past been varied and have included antiseptics and topical antibiotics. These are no longer considered appropriate for wound cleansing and should not be used (Cameron & Leaper 1988, Johnson 1988, Leaper & Cameron 1987).

Normal saline 0.9% is the cleansing solution of choice for most wounds. Although tap water can be used to cleanse wounds, it is generally only used on those that are colonized, i.e. leg ulcers, which need to be immersed or placed under running water. A study of leg ulcers by Eriksson et al (1984) suggested that sterility was not a prerequisite for healing. It is therefore unnecessary to remove all the bacteria and systemic antibiotic should only be given when clinical infection is present.

All acute wounds such as burns and surgical wounds must be irrigated with a sterile solution.

Normal saline for cleansing should be used at a temperature of 37°C to prevent a drop in temperature at the wound bed, which can delay the healing process. It should be remembered that each individual practitioner has a responsibility to ensure that the cleansing fluid is the correct temperature when it is applied to the wound. Patients receiving the treatment must also be made aware of this to aid compliance.

TREATMENT

- Dry, necrotic wounds require debridement.
- Wet, sloughy wounds require desloughing.
- Moist, granulating wounds require protection.
- Epithelializing wounds require protection.
- Clean, dry incisional wounds may be left exposed after 48 hours.
- Cavity wounds should be lightly filled with an appropriate dressing.
- Clinically infected wounds will require cleansing and systemic antibiotics.
- The wound dressing should be chosen by following an algorithm/flow chart based on the priorities of wound management.
- The use of wound management technologies should be considered if appropriate, e.g. larval therapy, use of negative pressure (VAC system), laser therapy, hyperbaric oxygen therapy.
- Ensure sufficient time has been allowed for the wound treatment to work.
- Progress of wound healing should be evaluated regularly and a change in management instigated if appropriate. Refer to local policy.
- Appropriate members of the multidisciplinary team should be involved where necessary.
- Prior to patients being discharged from hospital, sufficient dressings should be prescribed by the hospital and dispensed by the pharmacy for a minimum of 14 days following discharge. If a dressing cannot be prescribed by the GP, the community trust involved in the patient's care should provide the dressing required.

Specific types of wound will require additional treatment.

LEG ULCERS

The aetiology will need to be established and managed appropriately. A holistic assessment, including Doppler ultrasound to locate foot pulses and identify arterial sounds and recording of the Ankle Pressure Index (API) should be undertaken (RCN 1998). If venous hypertension is the main aetiology and arterial impairment has been ruled out, compression therapy should be applied.

Doppler assessment

> *A study in Oxford (Kulozic et al 1996) identified the misdiagnosis of some ulcers leading to inappropriate treatment. In order to diagnose the aetiology of a leg ulcer accurately it is essential to assess the Ankle Pressure Index using a Doppler. The Doppler uses a frequency of megahertz. A frequency of between 4 MHz and 8 MHz is required to detect blood flow in the superficial and deep vessels.*
>
> (Cornwall Ulcer Focus Team 1995)

Assessing the Ankle Pressure Index

This technique consists of determining the systolic blood pressure in the artery in the dorsum of the foot, the dorsalis pedis, or the posterior tibialis near the medial malleolus.

The patient needs to be lying for a minimum of 20 minutes prior to performing the Doppler test. During this time the nurse can take the relevant medical, social and familial history. (See Figs 19.1 and 19.2 for recording results and history.)

Procedure (Fig. 19.3)

1. Assess the brachial systolic pressure using the Doppler. Check this twice and record.
2. Palpate the dorsalis pedis pulse.
3. Place the cuff just above the malleolar area, covering the ulcer with Clingfilm to protect the cuff.
4. Measure the ankle systolic pressure in the same way as the brachial pressure.
5. To calculate the API, divide the ankle pressure reading by the brachial pressure reading.

The systolic pressure of the foot is expressed as a ratio of the brachial systolic pressure.

$$\frac{\text{Ankle Pressure Index mmHg}}{\text{Brachial Pressure Index mmHg}} = \text{API}$$

- Normal — API = 1.0 or >1.0
- Suspect arterial insufficiency — API = 0.9–1.0
- Mild arterial insufficiency — API = 0.8–0.9
- Mild/moderate arterial insufficiency — API = 0.7–0.8
- Moderate insufficiency — API = 0.5–0.7
- Severe ischaemia — API = 0.5 or >0.5

Patients with normal limb perfusion will have an ankle/arm ratio equal to or greater than 0.9; in other words, at least 90% of the brachial pressure is perfusing the leg. Patients with an API of 0.8 or greater may have compression bandaging applied.

DATE:

PATIENT DETAILS

SURNAME: ....

CHRISTIAN NAME: ....

DATE OF BIRTH: ....

AGE: .... SEX: ....

WEIGHT: .... HEIGHT: ....

OCCUPATION: ....

GP NAME: ....

CONCURRENT MEDICAL PROBLEMS

The following conditions may be predisposing factors to ulcers and impair the healing process. Record details:

DIABETES	**YES** ☐	**NO** ☐
ANAEMIA	**YES** ☐	**NO** ☐
RHEUMATOID ARTHRITIS	**YES** ☐	**NO** ☐
STEROID THERAPY	**YES** ☐	**NO** ☐
IMMOBILE	**YES** ☐	**NO** ☐
SMOKER	**YES** ☐	**NO** ☐
HYPERTENSION	**YES** ☐	**NO** ☐

VARICOSE VEINS:

ABSENT ☐ MODERATE ☐

MINOR ☐ SEVERE ☐

SKIN DISCOLOURATION:

PRESENT ☐ ABSENT ☐

INVESTIGATIONS

HAEMOGLOBIN: ....

BLOOD PRESSURE: ....

BLOOD/SUGAR: ....

OTHER: ....

ARTERIAL ASSESSMENT

In the presence of arterial insufficiency compression is dangerous.
Arterial assessment is strongly advisable.
Pressure readings should be taken after the patient has been resting for at least 10 minutes with patient seated with legs resting on stool (even a short walk will influence readings)

READINGS (mmHg) by Doppler

Brachial Artery Systolic Pressure= ☐ **Dorsalis Pedis Pressure=** ☐ ***OR* Posterior Tibial Pressure=** ☐

IF ANKLE PRESSURE LESS THAN ARM PRESSURE CONSIDER THE POSSIBILITY OF ARTERIAL INSUFFICIENCY

IN THE ABSENCE OF DOPPLER ASSESSMENT FOOT PULSES SHOULD BE CHECKED

FOOT PULSES ABSENT ☐ **PRESENT** ☐

ULCER DETAILS

DURATION: ....

WOUND TYPE (ref Wound Assessment Table)

....

....

CURRENT TREATMENT DETAILS

....

....

SITE: (please tick) LEFT LEG ☐ RIGHT LEG ☐

Indicate shape and position of ulcer:

Medial **Lateral**

RECOMMENDATIONS

CONTINUE CURRENT TREATMENT **YES** ☐ **NO** ☐

CHANGE TO..

....

....

REFERRED FOR FURTHER INVESTIGATION **YES** ☐ **NO** ☐

GP COMMENTS e.g. known allergies

....

....

....

....

....

SIGNATURE:..

Produced by the Primary Care Forum in association with Scholl, the experts in foot and leg care.

Figure 19.1 Patient record form.

Maximum dimensions should be recorded separately on the wound assessment chart

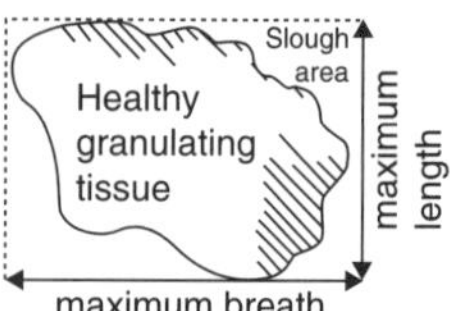

After the initial assessment and treatment the patient should be seen at least weekly to review progress. A tracing/measurement should be made monthly and details recorded below. Ensure all tracings are secured in the space provided (opposite).

	DATE OF APPOINTMENT	WOUND TYPE	TRACING REF	Dressing used/ Compression applied	SIZE MEASUREMENT	RESULTS/ COMMENTS
1.						
2.						
3.						
4.						
If there is no improvement in the ulcer after four weeks, a further assessment of treatment should be made with a view to possible referral.						
	Arterial insufficiency?		**Skin sensitivity?**		**Diabetes/anaemia?**	**Rheumatoid arthritis?**
5.						
6.						
7.						
8.						
9.						
10.						
11.						
12.						
13.						
14.						
15.						
16.						

Figure 19.2 Treatment assessment.

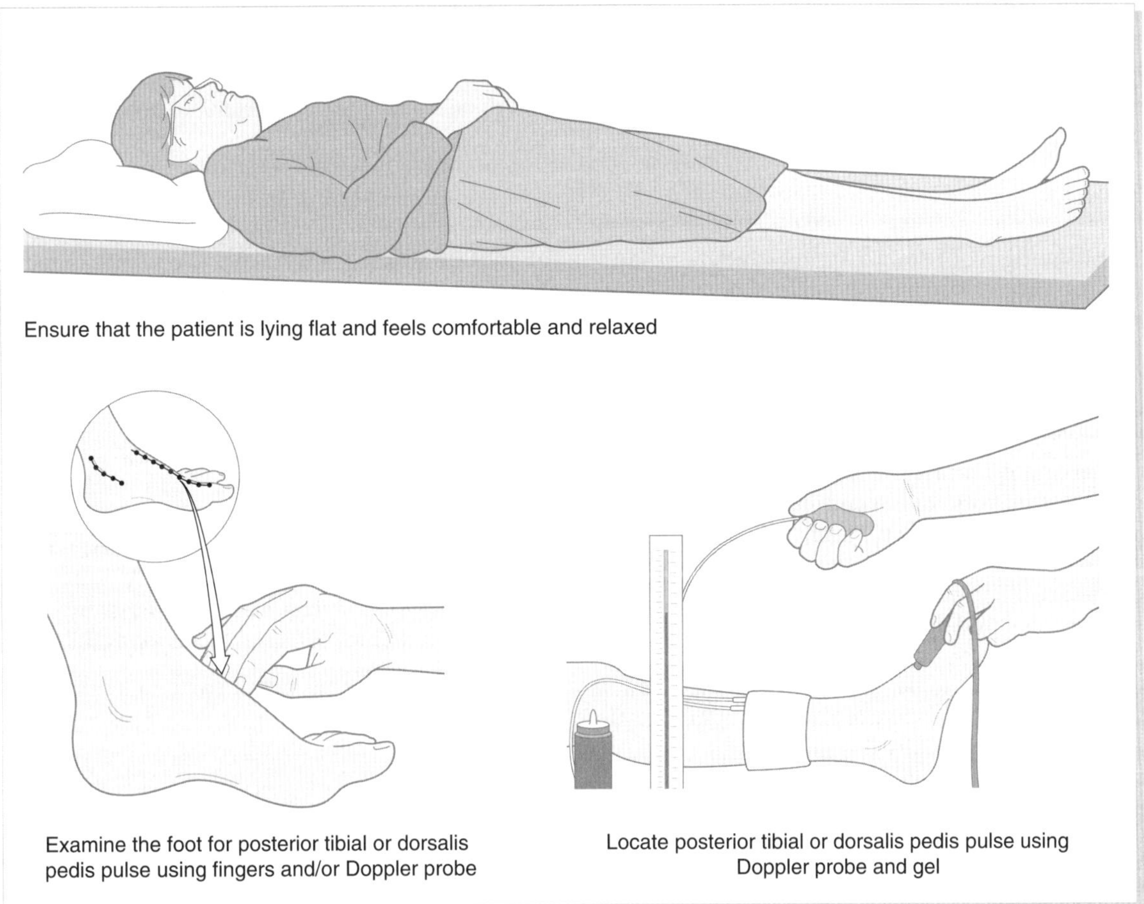

Figure 19.3 Procedure for recording Ankle Pressure Index.

All patients with an API of less than 0.8 should be referred to the GP who will refer on for specialist assessment. Patients with an API of less than 0.5 should be referred to a vascular surgeon.

Repeat Doppler assessment:

- if compression becomes painful
- with recurrence of ulceration
- on patients with borderline results
- routinely at 3-monthly intervals.

DIABETIC PATIENT WITH FOOT ULCER

The aetiology will need to be established by referral to the local podiatry department or diabetic foot clinic. Debridement of callus and necrotic tissue should only be undertaken by a podiatrist. Extreme care should be taken if the ulcer is on the plantar aspect of the foot to avoid shearing forces and rucking of the dressing. The wound should be inspected every day or on alternate days to check for signs of infection.

PRESSURE SORES

An appropriate risk score should be undertaken and documented, e.g. the Waterlow scoring system. The patient should be placed on an appropriate support surface, i.e. mattress and cushion, and position changed at regular periods.

SURGICAL WOUNDS

Monitor for signs of infection. Remove sutures, staples, etc. as appropriate.

TRAUMATIC WOUNDS

Monitor for signs of infection.

FUNGATING WOUNDS

Specific issues relate to the control of exudate and malodour, protection of surrounding skin and attention to altered body image.

FISTULAS

Establish origin of fistula. Control exudate production and protect surrounding skin. Contact stomatherapist if necessary.

BIOLOGICAL DEBRIDEMENT OF SLOUGHY/ NECROTIC WOUNDS

The larvae of *Lucillia sericata*, the green bottle fly, can digest necrotic tissue and pathogens and offer an extremely effective form of debridement (Thomas et al 1998, Young 1997). They are thought to produce a bactericidal enzyme and by the action of their jaws and movement in the wound, they stimulate the process of healing. The larvae used are specially bred to be 'germ free', so they cannot cause infection. They do not burrow under the skin or penetrate into healthy tissue.

The potential benefits resulting from the use of larvae are:

- rapid removal of dead tissue
- prevention of infection
- control of odour
- improved healing.

A hydrocolloid dressing with a hole the size of the wound protects the surrounding skin. The maggots are placed in the wound and may be left in place for 2–3 days, covered with a mesh dressing which is firmly sealed (Thomas 1996).

In the UK the sterile larvae can be purchased from the surgical materials testing laboratory at the Princess of Wales Hospital, Bridgend, Wales, and are delivered the following day.

The website for larval therapy is www.smtl.co.uk/VVMPRC/BioSurgery/Ordering, email maggot-info@smti.co.uk.

INFECTION CONTROL

All wounds are colonized with bacteria, but this does not necessarily indicate infection. Wounds therefore are a source or focus of organisms which could potentially cause infection so it is vital that prevention of cross-infection methods and techniques are always used. These are known as universal infection control measures. See Chapter 25 for details on these important aspects of wound management.

Hands are a major vehicle in the transmission of infection and hand washing is the single most important measure in infection control. Hands should be washed after general patient contact or handling potentially contaminated articles. All contaminated waste (with blood or body fluid) must be placed in yellow clinical sacks and left for incineration according to local policy.

CLINICAL SIGNS AND SYMPTOMS OF WOUND INFECTION

In a chronic wound the presence of bacteria does not necessarily mean it is 'infected'. A useful practical differentiation has been provided by Ayton (1986), who defines bacterial presence as follows.

- *Contamination*: presence of bacteria, with no multiplication.
- *Colonization*: multiplication, with no host reaction.
- *Infection*: the deposition and multiplication of bacteria in tissue, with an associated host reaction.

It is important to note, first, that colonization is the 'normal' situation in a chronic wound, and second, that any associated host reaction is the defining feature of an infected wound, not a positive wound swab result.

The host reaction may take a number of forms. The occurrence of any of the signs and symptoms in Box 19.1 on their own does not necessarily mean the wound is infected. Some of them may occur as part of the inflammatory response linked to the normal wound healing process. The likelihood of there being a wound infection, however, increases as more of the signs and symptoms are identified.

One difficulty for older people with chronic wounds is that they do not always mount a classic immune response, so the clinician or nurse needs to observe the patient closely for any or all of the symptoms in Box 19.1.

WOUND SWABBING

Wound swabs should only be taken to determine which antibiotic is necessary. It is unnecessary and

Box 19.1 Signs and symptoms of wound infection (Cutting & Harding 1994)

Painful redness around the wound
Swelling
The production of large amounts or increased amounts of exudate
Change in exudate/wound tissue colour
Malodour
A raised systemic temperature
Localized pain (or an increase in pain) and heat
Delayed or abnormal wound healing
Wound breakdown
Granulation tissue that is dull or darker than its normal bright red colour
Friable granulation tissue
Epithelial granulation tissue that covers some parts of the wound but not others (bridging)

unhelpful to swab chronic healing leg ulcers or pressure sores. As all wounds are colonized with bacteria, the microbiology laboratory will grow and report any bacteria found on the wound. Wound swabs should only be obtained once a clinical diagnosis of infection has been made and then the results of the wound swab will determine which antibiotic the causative organism is sensitive or resistant to.

A wound specimen should be obtained before the wound is cleaned and ideally before administration of antibiotics and must be taken from the suspected infection site, taking care to avoid the surrounding skin. It is preferable, whenever possible, to send samples of purulent discharge rather than a swab as pus is a much better specimen material for bacterial culture. Specimens of pus or exudate can be aspirated using a sterile syringe and sent to the laboratory in a universal container.

Requests for laboratory investigations are made by medical staff. It is vitally important that the specimen is labelled with the date and time of collection, the patient's name, date of birth and type and site of specimen and must be accompanied by a request form. This form must include identification, i.e. patient's name, date of birth and requester, so that the results can be returned easily. The other key area is *relevant* information; this needs to contain any antibiotic therapy, site of infection and any other medication which may be relevant.

It is also important that 'Danger of Infection' stickers are placed on any specimens from patients with known or suspected blood-borne viruses.

MANAGEMENT OF METHICILLIN-RESISTANT *STAPHYLOCOCCUS AUREUS*

> *Although* Staphylococcus aureus *is a common organism which colonizes many healthy individuals, it can be pathogenic in those whose health is compromised. Some strains of the organism have developed antibiotic resistance, making them difficult to treat, and therefore dangerous to patients.*
>
> (Kiernan 2000)

Staphylococcus aureus is a Gram-positive coccus, which is present on the skin of approximately 30% of the population (Gould 1995). It is a commensal, generally found in warm and moist parts of the body, such as the nose, throat, groin and axillae. Most patients affected by MRSA are colonized by the bacteria (Makoni 2002).

MRSA is mostly spread by contact with colonized hands of healthcare workers (Ayliffe et al 2000). It is therefore vital that all practitioners wash their hands before and after contact with patients.

Once a patient becomes colonized with MRSA they may carry it for years even though it does not cause an infection. In the community setting it is totally unnecessary to do any screening. It is, however, important that all the universal precautions are adhered to and if the patient is readmitted to an acute unit, the hospital is notified of a previous history of MRSA. As discussed above, chronic wounds, e.g. leg ulcers, pressure sores, will be colon-ized with many organisms. Even if it is known that MRSA was or is present then swabbing is totally unnecessary. If the wound is healing then the treatment plan will be unaffected by knowing which organisms are present.

PAIN MANAGEMENT

Assessment of pain that a patient is experiencing is a difficult concept for any nurse to grasp. Essentially a patient's experience of pain is affected by age, culture, sex, duration, pain type (chronic or acute, due to surgery, terminal illness or direct injury, continuous or intermittent); it can also be related to past experience with pain.

According to Sternbach (1968), pain is:

> *an abstract concept that refers to:*
> *A personal, private sensation of hurt*
> *A harmful stimulus, which signals current or impending danger*
> *A pattern of impulses, which operate to protect the organism from harm.*

A nurse will never know exactly what a patient is feeling, as pain is a complex condition which requires thorough and appropriate assessment.

It is because of the subjective nature of pain, and the fact that having a wound dressed can be a painful experience, that it is important to consider methods of reducing the pain whilst carrying out some dressing procedures.

Aspects to consider when assessing pain should include the following:

- patient's verbal report and communication skills
- language difficulty
- patient's dislike of discussing pain
- hindered verbal expression, due to illness or embarrassment
- chronic pain – expression difficult due to exhaustion
- type of pain and position – can clarify cause of pain
- severity – prolonged or intermittent
- observations – body language and clinical signs and symptoms
- personality, culture and emotion.

The aim of pain management is to ensure that the patient experiences as little pain as possible during a dressing change, whilst ensuring that the dressing applied causes as little discomfort as possible.

There are several different pain assessment tools available to assist nurses in helping the patient; these should ideally be short, accurate and take the minimum of administration time, whilst making no demands on the patient.

The most frequently used charts are visual analogue which allow the patient to indicate where, on a scale of 1–10 or from good to bad, their pain is; these tend to be most effective and can be used on almost anyone. Verbal indicators can often be misconstrued and rely upon individual patient interpretation of words.

The advantages of using such tools are an improved patient/nurse relationship, patient participation and empowerment as they are able to play an active role in their care. Patients also feel that their pain is taken seriously and as a result of this, effective analgesia is more likely to be administered.

Conversely there are disadvantages to using assessment tools. Patients may concentrate upon their pain, thus making it worse. Nurses may think that patients are overestimating pain and not provide adequate pain relief. Some charts can be time consuming and understanding what is required from the chart can often be arbitrary.

There is much evidence to support the fact that information about the procedure and the treatment a patient receives can reduce pain and anxiety so it is important that procedures and treatments are explained and agreed by both the patient and the practitioner.

Often medication taken prior to a dressing change can help because, taken at the right time, analgesia can be very effective.

ANALGESIA

For optimum pain relief analgesia needs to be prescribed:

- regularly
- for breakthrough pain
- if appropriate, as a slow-release preparation for night time
- for procedural pain.

If pain relief is required for dressings changes it is advisable to give the initial dose about 45–60 minutes before starting. The most frequently used medication for this purpose will be any one of or a combination of the following:

- paracetamol
- ibuprofen
- codeine.

Maximum doses

- Paracetamol: 4 g/24 hours; 500 mg–1 g to be repeated every 4–6 hours when required.
- Codeine: 240 mg/24 hours; 30–60 mg every 4 hours when required
- Ibuprofen: 1.2 g/24 hours in three or four divided doses.

Contraindications

- Paracetamol: avoid in patients with liver damage.

- Codeine: avoid in acute respiratory depression, acute alcoholism.
- Ibuprofen: avoid in patients with previous gastrointestinal ulceration, known sensitivity to NSAIDs and aspirin.

Side-effects

- Codeine phosphate can cause constipation, especially at high doses.
- Ibuprofen, like all NSAIDs, can cause serious gastrointestinal side-effects but has a low risk of these complications at the dose recommended above.

THE IDEAL DRESSING

Dressings are applied to wounds for a number of reasons. These include:

- the control and absorption of exudate
- the control of bleeding
- to achieve pain relief
- to clean and debride
- to protect newly formed tissue and to optimize the healing process.

The 'optimum' dressing should provide an environment in which wound healing can take place and cause the patient no harm.

The ideal method of wound care has been sought since the late 19th century when dressings such as the gamgee pad, sometimes impregnated with substances like iodine, were first used. Research into wound healing in the early 1960s by George Winter (1962), however, showed that occlusive dressings improved healing rates in the domestic pig, via increased cell division. This research led to the development of many new types of dressings, i.e. foams, films, gels, hydrocolloids, which have altered the treatment of all wound types.

Turner (1985) listed seven criteria for the ideal dressing:

- to maintain high humidity at the wound/dressing interface
- to remove excess exudate
- to allow gaseous exchange
- to provide thermal insulation
- to be impermeable to bacteria
- to be free of particles and toxic wound contaminants
- to allow removal without causing trauma to the wound.

MAINTAIN HIGH HUMIDITY

George Winter (1962) compared the effect of leaving superficial wounds exposed against the effect of using a semipermeable film dressing. His findings were that epithelialization occurred twice as fast on the wounds covered in film and concluded that this was due to the high humidity (Dealey 1995).

REMOVE EXCESS EXUDATE

Excess exudate can cause maceration of surrounding undamaged skin.

ALLOW GASEOUS EXCHANGE

Perrins (1967) found that epithelialization was speeded up in a hyperbaric oxygen chamber, thus indicating that gaseous exchange on the wound surface was advantageous. Knighton (1981), however, found that a lack of oxygen (tissue hypoxia) was required to stimulate angiogenesis.

Silver (1985) concluded that oxygen was essential for wound healing at all stages, which would mean that a wound does not rely on atmospheric oxygen alone. Gaseous exchange may be useful at some stages of wound healing but not others.

PRODUCE THERMAL INSULATION

A constant temperature of 31°C is required to promote macrophage and mitotic activity during granulation and epithelialization. Cooling of a wound during dressing changes can reduce the surface temperature by several degrees, thereby delaying the wound healing process by several hours.

BE IMPERMEABLE TO BACTERIA

A dressing should provide a barrier between the wound and the environment, first to prevent contamination by airborne microorganisms and second to prevent wound bacteria from escaping into the environment and hence possibly causing cross-infection. (Wet dressings provide an ideal climate for bacteria to travel in both directions.)

BE FREE OF PARTICLES

Gauze-type dressing pads often used to shed their particles into the wound. These particles have been shown to produce a prolonged inflammatory response.

ALLOW REMOVAL WITHOUT CAUSING TRAUMA TO THE WOUND

No dressing is of value if it causes trauma on removal. Damage occurs when dressings adhere to the wound surface, causing tissue disruption (of newly formed tissue) on removal. This can delay healing and cause a renewed inflammatory response.

ALGINATES

Alginates occur naturally as mixed salts of alginic acid. They are found primarily as the sodium form, in certain species of brown seaweed, including giant kelp, horsetail kelp and sugar kelp (Thomas 1996). Alginic acid contains both mannuronic and guluronic acid residues. Individual dressing characteristics are determined by the sodium and calcium ion content and the amount of mannuronic acid and guluronic acid residues.

- Form a gel when in contact with exudate from the wound.
- The gel formed provides a moist healing environment.
- Alginates are very absorbent and inappropriate for low exuding and dry wounds.
- Can be used and changed daily on infected wounds.
- Some alginates have haemostatic properties, e.g. Kaltostat.
- Require a secondary dressing.
- Should not overlap good skin.
- Can be easily removed by irrigation.
- Any fibres left in the wound are lysed.

KALTOSTAT

Description

Calcium alginate fibre, flat, non-woven, that reacts with wound exudate to form a strong viscous gel.

Indications

- Medium to heavily exuding wounds
- Leg ulcers
- Pressure sores
- Haemostat for bleeding wounds
- Cavity wounds
- Infected wounds
- Fungating wounds
- Diabetic foot ulcers
- Donor sites

How to use

- Cut or fold to the shape of the wound. Do not overlap onto good skin as this can cause maceration or adherence to the wound edges.
- Place in position and cover with a secondary dressing, e.g. gauze, hydrocolloid, foam or semipermeable film dressing.
- Remove by irrigation with warm tap water or normal saline at body temperature.

Contraindications

Do not apply to dry or necrotic wounds.

When to change the dressing

- Change daily if wound is infected or is a diabetic foot ulcer.
- Leave on other wounds for a maximum of 3–7 days.
- Change when maximum absorbency is reached or when strike-through occurs.
- If used as a haemostat, remove when haemostasis has occurred.

Presentation

- 5 × 5 cm
- 7.5 × 12 cm
- Cavity 2 g

IODINE-IMPREGNATED DRESSINGS

- For use on healing exuding wounds as well as on infected and sloughy wounds.
- Absorb moderate amounts of exudate.
- Reduce bacteria in wounds.
- Require a secondary dressing.
- Dressing change can be made between 1 and 7 days.
- Iodine is absorbed systemically when applied to large wounds. The amount of iodine applied must not exceed 50 g in a single dose or 150 g in 1 week.
- Not to be used on patients with iodine sensitivity and contraindicated in those patients

with thyroid disease, pregnant women and patients on lithium, sulphafurazoles and sulphonylureas.
- Should not be used on dry wounds.

IODOFLEX

Description

Cadexomer iodine paste, between two layers of gauze fabric that absorb exudate and simultaneously release iodine into the wound.

Indications

- Moderate to heavily exuding wounds
- Chronic infected or sloughy wounds

How to use

- Remove the gauze carrier from one side of the dressing and apply directly to wound.
- Remove the second layer of gauze and cover with a secondary dressing.
- The total amount of Iodoflex used in 1 week must not exceed 150 g.
- Treatment duration should not exceed 3 months.
- The dressing can be removed by irrigating with sodium chloride.

Contraindications

- Patients with known iodine sensitivity.
- Not recommended for use in children under 2 years.
- Patients with thyroid disease.
- Lactating or pregnant women.
- Dry or necrotic wounds.

When to change the dressing

- Dressing should be changed daily initially and then 2–3 times a week as exudate decreases.
- Iodoflex should be changed when the dressing has lost its colour.

FOAMS AND HYDROCELLULAR DRESSINGS

LYOFOAM

Description

A polyurethane foam dressing which is semi-occlusive, providing a warm and moist environment.

Indications

- Light to moderate exuding wounds
- Minor burns
- Overgranulating wounds
- Diabetic foot ulcers

How to use

- As a primary dressing.
- Allow 2–3 cm overlap around wound edges.
- Apply the smooth, shiny side of the dressing directly to the wound surface.
- Secure with an appropriate bandage or tape.
- Do not cover with an occlusive dressing as this affects its permeability.

Contraindications

- Dry, shallow wounds may produce adhesion of the dressing.
- Known Lyofoam sensitivity.

When to change the dressing

- Can be left in place for 1–7 days depending on exudate levels.
- Change daily on diabetic foot ulcers.

Presentation

- 7.5 × 7.5 cm
- 17.5 × 10 cm

LYOFOAM EXTRA

Description

Polyurethane foam film dressing with a highly absorbent layer.

Indications

- Heavily exuding wounds
- Overgranulating wounds
- Pressure sores
- Leg ulcers

How to use

- Mainly as a primary dressing.
- Apply with cream side onto the wound and pink side facing upwards.
- Overlap wound edge by 2–3 cm.
- Secure with bandage or tape.
- Do not cover with an occlusive dressing as this affects its permeability.

- Change to a more appropriate dressing when exudate decreases.

Contraindications

- Of limited use on necrotic or sloughy wounds.
- Known sensitivity to the dressing.

When to change the dressing

- Frequency of dressing change depends on the level of wound exudate.
- Can be left in place for 2–3 days.

Presentation

- 10 × 10 cm
- 17.5 × 10 cm
- 20 × 15 cm
- 10 × 25 cm

ALLEVYN CAVITY

Description

A hydrophilic cavity dressing. It consists of a low adherent polyurethane net, which comes into contact with the wound surface, and a central absorbent foam layer consisting of chips of Allevyn foam.

Indications

- Granulating cavity wounds

How to use

- As a primary dressing.
- Cover with an appropriate secondary dressing and tape in place.

Contraindications

- Of no use on necrotic wounds.

When to change the dressing

- Change when dressing is saturated.
- It can be left in place for up to 5 days.

Presentation

- 5 cm circular
- 10 cm circular
- 9 × 2.5 cm tubular
- 12 × 4 cm tubular

TIELLE

Description

A hydropolymer dressing, in which the 3D structure draws exudate into the dressing. As exudate is taken up into the dressing a soft bulge appears in the foam. It comes in several forms: Tielle Lite for minimally exuding wounds, Tielle for moderately exuding wounds, Tielle Plus for heavily exuding wounds and Tielle Plus Borderless for heavily exuding wounds with poor surrounding skin.

Indications

- Granulating wounds
- Finger tip injuries
- Leg ulcers

How to use

- Mainly as a primary dressing.
- Remove backing sheet and gently press into position.
- The dressing should extend at least 2 cm beyond the wound margins.

Contraindications

- Sloughy or necrotic tissue.
- Caution if patient has 'tissue paper' skin.

When to change the dressing

- Change when exudate reaches the edge of the dressing.
- Can be left in place for 4–7 days.
- Remove dressing by gently lifting the adhesive edge of the dressing and moistening with water, in order to break the bonding of the adhesive. Continue to do this until whole of dressing is removed.

Presentation

Tielle Lite

- 7 × 9 cm
- 11 × 11 cm
- 8 × 15 cm
- 8 × 20 cm

Tielle

- 11 × 11 cm
- 15 × 15 cm
- 18 × 18 cm
- 7 × 9 cm

- 15 × 20 cm
- 18 × 18 cm (sacrum)

Tielle Plus

- 11 × 11 cm
- 15 × 15 cm
- 15 × 20 cm

Tielle Plus Borderless

- 11 × 11 cm

HYDROCOLLOIDS

DUODERM EXTRA THIN

Description

A thin semipermeable hydrocolloid dressing.

Indications

- Superficial wounds
- Low exuding wounds
- Protection from shearing forces
- Reddened pressure areas
- Minor burns

How to use

- As a primary dressing.
- No secondary dressing is required.
- Adhesion is helped by warming between hands prior to application.
- Remove paper backing and lightly press into position.
- Ensure the dressing extends at least 2 cm beyond the wound edge.

Contraindications

- Moderate to heavy exudate.
- The presence of anaerobic infection.
- Known sensitivity to the dressing.
- Do not use on diabetic foot ulcers.

When to change the dressing

- Can be kept in place for 5–7 days or until wound is healed.
- Frequency of dressing change will depend on the amount of exudate.

Presentation

- 7.5 × 7.5 cm
- 10 × 10 cm
- 15 × 15 cm

GRANUFLEX

Description

A waterproof, semipermeable hydrocolloid dressing. The hydrocolloid particles react with wound exudate to form a gel.

Indications

- Low to moderate exuding wound
- Necrotic and sloughy wounds
- For general debridement of wounds
- Minor burns
- Granulating wounds
- Pressure sores

How to use

- As a primary or secondary dressing.
- A secondary dressing is not needed.
- Warm dressing between hands prior to application.
- Remove paper backing and lightly press into position.
- The dressing should extend at least 2 cm beyond the wound edge.
- A shower can be taken with the dressing in situ which is a great advantage to the patient.
- A bordered dressing is available.

Contraindications

- The presence of anaerobic infection.
- Diabetic foot ulcers.
- Known sensitivity to the dressing.
- If used inappropriately maceration can occur.

When to change the dressing

- Can be left in place for 5–7 days.
- When exudate has reached 2 cm from the edge of the dressing and when colour change has occurred.

Presentation

Granuflex Bordered

- 10 × 10 cm
- 10 × 13 cm
- 15 × 18 cm

Granuflex

- 10 × 10 cm
- 15 × 15 cm
- 15 × 20 cm
- 20 × 20 cm

COMFEEL PLUS

Description

A hydrocolloid dressing containing an alginate.

Indications

- Moderately exuding wounds
- Necrotic and sloughy tissue
- Granulating wounds
- Pressure sores
- Leg ulcers
- Patients with 'tissue paper' skin

How to use

- As a primary dressing.
- A secondary dressing is not required.
- Warm between hands prior to application.
- Remove paper backing and lightly press into position.
- The dressing should extend at least 2 cm beyond the wound margins.

Contraindications

- Heavily exuding wounds.
- Diabetic foot ulcers.
- In the presence of anaerobic infection.

When to change the dressing

- A change in the colour of the dressing to a near transparency indicates a dressing change is required.
- The dressing may stay in situ for up to 7 days depending on exudate levels.

Presentation

- 10 × 10 cm
- 15 × 15 cm
- 18 × 20 cm
- 20 × 20 cm

HYDROGELS

INTRASITE GEL

Description

A hydrogel made from 77% water, 20% propylene glycol and 3% modified carboxymethyl-cellulose polymer, which absorbs and retains significant volumes of exudate.

Indications

- Cavity wounds
- Debridement of sloughy or necrotic tissue
- Infected wounds
- To hydrate or soften eschar
- Fungating wounds
- Pressure sores
- Leg ulcers

How to use

- Apply directly to the wound to a depth of at least 5 mm.
- A secondary dressing is required, determined by the level of exudate, e.g. absorbent pad, hydrocolloid, paste bandage, semipermeable film or foam dressing.
- Remove by irrigation with warm tap water or normal saline.
- This product is for once-only use.

Contraindications

- Heavily exuding wounds, as can cause maceration.
- If anaerobic infection is suspected.
- Do not use in conjunction with iodine.

When to change the dressing

- Change daily on infected or malodorous wounds.
- Can be changed every 1–3 days.

Presentation

- Applipack of 8 g and 15 g

NU-GEL

Description

A hydrogel with alginate properties.

Indications

- Necrotic wounds
- Sloughy wounds
- Cavity wounds
- Fungating wounds
- Leg ulcers
- Pressure sores
- Infected wounds

How to use

- Introduce into wound to a minimum depth of 5 mm.

- Cover with an appropriate secondary dressing, e.g. Surgipad, hydrocolloid, semipermeable film or foam dressing.
- This product is for once-only use.

Contraindications

- Known allergy to the gel.

When to change the dressing

- Change daily if required, but can leave on for up to 3 days.

Presentation

- 15 g dispenser

IMPREGNATED DRESSINGS

INADINE

Description

Knitted viscose dressing impregnated with 10% povidone-iodine ointment.

Indications

- Traumatic wounds
- Superficial burns
- Infected wounds
- Minimal to moderately exudating wounds

How to use

- Apply directly to the wound.
- A secondary dressing is required, e.g. gauze, Surgipad or foam.
- No more than four dressings can be applied at the same time.

Contraindications

- Necrotic wounds.
- Sensitivity to iodine.
- Thyroid problems.
- Heavily exudating wounds.
- Use with caution in children and breastfeeding mothers.

When to change the dressing

- The dressing needs to be changed when the distinctive orange-brown colour changes to cream.
- Change every 2–3 days in infected wounds.

Presentation

- 5 × 5 cm
- 9.5 × 9.5 cm

SEMIPERMEABLE FILMS

OPSITE FLEXIGRID

Description

A thin semipermeable, hypoallergenic adhesive-coated film. It has a removable flexible carrier, which supports the film and incorporates a grid system for mapping wound size.

Indications

- Relatively shallow wounds
- Prophylactically on skin areas prone to friction, for protection
- Abrasions and lacerations
- Minor burns
- As a secondary dressing

How to use

- Ensure skin is dry before application.
- Remove backing paper and apply to area; can be cut to shape.
- Remove carrier and smooth down to ensure good adhesion.
- Allow an overlap of 4–5 cm beyond wound edges.
- Mark wound outline on grid carrier if a record is required.
- Remove by lifting a corner. Then, using a pull-and-release technique, stretch the film towards you and release.

Contraindications

- Incorrect removal can damage fragile skin.
- Do not use on infected wounds.
- Do not apply over third-degree burns.

When to change the dressing

- Change every 3–7 days.

Presentation

- 6 × 7 cm
- 12 × 12 cm
- 15 × 20 cm

TEGADERM

Description

A thin semipermeable, adhesive-coated film, which has a window border to assist in its application.

Indications

- Skin areas prone to friction
- Minor burns
- Abrasions and lacerations
- As a secondary dressing

How to use

- Remove backing paper and gently press into position.
- Once in position, remove paper border.
- Remove by lifting a corner of the dressing and gently stretching the film towards you, so breaking the bonding of the adhesive.

When to change the dressing

- Change every 3–7 days.

Presentation

- 6 × 7 cm
- 12 × 12 cm
- 15 × 20 cm

COMPRESSION BANDAGES

ROSIDAL K

Description

An inelastic 100% cotton bandage, tan in colour, with a high working pressure and low resting pressure.

Indications

- Venous ulcer, following full assessment and API reading between >0.8 and <1.2
- Management of lymphoedema
- Reduction of oedema in mobile patient

How to use

- Must only be applied by a suitably trained practitioner.
- Refer to the local Leg Ulcer/Wound Care Management Guidelines.
- Do not apply to a leg with an ankle measurement of <18 cm without full padding from toe to knee.
- Apply padding from toe to below the knee in a spiral manner.
- Secure bandage around the foot with a figure of eight around the ankle. Once past the ankle, apply full stretch with a 50% overlap in a spiral action, thus producing a compression of 40 mmHg at the ankle.
- Check for any extra pain, discolouration and tingling of the foot and toe and instruct the patient to remove the bandage immediately should this occur at a later time.
- Check the patient again the next day.
- Always remove the bandage if there is any doubt.
- Bandage may be washed according to the manufacturer's instructions and reused up to 12 times.

Contraindications

- Ischaemia.
- Diabetes.
- Known arterial disease.
- When a full assessment has not been carried out.
- Of limited use with immobile patients.

When to change the bandage

- Change 2–3 times weekly to avoid slippage.
- If using in the reduction of oedema, change daily until the oedema is reduced.
- Can be left for up to 1 week.
- Change on breakthrough of exudate.

Presentation

- 8 cm × 5 m
- 10 cm × 5 m
- 12 cm × 5 m

TENSOPRESS

Description

An elastic, high compression bandage.

Indications

- Venous ulcer, following a full assessment and API reading of between >0.8 and <1.2

- Varicosities
- As part of a multilayer system on limb circumferences >25 cm

How to use

- Do not apply without a full assessment and API reading <0.8.
- Must only be applied by a suitably trained practitioner.
- Apply over suitable padding to protect the limb from trauma.
- Apply in a spiral, toe to knee.
- Overlap the yellow line whilst maintaining a consistent extension of 50%.
- Cut any excess bandage.

Contraindications

- Ischaemia or API <0.8.
- Diabetic patients.
- Not suitable on ankle circumference <18 cm.

When to change the dressing

- Change on strike-through of exudate.
- Can be left in place for up to 1 week.

Presentation

- 7.5 cm × 3 m
- 10 cm × 3 m

MEDICATED PASTE BANDAGES

STERIPASTE

Description

Hypoallergenic cotton bandage impregnated with 15% zinc oxide paste.

Indications

- Eczema
- Lichenified skin
- Chronic dermatitis
- Leg ulcers
- Malodorous ulcers

How to use

- Apply bandage from base of toes to the tibial tuberosity, with the foot held at a right angle.
- A secondary dressing/bandage is required.
- Remove by unwinding the bandage.
- Wash limb in warm water.
- Observe for sensitivity reactions which can occur at any time following a course of treatment.

Contraindications

- Known sensitivity to the bandage constituents.

When to change the bandage

- Change when there is strike-through of exudate.
- Can be left in place for 1–2 weeks.

Presentation

- 7.5 cm × 6 m

ZIPZOC

Description

Rayon stocking impregnated with 20% zinc oxide ointment. It also contains white soft paraffin and liquid paraffin.

Indications

- Eczema
- Leg ulcers
- Dry skin conditions
- Chronic dermatitis

How to use

- Remove from pouch.
- Gather in hands and slide onto limb.
- Smooth out any folds or wrinkles.
- Any excess can be cut off.
- Apply secondary dressing and appropriate bandage.
- Can be used under hosiery.

Contraindications

- Known allergy to constituents of the bandage.

When to change the bandage

- Can leave in place for 7–14 days.
- Change when there is strike-through of exudate.

Presentation

- Single length 80 cm

Table 19.2 Taken from 'Joint Formulary' for Royal Hospital Trust, Cornwall Health Care Trust, Primary Care Group/Trusts and GPs within Cornwall and the Isles of Scilly. Dec 2000. (Permission granted)

Product	Choice	Sizes	Indications for use and comments
Adhesive island Mepore®	Primapore	8.3 × 6 cm 10 × 8 cm 15 × 8 cm 20 × 10 cm 25 × 10 cm 30 × 10 cm 35 × 12 cm	Dry postoperative wounds, for protection only, not waterproof or bacteria proof Non-stick island
Adhesive island	Opsite Post Op	5 × 5 cm 9.5 × 8.5 cm 23.5 × 8.5 cm 35 × 10 cm	Lightly exuding postoperative wounds Waterproof Bacteria proof
Perforated film dressing	e.g. Release®, Jeionet®, Skintact® not recommended, advise use of N-A Ultra or appropriate wound care product depending on assessment		
Non-adherent	N-A Ultra	9.5 × 9.5 cm 19.5 × 9.5 cm	Contact layer, use instead of Tricotex®, Jelonet® Superior non-adhesive dressing
Semipermeable film Cutifilm	Tegaderm	6 × 7 cm 12 × 12 cm 15 × 20 cm	Superficial wounds, skin protection, used as a secondary dressing and for securing syringe driver sites and venous lines Can remain in situ until edges wrinkle/roll, 7–14 days
Hydrocolloid Granuflex®	Comfeel	10 × 10 cm 15 × 15 cm 20 × 20 cm	Light to moderate exuding wounds, to aid debridement and granulation No animal products
	Comfeel plus	10 × 10 cm 15 × 15 cm 18 × 20 cm Sacral: 20 × 20 cm Contour: 6 × 8 cm 9 × 11 cm	Alginate included
Alginate ribbon Algisite® M Rope	Sorbsan ribbon	40 cm	Highly absorbent Pack sinuses and cavities loosely and irrigate dressing debris, probe included
Alginate packing Algisite® M	Sorbsan packing	30 cm × 2 g	Highly absorbent
Alginate flat sheet Algisite® M	Sorbsan	5 × 5 cm 10 × 10 cm	Highly absorbent
Alginate pad	Sorbsan plus	7.5 × 10 cm 10 × 15 cm 10 × 20 cm 15 × 20 cm	Highly absorbent Alginate with absorbent pad
Hydrogel Intrasite®	Purilon	8 g 15 g	Primarily used for wound debridement Single use application
Hydrogel sheet	Intrasite conformable	8 g 15 g 30 g	Primarily used for wound debridement Single use application Less wastage
Foam	Lyofoam	7.5 × 7.5 cm 10 × 10 cm 17.5 × 10 cm 20 × 15 cm	Light exudate Over granulation

Table 19.2 (*continued*)

Product	Choice	Sizes	Indications for use and comments
	Allevyn	5 × 5 cm 10 × 10 cm 10 × 20 cm 20 × 20 cm	Light to medium exudate
Foam, adhesive Tielle	Lyofoam extra adhesive	9 × 9 cm 15 × 13 cm 15 × 15 cm 22 × 22 cm 30 × 30 cm 22 × 26 cm	Moderate exudate
Allevyn Adhesive	Tielle plus	11 × 11 cm 15 × 15 cm 15 × 20 cm	Moderate to heavy exudate
Foam, shaped	Allevyn heel	Heel shaped: 10.5 × 13.5 cm	Longer wear time as remains in situ better
	Allevyn cavity	Round: 5 cm 10 cm Tubular: 9 × 2.5 cm 12 × 4 cm	For use in large cavities with heavy exudate
Combination dressing	CombiDERM adhesive	10 × 10 cm 14 × 14 cm 15 × 18 cm 20 × 20 cm 20 × 23 cm	High exudate management Combines 3 dressing products: Kaltostat® Aquacel® DuoDERM®
	CombiDERM non-adhesive	7.5 × 7.5 cm 14 × 14 cm 15 × 25 cm	
Charcoal dressing Actisorb Silver 220	CarboFLEX	10 × 10 cm 8 × 15 cm oval 15 × 20 cm	Malodorous wounds Benefits by having added absorption properties, hence longer wear time
Silicone	Mepitel	5 × 7.5 cm 7.5 × 10 cm 10 × 18 cm 20 × 30 cm	Restricted use where N-A Ultra is inappropriate Change weekly
Cadaxomer-iodine	Iodoflex	5 g 10 g 17 g	Primarily used for debridement, also antibacterial Change when it looks like wallpaper paste
Iodine tulle	Inadine	5 × 5 cm 9.5 × 9.5 cm	Restricted for palliative arterial/diabetic wounds Single layer use
Antimicrobial Actisorb Silver 220 has antimicrobial properties	Anabact	15 g 30 g	Malodorous wounds

(*continued*)

Table 19.2 *(continued)*

Product	Choice	Sizes	Indications for use and comments
Antibacterial	Flamazine	50 g 250 g 500 g	Primarily used in the initial treatment of burns (note 250 g and 500 g pots should be discarded 24 hours after opening)
Hydrofibre	Aquacel	5 × 5 cm 10 × 10 cm 15 × 15 cm 45 cm ribbon	Management of medium to heavy exudate Fibrous hydrocolloid
Barrier	3M Cavilon Foam applicator 3M Cavilon no sting barrier film pump	1 ml wipe 3 ml wipe 28 ml spray	Prevents maceration, general skin protection, ensure correct application One single application lasts 72 hours, do not overapply and ensure skin is touch dry prior to skin-to-skin contact
Biotherapy	Larvae		Wound debridement Authorization from tissue viability Requires funding, not on FP10
Enzymatic	Varidase	Combi-pack	Wound debridement
Emollient Oilatum	Hydromol	150 ml 300 ml 1000 ml	Dry skin conditions Dilute in water as prescribed
Skin hydration Aqueous cream	50/50, white soft paraffin & liquid paraffin	250 g	Soothes, smooths and rehydrates Diprobase® 500 g, useful in leg ulcer clinics
Wound irrigation	Steripod	20 ml	Irrigate wound ONLY if loose debris present Warm saline to body temperature
Atraumatic skin closure	Leukostrip	6.4 × 76 mm	For example skin flaps, trauma injuries Use in place of Steristrips
Surgical tape Micropore®	Scanpor	1.25 cm 2.5 cm 5 cm	Dressing and bandage retention

References

Andrews M, Gallagher-Allred C 1999 The role of zinc in wound healing. Advances in Wound Care 12(3):137–138

Ayliffe GAJ, Lowbury E 2000 Control of hospital infection, 4th edn. Arnold, London

Ayton M 1986 Wounds that won't heal. Nursing Times 81(46) (suppl):16–19

Cameron S, Leaper D 1988 Antiseptic toxicity in open wounds. Nursing Times 84(25):77–78

Casey G 2000 Wound care. In: RCN Practice Nurse Association handbook. Royal College of Nursing, London

Cornwall Ulcer Focus Team 1995 Guidelines for the Assessment and Treatment of Leg Ulcers. Cornwall Health Care Trust, Cornwall

Cutting K, Harding K 1994 Criteria for identifying wound infection. Journal of Wound Care 3(4):198–201

Dealey C 1999 The care of wounds, 2nd edn. Blackwell Science, Oxford

DoH 1998 A first class service. HMSO, London

Eckersley JRT, Dudley HAF 1998 Wounds and wound healing. British Medical Bulletin 44(2):423–436

Eriksson G, Eklaund A, Kallings I 1984 The clinical significance of bacterial growth in leg ulcers. Scandinavian Journal of Infectious Disease 16:175–180

Gould C 1995 Staph. aureus. A review of the literature. Journal of Clinical Nursing 4(1):5–12

Johnson A 1988 The cleansing ethic. Community Outlook February:9–10

Kiernan M 2000 Essential wound healing: MRSA. EMAP Health Care Ltd, London

Knighton DR, Silver IA, Hunt TK 1981 Regulation of wound-healing angiogenesis – effect of oxygen

gradients and inspired oxygen concentration. Surgery 90:262
Leaper D, Cameron S 1987 Antiseptic solutions. Community Outlook April:30–34
Makoni T 2002 MRSA: risk assessment and flexible management. Nursing Standard 16(28):39–41
McClaren SMG 1992 Nutrition and wound healing. Journal of Wound Care 1(3):45–55
Perrins DJ 1967 Influence of hyperbaric oxygen on the survival of split skin grafts. Lancet 1(7495):868–871
RCN 1998 The management of patients with venous leg ulcers. RCN Institute, London
Rollins H 1997 Nutrition and wound healing. Nursing Standard 11(51):49–52
Sternbach R 1968 Pain: a psychophysiological analysis. Academic Press, New York
Thomas S 1996 A prescriber's guide to dressing and wound management materials. Value for Money Unit, Welsh Office Health Department, Cardiff
Thomas S, Andrews A, Jones M 1998 The use of larval therapy in wound management. Journal of Wound Care 7(10):521–524
Turner TD 1985 Which dressing and why? In: Westaby S (ed) Wound care. Heinemann, London
Utley R 1992 Nutritional factors associated with wound healing in the elderly. Ostomy/Wound Management 38(3):22, 24, 26–27
Winter G 1962 Formation of the scab and the rate of epithelialization of superficial wounds in the skin of the young domestic pig. Nature 193:293–294
Young T 1997 Maggot therapy in wound management. Nurse Prescriber/Community Nurse September: 43–45

Resources

Useful addresses

Tissue Viability Society
Glanville Centre
Salisbury Hospital NHS Trust
Salisbury
Wilts SP2 8BT
Tel: 01722 336 262

Wound Care Society
PO Box 163
Huntingdon PE18 7PL
Tel: 01480 424401

European Wound Management Association
PO Box 864
London SE1 8TT
Tel: 020 7872 3436

Wound Healing Research Unit
University of Wales
Cardiff CR4 4XN
Tel: 02920 744 3720

Local contacts for advice

Pharmaceutical Advisor to the PCT
Tissue Viability Nurse

Chapter 20

Clinical procedures

Wendy K MacKinnon

CHAPTER CONTENTS

INTRODUCTION

The content of this chapter deals with a basic set of skills every practice nurse will need to possess. Some skills, such as blood pressure recording, are already familiar to nurses and some may be new skills to be learned. Although basic skills, their importance cannot be overestimated. The interpretation of investigations is one of the tools of general practice. When clinicians initiate or alter treatment they are reliant on the quality of the results.

The following provides a starting point for the newly employed practice nurse. The diversity of general practice dictates that it cannot be regarded as prescriptive and it is not intended to be so.

HEIGHT

Accurate height recording is becoming increasingly important because it is one of the factors considered in the diagnosis and treatment of osteoporosis.

- Patients should be measured without shoes.
- They should stand with feet together flat on the floor and heels against the wall. The back should be straight, with shoulder blades touching the wall.
- The head should be horizontal so that a line drawn between the eye and the upper margin of the entry to the ear canal is parallel to the ground (Fig. 20.1).

WEIGHT

- Patients should be weighed without shoes and outdoor clothing.

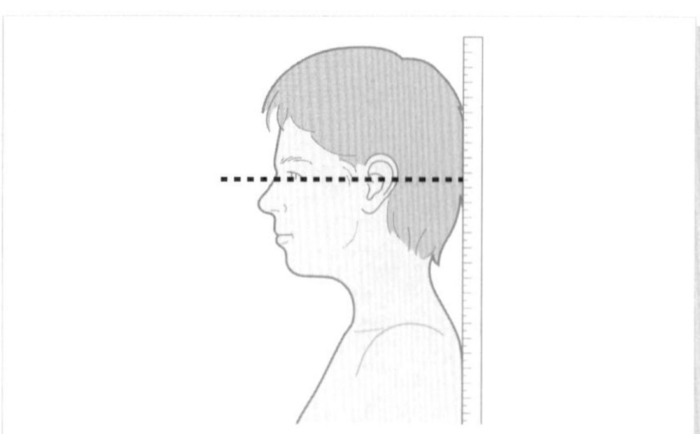

Figure 20.1 Height measurement. The patient should be standing straight with the line joining the eye socket and the top of the ear hole parallel to the ground.

- Check pockets for heavy items such as keys.
- Ask patients to look straight ahead.
- Record the reading when the needle settles.
- If monitoring weight loss/gain try to use the same set of scales and make a record of them in the notes.

BLOOD PRESSURE MEASUREMENT

Blood pressure measurement is a skill all nurses acquire during early training. As medicine and research progress there has been an increased emphasis on accuracy. There has also been a tightening up in the parameters and what was once regarded as a normal ageing blood pressure would now be treated aggressively. Obtaining an accurate reading is therefore more important so that treatment is not initiated or omitted unnecessarily. It is worth reviewing your technique if you discover that all readings miraculously end in zeros! The following information is based on the recommendations of the British Hypertension Society (O'Brien et al 1997).

PATIENT PREPARATION/ASSESSMENT

Most patients are familiar with the concept of taking blood pressure readings. However, an explanation and discussion of what to expect will help set them at their ease. Warn them that more than one reading will be taken and that the cuff may cause some discomfort as it inflates. Establish that you have the correct patient and notes, then check that the patient understands the reason and implications of this particular blood pressure measurement. If they are taking antihypertensive medication confirm that what they are taking matches what is recorded in the notes. It is not uncommon to find patients who stop taking their tablets once the course is completed. Agree with patients how their follow-up care will be organized or when a review should be arranged.

EQUIPMENT

There is an increasing array of equipment available to the practitioner wishing to record a blood pressure. The more common method until recent technological advancement was the mercury sphygmomanometer. This is still widely used although due to the health and safety concerns surrounding mercury and the risk of spillage, its use is on the decline.

Alternatives to the traditional machine are aneroid and automated devices. Aneroid devices are generally thought to give lower readings and require frequent recalibration, which is not practical in reality. Automated devices work in different ways: either a microphone detects the sounds or returning blood flow is picked up by ultrasound or vibration measurement. Microphones are sensitive to cuff friction and so most machines are now based on sensing the vibration of returning blood.

Whichever device is selected to record blood pressure, it should be used in accordance with the manufacturer's guidelines and have been independently validated. For further information see Resources.

NURSE PREPARATION

Ensure you are familiar with the device being used to record blood pressure. Most practices also have guidelines or protocols regarding what are considered normal or acceptable readings. When an unusually high or possibly low reading is recorded there should be clear instructions regarding when and to whom further referral is made.

TAKING A BLOOD PRESSURE READING

General

1. The patient may be seated or lying. (**Caution** – pregnant women should be seated if possible, due to possible low supine readings.)
2. The patient should have rested for a minimum of 3 minutes.
3. The arm should be supported.

4. Tight clothing should be removed.
5. Cuff depth should not be less than 12 cm and the bladder should cover 80% of the circumference. It is usual to have three cuff sizes, for children, adults and larger adults.
6. A minimum of two readings should be recorded at each visit with at least a minute's gap between them.
7. A note should be made if the patient appears stressed or anxious.

Recording with mercury sphygmomanometer

1. The manometer should be vertical, viewed at eye level and the zero should be at mid-thorax level.
2. The systolic pressure is estimated by inflating the cuff and palpating the radial pulse; the pressure is noted when pulsation stops. Allow the cuff to deflate fully.
3. Place the diaphragm of the stethoscope on the brachial pulse and inflate to 30 mmHg over the palpated systolic pressure.
4. Deflate slowly at a rate of 2 mmHg per second or heartbeat.
5. Systolic pressure is recorded when pulsating sounds begin and diastolic is recorded when they cease completely.
6. If pulsation continues to the bottom of the scale then diastolic is recorded at the point at which the sounds become faint.

Recording with automatic machines

1. Be familiar with the equipment you use.
2. Warn patients that the cuff may inflate tighter than they would normally expect.
3. Turn off any alarms that may sound.
4. Warn patients that the cuff may deflate and reinflate during the reading.
5. Ensure tubing is not kinked or damaged.
6. If it is the first time a patient has experienced an electronic recording then more reassurance is needed; it can be alarming to feel the cuff tighten and not be confident it knows when to stop.

HEALTH AND SAFETY ISSUES

Be aware of the dangers of using mercury and guard against spillage. Local guidelines should be in place for the action to be taken in the event of a spillage. A mercury spillage pack should also be available wherever mercury is used.

SPECIMEN COLLECTION

SWABS

Swabs are sent to microbiology to identify types of bacteria or virus that may be causing infection and to identify their sensitivity to antibiotics. The principle is that when the swab is in contact with the area of infection, bacteria/virus will pass onto the swab and be successfully cultured/identified within the laboratory. Due to varying storage conditions and transport times, the final result may be affected (Kingsley 2001). Local guidelines and policies should give guidance on swab type and medium depending on transport and storage facilities available.

Wound swabs

If wound cleansing is necessary the swab should be taken from the bed of the wound after cleansing. Wound edges and exudates may contain bacteria which are not actually responsible for the infection.

Nasal swabs

These very thin swabs should be gently swivelled against the moist mucosa of the patient's nasal passages. It is very irritating for the patient and cannot be tolerated for any time at all and usually results in a sneezing fit.

Throat swabs

The patient needs to be encouraged to tilt the head back and say 'aagh'. This helps to expose the back of the throat and a sample can then be taken from the nasopharynx. A tongue depressor may be needed. A hint is to be as speedy as possible; once the patient begins to think about it too much, it can be tricky to reach the correct area.

High vaginal swab

Ideally, a vaginal speculum should be passed so that the cervix can be visualized. The swab is then wiped in the area of the posterior fornix.

Chlamydia swab

This swab is taken to detect a virus and is therefore sent to the virology department. It is taken from the cervical os, having visualized the cervix as above. The swab should be held within the os for about 20 seconds to allow the transfer of infected cervical cells onto the swab. If a cervical smear is being taken the swab should be done first, although best practice advises against both investigations being done at the same time.

MIDSTREAM URINE SPECIMEN (MSU)

This is taken to detect infection. The patient should be advised to pass a small amount of urine into the toilet then collect some urine from the middle of the stream into the container provided and finish voiding into the toilet. This ensures that, providing normal hygiene standards prevail, an accurate result will be obtained and the specimen will not be contaminated.

EARLY MORNING URINE

These samples need to be the urine that has remained in the bladder overnight. Therefore it is important to stress to patients that if they get up at 5 am to urinate then that is the sample needed even if they are going back to bed.

STOOL SAMPLES

Stool samples are always collected by means of a scoop which screws into the transport container. They may be sent to microbiology or biochemistry depending on the investigations required. Faecal occult blood (FOB) specimens are usually collected from three consecutive stool samples in three separate containers and sent to biochemistry. Samples for investigation of diarrhoea are sent to bacteriology and only one is required, unless there has been an outbreak of infection, when serial samples are sometimes requested until the all-clear can be given.

SKIN SCRAPINGS

Skin scrapings are taken to diagnose infections so that correct treatment is initiated.

1. Equipment required: blade, transport box, card or Sellotape and slide.
2. Explain to the patient what you are about to do.
3. Check for the use of OTC products and take sample from untreated areas.
4. Using a scalpel blade (preferably rounded), hold the blade at right angles to the surface of the skin and scrape the edge of the lesion, where the disease process will be most active.
5. Send the scrapings to the local bacteriology department using the locally accepted method.
6. If the condition is affecting a hairy part of the body then scale and hair roots should be included in the sample.

NAIL CLIPPINGS

1. Ideally a chiropodist or podiatrist should take nail clippings.
2. Equipment needed: clippers, blunt-ended tool/probe, transport container.
3. To avoid bacterial contamination the nail should be swabbed with alcohol first.
4. Clippings are then taken, which should be full thickness.
5. The underside of the nail should be scraped with a blunt edge or probe and the scrapings included in the sample.
6. The sample is then placed in folded paper and sent in a sealed container. The local laboratory may provide commercially available paper especially for such clippings.

VENEPUNCTURE

Venepuncture, the withdrawing of blood from a vein, is a skill required by most practice nurses and as expertise develops there is much satisfaction in realizing that some time has passed since you failed to achieve your objective first time around.

As a beginner, keep your confidence, do not rush and always try at least once.

NURSE PREPARATION

Nurse training for venepuncture should be accessed according to local guidelines and should include guidance on how to deal with blood spillages and needlestick injury. Thereafter, it is the nurse's responsibility to remain up to date and ensure adequate practice to maintain skills.

EQUIPMENT

- Pair of gloves*
- Tourniquet
- Sterile wipe*

---

* The need for these items will depend on local guidelines and professional preference.

- Cotton wool balls
- Plaster/alternative if patient allergic
- Needle, collecting devices/tubes
- Specimen form
- Transport bags
- High-risk labels if needed
- Sharps disposal bin

PATIENT PREPARATION/ASSESSMENT

1. Identify the tests to be carried out and ensure that you have the correct patient.
2. Explain the procedure and obtain the patient's consent.
3. Enquire about the patient's previous experience of venepuncture and note any particular difficulties.
4. If it is the first time a patient has had blood taken it is advisable to get him or her to lie on a couch. Some people can faint automatically when the needle enters the vein, even though they are not generally nervous.
5. Depending on the investigations being carried out, check that patients are properly prepared, e.g. fasted, or if checking therapeutic drug levels, what time they last took their medication.
6. Explain how patients will receive the results of their tests; this will vary according to local circumstances. It is good practice to have systems in place that ensure that an abnormal result does not go astray.
7. Do not take blood from:
   - inflamed, scarred or bruised areas
   - limbs affected by stroke or oedema
   - the affected side of postmastectomy patients
   - limbs affected by disease.

PROCEDURE

1. *The tourniquet*. This is used to help fill the vein to make venepuncture easier. It is usual to apply it 10–15 cm above the intended puncture site. Experiment with different styles until you find the one that suits you best. It should not be applied too tightly in the first instance and should not be left longer than 2 minutes. It is acceptable to release the pressure and reapply after a few minutes' recovery time.

2. *Palpating the vein*. Easier said than done sometimes. (See Fig. 20.2 for names and position of suitable veins.) If the vein is visible press lightly with the fingertips to ensure it is full and large enough to take blood from. A good vein rebounds against the pressure of the fingertips. If no vein is visible feel across the elbow crease with the index fingertip for a vein beneath the surface. If you are uncertain that what you are feeling is a vein, release the tourniquet and the rebounding sensation will not be palpable any longer. (A tendon will feel the same with or without the tourniquet.)

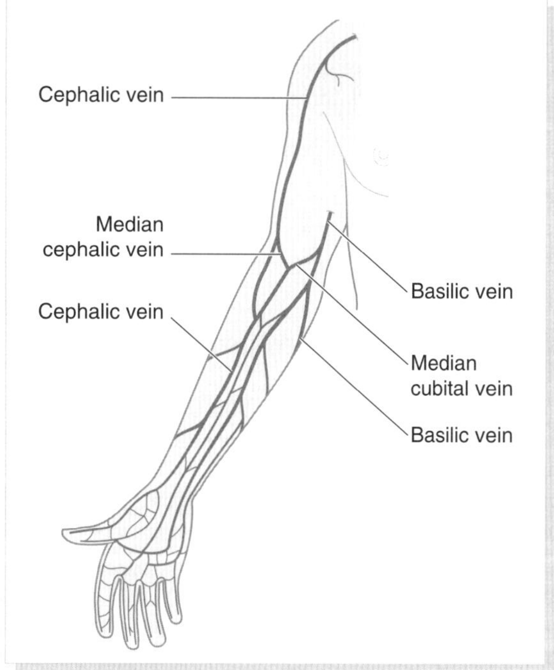

Figure 20.2 Veins suitable for venepuncture.

3. *Cleansing*. Opinions on methods and effectiveness of skin cleansing vary; it is therefore best to follow local guidelines.

4. *Needle insertion*. With the bevel side up, insert at an angle of 30–45°. A faster insertion results in less pain but may overshoot the vein so care is needed. Depending on the collection system being used, there may be a 'flashback' of blood. When this is seen insertion should stop and blood may be withdrawn. If there is no flashback, insertion stops when there is a slight 'give' in the insertion pressure as the needle enters the wall of the vein. The correct tubes are then connected in sequence.

5. *Tourniquet release*. This should be done immediately the needle is in the vein and collection begins.

6. *Needle withdrawal*. When collection is complete the tubes are disconnected, leaving only the needle in the vein. The cotton wall ball is then applied over

the wound immediately after the needle is withdrawn and pressure applied for about 1–2 minutes, keeping the arm straight.

7. *Needle disposal*. Straight away in the sharps bin without resheathing.

8. *Label tubes*. Immediately after disposing of the needle.

9. *Apply plaster/non allergic dressing* once bleeding has stopped.

TESTS AND LABORATORIES

When first sending tests to laboratories as a practice nurse, you may find the array of coloured tubes and forms daunting. There will always be the strange test you have never heard of before, no matter how long you have been in practice. The staff in laboratories usually have information available for practitioners giving details of what goes where and how much is needed. If in doubt, telephone; most patients would much prefer you got it right first time around.

RECORDING AN ELECTROCARDIOGRAPH

Recording and interpretation of an electrocardiograph (ECG) is a skill with which many nurses may already be familiar. The practice nurse will normally be expected to be able to record ECGs at short notice and as routine appointments. Urgent recordings are usually seen immediately they are taken for interpretation by the requesting clinician.

Routine recordings may also need urgent interpretation. Each practice will have its own system for dealing with such eventualities. It is therefore important that the nurse has some understanding of what the trace shows and how to identify abnormal patterns and their significance.

SIMPLIFIED EXPLANATION OF HOW THE ECG WORKS

Cardiac muscle contracts in response to an electrical impulse or signal, which travels through the heart. In a normal (disease-free) heart it always goes in the same direction. It starts at the sinoatrial (SA) node (Fig. 20.3) and travels across the atria, causing contraction. It then reaches the atrioventricular (AV) node where it pauses while atrial activity is completed. The AV node then initiates a signal that

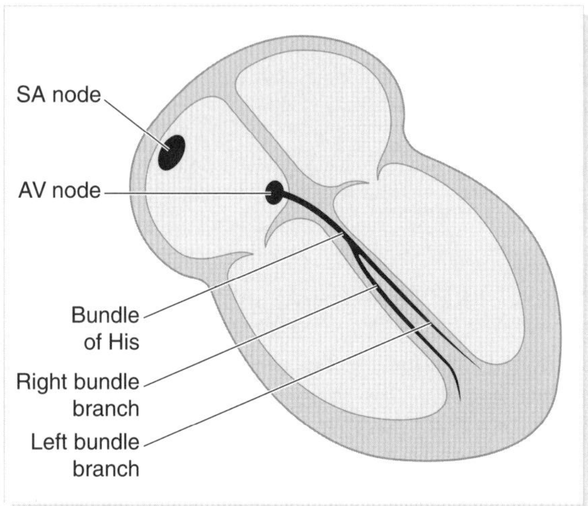

Figure 20.3 Structures of the heart.

travels across the ventricles (via the bundle of His) and causes ventricular contraction.

When heart muscle is diseased or damaged the signal cannot travel in the same uniform manner and takes diversions. Sometimes the initiation of the signal is delayed or altered and causes arrhythmias. If heart muscle is enlarged it needs a bigger signal to contract. It is these alterations away from the normal that can be detected in the electrical recording of heart muscle activity or ECG.

SIMPLIFIED EXPLANATION OF HOW THE SIGNAL IS FORMED

By placing electrical leads (electrodes) on a patient, it is possible to detect the signal as it travels across the heart. A needle moving over graph paper represents the signal picked up. The baseline (usually about the centre of the strip) represents no activity. If the needle moves up from the baseline then the electrode has detected a signal moving towards it and when the needle moves down, the signal is moving away from it. The electrodes are placed on the chest wall in such a way that different aspects of the heart may be 'viewed' in one recording.

A simplified normal complex is shown in Figure 20.4. The P wave represents atrial contraction. The PR interval represents the pause at the AV node. The QRS represents the ventricular contraction. The T wave is a recovery stage; after each contraction the heart muscle relaxes before the next contraction, an event called repolarization.

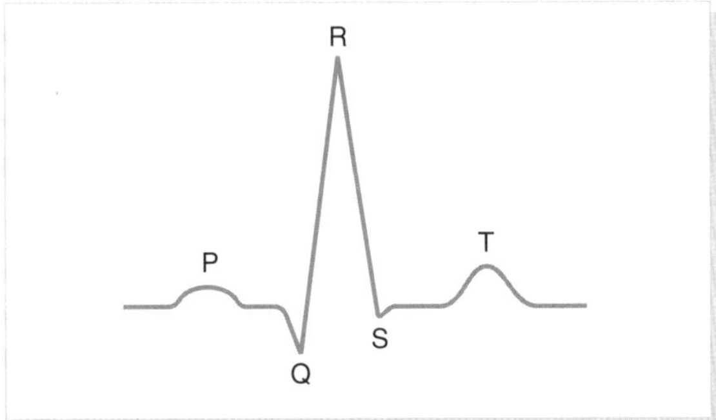

Figure 20.4 Simplified normal ECG complex.

PATIENT PREPARATION

A calm and reassuring manner helps put the patient at ease. Chest pain is a frightening experience and many patients will be anxious, wondering if they are having/have had a 'heart attack'. They should be asked/helped to remove top clothes and shoes/socks/stockings, so that their chest and ankles are bare. They are then made comfortable on a couch in a semi-recumbent position.

Explain that leads will be attached to their chest, arms and legs, that they don't contain electricity but simply monitor impulses within. Patients should keep still during the recording and breathe normally. (Excessive movement causes interference.)

ATTACHMENT OF LEADS

Leads are attached to each limb and the chest as follows (Fig. 20.5).

- V1 – 4th intercostal space right sternal border
- V2 – 4th intercostal space left sternal border
- V3 – between V2 and V4
- V4 – 5th intercostal space in the midclavicular line
- V5 – anterior axillary line (horizontal with V4)
- V6 – midaxillary line (horizontal with V4 and V5)

Many newer ECG machines now label the leads: RA = right arm, RL = right leg, C1, C2, etc.

A good connection is needed to ensure a good trace. If there is oil, sweat or hair on the skin the contact may be broken. In the case of oil or sweat, wiping with an alcoholic swab and drying will help. Parting and flattening the hair is sometimes sufficient but if not, shaving is necessary.

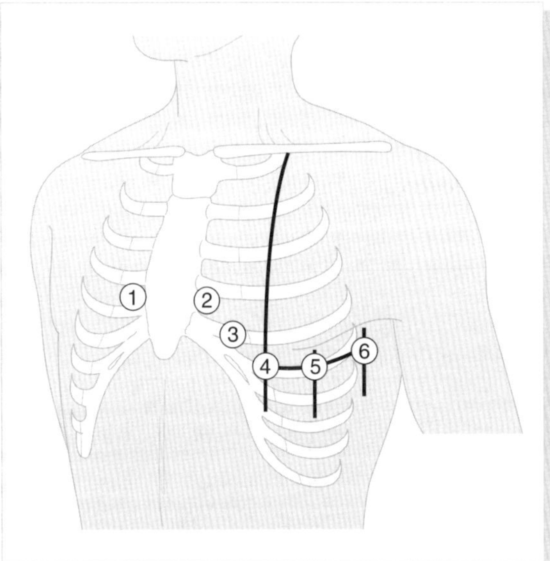

Figure 20.5 Attachment of ECG leads.

THE TRACE

The trace is normally recorded in the following order: I, II, III, AVR, AVL, AVF, V1–V6 (usually 3 complex per lead). A rhythm strip on II or V1 is also recorded. The nurse should label each lead if the machine does not do it automatically. Patient details and date and time of the recording should also be written on the trace.

INTERPRETATION OF THE ECG

Experienced practitioners are able to pinpoint what area of heart muscle is damaged following myocardial infarction, by interpreting the evolving changes. This level of skill is not generally expected of the practice nurse in primary care. There may be facilities locally for the faxing and interpretation of ECGs. A familiarity with the more common abnormalities will help nurses develop their professional practice. The clinician ordering the ECG should be aware of the skill of the practitioner carrying out the procedure and follow-up should be arranged accordingly.

If at any time the nurse is unsure what kind of trace she has recorded, the patient should be kept on the couch until a clinician has examined the trace.

Normal sinus rhythm (Fig. 20.6)

All parts of the PQRS complex are present and the rhythm is regular and each complex identical.

Sinus tachycardia (Fig. 20.7)

The PQRS complex is normal but very close together because the rate is fast, generally over 100 per minute.

Sinus bradycardia (Fig. 20.8)

The PQRS complex is normal but further apart because the rate is slow, generally less than 60 per minute.

Atrial ectopic beat (Fig. 20.9)

Most complexes are normal but there is an extra P wave because the atria have had an extra (ectopic) beat; the QRS that follows is normal. The P wave occurred just as the T wave was forming. The P wave is slightly pointy because it was generated from somewhere other than the SA node.

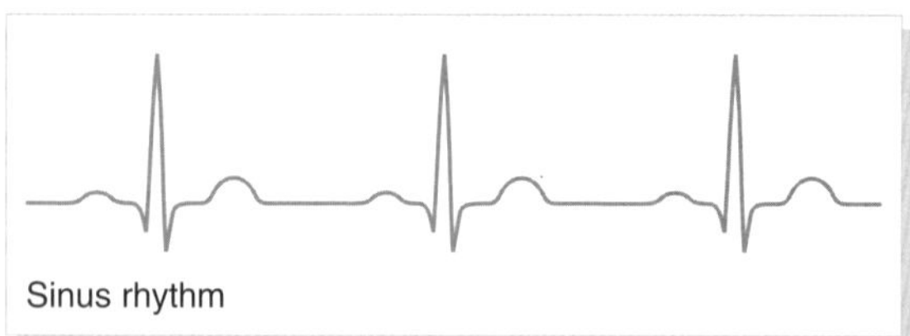

Figure 20.6 Sinus rhythm.

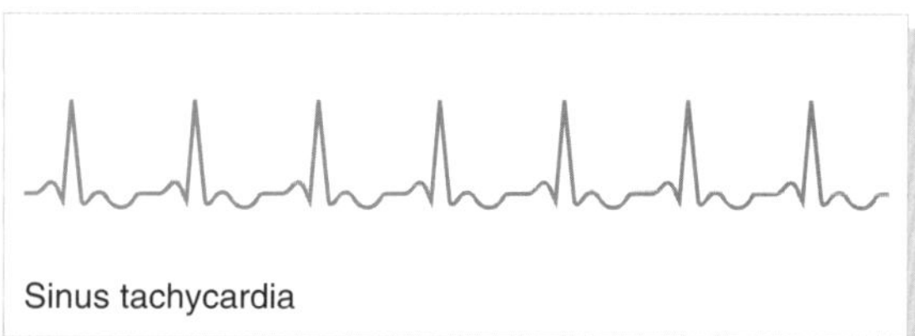

Figure 20.7 Sinus tachycardia.

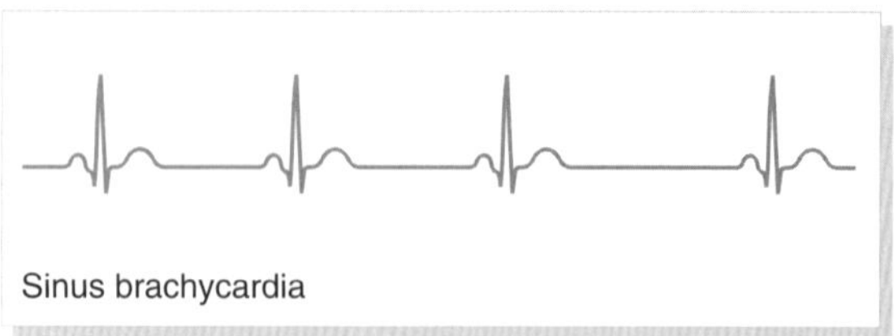

Figure 20.8 Sinus bradycardia.

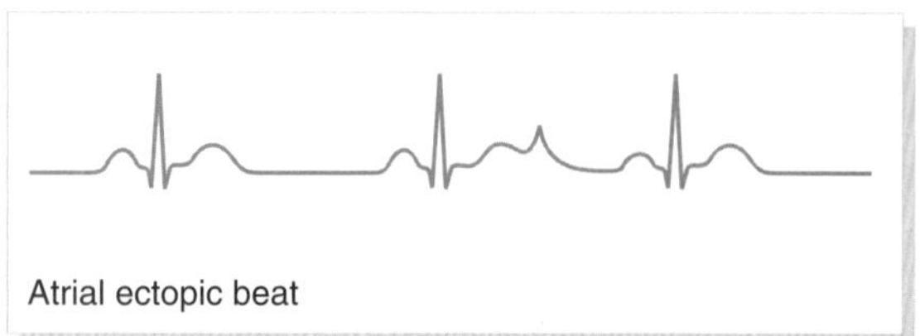

Figure 20.9 Atrial ectopic beat.

Ventricular ectopic beats (Fig. 20.10)

Several normal complexes with one unusual-shaped one. This is an extra beat (ectopic) of the ventricles that has been initiated away from the AV node; hence its bizarre shape. There is no P wave preceding it. There is often a prolonged gap after such a beat while the cardiac muscle recovers ready for a normal beat. An occasional ectopic is not considered harmful but if occurring at a rate of more than six per minute, it can induce ventricular tachycardia or fibrillation.

Atrial fibrillation (Fig. 20.11)

A wiggly baseline with normal QRS along it. The atria are twitching but not contracting in the normal way. The AV node is not getting normal signals from the SA node and so the ventricles beat but at a random rate. If the ventricular rate becomes greater than 100 per minute it can be dangerous.

ST elevation (Fig. 20.12)

There is deep Q wave and the QRS segment is distorted and does not return to the baseline. This indicates myocardial damage.

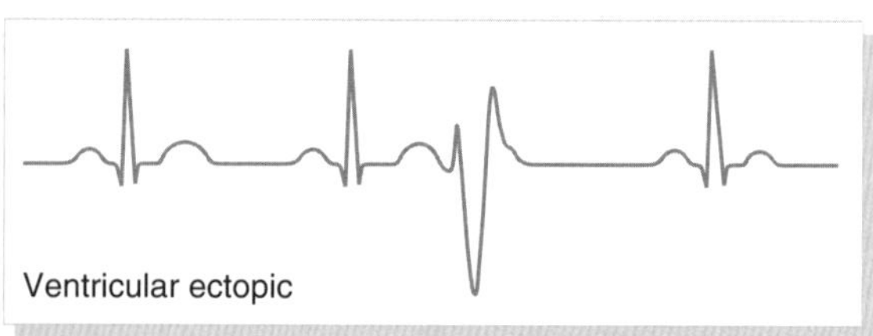

Figure 20.10 Ventricular ectopic beat.

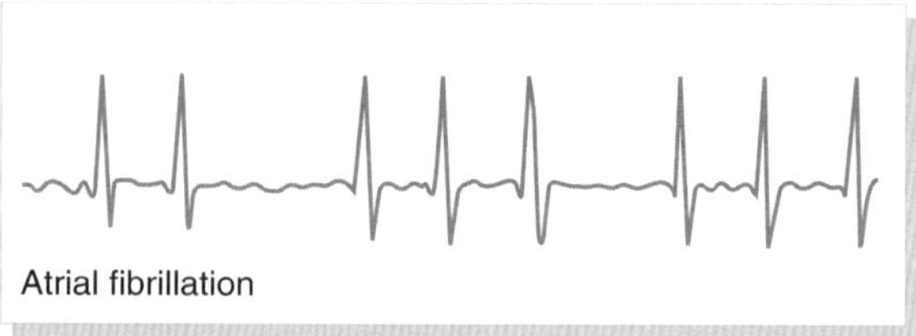

Figure 20.11 Atrial fibrillation.

ST depression (Fig. 20.13)

This time the QRS segment fails to reach up to the baseline. This indicates myocardial ischaemia.

Supraventricular tachycardia (Fig. 20.14)

The ventricular rate is fast because it is responding to an atrial rate that is so fast there is no recovery time. The QRS is a normal shape and therefore the pacemaker for this rhythm is arising from outwith the ventricles.

Ventricular tachycardia (Fig. 20.15)

The ventricles are contracting on their own, ignoring the usual pathway, and very fast. The QRS shape is bizarre because the pacemaker for this rhythm is arising within the ventricles. This is a serious condition needing medical treatment because there is a danger it may become ventricular fibrillation.

Ventricular fibrillation (Fig. 20.16)

No contraction, the ventricles are simply twitching. REQUIRES CPR.

Ventricular standstill (Fig. 20.17)

Little activity. REQUIRES CPR.

Asystole (Fig. 20.18)

No activity. REQUIRES CPR.

This is a very basic guide to ECG interpretation. Always be aware that a myocardial infarction may take some time to produce alterations in the ECG. It is a useful tool but should never replace clinical assessment, judgement and intuition.

Further reading and information sources are at the end of this chapter.

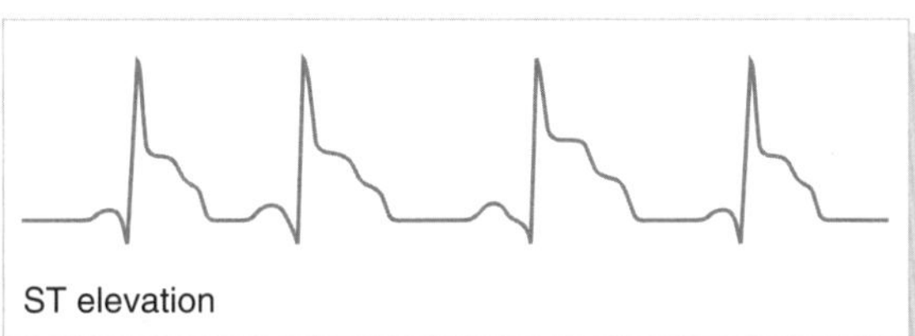

Figure 20.12 ST elevation.

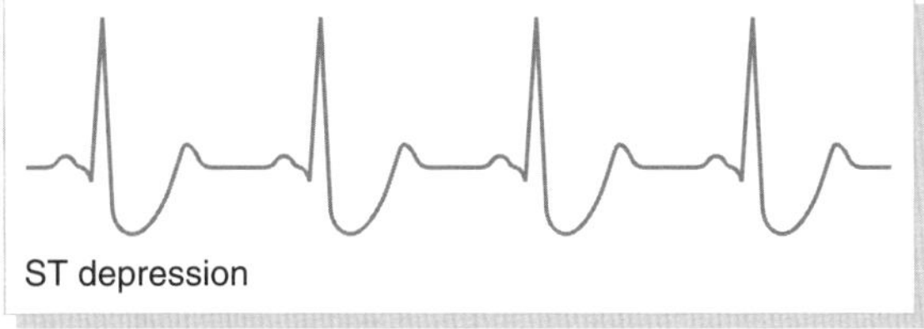

Figure 20.13 ST depression.

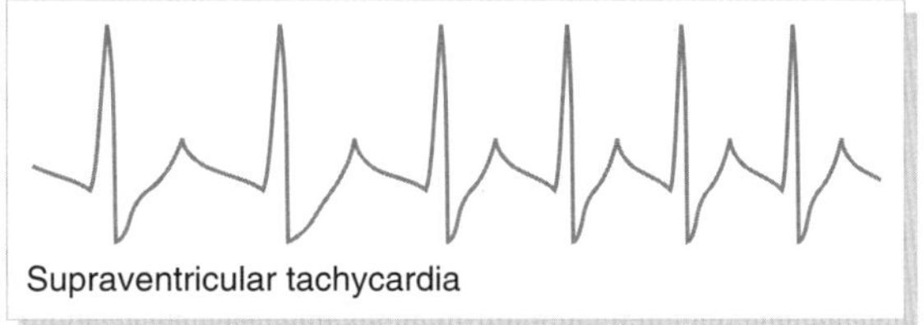

Figure 20.14 Supraventricular tachycardia.

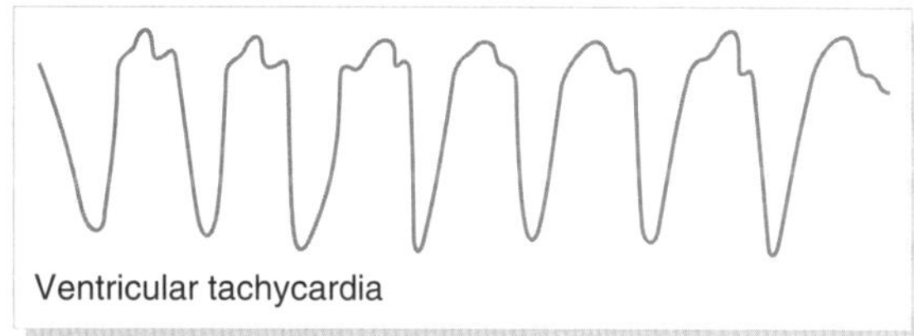

Figure 20.15 Ventricular tachycardia.

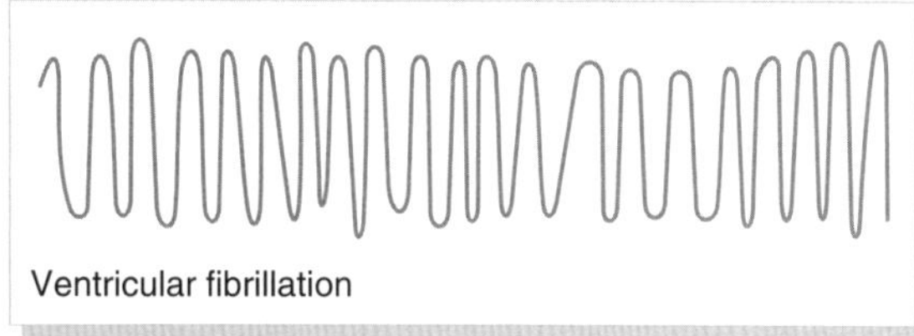

Figure 20.16 Ventricular fibrillation.

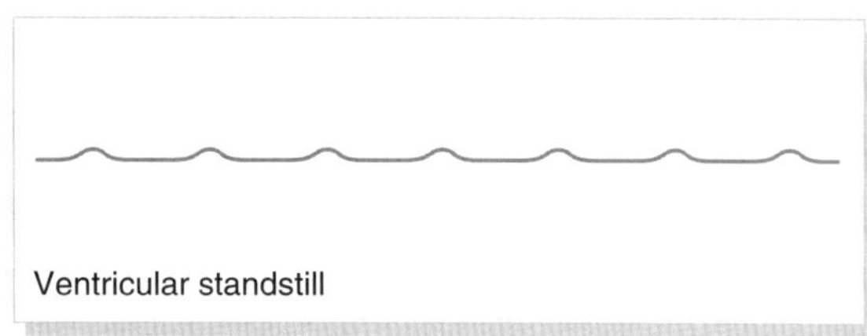

Figure 20.17 Ventricular standstill.

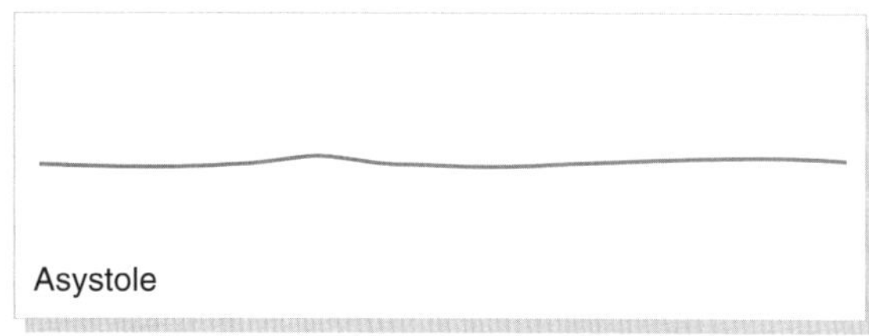

Figure 20.18 Asystole.

INJECTION TECHNIQUES

The practice nurse will be required to give many and varied injections. Vaccinations are probably the most common but there are now increasing numbers of treatments initiated in secondary care that need to be given in primary care.

A good technique will help avoid unnecessary complications and discomfort. The following is based on the booklet *UK guidance on best practice in vaccine administration* (Chiodini et al 2001).

SAFETY FIRST

It is commonplace for patients to present to the practice nurse with an injection collected from the chemist and ask for it to be administered.

1. Verify that the injection has been prescribed (except in the case of medications covered by patient group directions).
2. Ensure that you are familiar with the indications and contraindications for the particular injection.
3. Check the dose is correct and matches the original prescription.
4. Check the expiry date.
5. If you are uneasy in any way seek further advice.
6. Be prepared to deal with the possibility of anaphylaxis.
7. Record the type, dose, strength, location, batch number and expiry date of any injection given in the patient record.

PATIENT PREPARATION

In some cases patients will need a lot of reassurance due to previous bad experiences as a child. If they are likely to faint then the injection should be given whilst they are lying on a couch. Distraction techniques are effective, especially in children (e.g. asking a question at the very moment of needle insertion; they become so focused on thinking about the answer that they sometimes don't even feel it!).

1. Skin cleaning prior to injection has been found to be unnecessary except in unusual circumstances.
2. Ensure that the patient consents to the injection.
3. Identify the site to be used, remove clothing as needed and position the patient so that the muscle group to be used is relaxed.
4. Caution is required in those patients who suffer from serious bleeding problems. Seek expert advice.

CHOICE OF NEEDLE

In the UK there are three gauges of needle available for injections. The gauge is the diameter of the needle; the higher the gauge, the smaller the diameter. Each gauge is denoted by a different colour.

- Orange – the smallest size = 25 gauge; 10 mm, 16 mm, 25 mm lengths
- Blue – slightly larger = 23 gauge; 25 mm length
- Green – larger size = 21 gauge; 38 mm length

The choice of needle will depend on the site of the injection, the size and build of the patient and where the injection needs to be deposited.

Many injections are now supplied with a fixed needle. In these cases the medication should never be transferred to another syringe. If the needle is not appropriate for some reason another supplier may provide the medication in vials.

INTRAMUSCULAR INJECTION (IM)

The majority of injections in general practice are intramuscular, into the deltoid, the gluteal and thigh muscles. The choice of site will depend on the manufacturer's recommendations for the particular medication. When no recommendation is made then the deltoid is the more convenient site.

The injection is drawn up and a fresh needle used to give the injection. A blue needle is used for the deltoid muscle as the wider lumen has been shown to reduce pain and irritation (Chiodini et al 2001). A green needle is used for the larger muscles. The needle is inserted at 90° to the flat skin surface, up to three-quarters of the length of the blue needle and almost the full length of the green needle. Aspiration is performed to ensure that a blood vessel has not been penetrated. The injection should be given slowly (1.0 ml over 10 seconds) and then the needle is withdrawn smoothly and gentle pressure applied with a cotton wool ball.

SUBCUTANEOUS INJECTION (SC)

This type of injection is used mainly for insulin and patients with bleeding problems. The upper arms, abdomen and upper legs are all suitable for subcutaneous injections.

An orange or blue needle may be used. The skin is bunched up between the thumb and forefinger to lift up the adipose tissue from the underlying muscle. The needle is then inserted at 45° (90° for insulin needles) into the subdermal tissue. There is no need to perform aspiration since, in theory, there should not be any blood vessels close by; hence the suitability of this method for patients with bleeding problems. The injection is given slowly, as above, the needle withdrawn and pressure applied with cotton wool.

INTRADERMAL INJECTION

The most common reason for this type of injection to be given in primary care is for the BCG vaccine or rapid-schedule rabies vaccine (unlicensed use). Experience and training in the administration of this type of injection should be sought.

Any site suitable for subcutaneous injections is also suitable for intradermal injections. However, the BCG should specifically be given at the point of insertion of the deltoid muscle.

An orange needle is used. The skin is held taut and, with the bevel uppermost, the needle is inserted just under the skin for about 2 mm. The needle tip should just be visible under the skin. No aspiration is performed and when the injection is given a small bump should form just under the skin where the liquid has been deposited.

References

Chiodini J, Cotton G, Genasi F et al 2001 UK guidance on best practice in vaccine administration. Shire Hall Communications, London

Kingsley A 2001 A proactive approach to wound infection. Nursing Standard 15(30):50–58

O'Brien ET, Petrie JC, Littler WA et al 1997 Blood pressure measurement: recommendations of the British Hypertension Society, 3rd edn. BMJ Books, London

Resources

Further reading

Ernst DJ 1995 Flawless phlebotomy: becoming a great collector. Nursing 25(10):54–57

Hampton JR 1992 The ECG made easy, 4th edn. Churchilll Livingstone, Edinburgh

Mallett J, Bailey C 1996 Manual of clinical nursing procedures. Royal Marsden NHS Trust. Blackwell Science, Oxford

McGhee M 2000 A guide to laboratory investigations, 3rd edn. Radcliffe Medical Press, Oxford

Nash E, Nahas V 1996 Understanding the ECG: a guide for nurses. Chapman and Hall, London

Pollary C 1990 How to take blood. Practice Nurse 13(4):215–216

Stilwell B 1991 Venepuncture. Community Outlook 1(5):26–27

Workman B 1999 Safe injection techniques. Primary Health Care 10(6):43–49

Computer resources

Blood pressure measurement CD ROM. BMJ Books, London. Sometimes available from pharmaceutical company representatives.

www.hyp.ac.uk/bhs/ – to access a list of validated blood pressure machines.

www.ecglibrary.com/ecghome.html – history of ECG, examples of traces.

SECTION 4

Management and professional issues

SECTION CONTENTS

Chapter 21

The use of IT in primary care

Elaine Campbell

CHAPTER CONTENTS

INTRODUCTION

A glimpse into general practice of the foreseeable future will show one where Lloyd George notes are a thing of the past (stored only for retrieving historical data), receptionists no longer have to pull notes prior to appointments, with patient records being accessed from any terminal, dependent on the authorization status of the professional. Data entered directly into the electronic patient record (EPR) at the time of consultation (with no duplication in written form) is universally recognized by all computer systems, with information being transferred electronically between practices, hospitals and other healthcare providers (even in differing countries), simplifying referral procedures and saving hours of administration time. Audit is done at the touch of a button (almost!), with cost savings used directly to improve patient care.

Appointments are booked directly by the practitioner at time of referral or by the patients themselves from home or work. The ability to choose a convenient appointment time reduces the numbers who fail to attend. Information regarding waiting times for initial consultations and subsequent procedures is available from around the country so that referrals are made to a centre providing the quickest, most convenient appointment, with comparisons between centres given to ensure that the treatment is of a suitable standard.

Prescriptions are sent electronically to pharmacies with digital signatures having replaced the written form. From there, information on prescribing habits is sent directly to the Prescription Pricing Authority (PPA) which collects and analyses the data concerning individual prescribers. The pharmacist has access to information about the patient's status regarding exemption, or otherwise, from prescription charges, thereby reducing the fraud associated with this. All prescriptions are now legible and checked for accuracy and contraindications by the computer programs.

Requests for pathology tests or other investigations are generated and sent electronically, with results relayed back directly to the referee when complete. Those requiring 'action' are forwarded to the appropriate professional to implement and the status of that action remains highlighted until complete, thus ensuring appropriate follow-up. Referral letters are generated and sent by email, with appointment and discharge summaries returned the same way. Paper documents get scanned directly into the patient's record.

The clinical record stores visual images such as photographs of wounds at various stages of healing, ECG recordings and X-rays. These can be sent electronically to other professionals to enhance that individual's management. The patient's electronic health record (EHR) is accessible to authorized health professionals 24 hours a day to provide up-to-date information on health status and current medication, facilitating the delivery of safe and effective healthcare to that individual.

Communication between all the primary healthcare team (PHCT) members is enhanced by use of email. Those messages requiring more urgent action are added as 'alerts' to the consultation screen, reducing the need for interruptions. Recipients can then send a reply to the sender confirming the message has been received and action taken.

So what is stopping us? Much of this is already happening in individual areas but the use of up-to-date IT in primary care is piecemeal, highly dependent on the technology available and the desire of the professionals to make best use of it. There are those embracing the vision and driving forward the changes in practice to achieve it and there are others totally overwhelmed by even the most basic technological applications. How this influences the running of the practice will depend on whether the people willing to drive it forward are in a position of authority to do so.

This chapter aims to provide an insight into the use of IT in primary care, the political imperative driving it forward, the confidentiality and security issues and the benefits that can be achieved by the organization, the patient and the clinicians themselves if they increase their proficiency in this area.

ADDRESSING THE PROBLEMS

Many of the benefits are seen in terms of time saving, improved communications and having access to the information necessary to provide a high-quality service, yet no analysis of the benefits would be complete without acknowledging that there are barriers to achieving this. The problems include the following.

- Until we have the technology fully functioning we are operating a halfway house, often duplicating documentation.
- Change in working practice is costly in terms of time and resources, both of which are short in general practice.
- Some time-saving procedures are replaced with others more time consuming (especially in the early stages).
- Competition in the marketplace for the technology is necessary in order to drive the development forward and act as an incentive to the suppliers to provide a good service, yet this allows different systems to be used throughout the NHS which may not be compatible with one another.
- Terminology and coding are different amongst differing branches of care providers. Language needs to be developed that is universally adopted.
- When the technology fails the user loses confidence in it and reverts to previous practice.
- There are certain situations, for example home visits, where different technology is required.

These issues are being addressed by the government, the suppliers of the clinical systems and education providers. The NHS Information Authority (NHSIA) (www.nhsia.nhs.uk) oversees strategically critical IT-related programmes and has statutory public accountability.

GOVERNMENT POLICY

Government policy drives the use of IT in the health service, recognizing that its effective use is necessary for efficient working, reducing costs and monitoring performance. A carrot-and-stick approach has been used in general practice. The GP Contract of 1991 compelled GPs to provide the government with up-to-date demographic details of all registered patients, set targets for certain procedures such as cervical cytology and child immunizations, with payment linked to achieving these targets, and provided financial incentives to run health promotion and chronic disease management clinics. Computers facilitated the collection and management of the required data. The financial necessity to drive down prescription costs required generic substitution and close monitoring of prescribing habits. This, linked with the prescribing software in use and printed prescriptions, has undoubtedly improved safety and efficiency in this area.

Some of the resistance felt by the medical profession has been to do with the use of data by the government to monitor performance, reduce clinical freedom and impose standardization on working practices. This is undoubtedly true, yet it would have happened anyway due to consumer pressure and financial constraints. Computers have facilitated this process for both the government and the practice.

Government policies of the last 15 years have acknowledged the role of effective use of technology in reaching the desired goals. The more recent of these include the following.

The new NHS: modern, dependable (DoH 1997)

(www.doh.gov.uk/newnhs.htm)

- NHS Direct – easier and faster advice and information for people about health, illness and the NHS so that they are better able to look after themselves
- Connection of every GP practice to the NHSnet
- Investment in technology to support frontline staff

A first class service. Quality in the new NHS (DoH 1998a)

(www.doh.gov.uk/newnhs/quality.htm)

- Clinical governance. Monitoring standards
- Clinical effectiveness. Use of research and 'evidence'
- Lifelong learning
- IT strategy to support these objectives

Information for health: an information strategy for the modern NHS 1998–2005 (DoH 1998b)

(www.doh.gov.uk/ipu/strategy/summary/index.htm)

- Creation of electronic health records (EHR), which can be accessed 24 hours a day by any health professional needing to provide care to an individual. The EHR will be a summary of the clinical records of an individual and will be based in primary care
- Electronic transfer of records between GPs
- National Electronic Library for Health (NeLH)
- NHS Direct to be developed into a convenient home-based gateway to information and services for the general public covering the whole area of NHS activity
- Telemedicine and telecare to be developed to ensure specialist advice and support is more accessible to GPs and other professionals.

NHS Plan (DoH 2000)

(www.nhs.uk/nationalplan/)

- Telemedicine to be routinely considered in health improvement plans
- Financial investment in IT

PRACTICE NURSING AND IT

The development of practice nursing has occurred at the same time as the computerization of general practice and largely for the same reasons – consumer demands, GP Contract requiring targets to be met and incentives to run chronic disease management and health promotion clinics. Practice nurses, despite the majority being over 35 years of age and therefore trained before the era of computers, have shown a positive attitude towards computerization (Miller & Jeffcote 1997). They need to be able to use the practice computers as extensively as the GPs if the benefits of the effective use of the technology are to be achieved (Preece 2000). Yet 80% of nurses surveyed in a 1997 study (Miller & Jeffcote 1997) felt training had been either completely missing or inadequate. The nurses were using computers mainly for inputting and retrieving data and they perceived computers to have little use in helping to provide direct care. This lack of training has been demonstrated in a subsequent study (Russell & Alpay 2000) and it remains a challenge for the educators to improve the situation when there are competing needs for training, clinical systems suppliers' training is expensive and does not address the basic lack of IT skills of many nurses and in-house training is often inadequate and suffers from time and personnel constraints.

THE COMPUTER ON YOUR DESK

Since 1993 the clinical systems in use in general practice have had to conform to quality standards set by what is now the NHS Information Authority (NHSIA). The Requirements for Accreditation (RFA) are set 1 year ahead of their implementation date, after which reimbursement will only be given for the systems reaching that standard. This has had the effect of reducing the numbers of suppliers and encouraging conformity between them, the ultimate aim of which is to make them compatible with one another. At present the incompatibility between the systems prevents electronic data exchange, a key target in the NHS Plan. Older versions of systems and software continue to be supported by the manufacturers when they are no longer available to buy and this adds to the variety of applications currently in use. Changing the practice computer system causes huge disruption to smooth running of a practice. Keeping up to date with advances in technology is expensive in terms of financial outlay, interruptions to smooth working practice and staff training.

The main suppliers of clinical systems to general practice are:

- Egton Medical Information services (EMIS)
- Torex
- In Practice Systems (Vamp).

There are other smaller suppliers. Links to sites relating to these systems can be found at www.healthcentre.org.uk/hc/pages/gpcomputer.htm.

These suppliers have different systems to choose from. The result is that professionals moving between practices may need a working knowledge of many different systems. In reality, the level of training required to use a system competently is often not available and the practice's data recording suffers as a result. Nurses invariably have little input in the choice of computer package and make do with what is presented to them, whether it suits them or not.

Health professionals' confidence in their computer systems has been shown to be low (See Tai et al 2000). Concerns expressed include:

- not knowing how to use it
- difficulty with expressing complex situations/conditions adequately
- fear of losing information
- fear of messing up the system for others
- inability to troubleshoot when something goes wrong
- knowing how to manage when the technology fails
- security of the system
- dehumanizing the consultation
- increasing the length of consultations
- legality of computer records.

Not knowing how to use it

Many health professionals were educated in the era before widespread use of computers and therefore do not have the basic skills or level of understanding of how systems work in order to use them effectively. Until this is addressed, all the benefits will not be achieved. Large sums of money are allocated for IT training but finding both the time and inclination to seek out training remains a barrier. As personal computers become widely used within the home, familiarity with basic applications will improve.

Difficulty with expressing complex situations/conditions adequately

Data in a clinical record needs to sum up adequately all the relevant details that a health professional might need to know in a subsequent consultation. Some of that information might need to be easily identified for the practice's organization, for example identifying those with particular medical conditions for whom specific arrangements might be necessary. Some of the information might need to be submitted to the PCT, for example for local health needs assessment and planning. Critics of data inputting cite the frustrations of years of recording 'useless' data which is never acted on as a reason for not investing time and energy in compiling complete records. With the improvement in technology and the drive to develop EHRs, the rationale for compiling complete records should become more apparent. The saying 'rubbish in, rubbish out' is very relevant. Data will only be of use if it is recorded in a way that it is retrievable. 'Free text' allows practitioners to write as they would in a paper record, thereby satisfying the need to add the nuances of the consultation, but by recording significant data in 'Read Code' (see below) the record will become much more useful.

Fear of losing information or messing it up for others

It is important to remember that the robustness of the systems is improving all the time and with adequate back-up of data it is unlikely that crucial information will be lost. Crashes happen regularly and are not usually a disaster. All that is required is for the computer to be restarted and invariably you can pick up where you left off. The systems are designed for use by those with very basic computer skills – it is up to the programmers to make them user friendly.

Inability to troubleshoot when something goes wrong

Troubleshooting becomes much easier with experience and this increases as we become familiar with using computers both at work and at home. Within each practice there should ideally be an 'expert' readily available to help those having problems. The practice manager is often the ideal candidate for this role, being potentially more available than a GP and needing a good working knowledge of the system for the practice's administration. However, their knowledge of the clinical applications may be limited. The role of the expert user may need to be developed in the future if practices are to get best use out of their systems.

How to manage when the technology fails

There will be times when the technology fails but with a good maintenance contract with the supplier, faults will be rectified quickly. With the current methods of predominantly paper-based working, the 'system' still breaks down – communications get lost, notes are often not to hand or records incomplete or illegible. All information should be backed up. Reverting to 'old-fashioned' methods remains an option in some circumstances. Most information will be available through another source, e.g. a pharmacy keeps records of prescriptions generated, pathology labs have records of test results. Practices need to draw up contingency plans on how to manage incidences of technology failure and patients and staff will need to understand that some interruptions in service may happen from time to time. In a crisis you just have to do the best you can!

Security of the system

The greatest risk to security comes from human error. Examples include leaving a terminal with individual data visible to other patients, sending confidential information out by email to the wrong recipient, allowing prescription data to be seen by another individual when collecting prescriptions. These errors could happen with traditional methods and healthcare workers need to be aware of the consequences of their actions and take steps to prevent breaches in confidentiality. Further discussion of security issues occurs later in the chapter.

Dehumanizing the consultation

There are undoubtedly risks that computers will affect the consultation but this does not have to be in a negative way. Using the computer as a prompt that investigations or procedures are due can increase the efficiency of the consultation. Decision support software, such as prescribing packages or guidelines, may optimize the treatment offered. A study from Scandinavia (Risdale & Hudd 1999) suggests that patients feel the 'personal touch' is not lost if eye contact is maintained and the professional is not preoccupied with the computer. If the computer is regarded as a 'tool' it should not interfere with the doctor or nurse and patient relationship.

Increasing the length of the consultation

There is a risk of this happening, especially as we learn to use the systems and are duplicating documentation. Some recording of data is done after the patient has left the room in order to minimize disruption to the consultation, and inevitably takes time (See Tai et al 2000). A systematic review of published reports (Sullivan & Mitchell 1995) showed that on average a consultation took 90 seconds longer, the social and patient-initiated part of the consultation was reduced but the clinical performance of the doctor was increased. The review was based on studies performed prior to 1993, whilst the clinical systems were in their infancy, and was not concerned with the applications used in general practice management. The authors did not assess the length of nursing consultations, which may well be longer.

Legality of computer records

This has long concerned nurses who are required to keep accurate, signed records of consultations and procedures they undertake. The legality of EPRs was confirmed in 2000 providing certain good practice guidelines are adhered to (Bradley 2001). Personal log-ins with protected passwords replace a written signature. Nurses will need to ensure they protect their passwords and enter their own data.

WHAT ARE COMPUTERS CURRENTLY USED FOR?

A Department of Health survey (DoH 1998b) demonstrated that an improvement in the delivery of clinical care can be achieved, in terms of administration, management of clinical records, research and audit, by the use of computers. The majority of practices use their computers for prescribing, consultation records and searches (See Tai et al 2000).

The electronic patient record (EPR) is the computer version of the Lloyd George notes. Practices currently vary in their use of the EPR, from the basic recording of key information (such as childhood vaccination) to 'paperless' practices which aim to use the technology to the full, without the duplication of keeping a written record. The success of the system will depend on its ease of use by the health professional and a consistent approach to its use by all members of the team. Developments in software mean that using the EPR to replace paper records is becoming easier.

Electronic links for claims provide significant advantages to the practice over manual methods.

- Claims are generated at the time of consultation and therefore are less likely to be overlooked.
- Administration time is reduced as the claim procedure is so simple that it is easy for the professional to do.
- Computer reminders reduce the incidence of claims being overlooked by mistake and therefore practice income is maximized.

Personally administered drugs (PADs) are those bought in by the practice and which require reimbursement from the Prescription Pricing Authority (PPA). Computer-generated reports identify items requiring reimbursement and this, combined with crosschecking searches for items, ensures accurate requests. Some vaccines do not require individual prescriptions to be sent which has greatly reduced the paperwork associated with reimbursement. However, accuracy with recording the data is essential if costly items are not to be missed.

Prescribing is a significant process in general practice and one associated with safety issues. Practices vary in how they manage the process of repeat prescriptions but the basic principles remain the same.

- The prescription needs to be legible. Printed computer-generated prescriptions reduce interpretation errors by the pharmacist.
- Intervals between issuing prescriptions need to be monitored to assess if medication is being used appropriately.
- Time limits for reviewing medication need to be set. Review by a health professional or certain investigations may need to be undertaken within a set time frame.
- Safety of new prescriptions – interactions, contraindications and appropriateness for the individual need to be assured when authorizing a prescription.
- The volume of prescriptions generated nowadays would be extremely labour intensive if not automated in some respect.
- Generic prescribing is a necessity in many circumstances.

All of this is much more easily and safely managed using computerized prescription software and it is for this reason that repeat prescribing was the first widely accepted computer application in the UK. Drug databases are incorporated into all GP systems. 'Multilex' is most widely used, with 'Safescript' being an alternative package. Both provide monthly updates to ensure information is current. They check for interactions and contraindications with crossreferencing to the patient record, allow generic substitution, show the cost of the item and recommendations for usage. E-MIMS is supplied to NHS practices free of charge monthly and provides a wealth of information relating to the medications; for example, images of the tablets and access to manufacturers' websites.

Nurse prescribing does not currently allow for printed prescriptions. However, the issue of a prescription does need to be noted on the computer record. With the extension of nurse prescribing, nurses may use the prescribing software more extensively.

Digital photography and imaging makes it possible to store images in a clinical record. Nurses would find this particularly useful for documenting the progress of wounds and it would reduce the difficulties in describing a wound to another professional for ongoing treatment decisions. Other visual images that might prove beneficial include ECGs, spirometry and X-rays.

DECISION SUPPORT PACKAGES

These attempt to guide the health professional in the process of diagnosis and treatment of conditions according to protocols. There are various options available.

PRODIGY

Prodigy is decision support software funded by the Department of Health and has been largely viewed as an attempt to direct and control prescribing habits to keep costs down. It can be used with all GP clinical systems and there is the option of switching it on and off. When activated, it cuts in when a Read Code diagnosis is entered and guides the consultation, investigations and the subsequent prescription. Advice leaflets can be printed for the patient on the blank side of the prescription. Recommendations for treatment are based on information gleaned from 'reliable' sources such as the National Institute for Clinical Excellence (NICE) and the Cochrane Database. Information for patients can be printed off to enhance their understanding of their condition and treatment. Reports from some practitioners suggest it can be difficult to use but this should improve with modifications and experience.

SOPHIES, ISIS AND TEMPLATES

These are applications in the clinical systems that allow practices to customize the process of consultations and data recording according to their own protocols. They guide the user through stages, prompting certain questions or procedures. They can be adapted so that claims can be generated automatically or reminders given. Some allow patient advice sheets to be printed off. Protocols can be stored in the database for reference at the time of consultation. These are applications of particular use to nurses, providing structure to the consultation and ensuring the data required for management decisions, audit and recall is gathered and recorded correctly. Difficulties occur if the template does not allow for skipping data that is not available or allow the user to scroll up and down when entering data. In the natural course of a consultation information is gleaned according to the style of the professional, the way in which patients divulge information and the relevance to their circumstances. Some templates are too inflexible to cope with this and the user just switches them off, thereby losing the benefits.

Practices can share their templates/protocols with other users of the system either via the system suppliers or through user groups. Some of these user groups have websites for exchange of information. Links to these sites can be found at www.healthcentre.org.uk/hc/pages/gpcomputer.htm.

TRIAGE

Software packages such as those used in NHS Direct and walk-in centres are available for use by nurses in general practice for triage or nurse practitioner consultations. Whilst not yet widely used by practice nurses, possibly due to the cost of the software and the time taken to complete a patient interview, it is perhaps inevitable that as practice nurses increase their role in managing minor illness and triage, packages will be developed to support this role.

SEARCHES AND AUDIT

Being able to search the practice database to identify individuals with particular characteristics or medical conditions is essential in these days of clinical governance and financial restrictions, and impossible without computerization. Setting up searches can be time consuming and difficult to do, although the latest software is easier to use.

Searches can used for:

- compiling the practice's age/sex register
- identifying those with certain medical conditions requiring monitoring/interventions
- identifying who has/has not attended the practice for monitoring and therefore who needs a recall letter
- monitoring of workload including reason for patient attendance
- providing the figures to support purchasing decisions, e.g. personally administered vaccines
- auditing the result of interventions, e.g. improvement in test results.

In order to extract the data it is essential for it to be stored in a manner that makes it retrievable. Searches cannot be performed on free text. Codes need to be used that the search engine recognizes. Throughout the practice (and ideally throughout the locality) these codes need to be agreed and standardized to prevent data being missed or inaccurate.

READ CODES

Read Codes are the language used to store medical information in a computer system. They take their name from Dr James Read, a GP in Loughborough, who in 1982 devised the coding system to classify his own practice's patients with their medical conditions. From this grew an ever-increasing thesaurus of codes. The Secretary of State for Health purchased the codes in 1990, following recommendation by the Royal College of General Practitioners (RCGP) and the British Medical Association (BMA) that they become the standard for use in general practice, and potentially throughout the NHS. Continuing to update the codes is now the role of the NHS Centre for Coding and Classification (NHS CCC), in collaboration with the clinical professions. The coding system is 'dynamic' with updates being issued by the NHSIA 6 monthly (monthly for drugs). Any clinician identifying the need for a new code can ask for one to be added.

The main function of the coding system is to allow the storage and retrieval of clinical data. At present its use is predominantly for audit purposes but in future it will become the cornerstone of the EHR.

For most daily use it is only necessary to have a basic understanding of how Read Codes work. Each code has up to five characters, which means there are 600 million possible codes. The first character defines the broad class and the following characters define the subsets, each providing more information than the previous. For example, any circulatory system disease will begin with 'G', 'ischaemic heart disease' will be 'G3' and 'acute myocardial infarction' will be 'G30'. The more specific the code, the more possibilities there are for undertaking detailed searches and audit.

It is not necessary to know the codes themselves when entering data as this can usually be found by typing in the name of the condition or procedure. However, it is important to recognize that there may be a number of different codes for the same or similar things. The American coding system SNOMED is currently being amalgamated with the Read Codes.

MIQUEST

MIQUEST (morbidity information query and export syntax) is NHS software designed to extract data from the disparate GP clinical systems, in a manner that allows the data to be anonymized so that individuals cannot be identified outside the practice. It will be used predominantly by primary care organizations (PCOs) for clinical audit, needs assessment and commissioning. Individual practices receive information concerning management of its own patients, thereby auditing care and identifying areas for improvement. MIQUEST is supplied through the clinical system suppliers and all new systems need to be capable of supporting it for accreditation. Older systems may not be able to use it.

HEALTH INFORMATICS SERVICES (HIS)

To oversee the local implementation of the Information for Health strategy, each trust now employs HIS personnel. Their role is to manage all aspects of information management and technology (IM&T) within the organization, including business management, installation and support of networks, security, confidentiality, data quality, education, training, helpdesks and web design and maintenance.

PRIMIS (primary care information services) facilitators are being employed by some PCTs to assist practices in the collection and management of their data. PCTs have an interest in ensuring information is managed effectively as data are required for commissioning services, clinical governance and allocating resources. They will have a significant role in supporting practices to use their systems to the full potential.

THE ELECTRONIC HEALTH RECORD

The development of an EHR for everyone, which is capable of being accessed 24 hours a day by any authorized health professional, is the goal of the current IT strategy. How this will be managed is still under discussion and the infrastructure needs to be put in place to support it. Key considerations will be:

- confidentiality – ensuring authorization to access the information is restricted to only those needing to know
- standardizing language (coding) used to describe situations/conditions
- patient consent to personal information being stored and who is entitled to access how much of it
- protocols for adding or altering the information (Longstaff et al 2000).

SECURITY ISSUES

The computer systems throughout all branches of the NHS store vast quantities of confidential patient information. This information comes under the Data Protection Act 1983 and the amendments added in 1998 to bring it up to European standards. The Act covers all types of patient records – manual (paper), electronic (computer) or on a word processor – and practices need to register with the Data Protection Commissioner, setting out their policies and procedures for managing and protecting this data. Details of the Act can be viewed at www.hmso.gov.uk/acts/acts1998/19980029.htm and www.doh.gov.uk/dpa98/

THE CALDICOTT REPORT

Dame Flora Caldicott's committee published a draft document in 1997 www.doh.gov.uk/ipu/confiden/implemen/calcon1.htm, designed to build upon existing arrangements for safeguarding patient information following concerns about the amount of person-identifiable information being transferred throughout the NHS. Caldicott Guardians (senior managers within the organization) have been established and in primary care there is a Caldicott Guardian at PCT level. Whilst it remains the responsibility of individual staff members to keep information confidential, the Guardian identifies any lack of awareness by personnel or weaknesses in skills or protocols which must be addressed. NHS organizations are accountable, through clinical governance, for continuously improving confidentiality and security procedures governing access to and storage of person-identifiable information.

THE INTERNET

The Internet is a system that lets all computers in the world talk to each other (Levine et al 2000). It began life as an American military communications system for use in the event of a nuclear war and was adopted by the academic world before being taken over by commercial enterprise. The prime use of the Internet is for communication and it adds to, rather than replaces, traditional methods.

Connection to the Internet requires a computer with a modem and phone access. The time spent online (local phone call charges) and payment (if any) to an Internet service provider (ISP) determine the financial cost of using the Internet. Those spending long periods of time accessing the Internet often choose to pay a set fee for unmetered access. There is currently no cost to general practice for Internet use. Obtaining access to the Net at peak times may prove slow; the speed of the process depends on the modem in the computer, type of phone line (analogue, ISDN or broadband) and traffic using the Net at the time.

The enthusiasm for this medium by those who are comfortable with it is due to the fact that it allows access to information either not accessible elsewhere or at a much greater speed than would otherwise be possible – if you know how to find it and the technology doesn't let you down.

The Internet is anarchy at its best and worst (Levine et al 2000). It works by millions of individuals programming their computers to talk to each other, with the content of these communications being completely unregulated. This allows for freedom of expression away from governmental interference but it is open to abuse as well as being a source of great good. It is vulnerable to the technical failure of individual systems, yet as a whole is extremely robust.

Use of the Internet leads to specific concerns, of which the most common are:

- fear of what you might be exposed to – unsuitable material
- fear of hackers getting into your system and accessing confidential information
- fear of viruses disabling your system
- fear of being left behind if you don't learn how to use it fast
- cost in terms of time and phone calls accessing it.

The Internet is a window from your computer onto the world. You may or may not like what you see. You may let others see you and increase your vulnerability.

THE NHSNET

The NHS has vast quantities of confidential information stored on its computers. Allowing the outside world a route in could make it vulnerable to security breaches. In order to achieve the benefits of electronic communication whilst reducing this risk, organizations, including the NHS, have developed intranets, networks that can only be accessed from within the organization. However, the NHSnet needs access to the outside world in order to take advantage of sources of information and communication.

LOCAL AREA NETWORKS (LANs)

LANs can be set up within the NHSnet and are designed to allow access to a defined population, for example a PCT or hospital trust. They provide a secure environment for publishing protocols, policies and information pertaining to local services. Unfortunately those outside the organization are unable to access the data and therefore information published on a hospital intranet cannot be accessed by community staff and vice versa. This impedes the sharing of information unless it is published on both networks.

PROTECTION FROM OUTSIDE SOURCES

Whilst Caldicott Guardians try to address the confidentiality issues of personnel and procedures, there is also risk from the vandals (hackers and virus spreaders) who delight in finding access to the computer systems and spreading software that corrupts it. The Internet provides an entry point. Some protection is conferred by 'firewalls' (Fig. 21.2), software that allows information to be sent out from the network but scrutinizes any incoming information with specific exclusion criteria.

EMAIL

Electronic mail is the communication tool of the Internet. Major benefits include:

- speed – the message may reach the recipient within seconds
- convenience – the sender and recipient do not have to be available at the same time
- ability to send the same message to a group of people at the same time or forward a message to another interested party
- communication can be facilitated between people who would not otherwise make contact with one another
- documents can be sent in the form of attachments – more legible than faxes
- messages are stored in the computer system and therefore provide a record of the communication for future reference, if necessary.

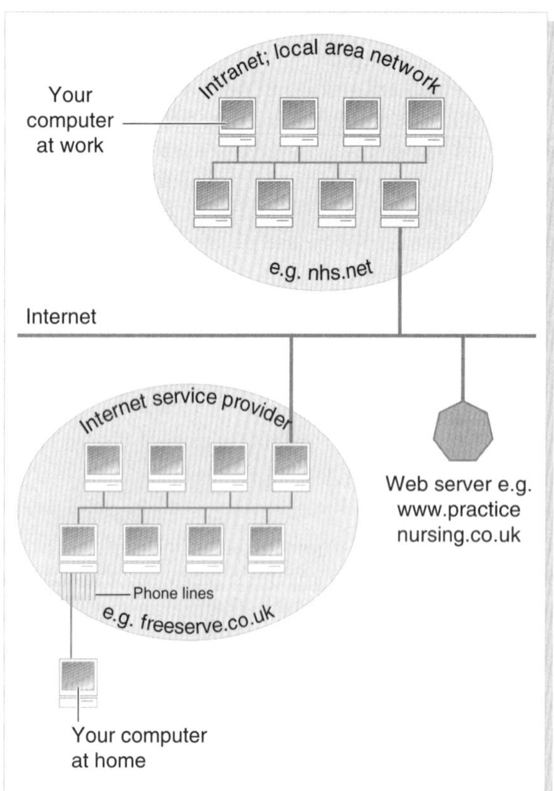

Figure 21.1 Local area networks connecting into the Internet.

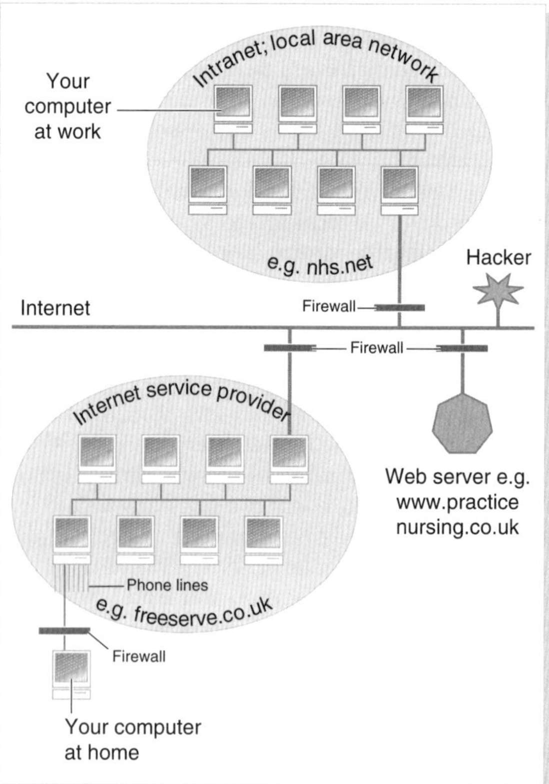

Figure 21.2 Local area networks connecting to the Internet with firewalls added for protection.

People will start to communicate with you via email once they are sure you will receive it. The recipient does need to log on in order to receive the message and therefore it is limited to those interested enough to use it.

Disadvantages

- The message remains in the In Box until the recipient is ready to receive it so it is no good in an emergency.
- There is a cost to the receiver of the message. Some attachments take a long time to be transferred to the recipient's computer.
- For the recipient to be able to read attachments their operating software needs to be compatible with that of the sender (unless an agreed format is used).
- Lack of privacy – the message passes through a number of systems and is available for reading by the system administrators and hackers.
- Lack of non-verbal clues – the message may be ambiguous and cause unintentional offence.
- Employers may have legal rights to see any emails sent or received at work.
- Viruses might be transported into your computer.
- There is no directory of email addresses, therefore you are unable to contact a person without first being given their address.
- Email addresses need to be accurate otherwise they will not be recognized.
- Junk mail (spam) is becoming more problematic.

Observing some basic rules helps to overcome some of these problems.

- Keep messages simple. Large attachments can be 'zipped' to compress them using zipping software, but the receiver requires software to un-zip them.
- Never send confidential information by email.
- Compose the message carefully. Always re-read it before sending to ensure it actually says what you want it to.
- Use up-to-date virus protection software on your computer (see below).
- The majority of email software has an address book feature. If set up efficiently the storage and retrieval of addresses can be very simple.
- Guard your email address carefully. It may be sensible to have a few different addresses to use according to whom you are communicating with. If you start receiving junk or obscene mail switch off that address and start using another. If you persistently get unsolicited mail from a particular source you can complain to their ISP. Another precaution is to be careful to tick relevant boxes refusing permission to pass your details on to other sources, otherwise you can be added to mailing lists.
- Do not pass on chain email – your address will be added to the list and forwarded to many others.

To use email it is necessary to be registered with an ISP who supplies you with a unique email address. This enables the message to reach your computer. The address may be case sensitive so it is essential to type it in correctly. Email addresses in general practice all relate to the practice's identifying code. If you know the address of one person within the practice you can invariably work out the address of everyone else. Equally home addresses can be personalized to reach the appropriate member of the household. Like personal car number plates, it is possible to rent an individual name, for example your family name or company name, for an annual charge. This can usually be arranged through some ISPs or companies set up to offer this service.

The end of the address denotes what sort of organization you are and the country you are in (with the exception of the USA). Examples include:

- .nhs – NHS
- .org – non-profit organization
- .ac – university
- .co – company
- .com – company.

ENCRYPTION

The lack of security when transferring information electronically is a concern for an organization with such a large volume of confidential data. One solution is to use encryption software (Kiley & Graham 2002). This translates the message into a series of numbers and letters that can only be deciphered if the recipient has the key to unlock it.

EMAIL DISCUSSION/NEWS GROUPS

There are many active discussion groups that utilize email to converse with others with similar interests. You can register to join the practice nurse egroup at http://groups.yahoo.com/group/practicenurse/ You do not have to join in conversations although the success of such groups depends on active participation by a significant number of members. This site has an associated website where members have posted information such as protocols and job descriptions that others may find useful.

VIRUSES

The scourge of the Internet is the destruction that can be caused to computers by the spread of viruses. These are programs devised by vandals intent on exploiting weaknesses in the software to cause damage. They can infect your system by being carried by email without the sender being aware that they are incubators of a bug. The greatest protection is conferred by use of good-quality anti-virus software, the best known of which are Macafee and Norton. Packages can be purchased that provide automatic updates.

Some viruses are spread in the form of attachments. There are some general rules for the opening of attachments which will offer some protection.

- Know who it comes from.
- Be expecting that person to be sending you something or have the reason for sending it to you explained.
- Ensure the content of the attachment is referred to in the main body of the email.

Viruses can be programmed to be sent to everyone in an address book – that person may not be aware that he has sent an infected message to you. It is important to make others aware so that they can rectify the problem within their own system.

If in doubt, do not open an attachment. Email the sender and ask them to confirm that it is safe to open. Saving it to disk does not confer any protection. It may only serve to delay the execution of the virus until it is opened.

Hoaxers can be equally destructive by feeding on fears and interfering with normal communication. You may be advised to perform a function which will cause damage to your system. Before doing anything it is advisable to search the anti-virus software manufacturers' websites as they post details of identified viruses or hoaxes as they are discovered and advise on action to be taken.

Firewall software is the last form of protection for your computer. It closes some of the ports through which hackers could gain access to your system. It is only really necessary for those spending long periods of time connected to the Internet. Some, such as Zone alarm, can be downloaded free from the Internet. More recent software such as Windows XP has firewall software incorporated into the package. Like anti-virus software, it is necessary to obtain updates to ensure continued protection.

THE WORLD WIDE WEB

The Web is a cross between a library, newspaper, bulletin board and telephone directory (and more) all on a global scale. The ability to post and store information on the Web is potentially infinite. We are led to believe that the answers to all questions can be found on the Web if only we look hard enough! This can be very helpful but it can also add to the feeling of failure if we can't find the answer. Searching through all this information can be soul destroying and ultimately fruitless if you don't look in the right place. Equally it requires someone to have posted the information that you are looking for in the first place. And why would they?

The main reasons why someone posts information on the Web are:

- *commercial* – there is money to be made through buying, selling or advertising on the Net
- *altruistic* – the idea of sharing something with others for no commercial gain
- *academic* – sharing of information and disseminating research
- *organizations* – set up and funded as part of a service.

It is essential to be critical about the sources of information you use. Ideally you should know who is funding the site and what they are trying to achieve. Anyone can post anything on the Web if they have the knowhow – it could be complete rubbish.

What you should know about a site:

- who is funding it
- who is the target audience
- who is posting the information
- when it was last updated
- what they are trying to achieve.

Features of a good site:

- easy to navigate
- up to date
- relevant.

Web browsers are the software facilitating access to the Internet. The best known are Microsoft's Explorer and Netscape's Navigator. Both allow the user to follow hyperlinks to other areas of the Web and both have a feature for making a directory of useful sites for future reference – called 'favorites' by Microsoft and 'bookmarks' by Netscape. Once a site has been visited some browsers save the visited pages onto disk, thereby allowing you to access the content (look under 'history') without having to go back online. Equally, it is possible to 'save' useful information into a file. Some documents are presented on the Web in portable document format (PDF). This makes them look exactly the same as they were published. The Department of Health publishes documents in this way. To download the information it is necessary to install Adobe Acrobat software from the Internet (free). You are usually given the option to do this when you are presented with a PDF file.

Search engines help you find what you are looking for. Perhaps the best known of these are Google, Yahoo and Lycos. Alternatively various people or organizations link sites of similar interest together in portals. In the UK, Rod Ward at Sheffield University grouped together nursing sites. This has since been amalgamated into Nmap, a gateway to Internet resources for nursing and allied health professionals (http://nmap.ac.uk/). Websites usually have 'links' sections with hyperlinks to other sites of potential interest. Following these hyperlinks can often lead you to the information you wanted to find.

Nursing websites

The majority of nursing websites are set up and moderated by professionals with an interest in providing a forum for communicating and sharing information with others in the same discipline. Some are commercial and rely on advertising or selling to generate income. Others are posted under the auspices of a larger organization, such as the RCN. There is a practice nursing website (www.practicenursing.co.uk) which includes an active discussion forum, links to sites of interest, a job page, forums for posting humour or information of potential use to others and a guestbook.

General practice websites

Some practices have set up their own websites. The benefits of doing this might be:

- selling the practice to the general public – someone looking for a new doctor would benefit from being able to access information about the practice before deciding whether to register
- publishing the practice leaflet and newsletters
- providing information about services and opening times – particularly useful during holidays
- potential to improve patient education and self-help – links can be set up to sites of interest such as NHS Direct online (McElhinney 2000).

It is envisaged that in the near future practice websites might become interactive, with patients ordering repeat prescriptions, or be a vehicle for email communication and telemedicine. At present their use is greatest in areas with a high population of Internet users but there is the potential for this to increase with digital television access in the future. Registering the practice's domain name will make it easier for the public to find the site.

A database with links to GP websites can be found at www.internet-gp.com/gpsites

TELEMEDICINE

The excitement about the use of telemedicine in healthcare is due to its potential to facilitate communication with either patients (to provide advice or help monitor conditions) or other professionals (to receive expert opinion) from afar. Telephone consultations, including triage, are already in common use. Use of NHS Direct and NHS Direct online is growing rapidly. It is not always either possible or necessary for patients to attend a medical establishment to receive the advice they need.

Videoconferencing is currently not a realistic option for most GPs as the technology is neither advanced enough nor affordable to be able to get any benefit from it (Bradley 2001). Where benefits could be more easily achieved is in the use of digital photography. The ability to attach a photograph to a referral letter may prevent the need for the patient to be seen by the consultant at all. The management of heart conditions could be greatly improved by the ability to send ECGs directly to cardiologists for interpretation where diagnosis is unclear or to A&E or CCU for assessment of changes in patterns. GPs and nurses could find that receiving digital images of X-rays and MRI scans with the radiologist's report might enhance their understanding of the patient's condition and preserve their skills in interpreting these images.

Home monitoring of patients with certain conditions is beginning to happen. Conditions ideally suited to this might include diabetes (blood glucose readings), cardiology (BP readings, ECGs), pregnancy (fetal heart rate and uterine tone recordings in preeclamptic toxaemia) and monitoring the frail newborn or elderly (more specialized equipment will be required for this).

Health professionals, including nurses, may find that an expansion in the use of telemedicine will impact on their roles and training requirements, some in ways still unimaginable at present.

SOURCES OF INFORMATION

Having access to sources of information is an essential component in being able to provide a high standard of care. It is equally important that the public has access to high-quality information. To be of use the information needs to be easily accessible and up to date. The Internet provides an ideal medium for this.

NATIONAL ELECTRONIC LIBRARY FOR HEALTH (NeLH)

In order to facilitate access to the wealth of medical information available on the Internet, the government, through the NHSIA, is overseeing the NeLH (www.nelh.nhs.uk). Its aim is to provide easy access to best current knowledge, improve health and healthcare, clinical practice and patient choice. Eventually there will be sections aimed at both health professionals and patients. All information accessible via the NeLH will be vetted for quality. Gateways will be provided to areas of special interest, e.g. primary care (www.nelh-pc.nhs.uk).

SOURCES OF INFORMATION FOR PRIMARY CARE

- *Medical libraries* – books and journals can be accessed or borrowed. CD-ROMs and online databases can be searched. Librarians provide help and training in searching the literature and accessing the Internet. Most can now provide remote access to these databases from the practice or home by supplying a password.
- *Journals* – either personal or practice subscription, through the library or via the Internet. Some now publish both abstracts and full text articles free online.
- *Internet* – including the NeLH, Department of Health and other government sites.
- *Disease-specific organizations*, e.g. Diabetes UK. Most now have websites and some have areas dedicated to health professionals.
- *NHS Direct* – can supply information on most aspects relating to health provision, including information leaflets for patients.

SOURCES OF INFORMATION FOR THE PUBLIC

Health professionals no longer have the monopoly on health information. The public now has access to medical information from many sources and may have more time than the health professional to find what they are looking for. They also have the luxury of being able to focus on a much narrower range of conditions. There are benefits to this as well as complications. Well-informed patients may be genuinely empowered to make treatment decisions, may have more realistic expectations and may reduce the demands on services by self-management of minor conditions (Kiley & Graham 2002). Equally their sources of information may be completely biased, providing them with unrealistic or dangerous expectations. They may present with information from other patients, sensationalist newspaper or magazine articles or information from dubious Internet sites. Health professionals need to be able to steer them to reliable sources of information including:

- health education leaflets from medical premises
- NHS Direct
- charitable/self-help organizations
- Internet – NeLH, local medical services sites, NHS site (www.nhs.uk).

Many professionals might find a 'well-informed' patient a threat. A strategy for managing the situation might prevent you feeling like this.

- Know where you get your information from and be able to explain that to the patient.
- Acknowledge your limitations in the subject.
- Ask them to provide you with references for you to interpret for yourself.
- Explain that not all treatment options are suitable for all patients.
- If you agree with their perspective then be prepared to follow it.
- If not, provide them with the evidence for why you disagree.

A useful resource for the practice library might be *The patient's Internet handbook* by Robert Kiley and Elizabeth Graham (2002). This book provides a concise critique of the pros and cons of accessing information from the Internet as well as pointing the way to reliable sources of information.

E-LEARNING

The Internet is set to revolutionize how we learn. As well as facilitating literature searching, it will be used for distance learning packages and online teaching. The benefits to the student would be:

- reduced travel time – less time required to be spent in universities
- less time taken out of the work environment
- ability to study at times convenient to you
- ability to study at a pace suited to you
- familiarization with using computer and Internet technology.

Disadvantages might be:

- pressure to study in your personal time
- the need for the technology to do it – especially if the work environment is unsuitable
- reduced peer support and networking
- it would cause difficulties for those uncomfortable with this medium.

It is likely that educational institutions will devise programmes with a mix of learning methods to gain the benefits from use of the new technologies without sacrificing the benefits of traditional methods.

LITERATURE SEARCHING

For nurses undertaking any study the two most useful features of computer technology are word processing and literature searching. Word-processing skills can be learnt from family members, friends, trial and error or one of the courses discussed below. Literature searching is best taught by a medical librarian.

Databases include:

- MEDLINE – medical and healthcare journals
- CINAHL – international nursing and allied health
- Cochrane Library – four databases covering the effects of interventions
- AMED – professions allied to medicine and alternative therapies
- ClinPsych – clinical and medical psychology journals
- BNI – British Nursing Index on CD-ROM; covers English language journals.

EDUCATION, TRAINING AND DEVELOPMENT

Central to the success of the government's Information for Health strategy will be the need to develop skills in the use of IT across the multiprofessional workforce. A large number of the clinicians working in primary care were educated before the widespread use of computers and some have little or no basic computing skill. Local groups need to identify training needs and provide education to meet them.

The European Computer Driving Licence (ECDL) is a national qualification set up by local education providers. NHS staff may be able to get this funded for free depending on local agreements. The ECDL consists of seven modules:

- basic concepts of IT
- using the computer and managing files
- word processing
- spreadsheets
- databases
- presentation
- Internet and email.

City and Guilds computer training courses are also usually available locally.

Information on ECDL, including local providers of training courses, can be found at www.ecdl.co.uk/nhs/index.htm and www.nhsia.nhs.uk/wowwi/pages/programmes/ecdl.asp

The clinical system suppliers provide training on the use of the practice's computer as part of the set-up agreement. However, this is frequently not adequate to ensure that all members of the practice fully understand how to use the various applications. Further training is expensive and not necessarily of a quality good enough to justify the expense. Practice nurses invariably rely on other staff members to teach them. With a multitude of different systems in use in one locality, it is not possible for one IT expert to be fully conversant with all them. Ways need to be found to address this problem. Ideally there should be an 'expert' user in each practice who could be trained to teach and support other staff members.

As part of the GP Connect project, many areas have employed facilitators to visit practices and provide in-house training on use of the Internet and email.

CONCLUSION

The increasing use of IT in primary care has already had an impact on the way services are managed and data is collected and utilized. There is huge potential to improve the delivery of healthcare further as technology advances and users become familiar with using it to its best advantage. Educating the workforce to achieve this is a challenge, particularly in general practice where there may not be the organizational structure or vision to support it. The government is investing huge resources in implementing its Information for Health strategy and it is hoped that the result of this investment will be improved communications between the differing sections of the NHS and social care and easy access to reliable, high-quality information pertaining to all aspects of delivering healthcare. Clinicians need to see the value of embracing the new technology and have good-quality training and support as they learn how to use it.

Acknowledgements

I would like to express my thanks to my husband Bernie for teaching me all I know about using computers and the Internet, and to Rachel Southon, Outreach Librarian at North Hants Hospital, for support and guidance.

References

Bradley S 2001 The paperless practice. Radcliffe, Oxford
DoH 1997 The New NHS: modern, dependable. Department of Health, London
DoH 1998a A first class service. Quality in the new NHS. Department of Health, London
DoH 1998b Information for health; a new IM&T strategy. Department of Health, London
DoH 2000 The NHS Plan. Department of Health, London
Kiley R, Graham E 2002 The patient's Internet handbook. Royal Society of Medicine Press, London
Levine J, Reinhold A, Levine Young M 2000 The Internet for dummies, 6th edn. IDG Books Worldwide, New York
Longstaff J, Capper G, Lockyer M et al 2000 EHR and EPR confidentiality based on accountability and consent: tools for the Caldicott Guardian. Health Informatics Journal 6:45–52
McElhinney A 2000 How useful are general practice websites? British Journal of Healthcare Computing and Information Management 17(1):20–22
Miller A, Jeffcote R 1997 Practice nurses and computing: some evidence on utilization, training, and attitudes to computer use. Health Informatics Journal 3:10–16
Preece J 2000 The use of computers in general practice, 4th edn. Harcourt, London
Risdale L, Hudd S 1999 What do patients want and not want to see about themselves on a computer screen? a qualitative study. Scandinavian Journal of Primary Health Care 15(4):180–183
Russell A, Alpay L 2000 Practice nurses' training in information technology: report on an empirical investigation. Health Informatics Journal 6:142–146
See Tai S, Donegan C, Nazareth I 2000 Computers in general practice and the consultation: the health professionals' view. Health Informatics Journal 6:27–31
Sullivan F, Mitchell E 1995 Has general practitioner computing made a difference to patient care? A systematic review of published reports. British Medical Journal 311:848–852

Resources

Websites

www.nhs.uk – NHS website
www.nhsia.nhs.uk – NHS Information Authority website
www.standards.nhsia.nhs.uk/other.htm – has links to sites under the auspices of the NHSIA
www.doh.gov.uk – home page of the Department of Health
www.nelh.nhs.uk – National Electronic Library for Health
www.nelh-pc.nhs.uk – primary care section of the NeLH
www.doh.gov.uk/nhsplanprimarycare/index.htm – the NHS Plan for primary care
www.nhsdirect.nhs.uk – NHS Direct online
www.nhsu.nhs.uk – NHS University

Further reading

Gilles A 2000 Information and IT for primary care. Everything you need to know but were afraid to ask. Radcliffe, Oxford
Kiley R 1996 Medical information on the Internet. A guide for health professionals. Churchill Livingstone, Edinburgh
Lock K 1995 Using computers to enhance care in a GP practice. Nursing Times 91(18):36–38
Nicoll L, Ouellette T 1997 Nurses' guide to the Internet. Lippincott, Philadelphia
Silagy C, Haines A 1998 Evidence based practice in primary care. BMJ Books, London
Thiru K, de Lusigan S, Hague N 1999 Have the completeness and accuracy of computer medical records in general practice improved in the last five years? The report of a two practice pilot study. Health Informatics Journal 5:224–232
Tyrell S 1999 Using the Internet in healthcare. Radcliffe, Oxford

Chapter 22

Accountability

Jeannett Martin

CHAPTER CONTENTS

INTRODUCTION

The aim of this chapter is to provide an overview of key aspects linked to professional accountability in relation to the law, record keeping, protocols, patient group directions and the management of patient complaints.

THE LAW OF NEGLIGENCE

The laws of tort are part of the civil law which provides for the rights and duties of individuals towards each other. The law will allow civil action to be taken to financially compensate the person who has suffered unwarranted harm, or damage, at the hands of another. Negligence is one of the most important torts and would enable patients who have suffered reasonably foreseeable harm, as a result of carelessness, to sue for financial compensation.

Negligence has been defined as the omission to do something which any reasonable man would do, or to do something which a prudent and reasonable man would not do. The case of negligence has to be proved by the claimant, not disproved by the defendant, and three elements must be satisfied. These are that:

- the defendant owed a duty of care to the claimant
- there was a breach of that duty of care
- harm resulted as a direct result of that breach in duty of care.

DUTY OF CARE

The legal test of whether a duty of care exists was established in the case of *Donoghue v Stephenson*[1] when a consumer bought a bottle of ginger beer which contained a decomposed snail. The judgment in this case held that the manufacturers had a duty to take reasonable care to avoid acts or omissions which could reasonably be foreseen as likely to injure the persons affected by the act or omission. This became known as the Neighbourhood Principle.

It would not be reasonable to expect a practice nurse to be available at all times to provide nursing services to friends and neighbours and therefore the nurse does not owe a legal duty of care to the whole population. However, the Nursing and Midwifery Council (NMC) may consider that the nurse owes a professional duty to provide help in life-threatening or emergency situations (NMC 2002, UKCC 1996).

Patients registered with a GP do not need to be referred by the doctor to the practice nurse, they are entitled to direct access by making an appointment. Therefore the practice nurse does owe a duty of care to patients registered at the practice who consult for nursing services.

BREACH OF THE DUTY OF CARE

The standard of care that the law would require was established in the case of *Bolam v Friern HCC.*[2] The standard required by law is the ordinary skill of an ordinary competent man exercising that particular art. This is known as the Bolam Test and is used to distinguish between errors of judgement and errors that fall short of the standard that could be expected.

The standard of care expected from a novice would be that of an ordinary practice nurse and not less because of inexperience, the assumption being that those who are inexperienced should take care to consult before they act. Therefore as the law stands at present, a practice nurse, even on the first day in the post, would be expected to be able to provide care for patients to the standard of an ordinary skilled practice nurse. This would apply to assessment, action taken and information and advice given. In providing vaccinations, for example, the accepted practice of the time is clearly laid out in the Green Book which is distributed free by the Departments of Health to all practices in the UK.

Should the practice nurse profess to be a specialist in a particular area such as asthma, then the nurse must be able to demonstrate the ordinary skill of that specialty. This would be likely to be in line with the knowledge and competencies of a practice nurse who had undertaken the Diploma in Asthma Management.

Ignorance is not a defence in law. If there has been a departure from accepted practice, for example in the choice of injection site, the defendant will need to justify this departure. This could be done by the testimony of expert witnesses who would agree that, in the same circumstances, they too would have acted in such a manner. However, in the case of *Bolitho v City & Hackney HA*[3] the judgment held that expert opinion needs to be 'responsible, reasonable and respectable'. The judge suggested that before the court accepted expert opinion, it should be clearly demonstrated that the experts have considered risks and benefits of the situation and can defend their conclusion.

The judge must decide what would be reasonable on the basis of probability. Records that were made at the time of the incident, that are accurate and complete, will be considered as important and persuasive evidence to enable the judge to make a decision. Practice protocols and policies can also provide a defence by illustrating the normal practice used.

HARM RESULTING FROM THE BREACH

It can be difficult for a claimant to establish a direct link and most cases that are unable to demonstrate causation are unsuccessful. This was illustrated in *Barnet v Chelsea and Kensington Hospital Management Committee*[4] where a night watchman had attended casualty complaining of stomach pains. He was not seen by the casualty officer and was sent home by the nurse; he died later that day due to arsenic poisoning. His widow's case was unsuccessful because, although the doctor clearly had a duty of care which he breached, the breach did not cause the death as it was clear that even if Mr Barnet had immediately been admitted to hospital and treated, he would have still died.

In the case of *Cassidy v Minister of Health*[5] it was held that employers can be liable for the consequences of the actions or omissions of their employees. When a GP agrees to allow a patient to register at the practice, implicit in that agreement is that the patient may use the services provided by the GP at the practice. The GP selects, appoints and employs the practice nurse and patients have no say in the selection process. If harm occurs as a result of the practice nurse's actions, the employer can be held liable for a nurse who does not provide the standard of care expected of an ordinary practice nurse or because the nurse was not provided with adequate facilities to do the job.

Because of vicarious liability for the consequences of the actions of a practice nurse, the General Medical Services Committee (GMSC) of the British Medical Association (BMA) issued guidelines to GPs on the training and delegation of duties to practice nurses (GMSC 1994). These guidelines make it clear that GP employers have a responsibility to ensure that the nurse is adequately trained and competent to carry out delegated activities but also that the activities delegated should be appropriate.

Finally, the nurse is bound by a code of conduct (NMC 2002) which is separate from any contract of employment and ensures that the nurse remains individually accountable for all actions. Even if an action for negligence is dismissed from the civil court, because of lack of causation, it can be referred on to a professional conduct committee of the Nursing and Midwifery Council or General Medical Council.

CONSENT

Obtaining consent has two functions. The clinical function is to foster trust and cooperation with patients, the legal function is to ensure that a person's right to autonomy has been addressed in order to prevent a charge of battery.

Cases heard in the civil courts have confirmed that individuals who have capacity to consent have the legal right to autonomy within decision making.[6,7,8] A person would be held to have capacity (competence) to consent if he was able to meet the three-stage test of being able to:[7]

- comprehend and retain the information
- believe it
- weigh it in the balance to make a decision.

ADULTS

All adults are assumed to have capacity unless it can be demonstrated that they do not meet the criteria outlined. Therefore unless a person is unconscious and in a life-threatening situation, consent must be obtained before any healthcare treatment is provided. It must be voluntary and not obtained under pressure or duress.

If an adult lacks the capacity to consent, the law does not allow for consent or refusal by one adult, e.g. a relative, on behalf of another. The decision to treat would be made by the health professional in charge of their care on the basis of the patient's 'best interests'. However, in more serious situations it is advisable to discuss the options with relatives as they may be able to give a view on what the patient would have wanted when he did have capacity to consent.

CHILDREN

The Children Act 1989 defines a child as a person under the age of 18 but a minor aged 16 or 17 would be assumed to have capacity to consent unless the criteria for capacity are not met. An adult with parental responsibility can decide on behalf of a minor who lacks capacity to consent.

The Fraser Guidelines outlined in the House of Lords judgment in the case of *Gillick v West Norfolk and Wisbech Area Health Authority*[9] held that a young person is competent to consent to contraception if:

- she understands the advice
- she cannot be persuaded to inform her parents or allow the doctor to inform her parents that she is seeking contraceptive advice
- she is likely to begin or continue having intercourse with or without contraceptive treatment
- her physical or mental health is likely to suffer unless she receives contraceptive treatment
- her best interests require the doctor to give contraceptive advice, treatment or both without parental consent.

This is known as Gillick competency and has since been applied to other aspects of healthcare. Therefore if a child under the age of 16 years can demonstrate competence to consent then that consent would be considered valid. However, an adult with parental responsibility for a child may be able to override a competent child's refusal, but this would then require that the health professional would be willing to proceed in these circumstances, which is likely to be a rare occurrence.

IMPLICATIONS FOR PRACTICE

Guidance from the DoH on consent is available at www.doh.gov.uk/consent. Statutory bodies (GMC 1999, NMC 2002) have advised healthcare professionals that to ensure consent is valid, patients must be given adequate information on which to base their decision to proceed or refuse treatment. Consent can be given verbally, in writing or implied.

The process of obtaining consent should have been the same whether the consent obtained is written, verbal or implied, e.g. holding out an arm to be vaccinated. For example, in relation to vaccination, before patients can make their decision they need to have a clear explanation and an opportunity to ask questions on:

- the need for the vaccine
- the vaccine/number of doses required
- the risks associated with the disease
- the risks/side-effects associated with the vaccine.

Written consent is not a legal requirement. However, depending on the construction of the form, it may have the advantage of being able to demonstrate what information was provided before consent was obtained and also that the patient had been given the opportunity to ask questions.

People are entitled to change their minds and withdraw consent. Therefore if an adult attends for a course of treatment, consent should be checked at each visit. Any refusal of recommended treatment should be recorded.

Parental consent for young children's vaccination also needs to be obtained at each visit and the practice should consider asking parents to provide a letter of authorization if they wish another adult to bring their child for vaccination. Management of parental refusal of child vaccination should be in line with local policy and may involve offering a parent the opportunity of a referral to the GP or community paediatrician in order to discuss their concerns.

CONFIDENTIALITY

Any individual with capacity to consent, regardless of age, can seek treatment from a GP or nurse in a general practice at which they are registered for general medical services. Part of the consultation will require that information be collected from the patient. Patients consider this information about themselves to have been given in confidence and that any sharing of this with others will not be undertaken lightly by health professionals (Bolton Group 2000).

The professional duty of confidentiality is central to establishing and maintaining a relationship of trust with an individual patient and patient confidence in this is considered to be the key to patients being open and honest with health professionals (Beauchamp & Childress 1989).

This duty of confidentiality relates to any patient, no matter what their age. It is their competence to consent which is the key principle so a young person under the age of 16 is as entitled as an adult to have information kept confidential if they can demonstrate capacity to consent.

The Data Protection Act 1998 relates to identifiable data on the physical or mental health, sexual life, racial or ethnic origin, religious or political beliefs of living individuals. It is based on eight core principles relating to protection of personal information which must:

- be processed fairly and lawfully
- be obtained for specified and lawful purposes
- be adequate, relevant and not excessive for the purpose
- not be used for other incompatible purposes
- be accurate and updated
- not be kept for longer than necessary
- be processed in accordance with the rights of individuals
- have security measures in place to prevent unauthorized processing and against accidental loss or destruction.

The Human Rights Act 1998 came into force in October 2000. It incorporates the European Convention on Human Rights into UK law. Article 8 establishes in law the right to respect for private and family life; confidentiality of medical information would be an integral part of this right. Disclosure would be judged against whether it was in accordance with law, necessary and proportionate.

DISCLOSURE

Professional codes such as the *Code of conduct* (NMC 2002) provide guidance as to when disclosure of identifiable information can be justified. Disclosure without consent should only take place if there is the potential for harm to an individual or a wider public interest.

The DoH Caldicott Report (NHSE 1999) recommends that a notice is displayed outlining what can be expected from the practice regarding patient information and when information may be released to external bodies, e.g. for research purposes or notification to appropriate organizations of notifiable diseases or adverse reactions to medicines.

Research involving information collected from or about NHS patients must be approved by local research ethics committees before it is undertaken.

Use of patient information for research purposes is an important part of ethical approval and will also have been considered during the peer review undertaken during applications for funding from national bodies such as the Medical Research Council (MRC).

In research projects involving an external body, the practice should register with the Data Protection Registrar to disclose information to their research collaborators.

As part of their Ethics Series, the MRC has recently published *Personal information in medical research* (2000), which provides guidance on access to patient information for research purposes. A copy of this document is available free by contacting the publications department at the MRC on 020 7636 5422 or at www.mrc.ac.uk/PDFs/PIMR.pdf.

Accidental disclosure can occur if:

- telephone conversations about patients are overheard
- computer screens are left displaying information from the previous consultation
- patient records or correspondence are left where they can be seen by visitors to the surgery, e.g. workmen.

If accidental disclosure does occur then an apology and explanation should be given to the patient and the surgery should review the incident to identify how it occurred and, if necessary, change practice systems to try to ensure that it does not happen again (RCGP 2000).

All health professionals are individually accountable for their own actions but in addition, practices have a responsibility to ensure that everybody employed by the practice understands the need for confidentiality and that systems and mechanisms to protect confidentiality are in place. The RCGP, with the support of the RCN and the BMA, have published a training pack on *Confidentiality and young people* (RCGP 2000) for use in general practice. This pack includes examples of a general practice confidentiality policy, staff confidentiality agreements (including a simplified version for staff such as contract workers) and a comprehensive training resource for staff training. A copy can be obtained from RCGP publications on 020 7823 9698.

COMPLAINTS

In April 1996 GPs' terms of service were amended and a new complaints system was introduced. This has been updated and revised guidance will apply from 2004. Patients who wish to make a complaint can now access a system which applies to all aspects of the NHS. It aims to satisfy the concerns of the complainant and to be:

- easy for the complainant to access
- quick and thorough
- fair to staff and complainant.

A complaint should normally be made within 6 months of the event or 6 months from the date that the matter came to the complainant's attention so long as it is not longer than 12 months from the date of the event itself. However, there is discretion for this time limit to be extended if it is still possible to investigate the facts of the case. Any matter which is the subject of litigation is not included in the local complaints procedure.

Each practice is required to set up its own local complaints system and to provide staff training. The practice system needs to be prepared to deal with a range of possible issues including clinical treatment, staff attitudes and administration matters. The system must include:

- the means of informing patients how and to whom complaints can be made at practice or primary care organization (PCO)
- publishing the procedure and time limits, e.g. by poster, practice leaflet
- appointment of a named person with responsibility for investigating all complaints
- a system, e.g. logbook or spreadsheet, to record all complaints and their outcome
- an initial response to a complaint within 2 working days
- a final written response with an explanation, apology if necessary and details of any change in practice policy in light of the complaint within 20 working days.

In addition, there is a designated person in each PCO who can:

- provide advice and assistance to practices
- act as an intermediary if the complainant feels unable to approach the practice directly.

Not all complaints will be resolved at local level and the system allows unsatisfied complainants to apply

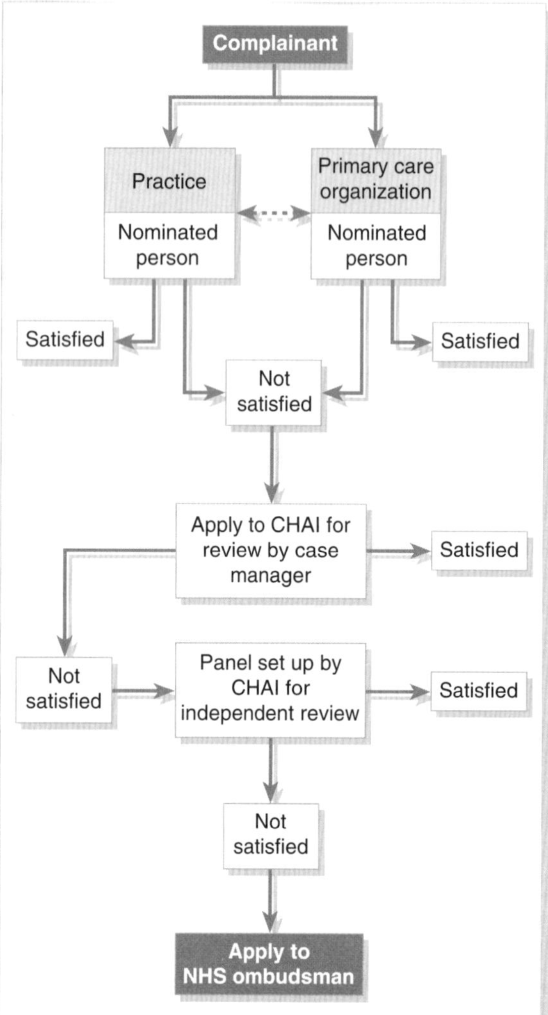

Figure 22.1 The NHS complaints system (due to be amended April 2004).

for an independent review of their complaint to the Commission for Health Audit and Inspection (CHAI). An independent review will involve individual interviews with the people involved and a report will be made based on the evidence collected.

Although any complainant can apply for an independent review, it is not an automatic right and cannot take place if there is an intention to proceed to litigation. The decision will depend on whether all practical action has already been taken and whether any further action is possible. If the complainant is refused an independent review or is unsatisfied by the outcome, he has the right to apply to the Health Service Commissioner (Ombudsman).

Further information on the complaints procedure can be obtained from www.doh.gov.uk/complaints

RECORD KEEPING

In general practice, where patient notes are shared between nurses and doctors, investigations or information gathered by one member of the team may be valuable when the patient consults another. Where information or actions taken are not clear patient care may be jeopardized and harm (negligence) may result.

We live and work in an environment of increasing litigation. The Health Service Commissioner (Ombudsman) is the official who investigates patient complaints if they have not been satisfied by a health authority tribunal. Between 1990 and 1992 complaints rose by more than 40%; poor communication was cited as the single most common problem. The Ombudsman noted that in many cases notes were often illegible, ambiguous, unclear, unsigned or undated.

The *Code of conduct* (NMC 2002) requires all registered nurses to ensure that no act or omission is detrimental to the interests of patients and in the document *Standards for records and record keeping* (UKCC 1993), which is abridged in Appendix 1, the UKCC states that 'keeping records is an essential and integral part of care and not a distraction from its provision'. The purpose of records is to:

- provide accurate information on the condition and care of patients
- record problems that arise and action taken
- demonstrate that nurses are meeting NMC requirements.

In general practice these standards are relevant to the following areas.

Assessment

- History and current situation
- Signs and symptoms
- Investigations and results
- Support or agencies involved

Action

- Care or action suggested, planned or taken
- Help or support offered
- Advice and information given

Patient response

- Agreement/refusal to suggested strategy
- Comments or information given

Referral

- Source of any advice sought and acted upon
- Referral to another member of PHCT
- Information on patient provided to other professional

Follow-up

- Planned return or recall
- Return as required by patient
- Appointment arranged with other agency or professional

Concerns

- Difficulty in obtaining advice/support/help and reason
- Missing or illegible notes
- Any concern expressed to other team members or to the patient

Should a nurse be required to account for actions or omissions months or even years after the event, accurate and complete records made at the time of the event would be necessary to justify the nurse's position. Records should focus on observations and facts rather than assumptions. For example, rather than recording in the notes that a patient was drunk, it would be more appropriate to state that the patient had an unsteady gait, slurred speech and that his or her breath smelled of alcohol. Poor records provide a poor defence, no records provide no defence.

Box 22.1 Summary of key points

Ensure records are:

- legible
- complete
- accurate
- focused on observations/facts
- dated
- signed.

PROTOCOLS

A protocol describes a sequence of activities which have been agreed beforehand. It does not outline a procedure for *how* to do something but instead describes the *why*, *what*, *where*, *when* and *by whom* involved in an area of practice.

Protocols can vary from surgery to surgery depending on the needs of the practice and the skills and resources available. They may take a variety of forms: they may, for example, refer to the assessment and diagnosis of self-limiting diseases, the review and management of chronic disease. In relation to the administration of prescription-only medicines, the authorization would need to be by means of patient group directions (NHSE 2000).

A protocol is not a document that is drawn up by one member of the team and then imposed on the others, although the initial draft for discussion may be delegated to an appropriate team member. It must then be negotiated and agreed to by all parties concerned, including nursing and medical staff. This negotiation allows a team to:

- set standards
- identify responsibilities
- define clear and agreed levels of competency
- support good practice
- plan appropriate training needs.

For example, a protocol for travel health will need to include:

- role of nurse and doctor
- risk assessment, e.g. date of travel, destination and stopovers, age, sex, medical history, medications, previous vaccinations, allergies, length of trip, reason for journey, etc.
- information source to be used
- health education advice to be given
- handouts to be used.

Once agreed, protocols can be used as a teaching tool for new staff and will improve record keeping. They should be reviewed annually and old protocols kept on file for 10 years as any complaint would be judged against usual practice and the practice protocol in use at the time. They also need to be reviewed and amended in response to new information or research evidence or if there is a change in circumstances such as staff changes. Protocols should be seen as an integral part of the audit cycle in that evaluation of the care given to patients may inform the planning of a protocol and will influence changes where necessary.

It is essential that nurses understand the implications of negotiating, agreeing and working to a protocol in relation to the NMC (2002) requirements on personal accountability, acknowledging any limitations in knowledge and competence and declining any responsibilities that exceed these.

PATIENT GROUP DIRECTIONS

The Medicines Act 1968 allows only doctors, dentists and vets to prescribe prescription-only medicines (POM). However, the Act allows others to administer POMs in accordance with the written or verbal direction of the medical practitioner. The law has been amended and the implications have been set out by the NHS Executive in Health Service Circular 2000/026 (NHSE 2000).

The legal term for group protocols for POMs is now patient group directions and health professionals who can supply or administer medicines under agreed patient group directions are nurses, midwives, health visitors, optometrists, pharmacists, chiropodists, radiographers, orthoptists, physiotherapists and ambulance paramedics. They can only do so as named individuals. The Medicines Control Agency will monitor compliance with amended legislation and failure to comply could result in a criminal prosecution under the Medicines Act (NHSE 2000).

HSC 2000/026 (NHSE 2000) has stated that black triangle vaccines may be included in patient group directions provided they are used in accordance with the schedules recommended by the Joint Committee on Vaccination and Immunization. Other black triangle drugs can be included in patient group directions as long as the use is justified by current best practice.

All parties involved in contributing to the care should be consulted and they should all sign a copy; a copy should then be available in the clinical setting in which it is used. The document should be dated and a review date set. The amendments to legislation have since confirmed the key aspects that must be included (Box 22.2).

It is possible to construct a proforma for the development of agreed protocols/patient group directions for the administration of POMs such as vaccines (see Box 22.3).

A review date of 2 years must be set after which the patient group direction will no longer be valid. Keep old copies on file in the practice in case of a patient complaint.

It can be useful to read through protocols on management of areas of care and patient group directions for administration and supply of POMs from other practices before constructing your own. However, as these may not reflect your practice's way of working, it is advisable to use them as examples rather than copying them.

Some practice nurses have lodged their protocols for areas of care such as asthma and patient group directions for POMs on the practice nurse email discussion list set up by Maresah Haines or the practice nurse website established by Elaine Campbell, for others to access and use as examples (see Chapter 21). There is also a useful website about protocols at www.groupprotocols.org.uk

Box 22.2 Particulars required for a lawful patient group direction

- Name of the business to which the direction applies
- Coming into force and expiry date
- Description of the medicine to which the direction applies
- Class of health professional to which the direction applies
- Signature of doctor or dentist and pharmacist
- Signature by appropriate health organization
- Clinical condition to which the direction applies
- Clinical criteria under which the patient is eligible for treatment
- Exclusions from treatment under the direction
- Circumstances in which further advice should be sought from a doctor or dentist and arrangements for referral
- Details of dosage, maximum dosage, quantity, strength, route, frequency and duration of administration
- Relevant warnings including potential adverse reactions
- Details of necessary follow-up action
- Record-keeping arrangements

Box 22.3 Example proforma patient group direction for a POM

Name and Address of Practice

Patient Group Direction for ....

1. Clinical situation

Clinical situation	
Aims and objectives	
National/local policies or guidelines	

2. Staff

Professional qualifications	
Additional training	
Continuing training	
Facilities and equipment available	

3. Patients

Inclusion criteria	
Exclusion criteria	
Action for excluded patients	
Action for those who refuse treatment	

4. Treatment

Name, dose, method, route of medicine	
Legal class (POM/P)	
Schedule	
Pt advice given pre or post vaccination (verbal and written)	
Follow-up treatment	
Identification and management of adverse reactions	
Reporting procedure of adverse reactions	
Arrangements for referral for medical advice	
Information recorded	

5. Management and monitoring

Date of protocol	
Review date	
Author of protocol	
Advice received from	
Authorized by: • PCT Clinical Governance Lead • HA Pharmaceutical Advisor • Dr All GPs	 Signed Signed
Agreed by: • Nurse All Practice Nurses	 Signed

Acknowledgement: this patient group directions proforma is based on an original protocol by Shelley Mehigan, Clinical Nurse Specialist in Family Planning, Berkshire.

References

Beauchamp TL, Childress JF 1989 Principles of biomedical ethics, 3rd edn. Oxford University Press, New York

Bolton Research Group 2000 Patients' knowledge and expectations of confidentiality in primary health care: a quantitative study. British Journal of General Practice 50: 901–902

General Medical Council 1999 Seeking patients' consent: the ethical considerations. General Medical Council, London

GMSC 1994 Practice nurses: training and delegation of duties. British Medical Association, London

MRC 2000 Personal information in medical research. Medical Research Council, London

NHSE 1999 The protection and use of patient information (Caldicott Report). NHSE, Leeds

NHSE 2000 Patient group directions (England only). HSC 2000/026. NHSE, Leeds

NMC 2002 Code of conduct. Nursing and Midwifery Council, London

RCGP 2000 Confidentiality and young people. RCGP/Brook, London

UKCC 1993 Standards for records and record keeping. UKCC, London

UKCC 1996 Guidelines for professional practice. UKCC, London

Law cases

1. Donoghue v Stephenson [1932] AC 562
2. Bolam v Friern HCC [1957] 2 All ER 582
3. Bolitho v City & Hackney HA [1997] 4 All ER 1151
4. Barnet v Chelsea and Kensington Hospital Management Committee [1969] 1 QB
5. Cassidy v Minister of Health [1951] 2 KB 343
6. St George's Healthcare NHS Trust v S: Rv Collins and Others ex parte S [1998] 2 FLR 728 CA
7. Re C (adult:refusal of medical treatment) [1994] 1 All ER 819
8. Re T (consent to treatment) 1992 2 FLR 458 CA
9. Gillick v West Norfolk and Wisbech Area Health Authority and another [1985] 3 All ER 402–437

APPENDIX 1 ABRIDGED VERSION OF THE DOCUMENT STANDARDS FOR RECORDS AND RECORD KEEPING (UKCC 1993)

This appendix is reproduced with the kind permission of the Nursing and Midwifery Council.

INTRODUCTION

1. The important activity of making and keeping records is an essential and integral part of care and not a distraction from its provision. There is, however, substantial evidence to indicate the inadequate and inappropriate record keeping concerning the care of patients and clients neglects their interests through:
   1.1 Impairing continuity of care.
   1.2 Introducing discontinuity of communication between staff.
   1.3 Creating the risk of medication or other treatment being duplicated or omitted.
   1.4 Failing to focus attention on early signs of deviation from the norm.
   1.5 Failing to place on record significant observations and conclusions.
2. For these reasons the Council has prepared this standards paper to assist its practitioners to fulfil the expectations it has of them and to serve more effectively the interests of their patients and clients.
3. To meet the standards set out in this document is to honour, in this aspect of practice, the Council's expectation (set out in the 'Code of Professional Conduct for the Nurse, Midwife and Health Visitor') (UKCC 1992) that:

   As a registered nurse, midwife or health visitor you are personally accountable for your practice and, in the exercise of your professional accountability, must:

   1. Act always in such a manner as to promote and safeguard the interests and well-being of patients and clients.
   2. Ensure that no action or omission on your part, or within your sphere of responsibility, is detrimental to the interests, condition or safety of patients and clients.

THE PURPOSE OF RECORDS

4. The purpose of records created and maintained by registered nurses, midwives and health visitors is to:
   4.1 Provide accurate, current, comprehensive and concise information concerning the condition and care of the patient or client and associated observations.
   4.2 Provide a record of any problems that arise and the action taken in response to them.
   4.3 Provide evidence of care required, intervention by professional practitioners and patient or client responses.
   4.4 Include a record of any factors (physical, psychological or social) that appear to affect the patient or client.
   4.5 Record the chronology of events and the reasons for any decisions made.
   4.6 Support standard setting, quality assessment and audit.
   4.7 Provide a baseline record against which improvement or deterioration may be judged.

THE IMPORTANCE OF RECORDS

5. Effective record keeping by nurses, midwives and health visitors is a means of:
   5.1 Communicating with others and describing what has been observed or done.
   5.2 Identifying the discrete role played by nurses, midwives and health visitors in care.
   5.3 Organising communication and the dissemination of information among the members of the team providing care for a patient or client.
   5.4 Demonstrating the chronology of events, the factors observed and the response to care and treatment.
   5.5 Demonstrating the properly considered clinical decisions relating to patient care.

STANDARDS FOR RECORDS – KEY FEATURES

6. In addition to fulfilling the purposes set out in paragraph 4, properly made and maintained records will:
   6.1 Be made as soon as possible after the events to which they relate.

6.2 Identify factors which jeopardise standards or place the patient or client at risk.
6.3 Provide evidence of the need, in specific cases, for practitioners with special knowledge and skills.
6.4 Aid patient or client involvement in their own care.
6.5 Provide 'protection' for staff against any future complaint which may be made.
6.6 Be written, wherever possible, in terms which the patient or client will be able to understand.

STANDARDS FOR RECORDS – ETHICAL ASPECTS

7. A correctly made record honours the ethical concepts on which good practice is based and demonstrates the basis of the professional and clinical decisions made.
8. A basic tenet of records and record keeping is that those who make, access and use the records understand the ethical concepts of professional practice which relate to them. These will include, in particular, the need to protect confidentiality, to ensure true consent and to assist patients and clients to make informed decisions.
9. The originator will ensure that the entry in a record that she or he makes is totally accurate and based on respect for truth and integrity.

STANDARDS FOR RECORDS – ESSENTIAL ELEMENTS

13. In order to fulfil the purpose stated in paragraph 4, to be effective and to meet the standards set out above, records must:
    13.1 Be written legibly and indelibly.
    13.2 Be clear and unambiguous.
    13.3 Be accurate in each entry as to date and time.
    13.4 Ensure that alterations are made by scoring out with a single line followed by the initialled, dated and timed correct entry.
    13.5 Ensure that additions to existing entries are individually dated, timed and signed.
    13.6 Not include abbreviations, meaningless phrases and offensive subjective statements unrelated to the patient's care and associated observations.
    13.7 Not allow the use of initials for major entries and, where their use is allowed for other entries, ensure that local arrangements for identifying initials and signatures exist.
    13.8 Not include entries made in pencil or blue ink, the former carrying the risk of erasure and the latter (where photocopying is required) of poor quality reproduction.
14. In summary, the record:
    14.1 Is directed primarily to serving the interests and care of the patient or client to whom the record relates and enabling the provision of care, the prevention of disease and the promotion of health.
    14.2 Will demonstrate the chronology of events and all significant consultations, assessments, observations, decisions, interventions and outcomes.
15. In hospitals or other institutions providing care, a local index record of signatures should be held. Where initials are regarded as acceptable for any purpose, these also should feature in the index, together with the full name in printed form.

THE 'PROCESS APPROACH' OR 'PLANNED INDIVIDUALISED CARE' APPROACH TO NURSING AND MIDWIFERY CARE

16. Given the nature of care plans and records associated with the planned individual care approach, this important aspect of records must satisfy the criteria specified in paragraphs 4–15 above. The 'process' approach assists a systematic approach to practice. It also provides a framework for the documentation of that practice. The term therefore describes the continuum of distinctly separate yet interrelated activities of practice, assessment, planning, implementation and evaluation of care.
17. Meticulous and timely documentation provides evidence of the practitioner's actions, the patient's or client's response to those actions and the plans and goals which direct the care of the patient or client.
18. The preparation and completion of care plans will, therefore, in addition to satisfying the criteria set out in paragraphs 4–15 above, demonstrate that each step in what is a continuing process has been followed and

provides the basis for further goal setting and actions.

19. The making of entries will be organised so that:
    19.1 A measurable, up-to-date, description of the condition of the patient or client and the care delivered can be easily communicated to others.
    19.2 The plan and other records complement each other.
20. The practitioner, in applying the process and using the plan, will distinguish between those matters which must be recorded in advance (such as planning and goals) and those which can only be current or slightly retrospective (such as observations and evaluation). Equally, the distinction must be made between entries on papers (for example, planning forms), which may not be locally retained, and other forms which are part of the clinical nursing or midwifery care records which record changes and events and must be retained.

THE LEGAL STATUS OF RECORDS AND ITS IMPLICATIONS

21. Any document which records any aspect of the care of a patient or client can be required as evidence before a court of law or before the Preliminary Proceedings Committee or Professional Conduct Committee of the Council (the UKCC) or other similar regulatory bodies for the health care professions including the General Medical Council, the comparable body to the UKCC for the medical profession.
22. For this, in addition to their primary purpose of serving the interests of the patient or client, the records should provide:
    22.1 A comprehensive picture of care delivered, associated outcomes and other relevant information.
    22.2 Pertinent information about the condition of the patient or client at any given time and the measures taken to respond to identified need.
    22.3 Evidence that the practitioner's common law duty of care has been understood and honoured.
    22.4 A record of the arrangements made for continuity of a patient's care on discharge from hospital.
23. Particular care will be exercised and frequent record entries made where patients or clients present complex problems, show deviation from the norm, require more intensive care than normal, are confused and disoriented or in other ways give cause for concern.
24. In situations where the condition of the patient or client is apparently unchanging, local agreement will be necessary in respect of the maximum time allowed to elapse between entries in patient or client records and the nature of those entries. All exceptional events, however, must be recorded and the Council will expect nurses, midwives and health visitors to exercise suitable judgement about entries in the record.
25. Ownership of the contents of a record would normally be seen as residing with the originator of any particular entry. In practice, however, where the professional practitioner is a salaried employee of the health services, the question of ownership turns on ownership of the document on which the record is made. Ownership does not rest with the patient or client, as the creation of law to grant patient or client access in certain circumstances clearly reveals.
26. Midwives must ensure that they are aware of and comply with the requirements in respect of records set out in the Council's 'Midwives' Rules'.
27. It is essential that members of the professions must be involved in local discussions to determine policies concerning the retention or disposal of all or any part of records which they or their colleagues make. Such policies must be determined with recognition of any aspects of law affecting the duration of retention and make explicit the period for which specific categories of records are to be retained. Any documents which form part of the chronological clinical care record should be retained.

PATIENT OR CLIENT HELD RECORDS

30. The Council is in favour of patients and clients being given custody of their own health care records in circumstances where it is appropriate. Patient or client held records help to emphasise and make clear the practitioner's responsibility to the patient or client by sharing any

information held or assessments made and illustrate the involvement of the patient or client in their own care.

31. Evidence from those places where this has become the practice indicates that there are no substantial drawbacks and considerable ethical benefits to be derived from patients or clients having custody of their records. This immediately disposes of any difficulties concerning access and reinforces the discipline that should apply to making entries in records.
32. A small number of instances will inevitably arise, where a system of patient or client held records is in operation, in which the health professional concerned will feel that her or his particular concerns or anxieties (for example about the possibility of child abuse) require that a supplementary record be created and held by the practitioner. To make and keep such a record can, in appropriate circumstances, be regarded as good practice. It should be the exception rather than the norm, however, and should not extend to keeping full duplicate records unless in the most unusual circumstances.

PATIENT OR CLIENT ACCESS TO RECORDS

33. With effect from 1 November 1991, patients and clients have had the right of access to manual records about themselves made from that date as a result of the Access to Health Records Act 1990 coming into effect. This has brought such records into line with computer held records which have been required to be accessible to patients since the Data Protection Act 1984 became operative.
34. These Acts give the right of access, but the health professional most directly concerned (which, in certain cases will be the nurse, midwife or health visitor) is permitted to withhold information which she or he believes might cause serious harm to the physical or mental health of the patient or client or which would identify a third party. The system for dealing with applications for access is explained in the 'Guide to the Access to Health Records Act 1990', published by the Government Health Departments (1990).
35. The Council fully supports the principle of open access to records contained in these Acts, and the guidance notes concerning their operation, and trusts that access will not be unreasonably denied or limited.
36. All practitioners who create records or make entries in any records must be aware of the rights of the patient or client in this regard, give careful consideration to the language and terminology employed and recognise the positive advantages of greater trust and confidence of patients and clients in the professions that can result from this development.

SHARED RECORDS

37. The Council recognises the advantages of 'shared' records in which all health professionals involved in the care and treatment of an individual make entries in a single record and in accordance with a broadly agreed local protocol. These are seen as particularly valuable in midwifery practice. The Council supports this practice where circumstances lend themselves to it and where relevant preparatory work has been undertaken. Each practitioner's contribution to such records should be seen as of equal importance. This reflects the collaborative and cooperative working within the health care team on which emphasis is laid by the Council in its 'Code of Professional Conduct for Nurse, Midwife and Health Visitor'. The same right of access to records by the patient or client exists where a system of shared records is in use. It is essential, therefore, that local agreement is reached to identify the lead professional to be responsible for considering requests from patients and clients for access in particular circumstances.

COMPUTER HELD RECORDS

38. The application of computer technology should not be allowed to breach the important principle of confidentiality. To say this is not to oppose the use of computer held records, whether specific to one profession or shared between professions. Practitioners must satisfy themselves about the security of the system used and ascertain which categories of staff have access to the records to which they are

expected to contribute important, personal and confidential information.

39. Where computer technology is employed it must provide a means of maintaining or enhancing service to patients or clients and avoid the risk of inadvertent breaches of confidentiality. It must not impose a limit on the amount of text a practitioner may enter if the consequence is that it impedes the compilation of a sufficiently comprehensive record. The case for it has to be considered in association with the questions of access, patient or client held records, shared records and audit. Local protocols must include means of authenticating an entry in the absence of a written signature and must indicate clearly the identity of the originator of that entry.

THE PRACTITIONER'S ACCOUNTABILITY FOR ENTRIES MADE BY OTHERS

40. Irrespective of the type of record or the form or medium employed to create and access it, the registered nurse, midwife or health visitor must recognise her or his personal accountability for entries to records made by students or others under their supervision.

SUMMARY OF THE PRINCIPLES UNDERPINNING RECORDS AND RECORD KEEPING

41. The following principles must apply:
    - 41.1 The record is directed primarily to serving the interests of the patient or client to whom it relates and enabling the provision of care, the prevention of disease and the promotion of health.
    - 41.2 The record demonstrates the accurate chronology of events and all significant consultations, assessments, observations, decisions, interventions and outcomes.
    - 41.3 The record and the activity of record keeping is an integral and essential part of care and not a distraction from its provision.
    - 41.4 The record is clear and unambiguous.
    - 41.5 The record contains entries recording facts and observations written at the time of, or soon after, the events described.
    - 41.6 The record provides a safe and effective means of communication between members of the health care team and supports continuity of care.
    - 41.7 The record demonstrates that the practitioner's duty of care has been fulfilled.
    - 41.8 The systems for record keeping exclude unauthorised access and breaches of confidentiality.
    - 41.9 The record is constructed and completed in such a manner as to facilitate the monitoring of standards, audit, quality assurance and the investigation of complaints.
42. Enquiries in respect of this Council paper should be directed to the:

    Registrar and Chief Executive,
    United Kingdom Central Council for
    Nursing, Midwifery and Health Visiting,
    23 Portland Place,
    London W1N 3AF

References

UKCC 1992 Code of Professional Conduct for the Nurse, Midwife and Health Visitor. UKCC, London

Government Health Departments 1990 Access to Health Records Act 1990: a Guide for the NHS. London

Chapter 23

Vulnerable adults and children

Tina Bishop

CHAPTER CONTENTS

INTRODUCTION

Over the past 25 years family violence has been recognized as a serious health and social problem. Traditionally some professionals have been regarded as more appropriately placed to identify and respond to the problem than others. Increasingly government policy now considers the abuse or mistreatment of any individual, irrespective of their age or status, as an issue of concern for society as a whole and all healthcare professionals in particular.

If we consider the fact that 97% of the population is registered with a general practitioner (Office of Health Economics 1994) it becomes apparent that the GP's list will include a substantial proportion of adults and children who are vulnerable and at risk of abuse by others.

GPs and practice nurses are actively involved with the practice population on a day-to-day basis. The role of practice nurses has expanded considerably in recent years and they now provide a comprehensive service to the practice population through baby clinics, screening, vaccination and immunizations, chronic disease management and health promotion clinics for all ages. Patients may be seen intermittently throughout their lives so trusting relationships can be built and maintained through this contact. There has been very little research examining the role of the practice nurse in recognizing and helping vulnerable people even though the potential is apparent.

The Department of Health has identified all health professionals as playing a key role in recognizing vulnerable individuals at risk of abuse and working in a multiprofessional way to meet their needs.

Family violence may be considered a public health issue requiring different ways of thinking about how we can help people to become and stay healthy. We can only estimate the numbers of people suffering, or at risk of, family violence due to the 'hidden' and 'silent' nature of the problem. Needs assessment and community profiling provide an opportunity for nurses to link with other professions, voluntary groups and the police to gain greater knowledge about the extent of the problem.

Clinical governance is the framework for health authorities and primary care trusts to identify health needs in order to develop appropriate, responsive services and interventions.

ROLE OF THE PRACTICE NURSE IN DEALING WITH VULNERABLE ADULTS AND CHILDREN

Practice nurses have traditionally focused on the practical hands-on approach to nursing care. However, all registered nurses, midwives and health visitors are personally accountable for promoting and protecting the interests of their patients/clients (NMC 2002).

Professional nursing encompasses a holistic approach to promoting health, which means acknowledging patients as individuals with a wide range of physical, emotional, social, cultural and spiritual needs. It is not enough to merely treat the results of abuse or mistreatment, nor is it acceptable to assume that recognizing victims of abuse is not part of the job and that somebody else, i.e. health visitor or social worker, is dealing with the problem.

CHILD ABUSE

Notions of the child and childhood have changed considerably over the years. In the Western world children no longer clean chimneys or work in factories and mills. Education and healthcare are freely available to all children in the UK. Attitudes and views concerning child rearing are influenced by many factors, not least our own childhood and family life. The family has also undergone tremendous change and various forms of parenting and family life are part of modern society. The family in whatever form can provide a loving, supportive and safe environment for children to develop and grow into mature and responsible adults. Many families provide this environment despite the stresses and strains of modern life. However, not all children are so lucky and many children are at risk of harm and/or neglect.

The National Society for the Prevention of Cruelty to Children reports that:

- each week at least one child dies following abuse and neglect. The vast majority of these children are killed by their parents or carers
- around 36 000 children are on child protection registers
- 26% of recorded rape victims are children.

There are many forms of child abuse and they are usually divided into four categories.

PHYSICAL ABUSE

Can range from overchastisement, slapping with the hand, a belt or any object, to shaking, punching or throwing a child across the room. Children have died as a result of deliberate physical injury by parents or other carers. This may also take the form of induced injury or fabricated illness (Munchausen's syndrome) by proxy.

NEGLECT

Can range from ignoring a child's development needs to not feeding, clothing or supervising him or her adequately.

SEXUAL ABUSE

The involvement of children or adolescents in sexual activities they may not understand, to which they cannot give consent and which are not acceptable to society. This includes inappropriate touching, obscene photographs and child pornography as well as attempted or actual sexual intercourse.

EMOTIONAL ABUSE

May include rejecting a child, refusing to show a child love or affection or deliberately making a child unhappy by continually belittling or verbally abusing him or her.

Although children witnessing domestic violence is not categorized as a form of child abuse:

> *Children who live in a battering relationship experience the most insidious form of child abuse. Whether or not they are physically abused by either*

parent is less important than the psychological scars they bear from watching their fathers beat their mothers. They learn to become part of a dishonest conspiracy of silence. They learn to lie to prevent inappropriate behaviours and they learn to suspend fulfilment of their needs rather than risk another confrontation. They expend a lot of energy avoiding problems. They live in a world of make-believe.

(Walker 1979)

RECOGNIZING ABUSE OR NEGLECT

Very few children get through childhood without occasionally falling over, falling off their bikes, etc. Cuts and bruises are usually seen on bony prominences such as foreheads, knees and shins. Practice nurses often provide treatment for minor injuries and should be aware of the possible indicators of non-accidental injuries and other signs of abuse.

Bruising

Uncommon sites for bruising include:

- back of legs and buttocks
- neck
- mouth, cheeks, ears and behind the ears
- stomach and chest
- under the arm
- genital and/or rectal area
- finger marks or bruising on the sides of the face, arms or chest.

NB: Mongolian spots, purplish blue markings commonly seen on the backs of black people, are not bruises.

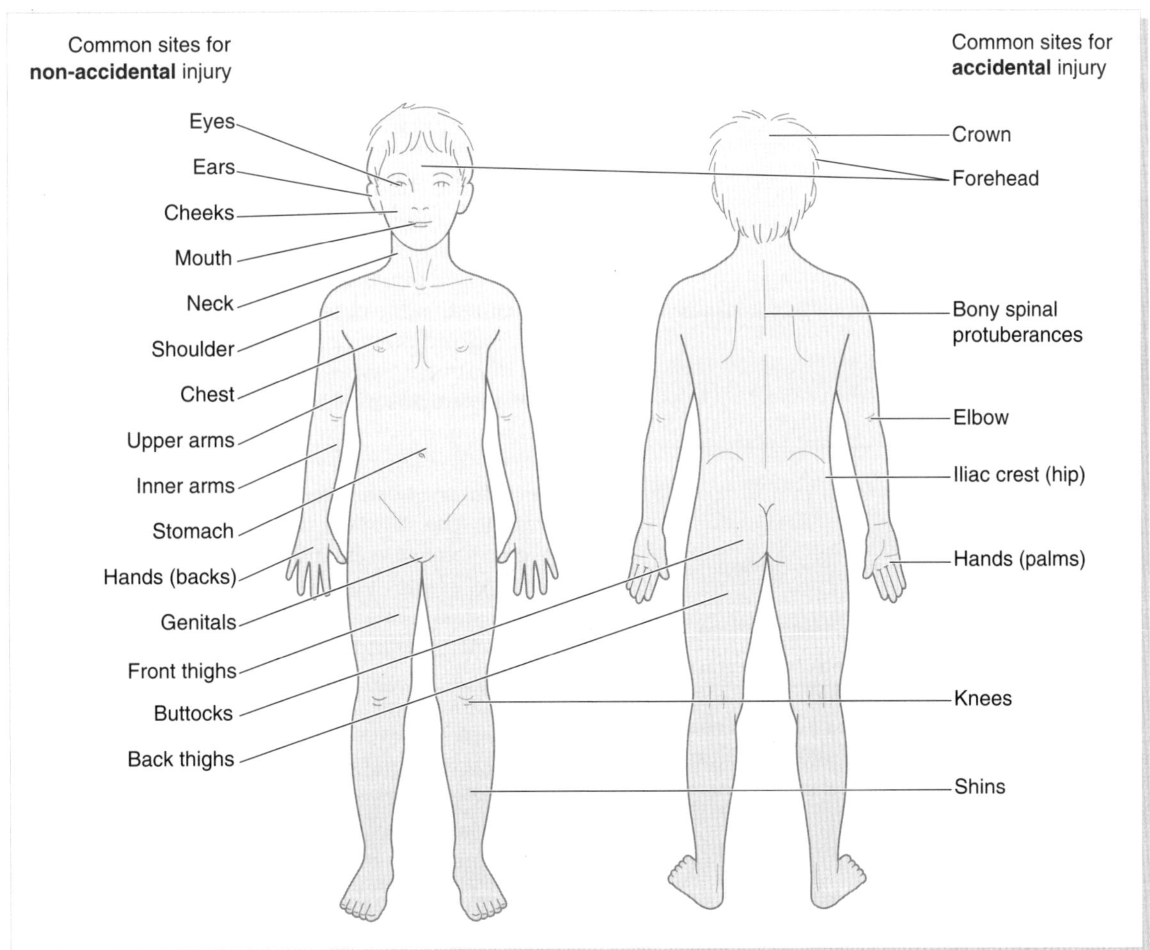

Figure 23.1 Common sites for accidental and non-accidental injury.

Bites

Human bite marks are oval shaped and can leave a clear impression on skin.

Burns and scalds

Splash marks are often accidental but lines may indicate non-accidental injury.

Fractures

It is very rare for a child under 1 year to sustain a fracture accidentally. X-rays may show old and/or multiple fractures.

Neglect

- Appears pale, listless and underweight.
- Regularly hungry.
- Evidence of poor hygiene, dirty, unkempt, dirty nappies or dirty clothes.
- Clothed inappropriately.
- Parents who fail to keep important appointments at school or at clinics.
- Developmental delay.

Sexual abuse

- Reluctance to undress or go to the toilet.
- Bleeding or soreness in the genital and/or rectal area.
- Knows a lot about sex for his or her age.
- Regressive behaviour such as bed wetting.
- Sad, withdrawn.
- Mood swings.

Emotional abuse

- Timid, withdrawn.
- Not putting on weight.
- Over- or underdemanding.

CHILD PROTECTION

The Children Act 1989 deals with the welfare of children. The Act does not use the term 'abuse' but introduces the concept of 'significant harm'. There are no absolute criteria on what constitutes significant harm.

The key principle of this Act is that the rights of the child are paramount.

Under S.31(9) of the Children Act 1989:

- 'Harm' means ill treatment or the impairment of health or development
- 'Development' means physical, intellectual, emotional, social or behavioural development
- 'Health' means physical or mental health
- 'Ill treatment' includes sexual abuse and forms of ill treatment that are not physical.

The local authority has a duty to make enquiries where it has reasonable cause to suspect that a child is suffering, or is likely to suffer, significant harm (DoH 1991).

The Department of Health document *Working together to safeguard children* (1999a) recommends that each primary care trust identifies a named doctor and a named nurse or midwife to take a professional lead within the trust on child protection matters. The doctor and nurse should have expertise in child welfare and child mistreatment and knowledge of the local arrangements for protecting children.

The document also states that GPs, practice nurses, practice managers and receptionists and any other staff should have training in child protection and have regular updates as part of their continuing professional practice. Marking the records of children who are on the at-risk register will raise awareness of members of the primary healthcare team. If practice nurses have suspicions or concerns about a child's welfare or a parent's or carer's ability to care for the child, they have a duty to report this to the GP and the appropriate named person who has responsibility for child protection.

It is good practice to develop a guideline/protocol to ensure that the necessary steps are taken to protect children and practice nurses should be familiar with this document.

Many nurses new to working in general practice will be unfamiliar with issues around child protection and regular joint meetings with other members of the primary healthcare team will be necessary to provide the support and development required to gain expertise in this sad and sensitive area of practice. Health visitors and social workers have a long history of working with child protection cases and joint training would offer the opportunity to develop interagency understanding of roles and responsibilities.

Communication and cooperation between professionals is essential to safeguarding children. Investigations into serious cases of child protection that have resulted in the death of a child reveal that communication between professional workers did not exist or had broken down (Marsland 1994).

The recent inquiry into the terrible suffering and appalling death of Victoria Climbié revealed that there were 12 occasions when local services had failed to intervene and protect her (HMSO 2002). The inquiry raised concerns that had previously been identified in other inquires, including:

- *poor communication and information sharing between professionals and agencies*
- *inadequate training and support for staff*
- *failure to listen to children* (RCN 2003).

Sharing information with other agencies can help to build a picture of what is going on.

RECORD KEEPING

Clear and concise record keeping is essential when undertaking a consultation concerning a child. Information recorded in children's notes should be straightforward accounts and descriptions; details where necessary can include drawings, measurements and other relevant information that may be disclosed. Records can be a source of evidence for an inquiry and may also be disclosed in court. Accurate record keeping can help professionals who have concerns about a child to track the course of events.

Box 23.1 Key points on child abuse

- Identify persons in the practice/primary care organization who take a professional lead in child protection.
- All practice nurses should receive education and training plus ongoing support and development in this area.

DOMESTIC VIOLENCE

In 1877 a man could beat his wife with a stick if it was no thicker than his thumb.

Domestic violence is usually defined as the physical, emotional or sexual abuse that occurs within a present or past relationship, usually (but not always) perpetrated by a man against a woman. In the past domestic abuse was not considered a violent act or a crime. Health professionals and the police considered that what goes on behind closed doors was private. Erin Pizzey challenged this notion in the 1970s when she opened a women's refuge for so-called 'battered wives' seeking safe shelter from a violent partner. The term 'battered wives' can be misleading; abuse may take many forms.

Table 23.1 Stages of healing in bruises

Colour	Age of bruise
Red to red-blue	Less than 24 hours
Purple to dark blue	1–4 days
Green to yellow-green	5–7 days
Yellow to brown	7–10 days
Disappearance	1–3 weeks

- *Physical*: pushing, shoving, punching, kicking, strangulation
- *Emotional*: threatening, humiliating, criticizing, verbal abuse, constant blaming or hectoring
- *Sexual*: rape/sexual assault, unacceptable sexual behaviour, being forced into sex without consent with partner or other
- *Economic*: withholding money, taking a woman's money, preventing financial independence

Some women may experience different forms of abuse on a frequent or infrequent basis. Domestic violence is a serious problem that can lead to fatal consequences. The statistics are staggering.

- Two women per week are murdered by a current or former partner (DoH 1999b).
- One in four women will experience domestic violence during their lifetime (DoH 1999b).
- Ninety percent of children in these households are in the same room or nearby when the violence occurs (DoH 2000a).
- One-third of children injured are trying to protect their mothers (Hughes et al 1987).
- Physical abuse often starts or is exacerbated when a woman becomes pregnant (DoH 2000a).

Myths surrounding domestic violence impede recognizing and dealing with the problem. Domestic violence occurs in any age, socio-economic and ethnic group (Mooney 1994).

Most victims of domestic violence do not report the problem to the police or the health services.

The Department of Health reports that a woman will consult health professionals 35 times before the abuse is revealed (DoH 1999) There are many reasons why women do not reveal domestic abuse, including shame, embarrassment, anxiety that their children may be taken into care, fear the situation may be made worse, guilty feelings that somehow they are responsible and feelings of helplessness that nothing can be done. The stigma attached to being a victim makes it hard for women to disclose their situation.

However, studies have shown that women consider general practice to be a safe place to discuss sensitive issues and that most women would talk about domestic violence if asked (DoH 2000a). Women will often present to A&E departments for help and studies have shown that staff training and the use of protocols can improve recognition of victims of domestic violence.

RESPONDING TO PATIENTS WHO SHOW SIGNS OF ABUSE

Women who experience domestic abuse may hint at or reveal their situation and any nurse has a duty to respond in the appropriate way.

Asking questions

In the US women are routinely questioned about domestic violence but this is not the case in the UK. Nurses may be reluctant to consider the possibility of domestic violence for numerous reasons.

- It may make the situation worse.
- Fear their suspicions may be unfounded.
- Personal knowledge of the victim and/or perpetrator.

Questions to ask women need to be developed locally within a multiagency framework to reflect regional and cultural needs (RCN 2000). The following questions have been suggested by the British Medical Association (1998).

- Do you ever feel afraid of your partner?
- Has your partner or ex-partner ever hurt or threatened you?
- Has your partner ever threatened or hurt your children?

It is not easy to ask questions about domestic violence, particularly if you do not know what you are going to do with that information. The Crime and Disorder Act 1998 expects the police, health authorities and other agencies to establish a local crime and disorder partnership in order to identify the degree of domestic violence at a local level. Recommendations are that all healthcare professionals should be given information and training about the nature and extent of domestic violence and the steps that should be taken to prevent further danger. Ongoing training should be specific to the practice in order to build up expertise in local arrangements and services. Multiprofessional/agency training is considered more likely to address the many dimensions of working with patients who are or have been victims of domestic violence.

The Department of Health (2000a) has produced a manual which outlines the issues of domestic violence, offers guidance on recognition of violence and makes recommendations on action.

Caution

Before practice nurses consider asking women about domestic violence, training, support, practice protocols and referral processes must be in place. Questioning by untrained staff, however well intentioned, may leave the women at risk of further violence.

Indicators of abuse

- Injuries to the breast, chest, abdomen and, particularly if pregnant, in the genital area.
- Multiple injuries in several areas including injuries to the head, neck and face.
- Bruising at different stages of healing which may indicate ongoing abuse.
- The woman may be nervous if her partner is present.
- Inconsistent accounts of injuries.
- Misuse of alcohol or drugs.
- Anxiety, stress or depression.
- Attempted suicide.
- Abused children.

What to do

Practice nurses have a professional duty to be competent in all aspects of their practice so increased knowledge of the subject is central to developing expertise. This may mean requesting training, updates and ongoing support in developing skills in this area of practice.

Ensure the practice promotes an environment where women can feel free to talk about violence.

- Display posters in women's toilets informing them they can talk about domestic violence to members of the practice team.
- Display posters that advertise where women can find support services, helplines, refuge centres, etc.
- Provide privacy for consultations; see the woman on her own.
- Listen carefully to what a woman has to tell you.

- Ask direct questions in a sensitive way.
- Reassure the woman about confidentiality; ask her permission before you share her story with others.
- Do not be judgemental and offer your own opinion about what you would do in a similar situation.
- If there are concerns about risks to children then the practice nurse has a professional duty to inform social services through practice protocols and guidelines.
- Ensure familiarity with your practice/trust guidelines/protocol. If none exist, then request that your practice develop a protocol.
- Consider the use of an interpreter and provide leaflets and posters in relevant languages.

RECORD KEEPING

Accurate and factual information should be recorded in the patient's notes. The date, time and signature should accompany all entries. The patient may decide to take action at some time in the future and accurate notes of past assaults and injuries would be beneficial to any legal proceedings.

Domestic violence can affect women in a number of ways and involve serious concerns affecting housing, finance, benefits and the police. It is unlikely that the practice nurse alone can offer the necessary ongoing support. Practice nurses are often isolated and support systems/clinical supervision may not be in place. Making decisions in this context may appear overwhelming. An agreed, structured, coordinating approach to identification and action for victims of domestic violence offers the opportunity to develop safe and effective practice.

Box 23.2 Key points on domestic violence

- Identify persons in the practice/primary care organization who have responsibility in this field.
- Request ongoing education, training and support.
- Identify local agencies and support groups in your area.

ELDER ABUSE

The abuse and mistreatment of elderly people gained prominence in the mid 1970s. Baker (1975) identified the existence of elder abuse, specifically as physical abuse to older women within the family. The term 'granny battering' was used to describe this violent action but it may be misleading. Elder abuse is defined by Action on Elder Abuse (1995) as:

'A single or repeated act or lack of action, occurring within any relationship where there is an expectation of trust, which causes harm or distress to an older person'.

Abuse of the older population does not appear to have attracted the same attention as other forms of abuse so reliable information on its incidence and prevalence is not available.

Older people are often viewed as a homogeneous group, stereotyped as powerless, dependent and needing help and support, with little to contribute to society. This negative view of older people can contribute to elder abuse through ignoring their needs and choices. Elderly people may share this negative view themselves which may prevent them reporting abuse.

The last UK national prevalence study was undertaken in 1992 and revealed that up to 5% of older people in the community were suffering from verbal abuse and 2% were the victims of physical or financial abuse (Ogg & Bennett 1992). Both men and women may be abused although the majority are female and many victims are physically and mentally frail.

Pritchard (2000) undertook a project in relation to the abuse of older women. She explored the needs of practitioners who work in this area and found that attitudes about working in this field were negative. Practitioners appeared to have insufficient knowledge about how to help patients. The tendency was for practitioners to 'rescue' victims rather than to consider other options.

Abuse may occur in many ways.

- *Physical*: hitting, pushing, slapping, restraining
- *Psychological*: shouting, swearing, frightening or humiliating a person
- *Financial*: the unauthorized use of the person's money, pension book or property
- *Sexual*: forcing a person into sexual activity without their consent
- *Neglect*: a lack of food, heating, clothing or comfort or essential medicine

The abuser may be a partner, child or relative, friend or neighbour, a volunteer worker, a health, social or other worker. The abuse may take place in the individual's own home, residential homes or hospital.

Demographic trends indicate a continuing rise in the number of older people. The 1990 Community Care Act, with the emphasis on caring for people at home, has put increasing pressure on some families to care for older people regardless of whether they can or wish to do so.

DEMENTIA

In 1998 it was estimated that 5% of the population aged 65 and over, and 20% of the population aged 80 and over, suffered from dementia. Dementia is a progressive disease of the brain, which leads to mental and physical disability. Individuals suffering from dementia can become increasingly disturbed. This can affect their behaviour in a number of ways, which include: confusion, aggression, forgetfulness, wandering, repetitive conversations, inappropriate behaviour and intolerance. Patients with dementia are among the most difficult and challenging people to care for.

The effects of dementia may mean a complete change of lifestyle for patients and their carers. The stress of caring for a person with dementia may be physically and mentally demanding and can contribute to the possibilities of mistreatment. Sleep may be disturbed, there may be a lack of time or opportunity for carers to do their own thing, physical abuse from the person who has dementia, feelings of isolation and guilt, lack of support. In addition, carers may be elderly themselves with health problems.

The Alzheimer's Disease Society suggests that the risk of mistreatment of these patients may be reduced if the condition is managed with openness and trust. Problems and difficulties should be discussed without judgement or prejudice with service providers.

Practice nurses will meet elderly patients for routine primary healthcare, over-75 health checks, flu vaccinations and chronic disease management. Providing over-75 health checks was a component of the 1990 GP Contract and this role has been undertaken by practice nurses in many instances. Routine screening for abuse or stress in elderly carers does not currently form part of this health check.

RECOGNIZING POSSIBLE SIGNS OF ABUSE

A wide range of indicators *may* suggest the possibility of abuse or neglect.

General signs

- Difficulty getting to see or interview the patient
- Repeated visits to general practice or A&E departments
- Request for help to different agencies or frequent transfers from one agency to another

Physical signs

- Bruising, particularly in well-protected areas, e.g. the inside of the thigh or upper arms
- Burns
- Unexplained fractures
- Unexplained/frequent falls or accidents

Psychological signs

- Depressed, sad, frightened, withdrawn, agitated
- Mood and/or behaviour change

Sexual signs

- Pain, itching in the genital or anal area
- Difficulty in walking or sitting
- Bruising or bleeding in genital/anal area

Signs of neglect

- Weight loss
- Unkempt appearance, dirty, poor hygiene
- Loss of or change to social activities

Recognizing abuse is the first step; the next is to determine the most appropriate intervention and who might provide this.

The National Service Framework for older people is an action plan to improve health and social services for older people. New national standards and models of care are set out for older people regardless of whether they live at home or in care. The focus is on:

- rooting out age discrimination
- providing person-centred care
- promoting older people's health and independence.

The *No secrets* document (DoH 2000b) advises that policies and procedures should be in place to protect vulnerable adults from abuse. Roles and responsibilities within and between agencies should be established. The need for practice nurses to work with other agencies is crucial to understanding the issues and developing practice and referral procedures.

Box 23.3 Key points on elder abuse

- Identify persons in the practice/primary care organization who have responsibility in this field.
- Request ongoing education and training.
- Establish multiagency links.

CONCLUSION

Protecting vulnerable adults and children from abuse involves the systematic collection and collation of data in order to assess the extent of the problem. Data from all agencies is essential so that a picture can be built across the locality. Many statutory and voluntary agencies have wide knowledge and expertise and have developed good practice guidelines and indicators. It would be foolish to ignore this expertise.

The appropriate training and supervision are required to integrate policy into practice. A well-planned and developed training strategy is a key requirement for promoting good practice. Training should extend from raising awareness right across to specialist courses to enable practice nurses to develop deeper and more specialist knowledge.

Primary care organizations have the responsibility of bringing together all agencies that can promote effective practice in this field. Practice nurses through their specialist knowledge can contribute to this ongoing development and should expect to be included.

References

Action on Elder Abuse 1995 Bulletin no. 11. Action on Elder Abuse, London

Baker A 1975 Granny bashing. Modern Geriatrics 5(8):20–24

BMA 1998 Domestic violence: a health care issue. British Medical Association, London

DoH 1991 Children Act: an introductory guide for the NHS. HMSO, London

DoH 1999a Working together to safeguard children. Stationery Office, London

DoH 1999b Living without fear: an integrated approach to tackling violence against women. Stationery Office, London

DoH 2000a Domestic violence: a resource manual for health care professionals. Stationery Office, London

DoH 2000b No secrets: guidance on developing and implementing multiagency policies and procedures to protect vulnerable adults from abuse. Home Office, London

HMSO 2002 The Victoria Climbié inquiry: report of an inquiry by Lord Laming. Stationery Office, London

Hughes H, Parkinson D, Vargo M 1987 Witnessing spouse abuse and experiencing physical abuse. Journal of Family Violence 4(2):197–209

Marsland L 1994 Child protection: the interagency approach. Nursing Standard 8(33):25–28

Mooney J 1994 The hidden figures: domestic violence in north London. Islington Council Police and Crime Prevention Unit, London

NMC 2002 Code of professional conduct. Nursing and Midwifery Council, London

Office of Health Economics 1994 Health information and the consumer. OHE briefing no. 30. Office of Health Economics, York

Pritchard J 2000 The needs of older women: services for the victims of elder abuse and other abuse. Policy Press/Joseph Rowntree Foundation, York

RCN 2000 Domestic violence: guidance for nurses. Royal College of Nursing, London

RCN 2003 Child protection – every nurse's responsibility. Guidance for nursing staff. RCN, London

Walker L 1979 Battered women. Harper and Row, New York

Resources

Child abuse – telephone helplines

Childline: 0800 1111
Children's rights: 0800 374860
NSPCC: 0800 800500

Domestic violence – telephone helplines

Rape Crisis:
National office: 020 7916 5466
24-hour helpline: 020 7837 1600
Women's Aid England:
National office: 0117 944 4411
24-hour helpline: 0845 702 3468
Women's Aid Northern Ireland:
National office: 028 9024 9041
24-hour helpline: 028 9033 1818
Women's Aid Scotland: 0131 475 2372
Women's Aid Wales:
National office: 02920 390874
24-hour helpline: 0870 599 5443

Elder abuse – telephone helplines

Age Concern: 0800 009966
Alzheimer's Disease Society: 020 7306 0606
Elder Abuse Response: 080 8808 8141

Websites

Action on Elder Abuse: www.elderabuse.org
Women's Aid: www.womensaid.org

Chapter 24

Employment issues

Josie Irwin Karen Didovich

CHAPTER CONTENTS

INTRODUCTION

Practice nurses work in a setting which is undergoing fundamental and radical change. The NHS Act 1999 introduced improvements to primary healthcare which are fundamentally altering the structure and characteristics of traditional community services. Ways in which primary care staff work are changing and so is the nature of their employment. Continuous change is more and more a feature of working in modern health services. This chapter describes the way practice nurses are employed currently, identifies employment issues and sets out best practice. It identifies changes in NHS structures and systems likely to impact on practice nurses and sets out some general principles for dealing with change in the workplace.

EMPLOYMENT WITH A GP PRACTICE

Practice nurses (PNs) are registered nurses. Most PNs are currently employed by general practitioners (GPs); some are employed by NHS trusts and a small minority are self-employed practitioners.

The number of PNs grew dramatically during the 1990s. Currently, about 22 041 PNs are employed in the UK. Many GP practices are therefore experienced in recruiting registered nurses. However, whether a GP practice has employed PNs already and is seeking to recruit to a vacant PN post or whether the practice is considering employing a PN for the first time, there is established good practice. This is set out below.

RECRUITING AND SELECTING A PRACTICE NURSE

DECIDING TO EMPLOY A PN

The first step for the practice is to determine what type of work will be required of the nurse and what facilities (equipment and space) the nurse will need to fulfil the role. Determining the activities required will assist in drawing up a job description and grading the post. It is a good idea to seek advice from other practices employing PNs, any PN already employed with the practice or the RCN.

The practice should consider the requirements of sex and race discrimination legislation. Advice on this can be sought from the Equal Opportunities Commission (EOC) or the Commission for Racial Equality (CRE), whichever is the most appropriate. Local offices of the Advisory, Conciliation and Arbitration Service (ACAS) also provide advice. The Department of Trade and Industry (DTI; website www.dti.gov.uk) is another useful source.

JOB DESCRIPTION

The information below is adapted from the RCN's *Guidance on the Employment of Nurses in General Practice*, April 1997.

A job description needs to be drawn up before advertising a post. This should identify the activities and tasks required from the person to be appointed and specify relevant experience and expertise. The job description is an important document as it ensures clarity for the PN about what may be expected of her and provides an important tool for reviewing performance for the manager.

The following points should be considered in formulating a job description:

- What is the job title? This should identify or 'label' the job appropriately.
- What is the purpose of the job? The objectives of the job should be stated in clear and unambiguous terms.
- What will the PN be expected to do? The activities involved and the way in which they are carried out should be detailed.
- What responsibilities will the postholder have? For example, responsibility for recommending or formulating policy in the practice or responsibility for managing resources, i.e. other staff or money.
- What are the work relationships for the post? Describe who the postholder will liaise with as she does her job. Who is she accountable to for her work?
- What are the conditions of employment for the job? What hours will the nurse be expected to work? What is the holiday entitlement? Practices will need to ensure that these conditions meet the requirements of the Working Time Regulations 1998. Many practices use the NHS terms and conditions handbook as a basis for the contract as this applies to nurses employed by NHS trusts. Details can be obtained from the Department of Health.

Once the job description has been prepared, it can be used to determine an appropriate grade and pay. It is important to remember that the job is graded, not the nurse. The current system used for most nurses is Clinical Grading (described below). A new system is currently being devised in the NHS under the heading Agenda for Change (this is also described briefly below).

GRADING AND PAY

In 1988, a new system of grading nurses was introduced nationally to ensure a fairer structure for determining nurses' pay. It is not a job evaluation scheme, however. The Clinical Grading scheme set out criteria which enable a nurse, midwife or health visitor's job to be placed on a scale which reflects the key attributes of that post, such as level of autonomy and skills required. While it has sometimes proved difficult to grade practice nurse posts according to the Clinical Grading criteria, as they were designed to be used within the NHS sector, Clinical Grading nevertheless provides a good general guide for grading nursing jobs. The RCN believes that practice nurse posts can be clinically graded, with most being F or G, with some nurses working at the higher H grade.

Key features of Clinical Grades F, G and H

Grade F PNs working at grade F will be able to assess the nursing needs of patients and provide appropriate care/treatment in conjunction with the GP or independently, as appropriate and according to practice policy, protocols, etc.

This nurse will be competent to deal with the general nursing care of the patient within the surgery.

Examples include wound care, ear syringing, eye washing, venepuncture, electrocardiography, management of skin disorders, recognizing mild childhood illnesses and giving immunizations and vaccinations.

The nurse will also assist in providing care to those patients with chronic diseases in addition to undertaking screening work such as cervical cytology.

The nurse will be able to document the assessment and care delivery processes. She will be able to evaluate the outcome of that care, making changes to the care plan for individual patients and modifying her practice with the patient.

PNs working at grade F will have a range of clinical skills developed through experience. They will undertake the delivery of nursing care in general practice as a self-directing practitioner, working with the GP to meet medical needs as appropriate.

Grade G PNs working at grade G will undertake similar activities to those described above. In addition, they could have the following responsibilities and attributes.

- Responsibility for meeting the nursing care needs of patients identified by the PN or identified by the GP and transferred to the PN.
- Responsibility for identifying care needs within the practice population by undertaking a practice profile or similar exercise and organizing work to best meet the needs identified.
- Ability to manage the nursing care of those patients with chronic disease, operating specific clinic sessions if needed, and maintaining an appointment and recall system for patients.
- Liaising with other members of the primary healthcare team and other agencies (such as local authority social services departments) to ensure that appropriate care is provided for the practice population.
- Involvement in policy development within the practice, and for overall practice management, providing the nursing input to any decision-making processes affecting the care of patients.
- Responsibility for teaching other PNs or other learners – for example, GP vocational trainers, new PNs, nursing students on a clinical placement, etc. – about care delivery from the perspective of an experienced nurse.
- Ability to demonstrate the rationale behind the various methods chosen to meet care needs of patients, to evaluate those methods and change them as necessary.

In summary, nurses working at grade G are responsible for ensuring that all nursing care delivered to the practice population is relevant, of a high standard and effective.

This nurse will work as a team member with the GP(s) to provide an optimum level of care delivery to patients, maintaining responsibility for the nursing components of that care.

This is a particularly appropriate grade for the nurse having expertise relevant to practice in the community.

Grade H PNs working at this level provide clinical advice and support to other professionals within the healthcare setting and to external agencies concerned with social issues. They provide clinical advice within the practice, participate in practice management and are responsible for developing clinical policies within the nursing field for the practice.

Responsibilities include making a specialist contribution to the teaching of other practice nurses; controlling admission to their own case lists; selecting, carrying out and interpreting the results of specific tests.

In addition, the nurse may qualify for H grade payments through carrying overall responsibility for the management of a number of localities where nursing care is delivered, for example several practices.

In this capacity, the nurse would demonstrate skills such as the development of care programmes, policy formulation, the supervision of nursing staff and ensuring high standards of care delivery.

In summary, the nurse would be seen as an 'expert' in nursing care delivery to patients in the practice. She will normally have direct clinical involvement in and extensive knowledge of a defined specialty, with evidence of postbasic study. She will be responsible for providing advice and support and liaising with other staff.

Pay

Once a job has been graded, it can be assigned a pay scale using the NHS pay scales, obtainable from the Department of Health. The RCN also reproduces the pay scales in leaflet form. Most GP practices pay their PNs the NHS rates including appropriate annual increments and uplifts.

Agenda for Change At the time of writing, work is ongoing to implement a new, modern pay system for the NHS. This is described briefly as the expectation that, as most GP practices pay PNs according to the NHS pay scales now, they will adopt the new pay and grading system once it is implemented. Discussions between primary care trusts and all NHS trade unions on implementation are ongoing.

There are certain elements of the package which are already widely accepted.

- There will be one single NHS job evaluation scheme to cover all NHS jobs with the exception of board-level posts. This means the Clinical Grading structure for nurses will be replaced and nursing jobs will be evaluated with reference to a new 16-factor job evaluation scheme. Unlike Clinical Grading, practice nurse posts have been tested within the job evaluation system and it will be possible to provide practices with an appropriate rank order for posts.
- There will be a set of 'core' NHS-wide conditions of service which will be the same for all staff. It is expected that as nurses form the largest group of staff in the NHS, terms and conditions will reflect those currently enjoyed by nurses.
- The new GMS contract will encourage practices to implement Agenda for Change.

Further details on how the RCN is supporting the implementation of Agenda for Change can be obtained from: www.rcn.org.uk/agendaforchange/

ADVERTISING PN JOBS

Using the nursing professional press, health service journals and/or the local press is recommended. To comply with equal opportunities good practice, posts should be properly advertised rather than by 'word of mouth'.

CONTRACT

A contract of employment exists as soon as a nurse starts work. An oral declaration of terms and conditions may have been made by the employer at interview and on taking the job the employee nurse and the employer are bound by those terms although it is far better for the particulars of a job to be written in a formal contract. In any case, the employee must by law (Employment Relations Act 1999) receive a written statement of the main terms of employment and an indication of disciplinary and grievance procedures within 2 months of starting work. Practice nurses who work part time have the same employment rights as those working full time.

ACCOUNTABILITY

MANAGERIAL ACCOUNTABILITY

There is a managerial relationship between the GP and a practice nurse – the nurse is accountable to the GP. This is managerial accountability and different from being professionally accountable. In carrying out instructions, the practice nurse should have regard to what is 'reasonable'. The nurse's judgement of what is reasonable should also include consideration of the professional code of conduct.

PROFESSIONAL ACCOUNTABILITY

Nurses have two main reference points for professional accountability. These are the *Code of professional conduct* and the *Scope of professional practice*. Both are issued by the Nursing and Midwifery Council (formerly the UKCC).

The Council is responsible for maintaining the standards of the profession and the *Code of professional conduct* is a binding document, which must be adhered to. Transgression can risk a finding of professional misconduct. Yet these documents are not intended to be a rule book but rather a framework for nurses to develop their practice in order to meet the needs of their patients/clients.

Nurses should remember that there is no such thing as vicarious professional accountability. The individual nurse, regardless of employment situation or geographical location, is responsible for her actions. It is for individual nurses to determine the scope of practice, the limits to the work they will take on and to be sure that they are actually competent to undertake that work.

If nurses are asked to undertake duties which they feel they have not been prepared for, then they must refuse to carry out such activities.

PENSIONS

Practice nurses were admitted to the NHS pension scheme on 1 September 1997. The NHS pension scheme provides an inflation-proofed pension. PNs have since gained the right to the same enhanced redundancy package enjoyed by other scheme members and the right to retire at 55 provided by special class status. The NHS pension scheme does not identify PNs separately so it is not known exactly how many PNs have joined but some 85 000–90 000 GP practice staff have joined the scheme to date. Details about the pension scheme can be obtained from the NHS Pension Scheme, which has offices in Fleetwood (England and Wales), Edinburgh and Belfast.

A contentious issue for PNs has been buying back added years at a reduced rate. PNs can buy back additional years in the scheme to make up for the years they were excluded but not at the reduced rate they would like and for which they have campaigned vigorously. The government opened the NHS pension scheme to GP practice staff as a special concession. To permit the 90 000 staff to purchase additional years at a special reduced rate would incur unacceptable costs to the Treasury.

EMPLOYMENT PRACTICE

Practices should be aware of the provisions of current employment legislation. ACAS and the DTI are useful sources of information and advice. Employees have rights, for example on disciplinary matters, which includes the right to be accompanied by a trade union official in a disciplinary investigation or formal hearing. There is a right to maternity leave, which has been extended from 14 weeks to 18 weeks, aligning it with statutory maternity pay, and a right to extra (unpaid) maternity leave of up to 40 weeks for those employed by an organization for 1 year or more. There is also an additional right to 'reasonable' time off for family emergencies.

It is good practice for an employer to have policies in place supporting:

- recruitment and selection
- health and safety
- pay and conditions
- equal opportunities
- grievance and disciplinary matters
- training.

Again, ACAS is a very useful source of practical guidance and model employment policies.

HEALTH AND SAFETY

Everyone has a right to a working environment that is safe and healthy and will not harm the staff, patients or other members of the public who are likely to use the premises. There is extensive legislation covering health and safety dating back to 1974 and the Health and Safety at Work etc. Act, which specified the duties of employers and employees. This all-embracing act has been extended by further regulations, many of which have been based on European Directives. Practice nurses as employees have rights and responsibilities in relation to health and safety, as follows.

- *A right to a safe working environment.* This extends to the physical and psychosocial aspects of the workplace. PNs have a right to work in a safe workplace. They also have a responsibility to ensure the workplace is safe, ensuring hazards are drawn to the attention of practice managers if they cannot deal with them. Physical hazards may be obvious, such as trailing leads that create a tripping hazard or exposure to chemicals such as glutaraldehyde. The physical environment also includes fire precautions, heating, lighting and ventilation. Psychosocial aspects are often associated with stress. Workloads and long hours should be reviewed regularly as they can lead to ill health.
- *A right to safe equipment, adequate for the job and properly maintained.* This could cover any equipment needed for patient handling, slides, autoclaves and electrical equipment. Health and Safety (Display Screen Equipment) Regulations 1992/2792 apply to workstations, screens and keyboards, aimed at preventing musculoskeletal and perceptual problems which could result from incorrect use of display screen equipment.
- *A right to safe systems of work.* There should be procedures for the safe disposal of clinical waste, including sharps, so that neither staff nor patients are put at risk. Procedures for spillages of substances such as mercury or body fluids should be defined. In dispensing practices, dispensers must be trained in health and safety aspects of formulation and if medication such as cytotoxic drugs are used, special handling precautions will be needed. Storage arrangements for medications, vaccines, specimens, food or other substances such as disinfectants must be made clear.
- *A right to free use of personal protective equipment when necessary.* Equipment must be fit for the purpose and must not create any additional risk for the wearer. Gloves provided to protect against infection must be powder-free latex gloves with a level of protein which is lower than 50 μg/g and where any residual accelerator is non-detectable. Powdered latex gloves are a hazard as they increase exposure to latex proteins and could lead to latex allergy (see Further reading).

- *Information about the practice safety policy.* Premises with more than five employees are required to have a written safety policy setting out a statement of intent and commitment to the protection of staff, patients and others on the premises along with the arrangements for achieving this.
- *First aid in the event of an accident.* Even though practices provide primary care, suitable arrangements must be in place for first aid. This includes having a nominated person to take charge in an emergency, a first aid box and a notice informing staff who the trained first aider or appointed person is and the location of the first aid box. The needs of patients must be considered so that staff know what to do in the case of sudden collapse of patients.
- *Welfare.* Legislation covers general well-being at work, requiring protection from exposure to passive smoking. It also covers access to occupational health advice. Practices need to consider how occupational health advice may be needed, particularly if the nurse is also a patient in the practice. Ensuring welfare also includes arrangements for immunization such as hepatitis B.
- *Consultation.* Nurses are entitled to be consulted about anything in the practice that has an impact on health and safety.
- *Accidents.* If an accident does occur, a record must be made in an accident book so that it can be investigated and remedial action taken to prevent a recurrence. Certain categories of accident must be reported to the Health and Safety Executive and these are defined in the Reporting of Injuries and Dangerous Occurrences Regulations 1995.

Risk assessment

A key aspect in managing a safe working environment is risk assessment. This is an important requirement of the Management of Health and Safety at Work Regulations 1992. Risk assessment provides a solid basis for safe systems of work and the elimination of hazards. PNs are likely to have a role in assessing risk in their workplace.

A basic risk assessment should cover the following which is not a comprehensive list but should provide a guide.

1. *Look for hazards.* These may be identified by inspecting accident records, personal observation and/or discussion with other staff. Possible hazards may exist because of the fabric of the building, worn flooring, heating or ventilation problems, for example. Security could be a problem because of uncontrolled access, particularly at times when there are few staff on the premises.
2. *Decide who might be harmed by any hazard and how.* The assessment should cover both staff and patients and others who may be visiting the premises, such as contractors. Patients may be more likely to trip in unfamiliar surroundings or because of their medical condition. Unguarded radiators could be a hazard for older people or children. Staff who go out on home visits may encounter problems in patients' homes, such as aggression from patients or relatives, hostile animals or unhygienic conditions.
3. *Evaluate the risks arising from the hazard.* An evaluation is likely to combine an assessment of the severity of damage that could occur and of the likelihood that it will occur. For example, if the flooring in the reception area is worn and causes people to trip up, then there is a high likelihood that an accident will occur and the injury could be substantial. The assessment would give this a high priority for action. Another example relates to systems of work – is the system for waste disposal adequate? Another example could be personal safety – are staff trained in dealing with aggressive patients?
4. *Record the findings.* This is a legal requirement if the practice has more than five employees. The record should show the identified hazards, who could be affected, the precautions to be taken or already in place and any further action required. A regular review and updating will be necessary to monitor progress and take any remedial action.
5. *Assess the effectiveness of risk control.* Risk assessment is an ongoing activity in maintaining safety standards. If accidents continue to occur then a reassessment is needed to eliminate the hazard or implement better control. Changes to the practice, such as new services, new equipment or new staff, should trigger a review.

Risk assessment is not an end in itself and it is likely that it will reveal weaknesses in the current systems and the working environment. There is an obligation to implement the results of the risk assessment and to have effective arrangements in place to plan, organize and control health and safety systems.

Other key requirements in the Management Regulations which are the duty of the employer are as follows.

- *Provide health surveillance where necessary.* This would normally be carried out by an occupational health practitioner with expertise in workplace conditions which can cause ill health.

- *Appoint one or more competent persons* to assist in meeting the requirements of health and safety legislation.
- *Provide employees with comprehensible and relevant information* on any risks to their health and safety and the measures that are being taken to control them.
- *Provide health and safety training* for new staff as part of their induction and if there is change, for example new equipment, new technology or new systems.
- A specific risk assessment is needed where *women of childbearing age or new or expectant mothers* may be at risk from either a physical, chemical or biological agent. If the risks cannot be controlled the employer must alter the working conditions or hours of work. If this is not possible the employee must be suspended but continue to receive pay.

PNs have duties as employees under health and safety legislation. They have responsibility not to put themselves or others at risk by any actions that they take or fail to take; they must cooperate with the employer by adhering to procedures that have been put in place. In addition, they must report to the employer if there are any situations of serious and imminent danger or any shortcomings in the arrangements for health and safety.

INSURANCE

GPs should carry insurance to protect themselves from mistakes made in the treatment of patients. This is usually provided by one of the medical defence organizations and may include the provision to indemnify employees of the GP. Additionally, practices should have employers' liability insurance which covers their employees for accidents at work. If a nurse takes on home visiting as part of her role, it must be clear that her workplace has been extended to include travelling to and visiting patients in their own homes.

CAR MILEAGE ALLOWANCE

Practice nurses may be required to make journeys on official business as part of their work. Car mileage rates are contained in the NHS terms and conditions obtainable from the Department of Health and issued by the RCN.

CHANGE AND GOOD PRACTICE

Continuous change is more and more a feature of working in modern health services. PNs may be required to work differently within a practice, for example in a team with different professions or with nurses and other professions from a primary care trust or local authority social services. Change is best achieved with the full involvement and participation of staff. PNs affected by change should be involved at the outset in planning and developing changes in practice.

If new ways of working require changes to a PN's terms and conditions of employment, for example longer or different working hours, employment law requires that a contract of employment cannot be changed without the agreement of the individual. This means if a practice proposes any change to terms and conditions, relevant staff must be consulted and must agree to the change. Failure to do this risks a claim for unfair dismissal at an employment tribunal. Staff are entitled to seek advice and representation from their trade union.

Change may involve a merger with other GP practices. In these circumstances, staff are protected by the Transfer of Undertakings (Protection of Employment) Regulations 1978 (TUPE). TUPE protections require both the transferor and transferee to consult transferring staff, who are entitled to retain their existing terms and conditions intact. Again, best practice shows that transfers are smoother if staff are fully involved and participate. PNs affected by merger and transfer should be involved at the outset in consultation.

Resources

Useful addresses

Advisory, Conciliation and Arbitration Service (ACAS), Brandon House, 180 Borough High Street, London SE1 1LW. Tel: 020 7210 3613.

Commission for Racial Equality (CRE), Elliot House, 10–12 Allington Street, London SW1E 5EH. Tel: 020 7828 7022.

Department of Health, Quarry House, Quarry Hill, Leeds LS2 7UE. Tel: 0113 545500.

Department of Trade and Industry (DTI). Tel: 020 7215 5000. Website: www.dti.gov.uk.

Equal Opportunities Commission, Overseas House, Quay Street, Manchester M3 3HN. Tel: 0161 833 9244.

NHS Pension Scheme, Hesketh House, 200–220 Broadway, Fleetwood, Lancs FY7 8LG. Tel: 01253 774774.

Nursing and Midwifery Council, 23 Portland Place, London W1N 3AF. Tel: 020 7637 7181.

Legislation

Employment Relations Act 1999

Health and Safety at Work etc. Act 1974

Health and Safety (Display Screen Equipment) Regulations 1992/2792

Reporting of Injuries, Diseases and Dangerous Occurrences Regulations 1995/3163

Management of Health and Safety at Work Regulations 1992/2051

Transfer of Undertakings (Protection of Employment) Regulations 1978 (TUPE)

Further reading

RCN 1997 Guidance on the employment of nurses in general practice. Royal College of Nursing, London

RCN 1998 Losing your touch? Avoid latex allergy. Royal College of Nursing, London

Chapter 25

Health and safety

Julia Lucas

CHAPTER CONTENTS

INTRODUCTION

There is now extensive legislation dating back to 1974 covering health and safety, which specifies the duties of employers and employees in ensuring a safe working environment. The Act in itself was comprehensive, but it has been further extended by regulations, many of which are based on European directives. The Health & Safety Commission and the Health & Safety Executive (HSE) are the bodies responsible for disseminating information and monitoring the implementation of the Act.

The Act imposes the following duties on employers.

- Ensure a safe system of work.
- Ensure safe premises for employees and visitors.
- Ensure the safe handling of medicines.
- Provide information, instruction and supervision for employees on health and safety measures.
- A practice with more than five employees must provide a policy statement for the staff.
- Staff must be trained properly to use the equipment.

In 1992 six further sets of regulations were added (HSE 1992).

- Health and safety management
- Work equipment safety
- Manual handling of loads
- Workplace conditions
- Personal protective equipment
- Display screen equipment

These came into force on 1 January 1993 and are in line with European Community directives on health and safety at work.

The working environment must be safe and healthy and ensure that neither staff, patients nor members of the public who use the premises come to any harm. Practice nurses as employees have duties under health and safety legislation not to put themselves or others at risk by any actions that they take or fail to take. They have a responsibility to adhere to procedures that have been put in place by the employer and must report to them any situations of serious or imminent danger or any shortcomings in the arrangements for health and safety.

RISK MANAGEMENT IN GENERAL PRACTICE

GENERAL PRINCIPLES OF RISK ASSESSMENT

All employers and self-employed persons are required to assess the risks to workers and any others who may be affected by their undertaking. Employers with five or more employees must also record the significant findings of that assessment.

Many employers already carry out de facto risk assessments on a day-to-day basis during the course of their work; they will note changes in working practice, they will recognize faults as they develop and they will take necessary corrective actions. However, the regulations require that employers should undertake a systematic examination of their work activity and that they should record the significant findings of that risk assessment.

A risk assessment should involve identifying the hazards present in any undertaking (whether arising from work activities or from other factors, e.g. the layout of the premises) and then evaluating the extent of the risks involved, taking into account whatever precautions are already being taken.

- *A hazard* is something with the potential to cause harm (this can include substances or machines, methods of work and other aspects of work organization).
- *Risk* expresses the likelihood that the potential harm from a particular hazard will be realized.
- *The extent of the risk* covers the population which might be affected by a risk, i.e. the number of people who might be exposed and the consequences for them.

PURPOSE OF RISK ASSESSMENT

The purpose of the risk assessment is to help the employer or self-employed person to determine what measures should be taken to comply with their duties under the relevant statutory provisions. This phrase covers the general duties in the Health and Safety at Work etc. Act 1974 (HSW Act) and the more specific duties in the various Acts and Regulations associated with the HSW Act.

- Identify hazards
- Identify those at risk
- Evaluate risks
- Decide on measures
- Record assessment

RISK IN THE GENERAL ENVIRONMENT

- Practice buildings
- Security of the building
- Audit of practice service
- Security
- Control of Substances Hazardous to Health (COSHH) Regulations
- Reporting of accidents and incidents in the workplace
- Occupational health and immunization programme
- Infection control, policies and protocols
- Compliance with HSW Act

EMPLOYER DUTIES

It is the duty of every employer to ensure, so far as is reasonably practicable, the health, safety and welfare at work of all employees. Included in this duty are:

1. the provision of systems of work which are safe and without risk
2. ensuring the safe handling, storage, transport, use of articles and substances, which may include:
   - handling of specimens
   - safe storage and use of disinfectants
   - guidelines and training on the use of sterilizers
   - safety when handling and administering vaccines
   - correct disposal, storage and ultimate incineration of clinical waste.

PATIENT-RELATED RISK

With the ever-increasing variety of services being provided by general practice today, there is also likely to be an increase in the risk exposures to the patient.

- Increasingly sophisticated procedures being performed in the surgery.
- An increase in the number of surgical wounds being seen in the practice related to the earlier discharge of patients from hospital.
- A greater number of patients with chronic health problems being treated in the surgery rather than in hospital.
- Requirements of the Patient's and Practice Charters.
- Handling complaints regarding high-quality clinical record keeping and secure storage of data to comply with the Data Protection Act.

HEALTH AND SAFETY POLICY

A further statement of policy specific to the practice should exist, signed by the responsible partner, which has been developed after discussion with all members of staff or their representatives, and which includes the following information.

1. The arrangements that have been made to:
   - identify hazards to health and safety
   - assess and control risks.
2. The person responsible for making the arrangements described above.
3. The person responsible for ensuring that the policy is implemented.
4. The intervals at which the policy is reviewed and updated.
5. The procedure for reporting accidents and dangerous occurrences.
6. How the policy is updated and by whom when circumstances change, e.g. new equipment.

ACCIDENT REPORTING PROCEDURE

All practices should have a system for the reporting and investigation of accidents and injuries in the workplace. This should comply with the Reporting of Injuries, Diseases and Dangerous Occurrences Regulations 1985 (RIDDOR) which came into effect in April 1986. Injuries, diseases and occurrences in specified categories have to be notified to the environmental health department of the local authority. Failure to do so is a criminal offence.

Notification of an event should be made immediately by telephone, if any of the following occur.

- Fatal injuries to employees or other people in an accident connected with the practice.
- Major injuries to employees or other people connected with the practice.
- Any of the dangerous occurrences listed in the regulations.

The notification should be followed by a written report within 7 days. Additionally a written report should be made of:

- any other injury to an employee which results in absence from work for more than 3 days, including days that would not normally be working days
- any of the following cases of ill health: exposure to toxic chemicals, occupational asthma, any illness caused by a pathogen.

EMPLOYEES

All practice staff must inform the practice manager or other nominated person of all accidents at work.

PROCEDURE

The reporting, recording and investigating of accidents, incidents and near accidents form an essential part of both good management practice and the legal responsibility of employers. From the information gathered, trends can be highlighted which may indicate the need for management intervention. Everybody has an important role to play in ensuring that accidents are eliminated. It is therefore important that all employees cooperate in the successful implementation of the accident reporting procedure.

1. When an accident or other untoward occurrence occurs the incident should be reported immediately to the employee's department manager/most senior colleague.
2. An accident form should then be completed by the department manager/most senior colleague.
3. The Health and Safety Officer should be notified.

4. An investigation should then be commenced in conjunction with the relevant health and safety nominee.
5. Report of investigation to the Health and Safety Officer.
6. Urgent action to be coordinated by the Health and Safety Officer.
7. Where appropriate, the Health and Safety Officer will report accidents as necessary to the HSE by the quickest possible means, confirming within 10 days on the appropriate forms.
8. All accident forms are discussed at the next health and safety meeting following the incident. A copy should be held on the personal file of the individuals concerned. An event such as this might be the topic of a 'critical incident meeting' at the practice.

A summary of the Reporting of Injuries, Diseases and Dangerous Occurrences Regulations 1985 (RIDDOR) is in Section 7 of the Health and Safety Handbook.

FIRST AID

Under the Health and Safety (First Aid) Regulations 1981, workplaces must have first aid provisions. These will depend on factors such as the nature and degree of hazards in the workplace. There is no obligation to have trained first aiders, particularly in a general practice setting where medical staff are normally close at hand. However, there should be a nominal appointed person to take charge of any accident, to ensure that an ambulance is called, if necessary, and that the accident is reported.

FIRST AID BOX

A first aid box should be provided, as it is not good practice to rely on treatment room first aid supplies. It should contain:

- a guidance card on resuscitation
- individually wrapped sterile adhesive dressings (various sizes)
- individually wrapped triangular bandages
- medium-sized individually wrapped sterile unmedicated wound dressings (approximately 10 × 10 cm)
- large sterile individually wrapped unmedicated wound dressings
- other wound dressings
- safety pins
- sterile eye pads with attachments.

First aid boxes should not contain medications of any kind.

A first aid record book should be kept with the box, together with a list of contents. The person responsible for first aid should check the contents of the box monthly and all practice staff must know where it is kept.

CONTROL OF SUBSTANCES HAZARDOUS TO HEALTH REGULATIONS

The Control of Substances Hazardous to Health Regulations 1994 (COSHH) set out a legal framework for the management of health risks from exposure to hazardous substances used at work. They aim to prevent occupational ill health by encouraging employers to assess and prevent or control risks from exposure to hazardous substances in a systematic and practical way.

The regulations apply to most hazardous substances. Those most likely to be encountered in the general practice setting include certain cleaning fluids, phenolics, formaldehyde and glutaraldehyde used as chemical disinfectants, clinical waste and pathological specimens containing pathogenic organisms.

The basic principles of occupational hygiene underlie the COSHH regulations. These include:

- assessing the risk to health arising from work and what precautions are required. This will usually need to be recorded in writing
- introducing measures to prevent or control exposure
- ensuring that control measures are used, equipment is properly maintained and procedures observed
- monitoring where necessary the exposure of employees and carrying out a suitable form of health surveillance where appropriate
- informing, instructing and training employees about the risks and the precautions to be taken.

VDU HEALTH AND SAFETY REGULATIONS

Working with VDUs can lead to musculoskeletal problems, eye fatigue and mental stress which can be overcome by good ergonomic design of equipment, furniture, the working environment and the task performed. The regulations cover employees who habitually use the VDU as a significant part of normal work.

- The VDU workstations should be assessed and risks identified and reduced.
- Workstations must satisfy minimum requirements set for the VDU itself regarding keyboard, desk and chair, working environment, task design and software.
- VDU work should be planned so that there are breaks or changes in activity.
- Information and training should be provided for VDU users.
- Eye and eyesight tests should be available if requested.

Display screen

- Check that the image on the screen is stable, with no flickering or other forms of instability.
- The brightness and/or contrast between the characters and the background must be easily adjustable.
- The screen must swivel and tilt easily.
- The screen should be free of reflective glare and reflections liable to cause discomfort.

Keyboard

- The keyboard is tiltable and separate from the screen.
- The space in front of the keyboard is sufficient to provide support for the user's forearms.
- The keyboard has a matt surface to avoid reflective glare.

Work desk or work surface

- The work desk or work surface should be sufficiently large, with a low reflective surface.
- The document holder should be stable and adjustable and positioned to minimize the need for uncomfortable head and eye movements.

Chair

- The chair must be stable and allow easy freedom of movement and a comfortable position.
- The seat should be adjustable in height.
- The seat back should be adjustable in both height and tilt.
- A footrest should be available.

Space requirements

The workstation should be designed to provide sufficient space to change position and vary movements.

Lighting

Room lighting and/or spot lighting (work lamps) should be satisfactory.

Reflection and glare

- Workstations are positioned so that sources of light, such as windows, cause no direct glare and, as far as possible, no reflections on the screen.
- The light from windows can be reduced by curtains or blinds.

Heat

Equipment belonging to the workstation must not produce excessive heat which causes discomfort.

Noise

Noise should be minimized.

Safety

No tripping hazards or other safety risks.

IMMUNIZATION OF STAFF

In August 1993, Health Circular HSG(93)40, 'Protecting health care workers from hepatitis B', was issued, strongly urging all general practitioners and practice nurses to ensure that they have immunity to hepatitis B. Vaccination should be offered to all staff, including cleaners, likely to be in contact with body fluids or clinical waste.

PREVENTIVE MEASURES

All practices should have a policy on the prevention of needlestick injuries and this is a clear requirement under the COSHH Regulations.

Preventive measures should include having a policy on hepatitis immunization for clinical staff and blood testing to check immunity levels. This should include action to be taken in the case of staff who do not develop adequate immunity after a standard course of immunization. (Serum should be tested for hepatitis B antigens and if staff are found not to be carriers then they should be given further immunization. If they are found to be carriers they should be counselled and excluded from invasive procedures.)

It is important that an immunization record card, including antibody titres, is kept for all practice staff. Staff coming into contact with antenatal patients should also be immune to rubella.

ENVIRONMENTAL WORKING CONDITIONS

The conditions of work should be such as to minimize hazard to health, inconvenience and discomfort, and maximize comfort and efficiency.

Checklist

- Ventilation
- Floors and traffic routes
- Temperature
- Windows/transparent doors/gates and walls
- Lighting
- Sanitary conveniences
- Cleanliness/waste

FIRE REGULATIONS

Measures for raising the alarm and dealing with a fire should be clearly understood by all members of staff. Fire drills should be held and all appliances checked regularly.

All staff have a duty:

- to prevent any causes of fire
- to be familiar with the actions to be taken in the event of fire
- to know the location of fire appliances and how to use them
- to ensure that fire exits and corridors are kept free from obstruction and available for use at all times.

Checklist

- A designated person or deputy responsible to meet the fire brigade on arrival.
- Regular fire drills for all staff, which should be recorded.
- Adequate extinguishers.
- Contract for inspecting/checking them.
- Fire alarm.
- Map of location of extinguishers.
- Fire instruction poster.
- Register of staff in the building, including attached staff, to be used as a role call in the event of a fire.
- The location of the main switches for electricity, gas and water.

MERCURY SPILLAGE

If there are mercury-filled sphygmomanometers and thermometers in the surgery there is always a chance that they will break and the mercury contained within them will be released.

Mercury is a toxic metal, which can cause ill health effects as a result of inhalation of the vapour and permeation of the skin. Do not touch mercury with bare skin and try not to breathe in the vapour.

Ensure that your practice has a mercury spillage kit available for use at all times. These can be obtained from:

- Mercury Safety Products. Tel: 0115 9213833
- SW Scientific. Tel: 0117 9354455
- Fisons/Fisher Scientific. Tel: 01509 231166
- Philip Harris. Tel: 029 207 32131

Mercury spillage kits contain:

- a sealable, disposable container partially filled with absorbent alloy wool in which the contaminated material should be placed
- one or two syringes or a foam pad
- protective gloves and face mask
- plastic scoop and brush.

If a spillage occurs:

- make an assessment of the severity of the spillage
- exclude people from the area if possible
- ventilate the area as well as you are able
- wear the gloves and mask provided in the kit and follow the instructions carefully
- use the syringe (or foam pad) provided to draw up the loose mercury and gather together any tiny globules with the scoop and brush
- seal the captured mercury in the container provided. DO NOT put any mercury-contaminated glass or other material in your normal sharps bin.

Local arrangements for the disposal of mercury and contaminated material vary from area to area but you will need to inform the company who usually collects your clinical waste.

Replace mercury-containing sphygmomanometers and thermometers with non-mercury versions (particularly sphygmomanometers because of the greater amount of mercury contained within them).

STORAGE OF MEDICAL GASES

Oxygen is the most likely gas to be found in general practice for use in emergencies and must be stored in a safe, well-ventilated area away from comustible materials and separated from cylinders of inflammable gases. It must, however, be readily available.

INFECTION CONTROL

Infection control comes under the remit of the HSW Act which imposes duties of care on both the employer and the employee.

Good infection control is important in primary healthcare to safeguard both patient and staff health. It is a key risk management strategy closely linked to clinical governance and plays a vital part in the provision of high-quality patient care.

Infection control precautions underpin routine safe practice and need to be carried out with all patients, regardless of perceived or known infection risk. This includes:

- hand washing and drying
- the use of protective clothing
- protection of open wounds
- safe disposal of clinical waste and sharps
- prevention of sharps injury
- safe handling of contaminated linen
- environmental cleaning
- decontamination of equipment.

HAND HYGIENE

Thorough and effective hand washing is the most important measure in reducing the spread of infection and is the responsibility of all members of the multidisciplinary team. Jewellery, except for plain wedding rings, including watches, should be removed since these items inhibit effective hand washing. Wash under running water – plugs are not required in hand basins. Wet all surfaces of the hands prior to applying soap. Lather all parts of both hands, cleaning beneath your wedding ring if you wear one. This should take 25–30 seconds. Pay particular attention to these areas most commonly missed (Fig. 25.1):

- thumbs
- backs of fingers
- backs of hands
- between the fingers and palms.

Rinse thoroughly and dry completely with paper towels, working from fingertips to the wrist in one direction. Dispose of the paper towels, making sure you do not recontaminate your clean hands, using elbows or by protecting your hands with a clean paper towel.

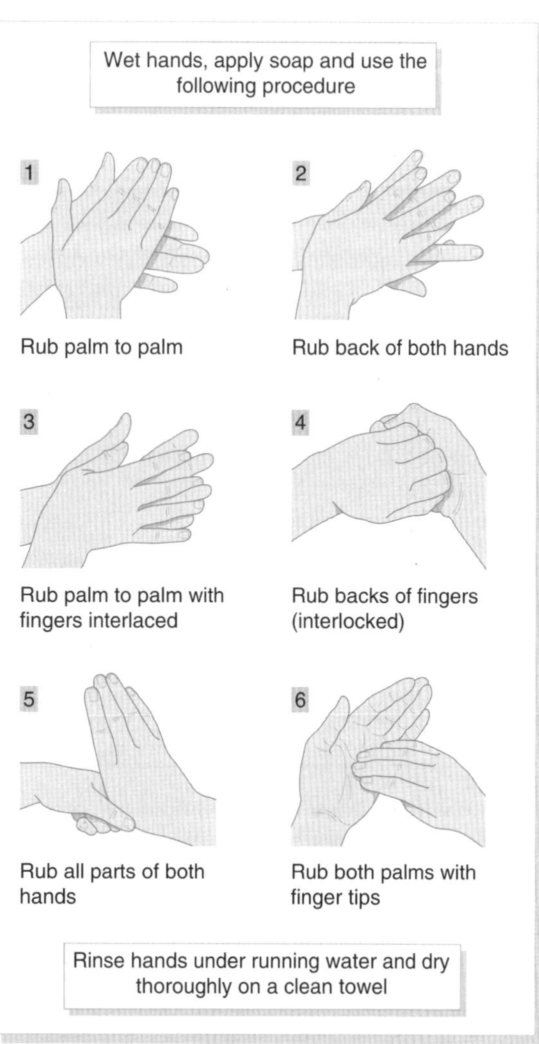

Figure 25.1 How to wash hands correctly and reduce infection.

Try to ensure that:

- hand-washing basins are available in all clinical areas
- liquid soap is available at all hand-washing basins in clinical areas
- paper towels are available at all hand-washing basins in clinical areas
- hand-washing basins in clinical areas are free from nail brushes
- clinical staff do not wear hand jewellery other than a plain, smooth wedding ring
- there are no cups or drinking facilities at hand-washing basins
- access to hand-washing basins is clear
- chlorhexidine or alcohol hand rub is available for use
- a poster demonstrating a good hand-washing technique is displayed by at least one sink
- elbow-operated mixer taps are available at hand-washing basins in clinical areas.

PROTECTIVE CLOTHING

To ensure that both staff and patients are protected from microorganisms, appropriate clothing is essential. The skin and mucous membranes must be protected from exposure to blood and body fluids. Uniforms must also be protected from contamination (HSE 1992, 1996, 1999). The following protective clothing should be available for use:

- disposable latex sterile and non-sterile gloves
- disposable plastic aprons
- eye and face protection.

Gloves should be worn whenever there might be contact with body fluids or mucous membranes or the skin is not intact, e.g. cuts. Gloves are not an alternative to hand washing.

Gloves should be changed after each procedure and hands washed after their removal. Gloves should be seamless, hypoallergenic, powder free and well fitting.

Staff with a latex allergy should be provided with latex-free gloves, made from a material such as nitrile (MDA 1996a).

Disposable plastic aprons

These should be worn when clothing might become contaminated and used for one procedure only and then disposed of, including minor surgical procedures.

Masks, visors, eye protection

If there is any likelihood that body fluids or substances might splash into the eyes, face or mouth, protection should be worn.

DISPOSAL OF CLINICAL WASTE

The disposal of waste is governed by the Environment Protection Act 1990. Producers of waste have a duty of care to ensure the waste is managed safely at all times until its final disposal.

Clinical waste

- *Description* – soiled dressings, swabs and contaminated waste from treatment areas, human tissues, blood
- *Disposal* – approved yellow clinical waste bag for incineration

Clinical sharps

- *Description* – discounted needles, cartridges, scalpels, stitch cutters, glass ampoules and sharp instruments
- *Disposal* – sharps bins which should conform with British Standard BS7320 and UN3291 and be assembled following the manufacturer's instructions. It is important that they are only two-thirds filled with no protruding sharps. The bins should be stored above floor level and safely out of the reach of children and visitors, using wall or trolley brackets

Household waste

- *Description* – uncontaminated waste, e.g. paper wrappings
- *Disposal* – black plastic waste bag

Pharmaceutical waste

- *Description* – prescription-only medicines, drugs or other pharmaceutical products
- *Disposal* – Special Waste Regulations 1996 and Misuse of Drugs Regulations 1997 may apply. Do not discharge into the sewer. Local collection should be arranged, e.g. Haul Waste

Cytotoxic waste

- *Description* – cytotoxic agents and anything which may be contaminated with a cytotoxic agent, e.g. used prefilled syringes, for example methotrexate

- *Disposal* – place in a special clinical waste bin for cytotoxic waste which is appropriately marked. Cytotoxic drug destruction kits can be obtained from DOOP Services, 53 Smugglers Lane North, Highcliffe, Dorset BH23 4NQ

Try to ensure that:

- there is a clinical waste policy and there are posters available
- there are foot-operated bins in clinical areas
- yellow bags are used for the disposal of clinical waste
- waste bags are less than two-thirds full, securely sealed/tied and labelled with source
- waste is stored in a designated area which is inaccessible to unauthorized persons prior to disposal
- glass, clinical and domestic waste is correctly segregated
- the storage area is visibly clear
- the collection of clinical waste is undertaken at least weekly by a registered company.

MANAGEMENT OF USED LINEN

Use single-use products such as paper roll for examination couches and disposable pillow cases if at all possible. If this is not possible place soiled linen in a leak-proof bag prior to laundering. Used linen must be laundered at 71°C for 3 minutes or 65°C for 10 minutes as a minimum (DoH 1991a, NHS Executive 1995).

ENVIRONMENTAL HYGIENE

Dust, dirt and liquid residues increase the risk of the transmission of infection and can be kept to a minimum by regular cleaning. Each practice should have in place a written cleaning schedule based on a COSHH assessment (HSE 1999).

The policy should stipulate the management of spilt body fluids and the regular removal of dust. It should also state the frequency of cleaning, the methods used with the expected outcomes together with the person responsible (ICNA 1999).

Try to ensure that:

- all general areas are clean and dust free
- clinical rooms are clean and free of extraneous items
- all sterile products are stored above floor level
- sluice areas are clean and free of extraneous items
- kitchens are clean and not used for specimen/medical equipment storage
- toys are in a good state of repair, clean, wipeable or machine washable
- examination/treatment couches can be cleaned using hot water and detergent
- disposable paper sheets are used to protect couches and pillows
- mops/buckets are clean, dry and stored inverted. Mop heads should be removable for frequent laundering
- separate cleaning equipment is available for kitchens/general areas/clinical area
- dressing trolleys are clean and in a good state of repair
- a written health and safety policy is available to all staff.

Managing blood or body fluid spills

Deal with blood and body fluid spills quickly and effectively (UK Health Departments 1998).

Hypochlorite method Use for body fluids such as blood.

- Protective clothing should be worn and excess fluid soaked up using disposable paper towels.
- Cover area with towels soaked in 10 000 parts per million of available chlorine, for example Milton or Haz Tabs, and leave for at least 2 minutes.
- Remove organic matter using the towels and discard as clinical waste.
- Clean area with detergent and hot water, and dry thoroughly.
- Clean the bucket/bowl in fresh soapy water and dry.
- Discard protective clothing as clinical waste.
- Wash hands.

Sodium dichloroisocyanurate (NaDCC) method

- Protective clothing should be worn.
- Cover spillage with NaDCC granules, for example Precept.
- Leave for at least 2 minutes.
- Scoop up the debris with paper towels and/or cardboard.
- Wash the area with detergent and hot water, and dry thoroughly.
- Dispose of all materials as clinical waste.
- Clean the bucket/bowl with fresh soapy water and dry.

- Discard protective clothing as clinical waste.
- Wash hands.

Detergent and water method Use for vomit or excreta.

- Wear protective clothing and mop up organic matter with paper towels or disposable cloths.
- Clean surface thoroughly using a solution of detergent and hot water and paper towels or disposable cloths.
- Rinse the surface and dry thoroughly.
- Dispose of materials as clinical waste.
- Clean the bucket/bowl in fresh hot, soapy water and dry.
- Discard protective clothing as clinical waste.
- Wash hands.

EQUIPMENT DECONTAMINATION

Equipment that is reusable must be decontaminated between each patient. Cleaning is the first step in decontamination and must be carried out before disinfection and sterilization to make these processes effective. The Medical Devices Agency in 1996 defined it as:

> *the process which physically removes contamination but does not necessarily destroy microorganisms. The reduction of microbial contamination cannot be defined and will depend upon many factors including the efficiency of the cleaning process and the initial bio burden.*

Thorough cleaning with detergent and warm water – maximum 35°C – will remove many microorganisms.

To clean by hand, a deep sink is needed to immerse the instruments completely. Precautions must be taken to prevent injury and splashing. Scrubbing can generate aerosols which may convey infective agents. Where possible use a washer/disinfector or an ultrasonic cleaning bath.

Disinfection

This is a process used to reduce the number of viable microorganisms but it does not inactivate all viruses and bacterial spores. Disinfection may not necessarily achieve the same reduction in microbial contamination levels as sterilization (MDA 1996b).

Disinfection methods used in general practice include the following.

1. *Chemical*. Chlorine-based chemicals such as hypochlorites, e.g. Domestos, Milton, and sodium dichloroisocyanurates, e.g. Precept, can be used on surfaces and for body fluid spills. Alcohol 79%, e.g. Levermed Alcohol Gel, can be used on surfaces, for skin and hand decontamination. Apply 5 ml of alcohol hand rub to socially clean hands for routine hand washing (two applications for surgical procedures) then rub until dry. This technique is only suitable if the hands are not visibly soiled; alcohol is ineffective in the presence of dirt.
2. *Hot water boilers*. May be unreliable and unsafe.
3. *Benchtop steam sterilizers*. The equipment should not be stored or used as sterile (MDA 1997).

Sterilization

'A process used to render the object free from viable microorganisms, including spores and viruses' (MDA 1996b). An autoclave which uses moist heat-saturated steam is the most efficient and reliable method of sterilization in general practice.

The purchase of presterilized single-use items avoids the necessity for resterilization. Increasingly practices are negotiating contracts with sterile supply departments to provide this service.

The Medical Device Agency provides written information on the installation, maintenance and operation of benchtop steam sterilizers (autoclaves) (MDA 1998).

A logbook which provides a permanent record of all testing, maintenance and repairs, and the actions taken in the event of a failed cycle or test, should be kept for each sterilizer.

It is necessary to:

- carry out daily testing and document the temperature achieved and its duration
- ensure that quarterly and annual testing is carried out by a qualified test engineer as advised in MDA DB9804
- ensure that operator training has taken place
- ensure that the legal and insurance aspects of ownership and use are understood.

Key points for sterilization in general practice

- If possible use a sterile supplies department which meets regulatory requirements.
- Keep dirty instruments separate from clean instruments.
- Confirm with the manufacturer that the steam sterilizer in use is suitable for processing the intended loads.

- Once installed, the sterilizer must be checked and tested by a qualified person who may be employed by the manufacturer or a contractor.
- Ensure training is given to the operator on the use and maintenance of the sterilizer.
- Ensure maintenance and quarterly and annual testing by a qualified engineer is carried out and documented. For further details on all aspects of testing consult HTM 2010 Part 3.
- Carry out daily testing in accordance with MDA DB 9605 and DB 9804.
- Report any fault immediately to the engineer and do not use until rectified.
- Wash instruments thoroughly with detergent and warm water (35°C) using an ultrasonic washer or at a dedicated sink. Rinse and dry instruments prior to sterilizing.
- Wear gloves, apron and eye protection when cleaning instruments.
- Only use sterile distilled or de-ionized water in sterilizers.
- Empty, rinse with sterile water and dry the sterilizer's reservoir and chamber when not in use. Refill daily. See HTM 2031 for details (NHS Estates 1997).
- Instruments should be sterilized for:
  - 3 minutes at 134–137°C or
  - 10 minutes at 126–129°C or
  - 15 minutes at 121–124°C.
- When loading instruments into the sterilizer, ensure they are dry and not touching.
- Place bowls and receivers on edge and leave hinged instruments open.
- Do not overload machine and baskets.
- Instruments must be **unwrapped and not in pouches** unless a vacuum steam sterilizer is used.
- For invasive procedures, use instruments immediately after being sterilized.
- For non-invasive procedures store instruments in a clean, dry, dust-free place.
- Do not soak instruments in disinfectants before or after sterilizing.
- Instruments with narrow lumens or wrapped instruments must not be sterilized in benchtop steam sterilizers. See Health Note 9503 (DoH 1995).
- Retain records for at least 11 years.

Single-use equipment

These items are intended only to be used once and then thrown away because there is insufficient evidence that it would be safe to reuse them. The MDA Bulletin MDA DB 2000 (04) states:

1. Devices designated for single use must not be reused under any circumstances.
2. The reuse of 'single use' devices can affect their safety, performance and effectiveness, exposing patients and staff to unnecessary risk.
3. The reuse of 'single use' devices has legal implications.
   a. Anyone who reprocesses or reuses a device intended by the manufacturer for use on single occasions, bears full responsibility for its safety and effectiveness.
   b. Anyone who reprocesses a single-use device and passes it to a separate legal entity for use, has the same legal obligations under the Medical Devices Regulations as the original manufacturer of the device.

Decontamination of specific items of equipment

Auroscope ear pieces Remove wax by cleaning thoroughly with general-purpose detergent and warm water (<35°C), using thin brushes to clean inside. Then immerse in 70% alcohol for 10 minutes.

Buckets for leg ulcers Line with plastic bin liner. After each use, clean with warm water (<35°C) and general-purpose detergent using disposable paper towels. Store dry.

Changing mats If possible line with paper. After use wipe with a solution of general-purpose detergent and warm water and dry thoroughly. Check integrity regularly.

Ear syringing machine Before use, flush system thoroughly with fresh tap water. After use:

- drain water from system. Flush system with 1% hypochlorite, dry reservoir with a paper towel
- clean tips with general-purpose detergent and water, rinse under running warm water. Soak in fresh 1% hypochlorite solution for 10 minutes.

Clean Jobson Horne probe with general-purpose detergent and water. Remove any wax using a new piece of pan scrubber. Rinse under running warm water. Soak in 70% alcohol for 10 minutes or autoclave.

ECG equipment Wash well with warm water (<35°C) or wipe with a damp cloth if non-immersible. Store dry.

Family planning equipment The DOH (1994) recommends that all items entering the vagina must be adequately decontaminated between uses. This can only be achieved by a heat sterilization method such as an autoclave.

Vaginal specula and IUCD instruments should be sterile, single-use items wherever possible. If reusable, soak in general-purpose detergent and sterilize after cleaning with warm water (<35°C).

Nail brushes Single use only.

Nebulizers Patients should have their own nebulizer mask and tubing, which should be washed with warm water (<35°C) and general-purpose detergent between uses or discarded. Store dry.

Suction equipment Disposable suction liners are recommended. For non-disposable bottles, ensuring appropriate staff protection, empty the contents into the toilet, rinse with cold water. Clean using warm water and general-purpose detergent, store dry.

Tubing should be single-patient use. Filters should be replaced when wet and at appropriate intervals in keeping with the manufacturer's instructions.

Thermometers Use disposable sheaths. Before and after each use, wipe with 70% alcohol swab. Store dry.

Trolleys (dressing trolleys) Clean top and all surfaces daily with warm water (<35°C) and general-purpose detergent. Dry thoroughly. Wipe with alcohol-impregnated wipes between cases. If trolley becomes contaminated between patient use, wash with general-purpose detergent and hot water again.

Weighing scales Line with disposable paper towel. Wash bowl of scales with general-purpose detergent and hot water or wipe with 70% alcohol wipes before next baby is weighed.

Key points for equipment decontamination in general practice

- Disinfectants are used at the correct dilution as per manufacturer's instructions.
- Chemical disinfectants are used only for heat-labile equipment.
- A deep sink separate from hand-washing facilities is available for washing items.
- Data sheets are available on detergents/disinfectants used (COSHH).
- Environmental surfaces are cleaned appropriately between patients.
- There is no evidence of single-use equipment being reused.
- Sterilizing equipment is maintained in accordance with HTM 2010.
- The sterilizing equipment cycle is checked and recorded daily.
- Instruments sterilized in equipment that does not have a vacuum cycle are unwrapped and not touching each other during the sterilization cycle.
- Staff are aware of the need for decontamination and a certificate prior to sending equipment for maintenance or repair.
- Clean and sterile instruments are stored in clean areas prior to use.
- Used equipment is stored out of patient areas after use.
- Examination equipment is either sterile single use or decontaminated appropriately between use.
- Surgical instruments are sterile prior to use.
- Suction equipment is clean and stored dry without catheter attached.

SPECIMEN HANDLING

Specimens in the clinical setting include any substance in liquid or solid state which has been removed from a patient so that it can be analysed. All staff who handle specimens should receive appropriate training and immunization which will require regular boosters.

- Specimens should be placed in an approved container immediately after collection.
- They should be stored in a cool place until collected.
- The outside of the container must not be contaminated.
- Specimens should be stored away from food and drink.
- The patient's details should be entered on both the container and the request form.
- A biohazard label should be attached to both the specimen container and the request form of any known or potentially high-risk specimen, e.g. hazard category 3 (ACDP 1995). This includes microorganisms such as hepatitis B and C and HIV. Although all specimens should be treated as high risk, highlighting these particular specimens helps to safeguard couriers, porters and laboratory staff.

VACCINES

Many pharmaceutical products and vaccines deteriorate if exposed to adverse environmental conditions. These are usually detailed on the product pack. In particular, it is vital that the temperature range for vaccines is not exceeded. Ensuring that these products are not affected by unacceptable elevation of temperatures is referred to as 'maintaining the integrity of the cold chain'.

STORAGE OF VACCINES

Vaccines are biological products that need to be stored under controlled conditions to maintain their potency and efficacy (DoH 1996a). They must be kept between 2°C and 8°C during transportation and delivery and must not directly touch ice packs. On arrival, vaccines should be checked to ensure the cold chain has not been broken and for signs of damage or leakage. A nominated person, who has received specific training in this field, should make sure vaccines are correctly stored and handled by staff.

Vaccines are prescription-only medicines and should be stored in a lockable refrigerator with access only by authorized staff.

Checklist

- Ensure strict stock rotation, with new vaccines being placed behind older stock.
- Discard expired vaccines safely.
- Prevent overstocking and allow air to circulate around all stock.
- Do not store in fridge door or in separate drawers in the bottom of the fridge as air cannot circulate.
- Vials and ampoules must not be removed from their original packing so that information such as batch numbers, expiry dates and advice on protection from light may remain available.
- Ensure systems are in place to prevent accidental disconnection of the electricity supply.
- Do not store items other than vaccines in the same fridge.
- Defrost and clean regularly, storing vaccines in an alternative fridge during the procedure.
- Store vaccines between 2°C and 8°C and not below freezing. Monitor fridge temperature using a minimum/maximum thermometer and record results, preferably daily.

Use reconstituted vaccine according to the manufacturer's recommendations, usually within 1–4 hours. Remove vaccines from the fridge for the minimum length of time before administration and discard any opened in error.

Do not allow oral polio vaccine (OPV) to remain at room temperature awaiting or following an immunization as this may decrease the potency of the vaccine.

Do not prepare vaccines in advance of immunization as this increases the risk of administering the wrong vaccine and may affect the temperature.

Prepare each vaccine for the individual who is to receive it. Unless the skin is visibly dirty, routine cleansing is unnecessary. If alcohol or other antiseptics are used, they must be completely dry otherwise the live vaccines may be inactivated.

Multidose vials may be used for one session only; discard any remaining vaccine at the end of the session. Dispose by heat inactivation or incineration. There are special precautions for the disposal of live vaccines (DoH 1996b).

Key points for vaccine storage and use

- Vaccines are immediately stored in a vaccine refrigerator after delivery.
- The vaccine refrigerator has a maximum/minimum thermometer.
- Temperature checks are performed and recorded daily (temperature range 2–8°C).
- The refrigerator is used for vaccine storage only (no food/specimens).
- The storage space for vaccines in the refrigerator is adequate – maximum 50% full.
- Prevention of accidental disconnection of the refrigerator has been ensured.
- Vaccines are checked as 'in date' before use.
- For immunization/vaccination sessions vaccines are transported in a 'cool bag' and removed from the bag/refrigerator only as required.
- Reconstituted vaccine is used within the period recommended by the manufacturers.
- Opened multidose vials are discarded at the end of immunization/vaccination sessions.

MINOR SURGERY

It is accepted practice that a room within the surgery where minor operations are performed will meet the following standards.

The room

- Floor area of at least 17.5 metres square with a clinical hand wash basin.

- The minimum equipment possible.
- Furniture, fixtures and fittings which are clean and in a good state of repair.
- Separate sink for cleaning.

Organization of the clinical area

Separate areas for clean and dirty procedures.

Flooring

- Sheet vinyl with welded seams for easy cleaning.
- Clean at least daily using detergent and water, preferably at the end of the session.
- Remove blood splashes as soon as possible.

Walls

- Paint preferably with oil-based eggshell finish paint.
- Clean when visibly soiled with detergent and water.
- Remove blood splashes as soon as possible.

Lighting

- Should allow easy cleaning and little dust build-up.
- Clean at the end of each day using detergent and water.
- Lighting used for patient examination/minor surgery should be fitted with a heat filter.

Mechanical ventilation

- Minimum standard is an electric extractor fan. Inspect monthly and clean every 3 months to prevent dust build-up.
- Do not open windows during surgery.

Central heating radiators

- Clean on a regular basis.
- Paint with oil-based, eggshell finish paint.

Fixtures and fittings, e.g. curtains, couches, etc.

- Must be easy to clean and in a good state of repair.
- Washed regularly, usually every 6 months or when visibly soiled.
- Use vertical blinds in preference to curtains.
- Use disposable paper sheeting for examination and operating couches.

Surgical instruments

- Should ideally be provided by a sterile supplies department.
- If not, there should be a high-quality system for cleaning and autoclaving in house.
- There must be adequate space for storage off the floor.
- Must be stored separately from dirty equipment.

Suction container

- Liners should be disposable and discarded as clinical waste.
- Replace suction tubing at the end of each session if used.
- Discard the contents of reusable jars into a sluice or toilet. To avoid splashing from aerosols, eye protection may be needed.
- Decontaminate the jar and store dry.
- Replace filters at regular intervals or whenever contaminated.

Surgical hand disinfection

- Keep hand wash basin separate from basin used for washing instruments.
- Fitted with an elbow-operated mixer tap.
- Keep liquid soap, antiseptic detergent dispensers and disposable paper towels next to the basin. Do not use reusable towels.

Skin sites

- Disinfect immediately before surgery.
- Preparation should be fast acting with a prolonged antibacterial effect. Alcoholic solutions of 0.5% chlorhexidine, 1% povidone-iodine or 0.5% triclosan are most frequently used.
- Skin reactions may occur with some products.
- Apply solution liberally to the site and surrounding area and allow to air dry.
- Hair removal is not always necessary. If required, use electric clippers rather than a razor.

Protective clothing

- Wear a new disposable plastic apron for each patient.
- Use sterile, non-powdered latex gloves for procedures involving contact with normally sterile areas of the body or mucous membranes.

- Wear eye protection if splashing is anticipated.
- Dispose of protective clothing after use as clinical waste.

Clinical waste

- Should be placed in a foot-operated waste bin.
- Remove yellow clinical waste bags at the end of each session/day. Appropriately tie and label and place in a secure designated holding area for clinical waste.
- Clean foot-operated bin on a weekly basis using detergent and hot water.

Records

- Must be maintained using an operations register for audit purposes and for medicolegal reasons.
- Should include the date/time of operation, patient's name and address, names of surgeon, procedure and anaesthesia given, name of assistant and whether histology or other specimens were sent to the laboratory. It is also important that the outcome of the histology report is recorded, together with the date on which the patient was informed.

References

ACDP 1995 Protection against bloodborne infections in the workplace: HIV and hepatitis. HMSO, London

Department of Health, Welsh Office, Scottish Office Department of Health, DHSS (Northern Ireland) 1996a Immunisation against infectious disease. HMSO, London

Department of Health 1996b Addendum to HSG (93) 40. Protecting health care workers and patients from hepatitis B. HMSO, London

DoH 1991 Decontamination of equipment, linen and other surfaces contaminated with hepatitis B and/or human immunodeficiency virus (HIV). HMSO, London

DoH 1994 Instruments and appliances used in the vagina and cervix: recommended methods for decontamination. SAB (94) 22. Department of Health, London

DoH 1995 Handpieces used in phaco microsurgical procedures and their re-usable accessories. HMSO, London

HSE 1992 Personal protective equipment at work: guidance on regulations. HMSO, London

HSE 1996 A guide to risk assessment requirements: common provisions in health and safety law. Health and Safety Executive, London

HSE 1999 Control of Substances Hazardous to Health Regulations. Health and Safety Executive, London

ICNA 1999 Glove usage guidelines. Infection Control Nurses Association, Edinburgh

MDA 1996a Latex sensitisation in the health care setting (use of latex gloves). Medical Devices Agency, London

MDA 1996b Sterilisation, disinfection and cleaning of medical equipment parts 1, 2 and 3. Medical Devices Agency, London

MDA 1997 The purchase, operation and maintenance of benchtop steam sterilisers. Medical Devices Agency, London

MDA 1998 The validation and periodic testing of benchtop vacuum steam sterilisers. Medical Devices Agency, London

NHS Estates 1997 HTM 2031. Clean steam for sterilisation. HMSO, London

NHSE 1995 Hospital laundry arrangement for infected linen. NHS Executive, London

UK Health Departments 1998 Guidance for clinical health care workers: protection against infection with blood-borne viruses. HMSO, London

Resources

Websites

www.decontamination.nhsestates.gov.uk/home.asp. NHS Estates website has information on decontamination of equipment.

www.icna.co.uk. Infection Control Nurses Association website; information on publications, conferences, courses and useful links.

www.phls.co.uk. Public Health Laboratory Service website; provides information and advice on communicable diseases and other infections.

Useful address

Health and Safety Executive. Information Centre, Broad Lane, Sheffield S3 7HQ.
HSE InfoLine: 08701 545500
HSE Books: 01787 313995

Further reading

British Medical Association 1996 Minor surgery in general practice. Royal College of General Practitioners. General Medical Services Committee, London

Department of Health 1990 Guidance for clinical health care workers: protection against infection with HIV and hepatitis viruses. HMSO, London

Department of Health 1993 Protecting health care workers and patients from hepatitis B. HSG (93) 40. HMSO, London

Department of Health 1998 A first class service: quality in the new NHS. DoH, London

Health and Safety Executive 1974 Health and Safety at Work Act. HSE, London

Health and Safety Executive 1981 Health and Safety (First Aid) Regulations. HMSO, London

Health Education Authority 1998 Health and safety in general practice: a guide to risk assessment for general practitioners and practice managers. HEA, London

Health Service Advisory Committee 1999 Safe disposal of clinical waste. HMSO, London

ICNA 1999 Guidelines for hand hygiene. Infection Control Nurses Association, Edinburgh

Medical device bulletins are available free of charge from the NHS, 210 Department of Health, PO Box 410, Wetherby, Yorkshire LS23 7EL. Fax: 01937 845 381. Quote title and reference number.

Medical Devices Agency 1995 The re-use of medical devices supplied for single use only. MDA, London

Moore R, Moore S 1995 Health and safety at work. Guidance for general practitioners. RCGP, Bishop Auckland, Co. Durham

Morgan D 1990 Decontamination of instruments and control of cross-infection in general practice. British Medical Journal 300:1379–1380

National Institute for Clinical Excellence 2003 Infection control: prevention of healthcare-associated infection in primary and community care. NICE, Oaktree Press, London

NHS Executive 1996 A national framework for the provision of secondary care within general practice. HSG (96) 31. NHSE, London

NHS Management Executive 1993 Decontamination of equipment prior to inspection, service or repair. HSG (93) 26. NHSME, London

Public Health Laboratory Services 1992 Transportable steam sterilisers: maintenance, inspection and insurance. Health and Safety Advice Note, SAB (92) 27. PHLS, London

RCN 2000 Good practice in infection control. Guidance for nurses working in general practice. Royal College of Nursing, London

Royal College of Nursing 1997 Hepatitis guidance from the Royal College of Nursing. RCN, London

Royal College of Nursing 1999 Working well initiative: latex allergy in healthcare settings. Employment Brief 25/99. RCN, London

Smith D, Dean J, Wheelhouse C, Bushell J 1995 Now wash your hands. Video. Southampton Teaching Support and Media Services, University of Southampton

Chapter 26

Research, evidence-based practice and audit

Jeannett Martin

CHAPTER CONTENTS

INTRODUCTION

The aim of this chapter is to outline the key aspects of research, evidence-based practice and audit and to provide practical information that can be used when undertaking these activities.

RESEARCH

Nursing research involves a systematic search for knowledge about the issues of importance to nursing, so that the care provided to patients can be improved. This section provides an overview of the recognized stages in the process of research and wherever possible, gives an explanation of the jargon that is often used in research.

Knowledge can be obtained from a variety of sources:

- tradition, which may or may not have been evaluated
- authorities or experts in a field whose knowledge is passed on and accepted by others
- trial and error where alternatives are tried successively until the problem is solved, but knowledge obtained is often unsystematic and unrecorded
- scientific approach when a specific problem or question is addressed.

The scientific approach to obtaining knowledge is the most sophisticated and will generally be more reliable than tradition, authority or trial and error in that it uses a systematic approach where the researcher progresses logically through a series of steps according to a plan of action. In addition, there will be checks and balances to minimize the possibility that bias or chance is responsible for the results. If a group of people work together to answer the question this is referred to as a *study;* if a single researcher is involved it is called an *investigation* or a *research project.*

The person doing the research is known as the *researcher, investigator* or *scientist.* When a study is undertaken by a research team the main person directing the investigation is known as the *principal investigator* (PI). The people who are being studied are often referred to as *subjects* or *participants.* If they provide information to the researcher, for example by questionnaire, they may be called *respondents.*

FORMULATE THE RESEARCH QUESTION

Decide on what you want to find out. This may seem an obvious statement but it is crucial to the success of the research project and is not always given sufficient consideration. A research question should not be longer than a sentence and must be easily understood. As part of the process of devising a research question, to generate ideas you might find it useful to brainstorm topics of interest that are significant to nursing and possible for you to research, and then create a question that relates to each area. Polit & Hungler (1995) suggest that it can be helpful to apply question stems to the topics you have identified, such as:

- what causes ....
- why do ....
- when do ....
- what factors contribute to ....
- how effective is ....
- what is the relationship between ....

LITERATURE SEARCH

The main purpose of a literature search is to determine what work has been done already in your chosen topic and then to review it to give you background for your study.

Decide on your major resources for the literature search. Most libraries now have computerized databases which you can use to search for and identify articles and journals by inputting key words. Librarians can be helpful with a literature search and can be of assistance if you require interlibrary loans. Internet search engines can also be a valuable source of information (see Chapter 21).

After you have gathered your articles and resources for the literature search, they will need to be read and critically reviewed. This may be very time consuming depending on how much research has been conducted around your topic. If it has been widely researched, it may be necessary to set limits to your literature review, e.g. for articles published in the last 5–10 years. If you do decide to do this you will need to explain and justify your decision when you write up your literature review.

REFERENCES

It is useful to keep an indexed reference system of what you have read. This should include an accurate reference of the article and a summary of the relevant points. This can be recorded on a manual card index system or on a computer system. A reference is a piece of written material, published or unpublished, which an author refers to. The purpose of it is to:

- allow the reader to locate the work and read more
- acknowledge another writer's work
- record your own reading for any future work you may do.

There are two reference styles that are most frequently used: the Harvard and Vancouver systems.

Harvard

The author's name and the year of publication appear in the main text in brackets next to the point of reference. The full reference will then appear in an alphabetical list at the end of your work.

Vancouver

A number is inserted above and to the right of the work that is referred to in the text. That same number is used throughout the essay or report if the same work is being referred to. Its full reference will then appear in a numerical list at the end of your work.

PREPARE A RESEARCH PROPOSAL

This is a detailed statement of your intended actions. It should outline why the research is necessary and how you intend to do it. Approval from your local research ethics committee (LREC) and primary care organization (PCO) is a requirement for any research that involves NHS patients. Each committee produces guidelines for presenting your research proposal at this stage. You may be required to attend a meeting of the committee to answer any queries they have about your proposal, but this should not be intimidating as members of these committees can have helpful suggestions. Your primary care organization will have contact details of your LREC.

Box 26.1 Information to be included in a research proposal

- Title of the research
- Aims and objectives
- Rationale for doing the research
- Brief literature review
- The population to be studied
- Research methodology
- Data analysis
- Ethical considerations, e.g. obtaining consent from participants, employers and LREC
- Name and designation of the researchers (include CV of researchers in the appendix)
- Supervisor if applicable
- Costs involved and resources required
- Timetable of events

SELECT AN APPROPRIATE METHOD

Certain methods of research will be more suitable than others, depending on the topic (see Appendix 1 for a description of research designs).

The choice of design may also depend on your experience and the resources available. It is advisable to perform a pilot study prior to the main research project. This will highlight any flaws in your methodology and you can then make changes.

Most research is either quantitative, i.e. concerned with generating data in numbers, or qualitative, i.e. concerned with generating data in words, although some studies can combine the two. The researcher should decide on which approach is the most suitable for the research to be conducted because this will influence the research method chosen.

DATA COLLECTION

The method used for data collection must be reliable and valid. Reliability refers to whether or not the method works consistently every time it is used and validity as to whether the method measures what it set out to measure. Both reliability and validity should be tested in a small pilot study before the main study is started. Methods of data collection commonly used include questionnaires, interviews and observation.

Sampling

It is usually impractical to collect data from the whole of a given population, e.g. all practice nurses in the UK, so it is necessary to identify a sample. The sample size and nature will depend on what you are researching but the selection process should be as unbiased as possible.

Questionnaire

This is probably the most common method of collecting data. It is relatively cost effective and can be used for collecting large amounts of data. Questionnaires are also easy to analyse. Questionnaires can guarantee anonymity, as the respondent has no personal contact with the researcher. This is important in certain topics of research, which may result in embarrassment for the respondent, and it helps to obtain more honest responses.

Two types of questions, closed or open, commonly appear in questionnaires and, depending on the type of data you wish to collect, a combination of both types of question can be used. A closed question encourages a straightforward response such as yes/no or a tick; this is useful for obtaining quantitative data. Open questions invite a more lengthy response, in which the respondent has to construct a reply.

A negative aspect of questionnaires is that they are difficult to construct. The guidelines given in Box 26.2 should be considered and the questionnaire should be piloted or tested on a small sample of people with similar characteristics to your intended study population.

Box 26.2 Constructing a questionnaire

- Make it as short as possible
- Are the questions really necessary?
- What response will each question generate?
- Keep questions simple, avoid jargon and technical words
- Avoid leading questions

- Do not irritate the respondent
- Avoid ambiguity
- Limit open questions which require a lengthy response
- Can the respondent answer the questions you have set?
- Devise a coding system for responses
- Ensure instructions are clear
- Ensure there is a logical progression
- Thank the respondent for their help

Interviews

These can be either structured or unstructured. In all cases interviews need to be piloted and rehearsed several times before being used in the main study. The main problem is preventing yourself from 'leading' the interview and influencing the responses.

Compared to questionnaires, interviews are more difficult to analyse and can be extremely time consuming if you have a large number of subjects, but they can provide more qualitative-type data. The major advantages of interviews are:

- response rate is relatively high
- will obtain in-depth responses
- respondents have greater difficulty in avoiding questions
- you can explore unplanned responses
- responses can be clarified.

Observations

There are two main types of observation: *participant*, where the researcher works alongside the people involved in the activity to be researched, and *non-participant*, where the researcher purely observes and records examples of behaviour or action but does not participate in the activity. However, the presence of an observer can influence the activity and behaviour of others.

DATA ANALYSIS

The aim of the analysis is to identify patterns or trends in the data that you have collected. This process must be valid and reliable. You must decide how you are going to analyse your data before you start to collect it, as it will be linked to your method of data collection. You may find it helpful to engage the help of a statistician for advice in this area. If you are dealing with quantitative data you may also require access to a computer statistics package (see Appendix 1 for definitions of some statistical terms).

MAKE CONCLUSIONS AND RECOMMENDATIONS

It is important that you do not try to make conclusions about your research project before you have the results. This will bias your work and you will not be open minded about the results. If the results are surprising then you can discuss the possible reasons for this in your discussion section.

Recommendations, if any, should be made as a result of the research and it is also useful to suggest further areas for study.

WRITING A DISSERTATION

A standard research dissertation should be set out in the following way.

Title page

- Name of university
- Name of department
- Title of research
- Name of author
- Qualification for which it has been submitted
- Date submitted

Abstract

A brief summary of the paper which should be understandable on its own so should include information on the problem, method, results and conclusions. This page is not numbered as it is considered separate from the dissertation.

Acknowledgements

Thank anyone whose help has been particularly valuable, e.g. respondents, supervisor.

List of tables and figures and their page numbers in the dissertation

List of abbreviations used in the text

Contents

Every page after this will be numbered 1,2,3, etc. Pages after the abstract and before the contents page should be numbered using Roman numerals, e.g. (i) (ii).

Introduction

Should explain the purpose of the research and clearly define its aims and objectives. This should be set in the context of background information about the topic. The introduction may also summarize the hypothesis, although this can be presented on its own.

Literature review

Organize, categorize and summarize references in the form of an essay so that they reveal the current state of knowledge on the selected topic. You should point out consistencies and contradictions in the literature then suggest possible reasons for these contradictions, e.g. different methodology. Identify any gaps in knowledge and demonstrate the need for further research such as yours.

Methodology

Explain how the research has been conducted and what design was used. This section should also summarize the pilot study and any changes that were made as a result of this. This section should be described in detail, so that a reader can replicate the work if so desired. The research tools used should be summarized and it is also useful to include copies of questionnaires, etc. in the appendix. This section should also address how the information was analysed and interpreted.

Results

Present a detailed and comprehensive analysis of the study. It may be appropriate to present the results as graphs, tables or diagrams.

Discussion

The results should be discussed and compared to the aims of the study and to other work.

Conclusion

Offer recommendations as a result of this study. Any limitations of the work should be identified and suggestions for future research can be made.

References

Alphabetical if you have used Harvard, numerical if Vancouver system used.

Appendices

Include examples of letters sent to respondents, LREC, PCO, questionnaires, consent form.

MULTICENTRE RESEARCH

The Medical Research Council (MRC) is a government-funded organization set up by Royal Charter to undertake and fund research with the ultimate aim of improving human health.

The MRC has established a General Practice Research Framework for research in primary care. Around 1100 practices across the UK are part of this framework and collaborate with the MRC on high-quality research into areas such as asthma, back pain, thrombosis prevention and the long-term risks and benefits of hormone replacement therapy. Each practice has a trial nurse, usually the practice nurse, who has day-to-day responsibility for the research. The time involved will vary depending on the type of project chosen by the practice. Training is provided for nurses before each project begins and support from study managers at the coordinating centre and a regional training nurse is ongoing throughout the study. Further details about the MRC General Practice Research Framework can be obtained from www.mrc/gprf.ac.uk or by writing to the Administration Manager, MRC General Practice Research Framework, MRC Clinical Trials Unit, Stephenson House, 158–160 North Gower Street, London NW1 2ND.

EVIDENCE-BASED PRACTICE

Evidence-based practice is the ability to track down, appraise and incorporate the growing body of evidence into one's clinical practice. Sackett et al (1997) described this as a five-stage process.

- Formulate the problem.
- Find the evidence.
- Appraise the evidence critically.
- Implement the results.
- Evaluate performance.

FORMULATE THE PROBLEM

This requires a question which focuses on whether one intervention is more effective than another or indeed than none at all. Generally the elements included in structuring a question are:

- *who* – the patient or problem being addressed
- *which* – intervention being considered, e.g. drug and comparison intervention if relevant

- *what* – outcome is desired as a result of the intervention from a clinical and patient perspective, e.g. reduced mortality or morbidity.

Box 26.3 Question: Does MMR triple vaccine reduce morbidity in children under 5 years?

Who	*Intervention*	*Counter intervention*	*Outcome*
Children <5 years	MMR triple vaccine	MMR separate antigen	Reduced risk of morbidity

FIND THE EVIDENCE – SOURCES OF INFORMATION

Textbooks

Textbooks can take up to 2 years to reach publication because of the time lag for writing, editing and production so information may be out of date. Textbooks are best for addressing facts which do not change quickly such as anatomy or disease characteristics, e.g. the incubation period for hepatitis A.

Journals

Deciding which journals to read regularly is an important aspect of continuing professional development. As well as the numerous nursing publications, general medical journals such as the *BMJ*, *Lancet*, *New England Journal of Medicine* and *JAMA* can be useful for nurses, as important advances in healthcare are often reported in these journals because of their large circulation.

Although journals are useful for identifying information about recent advances and new treatments they do have limitations, such as publication bias in that studies which have positive findings (either harmful or beneficial) are more likely to be published than those where no effect is shown. Also because of the huge numbers available it can be difficult to read all that is relevant. Sackett et al (1997) suggested that for general physicians to keep abreast of the journals relevant to their area of practice, they would need to read 19 articles a day, 365 days a year.

Distilled information sources

Evidence Based Medicine and *Evidence Based Nursing* are two journals which aim to summarize high-quality studies in a concise format, with an accompanying commentary from a clinician which links the study findings to practice.

Bibliographic databases

These provide access to citations, sometimes with abstracts for studies and reviews published in the healthcare literature. These include:

- MEDLINE – general-purpose database from the US
- CINAHL – general database from the US
- Embase – general-purpose database from Excerpta Medica in the Netherlands useful for almost everything!

Searches are undertaken by using terms that the authors have used in their titles or abstracts, often called textwords. This will generate a number of 'hits' which will provide the searcher with information on the title and source of each, sometimes with a short abstract on content. These can either be scrolled through or focused down even more if there are too many.

Consolidated information sources

Different studies can present conflicting data on the same topic. A systematic review attempts to consolidate these differences by synthesizing the findings of multiple studies on the same topic. A systematic review concentrates on a specific question and uses comprehensive sources and selects articles based on predetermined criteria and then critically appraises the selected studies. If judged to be sufficiently similar, the results of the studies may be combined using statistical methods. This type of systematic review is called a metaanalysis.

The NHS Centre for Reviews and Dissemination (NHSCRD) was established at the University of York by the NHS Research & Development programme in order to carry out and commission systematic reviews and to disseminate these to healthcare decision makers. Effective Healthcare Bulletins are produced by the University of York for this purpose and available free of charge throughout the UK.

The Cochrane Collaboration is an international network which produces systematic reviews of healthcare interventions. The Cochrane Library has four databases.

- Database of systematic reviews which contains the full text of more than 300 reviews and protocols for more than 300 planned or ongoing systematic reviews.

- Database for abstracts of reviews of effectiveness (DARE) is produced by the NHSCRD and contains >1500 records of systematic reviews published internationally.
- Review methodology database comprises references to articles on the theory and methods of systematic reviews and on critical appraisal.
- Controlled trials register is a database of citations of trials and has >150 000 entries.

The Internet

Provides access to information sources for both health professionals and patients. The quality of some sites may be poor so those searching should consider the source when deciding on how reliable or valid the information is. Some bibliographic databases such as MEDLINE can be accessed free via the Internet, as can some journals, e.g. *Nursing Standard* or *BMJ*. A postgraduate library may be able to provide you with access to a range of electronic journals.

APPRAISE THE EVIDENCE CRITICALLY

1. What question was it was designed to answer? Did it need to be done?
2. What type of study design was used and was it appropriate?
   - Primary research – randomized controlled trial, cohort study, case-control study, cross-sectional survey, case report
   - Secondary research – overview, systematic review, metaanalysis, decision analysis, guideline development
   - Qualitative – what was the researcher's perspective and has this been taken into account?
3. Whether the study was ethical
   - Informed consent
   - Was any harm caused?
4. The study design
   - Was the design appropriate? Greenhalgh (2001) described the use of study types for different areas of care (Box 26.4).
   - How were subjects selected?
   - Was the measurement tool appropriate?
   - Was there any quality control to ensure standardized data collection?
   - If a randomized controlled trial, was it truly random? Was assessment of outcome 'blind'?

Box 26.4 Appropriate study designs for different areas of care

Therapy	Randomized controlled trial*
Diagnosis	Cross-sectional survey* comparison with gold standard
Screening	Cross-sectional survey*
Prognosis	Cohort study*
Causation	• Cohort or case-control depending on rarity of condition • Case reports may be useful

*See Appendix 1 for definitions

   - Was the study large enough and continued for long enough to be able to provide reliable data?
5. Results
   - What method was used to analyse data?
   - Could the results have occurred by chance? Have the researchers provided 'p' values?
   - Could the results have been affected by bias or because a factor such as smoking acted as a confounder?
   - Have the researchers calculated the numbers needed to treat to obtain benefit?
   - Are the results transferable to your clinical setting?

IMPLEMENT THE RESULTS

Once high-quality evidence has been identified it can then be integrated into clinical practice. Sackett et al (1997) argued that to be of benefit to patients, evidence must be combined with clinical expertise, not replace it; without evidence, practice could become out of date but equally without expertise, practice could be tyrannized by evidence and a cookbook approach to care would be generated.

EVALUATE PERFORMANCE THROUGH AUDIT AND SELF-REFLECTION

One aspect of evaluation is individual self-reflection. This can be used to consider:

- how often the five steps of evidence-based practice are followed
- how successful the process has been in terms of identifying the evidence required
- the restrictions encountered, such as lack of library access.

Another aspect is to routinely use research evidence as the basis for clinical audit and in the development of agreed local protocols on which care is based.

CONCLUSION

Evidence-based practice is an important concept to ensure a scientific knowledge base for effective decision making and it is likely to be at the forefront of the way care is developed, commissioned and delivered to patients in the New NHS as envisaged by the government. However, it has also been argued (Mulhall 1998) that as nursing is an art as well as a science, trust, empathy and 'being there' also need to be encouraged and valued within nursing practice.

AUDIT

Audit is 'the method used by health professionals to assess, evaluate, and improve the care of patients in a systematic way' (Irvine & Irvine 1997). It became a requirement for all medical practitioners due to the NHS and Community Care Act of 1990. At that time medical audit advisory groups (MAAGs) were set up to facilitate audit within general practice and improve the quality of care delivered to patients.

The quality of healthcare has been described as consisting of three interrelated parts: structure, process and outcome (Donabedian 1966).

STRUCTURE

This relates to the physical aspects involved in the provision of healthcare such as the building, equipment, people and notes. The quality of structural aspects can impact on the quality of care provided; for example, practitioners with resuscitation equipment should be able to deliver better care in the event of anaphylaxis than those without.

PROCESS

This is the description of the care that the practitioner provides for the patient and will reflect attitudes, knowledge and skill. An example of a process audit would be whether known hypertensive patients had their blood pressure measured and what treatment was prescribed.

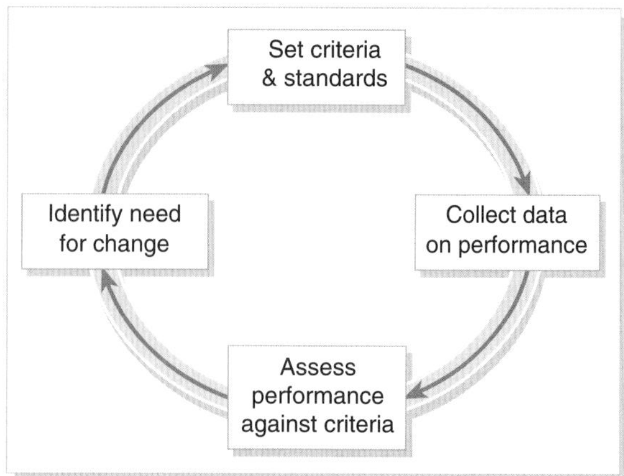

Figure 26.1 The audit cycle.

OUTCOME

This is the change in the patient's current and future condition that can be related to the care provided: for example, recovery, complications and mortality from a course of treatment. In theory most practitioners would want to measure outcomes but in reality these can be affected by factors other than treatment and long-term outcomes can be difficult to assess.

THE AUDIT CYCLE

Clinical audit can be undertaken on structure, process or outcome of care using the audit cycle (Fig. 26.1). Those involved should have the opportunity to agree the timescale, workload and to ensure that the results will be of benefit to their work.

Set criteria and standards

Criteria are definable and measurable items of healthcare which describe the quality expected. They are usually written in the form of statements and can be applied to structure, process or outcome. Standards describe the level of care to be achieved for each individual criterion, for example:

Criteria	Standards
Patients with heart failure:	
• should have received counselling and lifestyle advice	xx%
• should be on a diuretic	xx%
• should be on ACE inhibitors	xx%
• should have echocardiography	xx%

Box 26.5 Data collection sheet

Name	Age	Sex	Diuretic (if no, leave blank) Name	Dose	ACE (if no, leave blank) Name	Dose	Lifestyle advice Yes	No	Echo Yes	No

In order to carry out a successful audit which is not overambitious, it is best to concentrate on three or four criteria at the most. Published literature or clinical guidelines on an area of care can be used to identify criteria and then the standards that the practice would realistically expect to achieve can be agreed with all involved in the audit.

Collect data on performance

Decide how:

- many patients should be included in the sample, e.g. a practice with 2000 patients will have 25–40 with heart failure and in this case it would be practical to audit all of these patients
- the data will be collected, e.g. by computer or by manual note search
- the data will be recorded – a data collection sheet (Box 26.5) can be useful.

Compare performance against criteria and standards set

This may highlight areas which are not meeting agreed standards. Either the standards set were unrealistic or practice procedures may need to change in order to improve performance.

Identify the need for change

The practice team should attempt to identify reasons for any shortfall and an action plan can then be developed to implement change aimed at improving performance in order to achieve the original agreed standards. A review date should be set to repeat the audit to evaluate whether the change has had an effect.

Repeat the cycle

The purpose of audit is to improve quality, not just to collect numbers. Therefore a repeat audit is essential to see if it has led to change in practice and patient benefit.

NURSING STANDARDS AND AUDIT

Practice nurses must be safe and competent practitioners and are accountable for their actions and omissions. Accountability must involve some form of monitoring of quality and standard setting. Methods of assessing quality and standards within general practice nursing include:

- patient satisfaction questionnaires
- record, review or observe consultations
- self-assessment
- reflection of 'critical incidents'
- standard setting and audit.

Audit can be used as a tool to assess the standards set and maintain quality within practice nursing but it should be relevant to the nurses involved and not just another task to complete. Audit can be a powerful motivator for change in order to rectify deficiencies identified. This might require purchase of equipment or more nursing hours.

However, as audit can be threatening if it is seen as an outsider checking up on performance, it is of far greater value if the desire to improve standards and efficiency comes from within the nursing team itself. In addition, it is important to recognize that nursing audit should not be considered in isolation as within general practice a multidisciplinary approach to care is essential.

The National Service Frameworks will establish national standards in specific areas of care, e.g. coronary heart disease or mental health, that must be implemented and reviewed by primary care organizations such as primary care trusts.

The National Institute for Clinical Excellence has been established to give a strong lead on clinical and cost-effectiveness. It will produce clinical guidelines for dissemination throughout the NHS. In addition, the Commission for Health Audit and Inspection (CHAI) will undertake inspections within both primary and secondary care to review the quality of care provided to patients.

Audit within general practice will be a key aspect to ensure that the requirements of national policy are implemented. Many audit groups have become multidisciplinary and have taken a lead in the development and dissemination of local guidelines, which are based on national guidelines, e.g. for coronary heart disease, to enable and support evidence-based care. While research is concerned with identifying the 'right thing to do' and provides the evidence on which to base practice, audit is about ensuring that the 'right thing is done' (Balogh 1996).

References

Balogh R 1996 Exploring the links between audit and the research process. Nurse Researcher 3(3):5–16

Donabedian A 1966 Evaluating the quality of medical care. Millbank Memorial Fund Quarterly 44:166–204

Greenhalgh T 2001 How to read a paper, 2nd edn. BMJ Books, London

Irvine D, Irvine S 1997 Making sense of audit. Radcliffe Medical Press, Abingdon

Mulhall A 1998 Nursing, research and the evidence. Evidence Based Nursing 1(1):4–6

Polit D, Hungler B 1995 Nursing research; principles and methods, 5th edn. Lippincott, Philadelphia

Sackett D, Richardson W, Rosenburg W, Haynes R 1997 Evidence-based medicine. Churchill Livingstone, New York

Resources

Cochrane Collaboration, Summertown Pavilion, Middle Way, Summertown, Oxford OX2 7LG. www.cochrane.org/

NHS Centre for Reviews and Dissemination, University of York, York YO1 5DD. www.york.ac.uk/inst/crd/welcome.htm

University of Sheffield School of Health and Related Research (ScHARR). www.shef.ac.uk/~scharr/

Medical Research Council. www.mrc.ac.uk

Medical Research Council General Practice Research Framework. www.mrc/gprf.ac.uk

Bandolier – monthly newsletter that reviews the evidence base for areas of healthcare, free within the NHS. andrew.moore@pru.ox.ac.uk

Further reading

Clegg F 1987 Simple statistics, 4th edn. Cambridge University Press, Cambridge

Oglies M 1989 Reading research. Scutari Press, London

APPENDIX 1 GLOSSARY OF EPIDEMIOLOGICAL AND STATISTICAL TERMS (REPRODUCED WITH PERMISSION OF DR MADGE VICKERS)

Attributable (or absolute) risk The rate of a disease in exposed individuals that can be attributed to the exposure. It is derived by subtracting the rate of the outcome among the unexposed from the rate among the exposed individuals.

Case-control studies (see *observational studies*)

Chi-squared test (see *significance tests*)

Cohort studies (see *observational studies*)

Confidence intervals Show the range of values that will be expected to include the true population value. The statement 'the 95% confidence interval is from 5 to 15' means that we can be 95% certain that the true value will lie between 5 to 15 inclusive.

Confounding factor A factor that is associated with both the disease and the study factor, e.g. social class is associated with both coronary heart disease and diet. Such a variable must be controlled for to obtain an undistorted estimate of the effect of the study factor on risk.

Correlation The correlation coefficient measures the strength of the linear association between two variables. It lies between −1 and +1, where −1 and +1 indicate a perfect linear association and 0 indicates no linear association.

Pearson's correlation coefficient: uses actual values of the two variables, at least one of which must be normally distributed.

Spearman's correlation coefficient: based on the ranks of the values of the two variables and makes no asumptions about the distributions of the variables.

Crossover trials (see *randomized controlled clinical trials*)

Cross-sectional studies (see *observational studies*)

Double blind A double-blind trial is one in which neither the patient nor the observer knows to which treatment regime any patient in the trial is allocated.

Effectiveness The extent to which a specific intervention produces a beneficial effect on a defined population when used in normal practice.

Efficacy The extent to which a specific intervention produces a beneficial result under ideal conditions, e.g. during a randomized controlled trial.

Epidemiology The study of the distribution and causes of disease in specified populations and the application of this study to control health problems.

Factorial trials (see *randomized controlled clinical trials*)

Incidence The number of new cases of a disease in a defined population within a specified period of time.

Intention-to-treat analysis An analysis which includes all the persons randomized into a clinical trial in the group to which they were originally allocated, whether or not they complied with, or completed, the regimen under study.

Observational studies Studies in which certain features are observed in groups of individuals without any intervention being introduced other than the gathering of information. Observational studies can be used to investigate the diagnosis, causes and natural history of disease and to evaluate the process of care.

Case-control studies: a population of cases with the disease and a comparable population of controls are chosen. The two populations are then compared to determine any differences in past exposure to risk factors.

Cohort (longitudinal) studies

a) *prospective cohort*: a healthy population is followed for many years and disease incidence is observed. Prior exposure information can then be related to subsequent disease for each individual.
b) *historical cohort*: existing records about the health or other relevant aspects of a population at some time in the past are related to current (or subsequent) disease status.
c) *cohort analysis*: analysis of morbidity or mortality rates in relation to the ages of a specific group identified at a particular period of time and followed as they pass through different ages.

Cross-sectional studies: studies examining relationships between diseases and exposure variables as they exist in a defined population at one point in time.

On-treatment analysis Events in a trial are related to the treatment being received at the time.

Power The probability that a trial can detect a true difference between the intervention group and control group, if one exists. A power of 80% or above is usually acceptable for a clinical trial. (see *type II error*)

Precision

a) Precision is exact detail, i.e. a measurement is more precise if recorded to a greater number of decimal places.
b) Precision is the consistency of repeated measurements made to estimate the same variable (measured by the standard error).

A measured variable can be precise but inaccurate if there is bias in the measurement.

Prevalence The number of cases of a disorder present at a point in time in a defined population, as a proportion of the total population.

Prevention

Primary prevention: the prevention of new cases of the disease by removing a cause of the disease.

Secondary prevention: the prevention of overt recurrent (clinical) cases of a disease through screening and early detection followed by appropriate intervention.

Tertiary prevention: clinical treatment of a disease that prevents disability and pain resulting from that disease.

Probability (see *p-value*)

p-value The p-value is used to indicate the strength of the evidence for a true treatment effect. The smaller the p-value, the lower the probability that an observed difference between groups could have arisen by chance. p-values of 0.05 and lower are usually accepted as indicating significant differences.

Random error The variation of observed values from a true value which is due to chance alone. A large random error implies imprecision or poor repeatability. When random error occurs the estimate is equally likely to be above or below the true value.

Randomized controlled clinical trials Experiments in which interventions are evaluated for efficacy and safety in patients either with a specific disease or at risk of developing a specific disease. Patients are allocated at random to receive either the intervention or to be in a control group (receiving no intervention or placebo or an existing standard intervention).

Parallel group trials: patients assigned randomly to one of two (or more) interventions to try to achieve a fair, unbiased comparison through groups that are identical in all respects apart from the intervention.

Crossover trials: patients assigned randomly to one of two interventions and then after a set time transferred to the other intervention, sometimes after a washout period. The patients thus act as their own controls. This design is most suitable for treatments intended to provide rapid relief of symptoms in chronic disease.

Factorial trials: two (or more) treatments are used either alone or in combination to allow evaluation of the combined as well as the single effects of the different treatments.

Regression Statistical techniques (e.g. linear regression, logistic regression) commonly used to assess the effects of one factor on the outcome measure independent of its associations with other factors.

Relative risk The ratio of the risk of disease (incidence or prevalence) among the exposed to the risk among the unexposed. A relative risk of 1.50 indicates a 50% increase in risk among the exposed relative to the unexposed.

Repeatability (or reliability) Repeatability refers to the degree to which the same answer is obtained if a measurement is repeated under the same conditions.

Significance level (type I error (α)) Probability that an observed difference could have arisen by chance (i.e. a false-positive rate). (see *p-value*)

Significance tests Statistical tests to decide whether observed differences (i.e. between treatments) are true or could have arisen by chance.

Chi-squared (χ^2) test: used to test for a difference between proportions. The larger the value of χ^2, the smaller the probability (p) that the difference could have arisen by chance.

t-test

a) The two-sample or unpaired t-test is used to test whether the difference between two means obtained from two different groups of individuals is significant. The larger the value of t, the smaller the probability (p) that the difference could have arisen by chance.
b) The paired t-test is used to compare means of two measurements obtained on the same individuals, e.g. as in a crossover trial.

Analysis of variance (ANOVA): used to compare several means or two means after adjusting for other factors. The larger the value of F, the smaller the probability (p) that the difference could have arisen by chance.

Wilcoxon test: a test based on ranking values which can be used to test whether the difference between two medians obtained from two different groups of individuals is significant. Unlike the t-test, the Wilcoxon test can be used on data which are very skewed or based on few patients. The larger the value of Z, the smaller the probability (p) that the difference could have arisen by chance.

Standardized mortality ratio The ratio of the observed number of deaths in a study population to the number of deaths if a study population had the same specific rates as the standard population multiplied by 100.

Systematic error Systematic over- or undermeasurement of a variable related to the true value. Bias leads to estimates which are inaccurate even if precise and repeatable.

Possible types of bias include:
Confounding: the estimate of the association between an exposure and disease is mixed up with the real effect of another exposure on the same disease when the two exposures are correlated.

Recall bias: differences in accuracy or completeness of recall to memory of prior events, e.g. mothers whose children have leukaemia are more likely than mothers of healthy children to remember details of diagnostic X-ray examinations to which these children were exposed in utero.

Selection bias: cases or controls are included in or excluded from observational studies on criteria related to the factors under investigation.

t-test (see *significance tests*)

Type II error (β) Probability of failing to detect a real difference as statistically significant (i.e. a false-negative result). Power = 1 − β.

Validity Ability to measure what is claimed by the technique used.

Wilcoxon test (see *significance tests*)

Chapter 27

Writing for publication

Liam Benison

CHAPTER CONTENTS

INTRODUCTION

> *...writing is not just the last stage of a research process but from its beginning a guide to critical thinking* (Booth et al 2003)

Government guidelines require nurses to practise research-based care but, for many nurses, researching and writing may seem remote from the activity of caring for patients. It is a powerful perception that writing is a mysterious, lonely, arcane process, which is the preserve of scientists or hermits (or of nurses with a desire for self-aggrandizement). This is unfortunate for two reasons.

Nurses have much to share with their colleagues in the health professions about what they have learnt about nursing problems and the needs of patients. Publishing is an effective way to share insights with colleagues and extend your knowledge.

Like nursing, writing is a discipline that requires a balance of critical thinking, intuition and care. Writing for publication demands the application of critical thought to solving a defined problem that you agree to write about for a journal and its audience. Just as it is necessary to choose your words carefully to put a patient at ease or convey a difficult message sensitively, so writing requires care and intuition to gauge the most explicit way to relate a complex message.

If writing is 'a guide to critical thinking', as Booth and colleagues say, likewise, it can guide reflective practice. The stages of researching an article idea, submitting it to a journal and revising it with the help of an editor can provide an effective way to think critically about nursing problems and arrive at conclusions that can be applied to the care of patients.

FORMULATING A TOPIC

If you are going to write, you need to have something to say. You also need the patience to think through ideas carefully and the persistence to find the right words for what you want to say. Most advances in knowledge proceed by small incremental steps; that is, by individuals carefully applying what they already know to solving a small but important problem. You will come across the raw material of potential topics in everyday problems and questions that arise in practice: questions that nobody seems to know the answer to, difficult questions that patients ask or questions or ideas for further research that are suggested in journal articles and books.

You might keep a notebook to record questions as they occur to you. Florence Nightingale expressed her belief in the value of recording notes.

> *Do we look enough to the importance of ... keeping careful Notes of Lectures, of keeping notes of all type cases ... so as to improve our powers of observation: all essential if we are in future to have charge? ... Many say: 'We have no time; ...' But it is so easy to degenerate into a mere drudgery ... when we have goodwill to do it and are fonder of practical work than of giving ourselves the trouble of learning the 'reason why'* (Dossey 2000)

If you keep regular notes and reflections, you will have plenty of material to choose from to write about. Choose a question or idea you think is especially relevant and important to your work with patients. Discuss your ideas with colleagues and read the literature to see if you can extend your ideas further.

A notebook is also useful for recording things to chase up later, e.g. reference checks you need to do somewhere else, ideas that are not relevant to your immediate question but would be worth following up later, other references to check out, ideas for an article on a related topic.

Sometimes an article can be written about a protocol that you have written with a colleague or about procedures or clinics you are running. The process of writing will force you to compare your work with what others have written about the topic and help answer the question, what does your project contribute that is new?

WRITING AN ABSTRACT

Once you have thought about your ideas and collected some articles and information, you need to narrow down your thinking to a question that can be answered in a specific piece of writing. This should be done as soon as possible. Your first abstract is unlikely to be the proposal you submit to a journal editor. The discipline of writing an abstract should help you clarify your ideas, what you know and which questions you need to answer.

An abstract is a succinct and explicit idea of what your article will investigate and what you hope to achieve by writing it. An abstract needs to do three things.

1. State your question or hypothesis.
2. Place your question in the context of what is already known.
3. State why your question needs to be answered or discussed and what it can add to current knowledge.

Your abstract should tell the editor of the journal in which you intend to publish your article why that journal's readers need to know what you have to say and what you can tell them that is new. Show your abstract to colleagues or a university supervisor and ask for criticism. It is safer to refine your work from feedback from people you know, rather than have your efforts rejected out of hand by an editor.

You are now ready to do more detailed research and begin writing. Once we have looked at the requirements of good research and writing we will consider how to approach an editor with a proposal and explain the stages of the publication process after submitting your work.

REFERENCES AND RESEARCH

References are crucial to good research and writing. They should not be regarded as a waste of time that can be left to the last few hours before submission. Respect for referencing guarantees sound research and saves you time searching for that elusive reference that you 'just know' you put back on the shelf.

When you read each potential reference for your article, ask if it is relevant to your research questions. Does it contain any leads to other sources of relevant information? If the answer is no, discard the reference. If yes, record the details of the source as shown in Box 27.1.

> **Box 27.1 What to record for each reference you consult**
>
> *Author.* If the article or book has many authors, do not cut corners by recording the first one plus 'et al'. Record them all. It is much easier to take out the extra authors later than go searching for the item or its reference again.
> *Title.* Record the full title exactly as it appears. Only use abbreviations or acronyms if they are used in the title.
> *Chapter.* If the article is a chapter in a book, record the title and authors of both the chapter and the book and the page numbers of the chapter.
> *Journal.* If the article appears in a journal, record the journal's title and the publication date, volume and issue numbers, and page numbers.
> *Publication details.* For books, record the publisher, the place of publication and the date. And the number of the edition (if necessary).
> *Shelfmark.* Record where you found the source: the Library's shelfmark number or the Internet address for a document on the web.
> *Edition.* Also, check that the book is not available in a more up-to-date edition. This can be done by checking the catalogues of the British Library (www.bl.uk) or, for works published in the USA, the Library of Congress (www.loc.gov).

When quoting a source, ensure you quote accurately and record the page number. Ensure you distinguish quotes from paraphrases and summaries. Always record your own thinking about the notes you have taken and ensure these thoughts are also distinct from the summaries, quotes and paraphrases.

The science of medicine and health changes rapidly and references get out of date very quickly. Ensure you have at least two (relevant) references that have been published within the last year. If you are citing guidelines or frequently updated data from the Department of Health, the World Health Organization or other organizations, ensure they are the latest update.

Ensure when you quote or paraphrase from a source that you do so fairly and accurately. It is misleading and embarrassing to claim that someone said something they did not. Booth and colleagues (2003) give the example of the reviewer who attacked an article called 'Novels must be realistic'. The reviewer failed to read beyond the headline and did not know that the author's argument disagreed with the headline. This is an extreme case. The more common error is to take an author's statement out of context or to exaggerate what an author says in order to suit your own argument. This should be avoided. This is a danger particularly when reading the concluding statements of primary research articles, where writers usually qualify definitive statements very carefully.

It is also important not to take quotations from your source out of context. This is another way to misinterpret the text. Read the entire text so that you understand the way in which the quotation contributes to the author's overall argument. The context of the quote can sometimes be more significant than its content.

WRITING THE INTRODUCTION

The introduction should say what you are doing and why. It should state the problem that the article investigates and why this problem needs to be addressed. Many introductions are overlong and recount a series of statistics and references without explaining why these facts are important. The first sentence is especially important. Consider this example:

> *Although it also costs the NHS £500 million a year (Bellamy & Booker 2000) and 30 000 people per annum die of the condition every year (Royal College of Physicians of Edinburgh 2001), given the suffering that it causes, chronic obstructive pulmonary disease (COPD) does not receive the attention it deserves.*

Excessive statistics and references are not the only obstacle to clarity here. It is almost never appropriate to begin your first sentence with 'although' or another word that introduces a modifying clause. This forces the reader to wait to discover the subject of the sentence. This writer has tried to include too much in the first sentence. Here is a better example:

> *Multiple sclerosis (MS) is a chronic neurological disease that appears rarely in general practice. A GP sees a new case of MS only once in every 100 000 patient contacts (Keen 2000). However, diagnosis is a lengthy, complex and distressing process, in part because symptoms may have many other causes. Therefore, it is important for GPs to consider the information and referral needs of the two or three patients in their care who have diagnosed or suspected MS.*

The writer gives a simple definition of MS and explains the problem succinctly. The use of statistics is sparing and the last sentence indicates the direction of the rest of the article without using the tired phrase, 'this article will ...' The term 'MS' is used three times and the writer wisely refrained from substituting 'the condition' or 'the disease'. Evans (2000) has warned against excessive 'monologophobia', i.e. the avoidance of repetition at all costs. If you are discussing MS, call it MS.

DEVELOPING THE ARGUMENT

As you begin, it is important to hold two things in mind: the audience you are aiming to convey your message to and the type of article you are writing. These will limit the kinds of things you will say and the way you say them.

Writing and researching is like conversation. Just as you assess what another person is saying before you answer, in research you critically appraise the writing of other researchers and respond in your writing. As you begin to write, it may be helpful to imagine you are writing a letter to a friend who wants to know all about your topic. When you write a letter, you imagine the person you are writing to, whether it is a friend or an official you have never met. You adjust your style accordingly and choose your language to get the response you want. It is a two-way process; if you do not say what you mean, your letter may be ignored. Therefore, you must judge who your readers are, what they already know about your topic and how best to explain it to them.

As you begin to write, continually ask questions of your writing. For example: 'What am I trying to say?', 'How does this paragraph (or sentence or word) contribute to my argument?', 'How does it lead the reader from the last point to the next?'. Use everyday words and short simple sentences. This is especially important when discussing a complex idea. As Goodman & Edwards (1997) say, a phrase such as 'maternal parent' 'is no more precise [a] way of expressing the idea of a female parent than the word *mother*'. Every sentence and every word should have a purpose that carries your argument forward. Convoluted language usually indicates convoluted logic or a lack of reasoning. Don't be lazy; if you are struggling to express what you want to say, don't gloss it over with woolly language. Take the time to put your point in precise language.

Your conclusion should summarize your key argument and state what you have concluded by investigating your key question through the article. It should say what your article has added to knowledge about the topic of investigation. It is useful to readers to recommend ways in which your conclusions might be put into practice or suggest further research that is required to take your conclusions further.

APPROACHING A JOURNAL

Once you have done some research, gathered references and written an abstract, choose an appropriate journal to approach. Choose carefully. (You can submit an abstract to only one journal at a time.) You need to consider:

- *The audience* – who will want to read your article? Who should read it?
- *Length* – how much do you have to write? The average length of a journal article is 3000 words, but this varies depending on the journal.
- *Article type* – which journal publishes the kind of article you have in mind? Is your article the results of research (e.g. a study of how a new asthma clinic has altered patients' medication), a review of current research (e.g. a review of the latest guidelines for treating TB), a news report (e.g. on a conference you have attended) or a viewpoint on a contentious issue (e.g. the safety of the MMR vaccine).

The aims of your article and your intended audience need to match the aims and audience of the journal. Compare nursing journals and decide which would be the most appropriate place for your article.

It is a good idea to contact the editor by telephone. This way you will find out how interested the editor is in your topic and whether it is worth submitting a proposal and in what format. Some editors may send you instructions for authors and ask you to submit a draft of your entire article. Others will insist on a proposal first, together with a reference list.

If an editor rejects your proposal, ask why. It may be that your proposal is a good one but that it is unsuited to the journal's audience or that the journal has recently covered your topic in detail. When an editor invites you to submit an article, ensure you receive instructions for authors and clarify any queries with the editor.

Before you submit, re-read the instructions for authors and ensure that you have followed them precisely. If the editor can see that you have read the instructions for authors and followed them, it indicates that you are a careful reader who will probably also have recorded your research and thinking carefully. Before submission, it is wise to have your work read by a colleague or a representative of your intended audience.

PEER REVIEW AND EDITING

Writing for publication is a collaborative effort, more like making a film than writing your novel on a remote Scottish island. Once your work is submitted it will be read by an editor, perhaps two or three peer reviewers and a subeditor. These people all contribute comments and suggestions, which you will be obliged to consider seriously.

You do not have to accept everything the editor and reviewers say. You should take the time to evaluate their comments critically and argue against them if necessary. Sometimes changes are suggested that distort your intended meaning. It may be, however, that your intended meaning was unclear in the way you originally expressed it. Look at this example:

The majority of children who have HIV infection have acquired the infection from a mother who is infected with the virus either during pregnancy, at the time of birth or during subsequent breastfeeding.

Subeditor's change
The majority of children with HIV acquired the virus from a mother who was infected either during pregnancy, at birth or during subsequent breastfeeding.

The subeditor assumed, naturally enough, that 'during pregnancy' referred to the mother. However, the author intended to specify when the children were infected, not when the mother was infected. If the author had included a comma after 'virus' the sense may have been less ambiguous. Once the author pointed out the misunderstanding, the text was amended as follows:

The majority of children with HIV acquired the virus from their mothers, either in the womb, at birth or during breastfeeding.

This example highlights the importance of using the right words for what you intend to say and shows how punctuation clarifies meaning. Fewer words are usually clearer. The author's original phrase which caused the misunderstanding, 'who is infected with the virus', is superfluous. If the children got the virus from their mothers, it is impossible that the mothers were not infected by the virus. The final version also uses the simple past tense ('acquired') instead of the present perfect ('have acquired'). The present perfect is unnecessary because it is clear that the children were infected by the virus at a single point in the past.

Peer reviewers will ask if your argument is clear and adequately substantiated by appropriate evidence and by relevant, up-to-date references. The peer review process varies among journals. The most common is 'double blind' (where the author remains anonymous to the reviewer and vice versa). Some journals only keep reviewers anonymous to authors.

Subeditors may not be specialists in the field. Their skill is in assessing if your argument and meaning will be intelligible for the audience. They amend grammar and spelling and make other changes so that the text conforms to the journal's 'house style'. This may include conventions of spelling (e.g. English, American), of word choice (e.g. 'although' instead of 'though') and of symbols and abbreviations (e.g. '%' for 'per cent'). If you use abbreviations, they must be spelt out at the first occurrence with the abbreviation in brackets. Thereafter the abbreviation only should be used.

When your manuscript has been peer reviewed and subedited, you will receive an edited manuscript along with reports from the reviewers. The editor includes instructions for revision in a letter to you and may indicate which of the reviewers' comments it is most important that you respond to.

Don't be discouraged if your manuscript returns littered with red marks. Sometimes reviewers' comments seem unkind. The editor decides what will be published and will tell you what needs to be modified to satisfy the journal's requirements for publication. Few of us like criticism, especially if it seems to question our ability to express ourselves in our own language. The author who sobs that, despite the reviewer's comments, her grammar is perfect because she went to school in the 1950s needs to recall that writing is a difficult and precise art. However much we think we know, most of us received only the sketchiest instruction in grammar at school, regardless of our age. The experience of receiving feedback on our writing is invaluable if only to reveal what we can still learn about how to express ideas more precisely.

Although some reviewers may criticize your article to promote their own agenda, most volunteer their time because they are interested in what others have to say about their field. Spelling and

Box 27.2

Why articles are rejected

1. Not relevant to the journal and its audience.
2. Contain grammatical, spelling and typographical errors.
3. Written unclearly, containing jargon that makes it difficult for the reader to understand what the writer wants to say.
4. Unfocused: the introduction fails to direct the reader and convey the author's argument and approach. (The author appears to be confused by the topic and does not know what she wants to say.)
5. Based on inaccurate research or biased argument.
6. Article fails to say anything new.

Why articles are accepted

1. Relevant to the journal and targeted for its audience.
2. Well written, with the author's argument presented simply and directly, with each point following logically and claims supported by evidence.
3. Contains accurate grammar and spelling.
4. Introduction sets out the argument succinctly and indicates what is to come. (The author knows what she wants to say and how to say it.)
5. Research is critically appraised and well referenced.
6. Adds something new to the topic.

grammatical errors that distract their attention and make your ideas difficult to understand only irritate them and make them less inclined to review your work favourably. Box 27.2 lists some reasons why articles are accepted or rejected.

CONCLUSION

This guidance to writing for publication is intended to be useful for whatever critical study you undertake, whether you apply it to article writing, reflective practice, solving nursing problems, improving patient care or furthering your career aspirations. The strategies discussed here are designed to ensure accurate research, clear expression of ideas and effective ways to draw conclusions about complex problems. Writing demands care for detail and accuracy, checking to ensure that quotations and references are correct and the persistence to find the best words to express what you want to say. You may find that the practice of writing has more in common with the practice of nursing than you initially thought.

Acknowledgement

I would like to thank Diana Saunders MSc RGN for her kind assistance and helpful suggestions.

References

Booth WC, Colomb GG, Williams JM 2003 The craft of research, 2nd edn. University of Chicago Press, Chicago

Dossey BM 2000 Florence Nightingale: mystic, visionary, healer. Springhouse, Pennsylvania

Evans H 2000 Essential English for journalists, editors and writers (revised Gillan C). Pimlico, London

Goodman NW, Edwards MB 1997 Medical writing: a prescription for clarity, 2nd edn. Cambridge University Press, Cambridge

Further reading

Read widely to pick up helpful hints on the process of writing and research from the many books and articles on this topic. *Hospital Medicine* runs a regular series of articles on research. *Practice Nursing* publishes articles on research from time to time.

Index

NB: Page numbers in *italics* refer to the Plate section.

A

C

D

F

G

H

I

J

K

L

P

T

U

V